HEALING IMAGES
The Role of Imagination in Health

Edited by
Anees A. Sheikh
Department of Psychology
Marquette University
and
Department of Psychiatry and Behavioral Medicine
Medical College of Wisconsin

Imagery and Human Development Series
Series Editor: Anees A. Sheikh

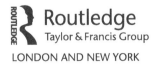

Routledge
Taylor & Francis Group

LONDON AND NEW YORK

First published 2013 by Baywood Publishing Company, Inc.

Published 2017 by Routledge
2 Park Square, Milton Park, Abingdon, Oxon OX14 4RN
711 Third Avenue, New York, NY 10017, USA

Routledge is an imprint of the Taylor & Francis Group, an informa business

Library of Congress Catalog Number: 2002071675
ISBN 13: 978-0-89503-226-3 (pbk)
ISBN 13: 978-0-89503-208-9 (hbk)

The Library of Congress has cataloged a previous printing as follows

Healing images : the role of imagination in health / edited by Anees A. Sheikh.
    p. cm. - - (Imagery and human development series)
Includes bibliographical references and index.
  ISBN 0-89503-208-2 (cloth) - - ISBN 0-89503-226-0 (pbk.)
  1. Imagery (Psychology)--Therapeutic use. 2. Imagination--Therapeutic use. 3. Visualization--Therapeutic use. 4. Mind and body. 5. Medicine and psychology. I. Sheikh, Anees A. II. Imagery and human development series (Unnumbered)
  RZ401 .H33 2002
  616.89'14--dc21

                            2002071675

I can give you nothing that has not already its being within yourself. I can throw open to you no picture gallery but your own . . . I help you to make your own world visible. That is all.

Hermann Hesse

To My Beloved Family:
My Wife
KATHARINA
My Daughter
SONIA
My Sons
NADEEM and IMRAN

Table of Contents

Preface

> You must give birth to your images. They are the future waiting to be born . . .
> fear not the strangeness you feel. The future must enter into you long before
> it happens. . . . Just wait for the birth . . . for the hour of new clarity.
>
> Rainer Maria Rilke (cited in Brigham, p. 329)

"Come on in—the water is fine" (Holt, 1964). This frequently quoted invitation to investigators by Robert Holt in 1964 did not fall on deaf ears. In the course of the last 35 years, an ever-increasing number of scientists and clinicians have enthusiastically answered Holt's call, and by their tireless efforts, imagery has become recognized as a legitimate and fruitful area of inquiry and as an effective therapeutic tool. This book celebrates the coming of age of the once ostracized.

To my knowledge, *Healing Images* is the first comprehensive attempt to reflect the current state of knowledge concerning the role of imagination in health. All chapters are written by internationally or nationally known experts or in collaboration with them. This work consists of 22 chapters and discusses theory, research, and clinical applications. It presents a brief history of the use of imagery for healing in both Eastern and Western traditions, a review of research that deals with the physiological consequences of imagery and related approaches, and an explanation as to how images lead to such bodily changes. *Healing Images* covers the latest theory and research on the relationship between imagery, cerebral laterality, and healing. An attempt is also made to integrate modern systems theory and concepts of information and energy, which disclose the role of imagery and love in health. Imagery and music in health are also discussed.

Healing Images examines how and why mental images help in connecting with our inner wisdom and covers in detail applications of imagery in pain management, smoking cessation, weight management, sex therapy, and in the treatment of phobic disorders, eating disorders, and cardiovascular disorders, depression, trauma, and cancer. This volume also explores imagery in intuition and spiritual development and includes a discussion of transpersonal and death images along with their implications for health and growth.

I am delighted that His Holiness, the Dalai Lama has taken the time to adorn this book with a few words of wisdom. It is a brand of wisdom which has molded him into a consummate human being, a beacon of love, compassion, and understanding. The endorsement of the efficacy of imagery by a man who is a profound scholar and who has thoroughly explored the far reaches of the human mind by meditation, undoubtedly will be an inspiration to many researchers.

In conclusion, I cordially thank all contributors. Each chapter uniquely elucidates many questions, poses new ones, and enriches the debate. Also I am grateful to the staff of Baywood Publishing Company, especially to its president, Stuart Cohen, and Bobbi Olszewski, Julie Krempa, and Joi Tamber-Brooks, for their patience, cooperation, and valuable guidance. At the Marquette University Department of Psychology, I am indebted to Sherri Lex for her expert help, and particularly to Sue Farrell for her cheerful, generous, and conscientious assistance and her kind support throughout the preparation of this volume. Also, I would like to express my sincere appreciation to Marquette University for the assistance provided to me through its sabbatical leave program.

Finally, I would like to take this opportunity to lovingly acknowledge the valuable assistance and encouragement provided by my wife, Katharina, not only throughout this project, but also during the numerous other imagery-related endeavors over the last many years. Without her generous help and support, I know I would not have been able to accomplish even half as much as I did.

Anees A. Sheikh
Milwaukee, Wisconsin

REFERENCES

Brigham, D. D. (1994). *Imagery for getting well.* New York: Norton.
Holt, R. (1964). The return of the ostracized. *American Psychologist, 19,* 254-264.

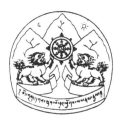

Foreword

The reality of human existence includes our experience of illness, suffering, and death. Pretending that we are not sick when we are, or that we will never die, would be as foolish as to deny the possibility of ever getting well.

As living beings, we all wish for happiness and seek to avoid suffering. One of the major factors here is our mental attitude. Physical health is closely related to our state of mind. Scientific experiments have shown that if the mind is stable and calm, basic physical functions like digestion and sleep improve. On the other hand, when someone is mentally distressed, even the presence of friends, comfort, and wealth will not make them happy.

This book, *Healing Images,* deals exhaustively with the role imagination can play in health. I have no doubt that an important factor even in matters of physical health is to train the mind. On the one hand this means cultivating a sincere compassionate motivation and performing positive actions. On the other, it means calming and controlling the mind, which may involve structured use of the imagination and is a more profound way of preparing for the future. Moreover, by identifying negative states of mind like anger, hatred, frustration, jealousy, and pride, we can work to eliminate them. At the same time we can cultivate positive attitudes like compassion and love, tolerance, and contentment. Training the mind in this way is both useful and realistic. Positive attitudes are a source of health and happiness for ourselves and others.

In the practice of healing, a kind heart is as valuable as medical training because it is the source of happiness for both oneself and others. People respond to kindness irrespective of whether medicine is effective or not, and in turn culti-vating a kind heart is a cause of our own good health. Helping others wherever you can according to their need is the true expression of compassion. I have no doubt that employing the imagination in a positive way, and this book describes many different ways of doing so, can have a significant impact on improving our physical and mental health and well-being.

Tenzin Gyatso
The 14th Dalai Lama

December 15, 2001
Dharamsala, India

Theory and Research

CHAPTER 1

Healing Images: Historical Perspective

ANEES A. SHEIKH, ROBERT G. KUNZENDORF,
AND KATHARINA S. SHEIKH

> *I dream the world, therefore the world exists as I dream it.*
> Gaston Bachelard (1969, p. 158)

The ancient literature of numerous cultures abounds with accounts of spectacular cures resulting from the imaging process. These accounts are now being corroborated by a growing body of clinical and experimental evidence. The effectiveness of mental imagery in the treatment of a wide variety of problems has been documented (Epstein, 1989; Naparstek, 1994; Sheikh, 1983). These include: obesity (Bornstein & Sipprelle, 1973), insomnia (Sheikh, 1976), phobias and anxieties (Habeck & Sheikh, 1984; Meichenbaum, 1977; Singer, 1974), depression (Schultz, 1984), sexual malfunctions (Singer & Switzer, 1980), chronic pain (Jaffe & Bresler, 1980; Korn & Johnson, 1983; McCaffery & Beebe, 1989), fibroid tumors (Pickett, 1987-1988), cancer (Hall, 1984), and a host of other ailments (Sheikh, 1984, 2002; Sheikh, Kunzendorf, & Sheikh, 1996).

This chapter will outline the use of imagery in various ancient traditions, as well as in Western medical practice, and it will review current imagery-based therapeutic approaches.

HEALING IMAGES: ANCIENT WISDOM

Many believe that in the beginning our universe was completely sacred and that humans were an integral part of it (Eliade, 1959; Samuels & Samuels, 1975). Their existence consisted of participating in the endless dance of creation, carefully examining its steps, resonating with its rhythm, and exploring its many meanings. Humans sought solitude to contemplate the multiple facets of the self and they also sought companionship. They intuitively understood that humans and all other aspects of the universe, the animals, plants, minerals, and stars, issued from the same spring and were one. They knew life and death but did not

3

distinguish between them. Consciousness was not restricted to the self, but echoed the heartbeat of the entire universe. Within this context, health consisted simply of being in harmony with creation (Scholem, 1961).

Over time, this sense of unity with the universe was lost; the feeling of the interrelation and interdependence of all things faded from human consciousness. There now was an abyss separating individuals from God, or, in Judeo-Christian terms, they had been driven from the Garden of Eden. They experienced loneliness and anxiety; their quest for a return to the state of grace is called "mysticism" (Scholem, 1961).

The basic means that mystics have used to regain the state of unity and to experience the ecstasy produced by it are ascetic practices and visualization. Shamanism is an ancient form of mysticism.

Shamanism and Imagery

Shaman is derived from the Russian *saman*, which means "ascetic." The concept of the shaman, which encompasses the notions of priest, healer, and magician, is ancient and is found among the people of all continents. Also, shamanistic practices are remarkably similar across cultures (Achterberg, 1985; Noll, 1987). Basically they consist of healing by imagination or, more specifically, by using visualization to bridge the gulf between the individual and the universe. Eliade (1964) has called the shaman "the great master of ecstasy" and has defined shamanism as the "technique of ecstasy."

In primitive societies, where shamanism flourished, sacred and secular aspects of life were thoroughly integrated. Hence the shamans were equally involved with such diverse affairs as raising crops, waging war, performing marriages, and providing spiritual guidance. In short, they used their power to assist the community in whatever area a need arose (Desjarlais, 1992; Kripner, 1993).

The shamans were both priests and doctors. They were concerned both with the spirit and with the body because they considered the two to be aspects of one integrated organism. Obviously, the current dominant belief among Western physicians that mind and body are separate entities stands in radical opposition to the shamanic stance. Modern scientists generally look upon the body independently of the spirit. Disease is an external agent, something against which one should protect oneself; failing that, disease is something that should be removed or destroyed through technological intervention. The shamans not only knew of no reason to isolate the spirit from the body, but they even recognized the danger of doing so. In their view, the primary problem was not the pathological change in the body but the decrease in personal power that led to the intrusion of disease. In other words, disease was a concrete manifestation of a spiritual crisis. Hence the shamans' first course of treatment for all ailments consisted of an attempt to build up the patient's power; only then would they begin to deal with the bodily symptoms. For instance, among the Navaho Indians, elaborate concrete visualizations are used to bolster the patient's spiritual resources. This rite, in which a number of people participate, encourages the patient to visualize himself or herself as healthy, and it aids the healer to visualize the patient regaining a harmonious place (Achterberg, 1985; Samuels & Samuels, 1975).

The shamans' primary focus was not bodily well-being but spiritual health. They were not primarily concerned with prolonging life, but rather with improving its quality by restoring harmony. Their interest in disease sprang from their belief that illness pointed to a spiritual crisis. If it was handled incompetently, it could be destructive; however, it also could become the springboard for personal growth and vision. According to shamanic tradition, a person's reason for being is to be initiated into the realm of the spirit and thereafter to live in harmony with the rest of the universe. The ultimate disaster is the loss of one's soul, for it robs life of all meaning forevermore (Achterberg, 1985; Grossinger, 1980; La Barre, 1938, 1979).

The shamans' primary mission was to nurture the soul and to protect it from going astray; thus they often described their role in the health process as making an imaginary journey in a quest of the sick person's soul, finding it and returning it to its owner. Although the shamans were active in many facets, their own cultures rated them primarily on their skill as "technicians of the sacred" (Rothenberg, 1968).

A closer look at some shamanic healing procedures would be appropriate. Spiritualistic methods predominated, but a variety of other approaches also were used widely, and many of these were imagery based. A four-step training process developed by the Kahuna healers of Polynesia and described by King (1983) well serves as our example. It involves 1) awareness of thoughts *(ike)*, 2) establishing goals *(makia)*, 3) changing *(kala)*, and 4) directing energy *(manawa)*.

The Kahunas maintain that before you can proceed to change attitudes and assumptions, you must be aware of the ones you have *(ike)*. Therefore, the Kahuna may begin by encouraging the patient to note habitual patterns of speech, internal dialogue, and imagery themes. A patient who is accustomed to suppressing negative thoughts often requires considerable help to bring them to consciousness. Toward this end, the Kahuna attempts to stimulate *makahu* imagination, which is spontaneous or stimulated imagination that reveals belief patterns; the means is guided imagery. Sometimes the mere awareness of the counterproductive habits of thought or speech suffices to bring about immediate changes in attitude, but generally awareness alone does not lead to any change. The Kahunas feel that this is so because all current experience is supported by habits, and their way of dealing with a bad habit is replacing it with another desirable habit. This leads to the next step, *makia* (establishing goals).

Goals would include adopting new beliefs and habits and making plans for the future. The Kahuna nudges the patient toward clear ideas of his or her target state of health, personality, and environment and toward the realization of what he or she will need to do to achieve the goals. An important technique used in *makia* is *pa laulele* ("see and be"). It consists of clearly visualizing a desired circumstance and then adding oneself to the picture with all one's senses. In other words, one is aiming for the mind set of a mime during his or her act. This exercise pretrains the subconscious and the body in preparation for the new experience. Another technique in *makia* is the repetition of short, emotionally laden affirmations. These must be chosen with care in order to ensure that they are fostering the desired condition and not merely suppressing unwanted material. Affirmations that are believable are generally more effective than those that are not. Maintaining the affirmation "I am healthy" when one is ill, is effective with only a few.

Many patients display considerable subconscious resistance to change. This will prompt the Kahuna to proceed to the next step, *kala* (changing). The word *kala* means "release, freedom, and forgiveness," and also "changing one's path" (King, 1983, p. 127). In order to be successful in this phase, the patient must recognize his or her inner conflict with respect to the negative habit, and he or she must be consciously willing to relinquish old ways and adopt new ones. The Kahuna will encourage the patient to replace the undesirable thought, feeling, or action with a desirable one, stressing replacement rather than suppression followed by substitution. To facilitate the task, the healer may use a variety of techniques. The Kahuna may instruct the patient in muscle relaxation, since negative thoughts and emotions do not develop in a relaxed state. The healer may decide to lead the patient in an exploration of his or her memory with the aim of reinterpreting or even altering past experiences. But the Kahuna's main technique for dealing with negative habits is *laulele,* or deliberate imagination. It is an imagery pattern to direct thoughts, emotions, and actions into new directions. With practice, this pattern becomes a habit. This process involves the step of *manawa* (directing energy).

The word *manawa* means "directing *mana*" (energy, life force). *Manawa* involves the establishment and maintenance of positive habits, and this can be accomplished only through practice. The patient may use anything that contributes to reinforcing target habits, such as reading material, symbolic pictures and objects, rituals, physical surroundings, and the company of role models.

The Kahunas stress the final step. They maintain that ideas are ineffective unless they are part of the *Ku* mind (the subconscious). Knowledge that is merely intellectual is just an opinion, and, as such, is incapable of affecting the individual's life. Hence another Huna word for enlightenment is *ná auao,* which means "gut knowledge."

This is a very cursory outline of some shamanic healing practices involving imagination. A closer look would reveal their intricacies and sophistication.

Imagery in Judaism, Christianity, and Islam

The ecstasy states and the powers that accompany them, which have been described by the shamans, were echoed by the disciples of the evolving religions of India, the Middle East, and Europe. As the modern religions of

Judaism, Christianity, and Islam developed, they became more institutionalized—that is, they elaborated doctrines and policies that were based on reason and emphasized the authority of the institution. Also, they established priests as mediators between the individual and God, thus curtailing direct experience of God (Samuels & Samuels, 1975).

But visualization continued to play a role in these institutionalized religions. It could not be otherwise, for all religions involve the notion of a spiritual universe that cannot be verified in the physical world. Biblical Jews rejected idols, which are externalizations of inner images, but the Old Testament and the New Testament are replete with visions and dreams. These visions are unique in that they come and go unbidden, often are extremely vivid, and generally exert a profound effect. A familiar example is the dream of the Egyptian pharaoh of seven fat cows being devoured by seven gaunt cows, and seven full ears of corn being swallowed up by seven thin ears. Joseph's interpretation that 7 years of plenty would be followed by 7 years of famine would prove to be correct.

In addition to textual examples of visualizations, the rituals of these religions rely heavily on imagery, for it has proven itself to be an effective technique in helping the faithful attain their spiritual goals. Visualization translates an abstract idea into a concrete experience and thus clarifies and intensifies it (Samuels & Samuels, 1975). The Christian Communion service is an eminent example. As participants in the ceremony partake of bread and wine, they visualize the Last Supper, which Christ shared with his disciples, and are purified by it. Furthermore, Roman Catholics believe that the bread and wine *become* the body and blood of Christ; that they are transmuted, transubstantiated in the ceremony.

Throughout history, many rich mystical traditions have coexisted with the institutionalized forms of Judaism, Christianity, and Islam. The mystics sought a personal experience of God, or ecstatic states, and their methods to achieve their goal generally involved visualization.

Kabbalah is a Jewish mystical tradition that began in Biblical times and is still alive today. In early times, it was regarded to be heretical by mainstream Judaism, and hence its teachings were spread secretly (Scholem, 1961).

Kabbalistic mysticism involves the use of symbolic doctrines, magic, and ascetic rites. The latter relied heavily on visualization. The practice of the Kabbalistic mystics of the period between the 1st century B.C. and the 10th century A.D. will serve as an example. They aspired to the ascent of their soul from earth, past hostile rulers of the cosmos, to its ultimate home in God's light. To bring about this ascent, the devoted fasted, whispered hymns, and sat with their heads between their knees. Then they visualized the seven palaces of the hostile rulers and entered one after the other. They saw the rulers of the palaces and used armor, weapons, or secret names to pass through. Then they experienced the burning of their body, and finally they came into the presence of God. This visualization may not have originated with the Kabbalistic mystics, for it can be traced to Greek texts and to earlier papyri written in Egypt (Samuels & Samuels, 1975; Scholem, 1961).

The Christian Gnostic tradition is very similar to the Kabbalistic one. The Christian mystics speak of a detachment from external sensations, symbolism and magical rituals, intense concentration, visualizations of ascent and descent to other worlds, and direct experiences of God. A manual of spiritual exercises written in the first century A.D. by St. Ignatius, one of the church fathers, illustrates the practices of this tradition. St. Ignatius instructs the reader to imagine a graded series of holy scenes leading up to a visualization of Christ, which fully absorbs the mind. St. Ignatius also wrote about personal mystical experiences: He reports that, upon one occasion, he distinctly saw the divine plan in the creation of the universe and that at another time he was allowed to contemplate, in images suited to man's feeble understanding, the mystery of the Holy Trinity (James, 1963; Jonas, 1958; Samuels & Samuels, 1975).

Another prominent example of the use of imagery within Christianity is provided by a relatively recent development. In the late 1800s, Mary Baker Eddy founded Christian Science, which rests on the concept that God is an infinite, divine mind. Disease is essentially a human product, and deep prayer causes the power of the Divine Mind to focus on the disease and to bring about healing. Mary Baker Eddy (1934) described this procedure:

> To prevent disease or to cure it, the power of Truth, of divine Spirit, must break the dream of the material senses. To heal by argument, find the type of the ailment, get its name, and array your mental plea against the physical. Argue at first mentally, not audibly, that the patient has no disease, and conform the argument so as to destroy the evidence of disease. Mentally insist that harmony is the fact, and that sickness is a temporal dream. Realize the presence of health and the fact of harmonious being, until the body corresponds with the normal conditions of health and harmony. (p. 412)

The importance of imagination has been recognized also in Sufism, the mysticism or inward aspect of Islam (Corbin, 1970). Sufi literature presents a clear inner road map for spiritual awakening. In Sufism, "love is the underlying principle of morality. It springs from self-denial and expresses itself in service to others. It can reconcile all differences and heal all wounds" (Arasteh & Sheikh, 1996, p. 148). The major emphasis in Sufism is on self-knowledge which eventually evolves into knowledge of God. There are several Sufi meditative techniques in which imagery inevitably plays a role. These include: 1) *zekr*, a contemplation on the 99 names or attributes of God; 2) visualization of the spirit of a saint; 3) *takhliya*, a meditation aimed at obviating one's moral weaknesses; and 4) *tahliya*, a meditation designed to strengthen one's virtues so that vices become weak and ultimately die (Ajmal, 1986).

Imagery in the Hindu/Buddhist Tradition

Although most of the religions of the world employ imagery techniques for healing and spiritual growth, the Hindu/Buddhist traditions—in particular the Indian Yogic practices and the Tibetan Buddhist medical systems–display the most highly developed forms.

Imagery In Yoga. Indian yogic practices have included visualization for thousands of years. Although the *Yoga Sutras* of Patanjali was written approximately 200 B.C., the ascetic practices it contains had been in use in India for millennia. Some of the main yogic practices described are *dharana,* or riveting one's attention on a specific place inside or outside the body; *dhayana,* or sustained focus of attention supported by helpful suggestions; and *samadhi,* or the union of the object of concentration and the person focusing upon it. According to the *Yoga Sutra,* when an individual achieves this union, he or she grasps the truth of the object and attains a state of bliss (Eliade, 1958, 1964; Mishra, 1973).

Tantric yoga is the most sophisticated system of holding images in the mind for a specific purpose. *Tantra* means "that which extends knowledge." It arose in India and Tibet around 600 A.D., and it became a dominant religious and philosophical force because it provided an answer to the increasingly common belief that humans had lost direct contact with truth. Tantra offered a series of complex methods by which the individual could attain truth once more (Samuels & Samuels, 1975).

Like other religions, Tantra distinguishes between the ephemeral world of matter and the real world of the spirit. According to Tantra, the entire cosmos is *maya,* or cosmic illusion—that is, the physical world of the senses as well as the mental realm of thoughts and dreams are *maya.* Beyond matter and mind lies absolute reality, which is eternal and permanent. A primary goal of Tantrism is liberation from the illusion that the physical world, as perceived by the senses and the mind, is real (Eliade, 1958).

In order to achieve this goal, the aspirant must transcend the ego, that is, both the "I" of the conscious reality of the senses and the "I" of subconscious tendencies and realities. He or she must stop regarding himself or herself as matter and learn to identify with the absolute (Samuels & Samuels, 1975).

This is accomplished not by means of theoretical learning but through personal experience or, more precisely, by learning to concentrate, to control the mind, and to ignore the distractions offered by the senses. The basic techniques for changing the focus from the physical world to the spiritual realm are visualization and meditation. The master may instruct the yogi to visualize a certain god or an object, and the yogi will focus repeatedly upon this image until it is very clear, which may take years (Eliade, 1958).

After the yogi has succeeded in developing a vivid image of the deity, the master may direct him or her to identify himself or herself with this deity. This technique of visualization and identification is not just a mental exercise; it serves to awaken the divine nature within the practitioner and thus helps him or her to go beyond *maya* to ultimate reality (Samuels & Samuels, 1975).

In the book *Tibetan Yoga and Secret Doctrines,* Evans-Wentz (1967) includes a number of visualizations taken from ancient Tantric texts. One example follows:

> Imagine thyself to be the Divine Devotee Vajra-Yogini (a goddess of intellect and energy); . . . the right hand holding aloft a brilliantly gleaming curved knife and flourishing it overhead, cutting off completely all mentally disturbing thought-processes; the left hand holding against her breast a human skull filled with blood (symbolizing renunciation of the world) . . . with a tiara of five dried human skulls (symbolizing highest spiritual discernment) on her head; wearing a necklace of fifty blood-dripping human heads (symbolizing severance from the round of death and re-birth); her adornments, five of the Six Symbolic Adornments (the tiara of human skulls, the necklace of human heads, armlets and wristlets, anklets, the breastplate Mirror of Karma), the cemetery-dust ointment (symbolizing renunciation of the world and conquest of fear over death) being lacking, holding in the bend of her arm, the long staff, symbolizing the Divine Father, the Heruka (the male power); nude, and in the full bloom of virginity, at the sixteenth year of her age (unsullied by the world); dancing, with the right leg bent and foot uplifted, and the left foot treading upon the breast of a prostrate human form (treading upon ignorance and illusion); and flames of wisdom forming a halo about her.
>
> (Visualize her as being thyself), eternally in the shape of a deity, and internally altogether vacuous like the inside of an empty sheath, transparent and uncloudedly radiant; vacuous even to the fingertips, like an empty tent of red silk or like a filmy tube distended with breath. (pp. 173-175)

In other visualization exercises commonly used by Tantric yogis, a mandala is the concentration device. A mandala is a complex circular design composed of concentric geometric forms that may contain images of deities or objects. The contents symbolize principles of the universe, such as tension, action, receptivity, and wholeness, as well as Tantric doctrines, such as the eradication of ignorance. Concentration upon the mandala, again, is not just a mental discipline; it eventually leads to identification with the principles depicted (Mookerjee, 1971).

Healing and salvations also are promoted by *mantras,* or mystic syllables. The energy of the body produces vibrations. The vibrations of the diseased body produce a discordant sound, but the recitation of *mantras* can restore harmony.

Tantric yogic practices involving visualization were extensively incorporated and developed by the Tibetan Buddhist medical tradition.

Imagery in Tibetan Buddhist Medicine. Religion, mysticism, psychology, and scientific medicine have come together in Buddhist Tibetan medicine to produce a highly complex tradition. To the Westerner steeped in scientific materialism, the study of this product of an ancient and sacred culture is baffling but also richly rewarding. It offers carefully elaborated and relevant models of holistic medicine, of psychosomatic medicine, of mental and psychic healing, of the role of the healer, and of the use of illness to develop wisdom. Tibetan medicine, like most traditional systems, is holistic. It recognizes the link between mind and body and also between humans and the cosmos. The Tibetan approach also shares with other ancient medical systems the view that health is a matter of balance; however, the Tibetans have presented the most refined version of this concept. They propose that illness is brought on by imbalance or disharmony within the microcosm or between the latter and the macrocosm (Epstein & Rapgay, 1996). The root cause is the delusion of the ego's self-existence; thus, the ultimate cure lies in enlightenment. The various aspects of Tibetan medicine are tightly integrated; however, in order to facilitate study, it is useful to separate them into three areas (Clifford, 1984).

1. *Somatic medicine* has its roots primarily in the Indian Ayurvedic system. It relies on naturopathy (e.g., massage and controlled diet), herbal medicines, acupuncture, and other techniques.
2. *Dharmic (or religious) medicine* utilizes spiritual and psychological practices, such as meditation, moral development, and prayer, in order to fathom the nature of the mind and to control negative emotions.
3. *Tantric (or yogic) medicine* contains elements of both the mental and the physical approach. It relies on psychophysical practices to direct the body's energy toward healing.

Both the dharmic and the tantric aspects of Tibetan medicine utilize meditation and visualization extensively. One widely used visualization involves the mandala of the medicine Buddha. At the center of the mandala, a radiant Buddha sits in lotus position on a 1,000-petaled lotus, which in turn is perched on a jeweled throne. In his right hand he is holding the myrobalan plant, and in his left hand a begging bowl filled with healing nectar. In this exercise, one imagines that one is sitting in a beautiful landscape and offering to the Buddha all that is precious. Now one asks him to bless one's being and to sit on the top of one's head. Then one senses the Buddha's rays of a brilliant light stream into the body, dissolving illness and suffering.

A variation is to visualize oneself as the medicine Buddha and the outer world as the outer part of the mandala. Thus one generates the healing light of the Buddha and thereby one's view of the self and of the world is purified.

The visualization of light plays a large part in tantric healing. One images brilliant light, generally white or blue, radiating from the deity and flowing through one's being, purifying it both mentally and physically. If the meditation is used for a personal ailment, the light is directed to the diseased area; if the exercise is used for the healing of others, the light is sent out into the universe. A variation of this exercise is to merge with the deity's light after it has entered one's being and to become light oneself. This light eradicates dualistic concepts; consequently, one enters a state of blissful emptiness. After coming out of this meditation, one is still identified with the deity and can focus one's healing light on disease in oneself or in someone else (Birnbaum, 1979).

Another healing meditation involves Buddha Vajrasattva, a deity of purification. He is white, sitting in lotus position, holding in his right hand a *vajra*, representing skillful means, and in his left hand a bell, representing wisdom. One imagines him to be sitting on the top of one's head and confesses one's transgressions to him. Then by the strength of one's promise to avoid further wrongdoing and due to Vajrasattva's vow to purify, his light streams into one's head and descends into the body illuminating it. All one's mental and physical ailments dissipate and exit one's being in the form of blood, pus, smoke, or insects.

Mantras are also widely utilized to promote well-being. They may be used alone but generally are used in combination with other techniques. One can visualize a healing *mantra* as a mandala. This mantric mandala can be imagined to be in one's own hand, conferring upon it a healing touch, or in the heart of the individual to be cured. Or one can repeat a *mantra* at the same time as one is doing the imagery of healing light (Clifford, 1984).

It is obvious that according to the Tibetan tradition disease originates in the spirit and thus the potential for recovery likewise lies in the spirit; cure cannot be wrought by mere external intervention. Unlike modern Western physicians, the Tibetan healer does not merely diagnose the ailment and prescribe treatment; he or she interacts with the patient and nurtures him or her back to health. Since this is a spiritual undertaking, the healer's moral quality is believed to play an important role in the cure. No matter which type of medicine the healer uses primarily, he or she also will be practicing some mystic healing exercises. Their potency is believed to be directly affected by the state of his or her consciousness—the purity of intention and by the powers of concentration.

The ultimate goal of the healer is not to bring about relief from symptoms but to put the patient back on the path that leads to enlightenment—life's ultimate goal. Disease must be regarded as a blessing, for it lets the patient know that he or she is harboring a fundamental disharmony—that he or she is out of balance. This awareness is the first step in making necessary adjustments in life and thus progressing toward enlightenment (Blofeld, 1970; Burang, 1974; Clifford, 1984).

HEALING IMAGES: A HISTORICAL OUTLINE OF THEIR USE IN THE WESTERN MEDICAL TRADITION

To Westerners of the 20th century, it might appear that the use of imagination in healing is not part of our culture. Yet, this is untrue. In fact, the ethical code of honor accepted by all physicians today pays tribute to the mythical founding family of medicine who contributed a method for healing by the imagination. The oath begins: "I swear by Apollo, the Physician, by Asclepius, by Hygeia and Panacea and by all the Gods and Goddesses, making them my witnesses, that I will fulfill according to my ability and judgement this oath and this covenant."

As we have already noted, dreams and visions universally have been the most common method of diagnosis and treatment. But it was during the Grecian era, a time when the art of medicine flourished, that imagery-based diagnosis and therapy were systematized and incorporated into the standard approach to disease (Achterberg, 1985).

The figurehead of this movement was Asclepius. He probably was a mortal, but in the *Iliad*, Homer presents him as the son of Apollo who was brought into heaven by Zeus as a demigod. Asclepius's immediate family shared in his healing power. His wife, Epione, soothed pain; his daughters, Hygeia and Panacea, were regarded as deities of health and treatment; and his son, Telesphores, represented convalescence or rehabilitation.

Asclepius became the patron of healing for centuries, and his influence extended far beyond the borders of Greece. Asclepius seemed to satisfy the need for a personal, compassionate divinity; hence, wherever he was introduced, he replaced or merged with the local healing deity. The legend of Asclepius merged with that of the Egyptian god of healing, Imhotep, and with the god Serapis of the Ptolemics. Within Christianity, Saints Damian and Cosmos carried on the healing traditions of Asclepius (Lyons & Petrucelli, 1978).

A testimony to the influence of Asclepius is found in the over 200 temples, or Asclepia, which were built throughout Greece, Italy, and Turkey both to pay tribute to him and to foster the practice of medicine. These Asclepia were the first holistic treatment centers. They were located in picturesque areas and contained baths, recreational facilities, and places of worship. All who sought treatment were admitted, regardless of their ability to pay, for Asclepius taught that a physician was primarily someone to whom anyone who was suffering could turn.

At the Asclepia, dream therapy or divine sleep, which later was renamed incubation sleep by Christian practitioners, was perfected as a diagnostic and therapeutic tool. Most of the patients who underwent this treatment were seriously ill and had not responded to other treatments. In preparation for dream therapy, the patient fasted for one day and did not consume wine for three days; thus attaining spiritual clarity to receive the divine message. Then the patient went to the temple to await the gods. Insight and consequently healing occurred during the state of consciousness immediately preceding sleep, when images appear unbidden. At this time, the image of Asclepius would emerge—a gentle but powerful healer, carrying a rustic staff entwined by a serpent—and he would either cure or prescribe treatment (Achterberg, 1985).

Many cures have been ascribed to Asclepian dream therapy: the blind, deaf, lame, impotent and barren, and those afflicted by innumerable other diseases have left stone images or written accounts of their cures on the temple walls.

Aristotle, Hippocrates, and even Galen have their roots in the Asclepian tradition and were convinced that imagination played a central role in health. Aristotle proposed "that the emotional system did not function in the absence of images. Images were formed by the sensations taken in and then worked upon by the *senses communis* or the 'collective sense.'" Also, he felt that images of the dream state deserved special notice. In *Parva Naturalia*, he advises, "Even scientific physicians tell us that one should pay diligent attention to dreams, and to hold this view is reasonable also for those who are not practitioners but speculative philosophers" (see Achterberg, 1985, p. 56).

But it was Galen who was the first one to provide a detailed outline of the relationship between mind and body. He proposed that the patient's images or dreams provide valuable diagnostic information. For instance, images of loss, grief, or disgrace indicate an excess of melancholy (black bile), and images of fear or fighting reveal an excess of choler. Galen was aware of the vicious circle created by an excessive humor that produced corresponding images, which then exacerbated the humor; and he stressed that the cycle had to be broken in order to regain health (Binder, 1966; Osler, 1921).

The Asclepian tradition and the art of healing through imagination survived the gradual ascendancy of the Christian Church and its purge of pagan gods. Statues of the Asclepian family, the caduceus symbol, and the Hippocratic oath have endured perhaps because they stand for a value inherent in the art of medicine—respect for humanity. As Hippocrates said, "Where there is love for mankind, there is love for the art of healing" (see Achterberg, 1985, p. 57).

Within Christendom, however, the miracles of healing were no longer ascribed to the Asclepian family but rather to Saints Cosmos and Damian. These two men worked tirelessly to provide medical care until they became victims of the Diocletian persecution (278 A.D.). Churches dedicated to them were always open to the sick. The primary method of diagnosis and therapy in use was incubation sleep, a variation of the Asclepian divine sleep (Lyons & Petrucelli, 1978). During the state of drowsiness preceding sleep, the patient would have images of Saints Cosmos and Damian, who would offer a diagnosis and a cure (Achterberg, 1985).

Imagination continued to play an important role in the Western healing traditions well into the Renaissance. For instance, Paracelsus, a famous physician and the founder of modern chemistry, restated a theme common among the ancient Greeks—that is, the individual comprises three elements: the spiritual, the physical, and the mental. He reportedly said:

> Man has a visible and an invisible workshop. The visible one is his body, the invisible one is imagination (mind). . . . The imagination is the sun in the soul of man. . . . The spirit is the master, imagination the tool, and the body the plastic material. . . .   The power of the imagination is a great factor in medicine. It may produce diseases . . . and it may cure them. . . . Ills of the body may be cured by physical remedies or by the power of the spirit acting through the soul. (Hartman, 1973, pp. 111-112)

Paracelsus also maintained, "Man is his own healer and finds proper healing herbs in his own garden, the physician is in ourselves, and in our own nature are all things that we need" (Stoddard, 1911, p. 231).

Physicians of the Renaissance still considered health to be a matter of equilibrium, and their therapy consisted of adjusting imbalance. Hence they prescribed arousing images for the phlegmatic personality and used joyful images to combat melancholy. Shakespeare reflects this view in the introduction to *The Taming of the Shrew*.

> For so your doctors hold it very meet:
> seeing too much sadness hath congeal'd your blood,
> And melancholy is the nurse to frenzy:
> Therefore, they thought it good you hear a play,
> And frame your mind to mirth and merriment,
> Which bars a thousand harms and lengthens life.
>
> (Act I, Scene I)

This holistic approach prevailed until the 17th century when René Descartes (1596-1650) proposed a revolutionary view. He defined the mind as a separate entity. He maintained that the mind or soul, terms he used interchangeably, is "entirely distinct from the body . . . and would not itself cease to be all that it is, even should the body cease to exist" (McMahon & Sheikh, 1984, p. 13). This dualistic view, which gradually won over Western thinkers, quite radically changed the approach to disease.

Imagery in Pre- and Post-Cartesian Medicine: A Comparison

In the pre-Cartesian period, no mind-body problem existed. Both mental and physical events had their roots in a common substrate, a biological soul. But Descartes proposed that mind and body are mutually exclusive entities. Therefore, mechanistic physiopathology became the dominant approach to disease (McMahon, 1976).

In the holistic era, imagination—a faculty of the biological soul—was considered to be a very significant psychophysiological variable. Aristotle had proposed, "The soul never thinks without a picture" (Yates, 1966, p. 32). He also felt that the emotions always were activated by imagery. Of course, the images were believed to provoke certain physical effects. That is, when the imagination conceived an image, spirits activated the brain and then aroused the heart, and the vividness and persistence of the image determined the extent of its impact on bodily functions. It is interesting to note that imagination was considered to be more powerful than sensations; therefore, dread of an event was viewed more harmful than the event itself. Images were considered sufficiently potent to be used to gain conscious·control over autonomic or involuntary functions, and it was thought that images could even imprint traits on embryos in the womb. Charron stated in 1601 that imagery "marks and deforms, nay, sometimes kills embryos in the womb, hastens births, or causes abortions" (McMahon, 1976, p. 180).

The key to a correct evaluation of the role of the imagination in the pre-Cartesian period lies in realizing that imagery was regarded to be as much a physiological phenomenon as a psychological one. It was believed that a vivid and persistent negative image spread throughout the body and wrought its mischief, which soon became manifest in physical symptoms. Since healers of this period believed images to be capable of causing disease, it follows that they also looked to images for their therapies (McMahon & Sheikh, 1984; Sheikh, Richardson & Moleski, 1979).

After Descartes's dualism had taken roots in the Western mind, imagination was stripped of its role in disease and wellness. During the 18th and 19th centuries, several protests were voiced, but the dualistic trend prevailed.

HEALING IMAGES: PSYCHOTHERAPEUTIC USES

When psychology emerged as a separate science in the late 19th century, interest in the arousal function of imagery became apparent, and William James's theory of "ideo-motor action" was received very favorably. It seemed that the time was ripe for a renaissance of Aristotelian theory. But this was not the case. The behaviorists successfully eliminated all mentalistic concepts from the arena of serious research (McMahon & Sheikh, 1984). Watson (1913) regarded mental images as mere ghosts of sensations with no functional significance whatsoever. Klinger (1971) notes that from 1920 to 1960, there was a moratorium in North American psychology on the study of inner experience, and not even one book on the topic of mental imagery was published. However, in Europe the situation was not quite the same. European clinical psychologists and psychiatrists continued to evince significant sensitivity to the inner realm of imagery and were relatively unperturbed by the rapidly increasing influence of behaviorism in America. Several factors aided the continuation of this largely subjective approach to imagery in Europe: 1) many experimentalists left Europe during the two World Wars; 2) German and French phenomenology influenced European clinical and scientific systems; 3) the subjective approaches to the investigation of various aspects of the inner experience, proposed by Jung, affected many European practitioners; and 4) Europe had been influenced by subjective Eastern psychology (Jordan, 1979; McMahon & Sheikh, 1984; Sheikh & Jordan, 1983). It must be noted, however, that although European clinicians were successful in escaping the stranglehold of behavioristic formulations, until very recently, they were unable to elude the powerful influences of Cartesian dualism. Consequently, with a few exceptions, the use of imaginative skills was confined to the treatment of only the so-called psychological problems and was not applied to physical ones.

European Contributions in the 1900s

The notable contributions to the clinical use of images in the early 1900s include the work of Pierre Janet, Alfred Binet, Carl Happich, Eugene Caslant, Oscar Vogt, Johannes Schultz, Ludwig Frank, Sigmund Freud, and Carl Jung (see Sheikh & Jordan, 1983, for a review). Of all these, Jung's contribution played the most significant role in the imagery movement in psychotherapy. He regarded mental imagery as a creative process of our psyche to be employed for attaining greater individual, interpersonal, and spiritual integration (Jordan, 1979). Jung stated:

> The psyche consists essentially of images. It is a series of images in the truest sense, not an accidental juxtaposition or sequence but a structure that is throughout full of meaning and purpose; it is a picturing of vital activities and just as the material of the body that is ready for life has a need of the psyche in order to be capable of life, so the psyche presupposes the living body in order that its images may live. (Jung, 1960, pp. 325-326)

By recognizing the reciprocity of the psyche and the body, Jung indicated his belief in the mind-body unity as a life process and proposed that imagery is a vehicle of perceiving and experiencing this life process (Sheikh & Jordan, 1983). Jung remarked that when we "concentrate on a mental picture, it begins to stir, the image becomes enriched by details, it moves and develops . . . and so when we concentrate on inner pictures and when we are careful not to interrupt the natural flow of events, our unconscious will produce a series of images which makes a complete story" (Jung, 1976, p. 172). Jung's therapeutic use of imagery is best represented by the method he termed "active imagination." For details of the method, the reader is referred to other sources (Jung, 1960; Sawyer, 1986; Singer & Pope, 1978; Watkins, 1976).

More recently, several French, German, and Italian clinicians, all significantly influenced by Jung, have investigated the potential use of imagery as a method of psychotherapy. The most prominent of these approaches include Desoille's (1961, 1965) *Directed Daydream,* Fretigny and Virel's (1968) *Oneirodrama,* Leuner's (1977, 1978) *Guided Affective Imagery,* and Assagioli's (1965) *Psychosynthesis.* The first three of these four approaches have some basic similarities. The term "oneirotherapy" (from the Greek *oneiros* meaning "dream," hence also known as "dream therapy" or "waking-dream therapy") has been used to describe all three therapies (Much & Sheikh, 1986; Sheikh & Jordan, 1983).

1. All three oneirotherapies employ *extended* visual fantasies in *narrative* form to obtain data concerning the motivational system of the client. These fantasies are generally preceded by an attempt to induce relaxation.
2. Products of visual imagination are used in conjunction with associations, discussion, and interpretation.

3. Generally, the client is presented with certain standard symbolic scenes as the starting images. These scenes are presumed to reflect common areas of conflict.
4. With respect to assumptions and interpretations, all oneirotherapeutic procedures are psychodynamic in nature. These methods rest on the belief that the symbolism inherent in visual imagery constitutes an affective language that expresses unconscious motives without fully imposing them on conscious recognition. Therefore, it is assumed that the participant will show less resistance to the expression of the underlying motives (Sheikh & Jordan, 1983).

In general, these methods have been reported to be effective in uncovering the structural details of the client's personality, in discovering the nature of the affective trauma, and in quickly ameliorating the symptoms. Fretigny and Virel (1968) mention a few other advantages of their use of imagery, which can be applied to all three approaches. They claim that: 1) mental imagery can be used with persons who find systematic reflection difficult due to their low level of sophistication; 2) the use of imagery circumvents the snares of rational thinking; 3) this approach discourages sterile rumination; and 4) mental imagery aims directly at the individual's affective experience (Sheikh & Jordan, 1983).

Compared to most European approaches, Assagioli's psychosynthesis is more holistic and eclectic. One of the goals of psychosynthesis is to enhance the personal and spiritualistic potential of the individual. To achieve this goal, Assagioli and his followers have employed Western analytic, behavioral, and humanistic procedures along with Eastern meditative techniques. In psychosynthesis, the human personality is considered to have a number of layers of awareness. The goal "is not only the explication of these various levels of awareness and the relief of personal difficulties. Rather, its goal is a thorough reconstruction of the total personality, exploration of the various levels of personality, and eventually the shift of personality to a new center through exploration of its fundamental core" (Singer, 1974, p. 109).

Mental imagery is only one of the many methods employed in psychosynthesis. Assagioli uses several imagery procedures that reflect the principles discussed by Jung, Desoille, and Leuner, along with conditioning and cognitive restructuring techniques. In interpreting the images, accompanying verbal associations and other relevant information are utilized. Every element of the image is believed to represent, at one level or another, a personality trait, albeit distorted, displaced, or projected. Identification with all aspects of the image drama is regarded as a means of assimilating repressed material in socialized form and expanding the boundaries of the self (Sheikh & Jordan, 1983).

One must credit the European clinicians not only for keeping alive the clinical use of images in the wake of behaviorism but also for providing a rich heritage of therapeutic procedures, for keeping us in touch with the unavoidably phenomenological nature of perception, and for building a bridge between Eastern and Western approaches to the understanding of the nature of human consciousness (Jordan, 1979; Panagiotou & Sheikh, 1977; Sheikh & Jordan, 1983).

Current American Approaches

During the last two decades, imagery has risen from a position of near disgrace to become one of the hottest topics in both clinical and experimental cognitive psychology. Experimental and clinical psychologists of varied persuasions have made imagery the subject of their inquiry, and they have produced a considerable body of literature documenting that images are indeed a powerful force.

Due to space limitation, it is not possible to present a detailed discussion of various American imagery approaches to psychotherapy. Interested readers are referred to other sources (Sheikh, 2002; Sheikh & Jordan, 1983; Singer, 1974; Singer & Pope, 1978). However, it is possible to categorize the numerous existing imagery approaches in America into the following six broad groups.

1. A number of imagery approaches that are based largely on the Pavlovian and Skinnerian models constitute the first group. They highlight the surface relationship between images and emotional responses as well as the ability of images to act as powerful stimuli. These procedures consist of several variations of counterconditioning and emotional flooding (Sheikh & Jordan, 1983; Sheikh & Panagiotou, 1975). They include systematic desensitization (Wolpe, 1969), implosion therapy (Stampfl & Lewis, 1967), covert conditioning (Cautela, 1977), coping imagery and stress innoculation (Meichenbaum, 1977), and many others.

2. The second category is composed of the procedures advanced by a number of clinicians who believe that mental images effectively give us a clear understanding of our perceptional and affective distortions. Unlike the cognitive behavior therapists, proponents of these approaches do not resort to explanations in terms of conditioning principles. Beck (1970), for example, explains the conditioning effects of repetitive fantasy in cognitive terms. He states that the repetition of images provides important information and clarifies cognitive and affective distortion for the client. Gendlin and his associates (Gendlin, 1978, 1996; Gendlin & Olsen, 1970) employ "experiential focusing" to clearly comprehend all aspects of the feeling. They claim that emergence of an image frequently moves the client from a "global sense of feeling to a specific crux feeling." This image, "typically becomes quite stable as the feel of it is focused on and even refuses to change until one comes to know what the feeling it gives one is. Then one feels not only the characteristic release, but the image then changes" (Gendlin & Olsen, 1970, p. 221). Morrison (1980) emphasizes "the value of retracing early developmental experiences in order to apply the adult's more

adequate construct system" and thus to better understand those experiences (p. 313). In Morrison's emotive-reconstructive therapy, images are the primary therapeutic agent.

3. The third class includes a number of approaches that basically consist of imagery rehearsal of physical and psychological health (Achterberg, Dossey, & Kolkmeier, 1994; Naparstek, 1994). The client may be asked to image a malfunctioning organ becoming normal or to practice in imagination a healthy, interpersonal relationship. No complicated theories are offered except the assumption that sane imagination will eventually lead to sane reality (McMahon & Sheikh, 1984). No one can claim credit for developing these procedures, for they have been around for centuries (Sheikh, 1984, 1986, 2002).

4. The fourth group consists of image therapies with a psychoanalytic orientation. Prominent among these approaches are "emergent uncovering" (Reyher, 1977) and "psycho-imagination therapy" (Shorr, 1978). Mardi Horowitz (1978) is another psychoanalytically oriented clinician who has made important contributions to the study of the role of mental images in clinical practice.

It is noteworthy that Freud was well aware of the spontaneous images experienced by his clients, and he apparently used imagery extensively prior to 1900. But he later abandoned it in favor of verbal free association. Yet, although Freud and his followers tended to avoid the explicit uses of mental images in therapy, several characteristics of the psychoanalytic setting encourage the production of imagery. These include: reclining in a restful position, low level of sensory stimulation, use of free association, and emphasis on dreams, fantasies, and childhood memories (Pope, 1977; Sheikh & Jordan, 1983; Singer & Pope, 1978).

5. The fifth class includes the "depth" imagery procedures in which emphasis is on healing through "magical" or "irrational" methods as opposed to rational or reflexive techniques. A prime example of this group is "eidetic psychotherapy" (Ahsen, 1968; Sheikh, 1978, 2001; Sheikh & Jordan, 1981), which relies on the elicitation and manipulation of eidetic images. Every significant event during our development is considered to implant an eidetic in the system. The eidetic is seen as a tridimensional unity. The visual component, the *image,* is always accompanied by a *somatic pattern*—a set of bodily feelings and tensions, including somatic correlations of emotions—and a cognitive or experiential *meaning.* This triadic unity is considered to display certain lawful tendencies toward change that are meaningfully related to psychological processes.

6. Recently, a sixth category of imagery approaches has been attracting increasing attention among health professionals. These approaches have resulted from the advent of the "third force," or humanistic psychology, and of the "fourth force," or transpersonal psychology. Both of these put emphasis on greater access to experience, on a variety of states of consciousness, and on increasing realization of our potentials. This orientation has led to the emergence of numerous novel imagery methods, which are derived from European oneirotherapies, psychosynthesis techniques, autogenic training, Jungian active imagination, and from

Eastern meditative practices (Perls, 1970; Progoff, 1970; Sheikh & Jordan, 1983; Singer, 1974). These methods include taking an imaginary inventory of the body, having an imaginary dialogue with internal parts of oneself, creating and interacting with an inner advisor in one's imagery, dying in one's imagination, visualizing communication between the two hemispheres of the brain, crawling into various organs of the body for observatory or reparatory purposes, exorcising the parents from various parts of the body, and regressing into the "previous life" (Sheikh, 1986, 2002; Sheikh & Shaffer, 1979; Sheikh & Sheikh, 1996).

CONCLUDING REMARKS

It is obvious that imagery is generally perceived as an extremely effective therapeutic tool. Researchers have ascribed the clinical efficacy of images to a variety of mechanisms. Singer (1974) believes that the effectiveness of imagery essentially depends on: 1) the client's clear discrimination of his or her ongoing fantasy processes; 2) clues provided by the therapist regarding alternate approaches to various situations; 3) awareness of usually avoided situations; 4) encouragement by the therapist to enter into covert rehearsal of alternate approaches; and 5) consequent decrease in fear of overtly approaching the avoided situations. Meichenbaum (1978) has suggested further simplification. He believes that the key to the effectiveness of the images lies in: 1) the feeling of control that the client gains from monitoring and rehearsing various images; 2) the modified meaning or changed internal dialogue that precedes, accompanies, and succeeds instances of maladaptive behavior; and, 3) the mental rehearsal of alternative responses that enhances coping skills (Sheikh & Jordan, 1983).

In addition to the processes outlined by Singer and Meichenbaum, numerous other characteristics of the imagery mode have been credited with contributing to its clinical effectiveness.

1. Experience in imagination can be viewed as psychologically equivalent, in many significant respects, to the actual experience; imagery and perception seem to be experientially and neurophysiologically similar processes (Klinger, 1980; Kosslyn, 1980; Richardson, 1969, 1994; Sheikh & Jordan, 1983).
2. Verbal logic is linear, whereas the image is a simultaneous representation. This trait of simultaneity gives imagery greater isomorphism with perception and, therefore, greater capacity for descriptive accuracy (Sheikh & Panagiotou, 1975).
3. The imagery system fosters a richer experience of a range of emotions (Singer, 1979).
4. Mental images lead to a variety of physiological changes (Richardson, 1984; Sheikh & Kunzendorf, 1984; Sheikh, Kunzendorf, & Sheikh, 1996; White, 1978).

5. Images are a source of details about past experiences (Sheikh & Panagiotou, 1975).
6. Imagery readily provides access to significant memories of early childhood when language was not yet predominant (Kepecs, 1954).
7. Imagery appears to be very effective in bypassing defenses and resistances (Klinger, 1980; Naperstek, 1994; Reyher, 1963; Singer, 1974).
8. Imagery frequently opens up new avenues for exploration, after therapy has come to an impasse (Sheikh & Jordan, 1983).
9. Images are less likely than linguistic expression to be filtered through the conscious critical apparatus. Generally, words and phrases must be consciously understood before they are spoken—that is, they must pass through a rational censorship before they can assume a grammatical order. Perhaps imagery is not subject to this filtering process; therefore it may be a more direct expression of the unconscious (Panagiotou & Sheikh, 1977; Sheikh, Kunzendorf & Sheikh, 1996).
10. The failure to think imagistically creates disharmony in the mind and body (Ahsen, 1978; Schwartz, 1984).

In the light of the foregoing characteristics of imagery, it seems reasonable to believe that images hold enormous potential for healing, and it is not surprising that extensive claims about the promise of imagery for therapeutic benefits have been made. A large body of recent scientific research on imagery indicates that these claims are justified. However, direct systematic research on the therapeutic outcome of imagery approaches with clients suffering from a variety of ailments has started to receive attention only recently and further work is urgently needed.

REFERENCES

Achterberg, J. (1985). *Imagery in healing.* Boston: Shambhala.
Achterberg, J., Dossey, B., & Kolkmeier, L. (1994). *Rituals of healing: Using imagery for health and wellness.* New York: Bantam.
Ahsen, A. (1968). *Basic concepts in eidetic psychotherapy.* New York: Brandon House.
Ahsen, A. (1978). Eidetics: Neural experiential growth potential for the treatment of accident traumas, debilitating stress conditions, and chronic emotional blocking. *Journal of Mental Imagery, 2,* 1-22.
Ajmal, M. (1986). *Muslim contributions to psychotherapy and other essays.* Islamabad, Pakistan: National Institute of Psychology.
Arasteh, A. R., & Sheikh, A. A. (1996). Sufism: The way to universal self. In A. A. Sheikh & K. S. Sheikh (Eds.), *Healing East and West.* New York: Wiley.
Assagioli, R. (1965). *Psychosynthesis: A collection of basic writings.* New York: Viking.
Bachelard, G. (1969). *On poetic imagination and reverie.* Boston: Beacon.
Beck, A. T. (1970). Role of fantasies in psychotherapy and psychopathology. *Journal of Nervous and Mental Diseases, 150,* 3-17.
Binder, G. A. (1966). *Great moments in medicine.* Detroit: Park-Davis.
Birnbaum, R. (1979). *The healing Buddha.* Boulder, CO: Shambhala.

Blofeld, J. (1970). *The Tantric mysticism of Tibet.* New York: Dutton.

Bornstein, P. H., & Sipprelle, C. N. (1973, April). *Clinical applications of induced anxiety in the treatment of obesity.* Paper presented at the Southeastern Psychological Association meeting.

Burang, T. (1974). *The Tibetan art of healing.* London: Robinson and Watkins.

Cautela, J. R. (1977). Covert conditioning: Assumptions and procedures. *Journal of Mental Imagery, 1,* 53-64.

Clifford, T. (1984). *Tibetan Buddhist medicine and psychiatry.* New York: Samuel Weiser.

Corbin, H. (1970). *Creative imagination in the Sufism of Ibn 'Arabi* (R. Manheim, Trans.). London: Routledge & Kegan Paul.

Desjarlais, R. R. (1992). *Body and emotion: The aesthetics of illness and healing in the Nepal Himalayas.* Philadelphia: University of Pennsylvania Press.

Desoille, R. (1961). *Theorie et pratique du rêve éveillé dirigé.* Geneva: Mont Blanc.

Desoille, R. (1965). *The directed daydream.* New York: Psychosynthesis Research Foundation.

Eddy, M. B. (1934). *Science and health with key to the scriptures.* Boston: First Church of Christ Scientist.

Eliade, M. (1958). *Yoga: Immortality and freedom.* New York: Pantheon.

Eliade, M. (1959). *The sacred and the profane.* New York: Harper & Row.

Eliade, M. (1964). *Shamanism: Archaic techniques of ecstasy.* New York: Pantheon.

Epstein, G. (1989). *Healing visualization.* New York: Bantam.

Epstein, M., & Rapgay, L. (1996). Mind, disease, and health in Tibetan medicine. In A. A. Sheikh and K. S. Sheikh (Eds.), *Healing East and West.* New York: Wiley.

Evans-Wentz, W. Y. (1967). *Tibetan yoga and secret doctrine.* London: Oxford University Press.

Fretigny, R., & Virel, A. (1968). *L'imageri mentale.* Geneva: Mont Blanc.

Gendlin, E. T. (1978). *Focusing.* New York: Everest House.

Gendlin, E. T. (1996). *Focusing-oriented psychotherapy: A manual of the experiential method.* New York: Guilford Press.

Gendlin, E. T. & Olsen, L. (1970). The use of imagery in experiential focusing. *Psychotherapy: Theory, Research and Practice, 7,* 221-223.

Grossinger, R. (1980). *Planet medicine: From stone age shamanism to post-industrial healing.* New York: Doubleday.

Habeck, B. K., & Sheikh, A. A. (1984). Imagery and the treatment of phobic disorders. In A. A. Sheikh (Ed.), *Imagination and healing* (pp. 171-196). Amityville, NY: Baywood.

Hall, H. R. (1984). Imagery and cancer. In A. A. Sheikh (Ed.), *Imagination and healing* (pp. 159-169). Amityville, NY: Baywood.

Hartman, F. (1973). *Paracelsus: Life and prophecies.* Blauvelt, NY: Rudolf Steiner.

Horowitz, M. J. (1978). Controls of visual imagery and therapeutic intervention. In J. L. Singer & K. S. Pope (Eds.), *The power of human imagination.* New York: Plenum.

Jaffe, D. T., & Bresler, D. E. (1980). Guided imagery: Healing through the mind's eye. In J. E. Shorr, G. E. Sobel, P. Robin, & J. A. Connella, (Eds.), *Imagery: Its many dimensions and applications.* New York: Plenum.

James, W. (1963). *The varieties of religious experience.* New York: University Books.

Jonas, H. (1958). *The Gnostic religion.* Boston: Beacon Press.

Jordan, C. S. (1979). Mental imagery and psychotherapy: European approaches. In A. A. Sheikh and J. T. Shaffer (Eds.), *The potential of fantasy and imagination.* New York: Brandon House.

Jung, C. G. (1960). *The structure and dynamics of the psyche* (R. F. C. Hull, Trans.). (Collected works, Vol. 8). Princeton: Princeton University Press. (Original work published 1926.)

Jung, C. G. (1976). *The symbolic life* (R. F. C. Hull, Trans.). Collected works, Vol. 18). Princeton: Princeton University Press.

Kepecs, J. G. (1954). Observations on screens and barriers in the mind. *Psychoanalytic Quarterly, 23,* 62-77.

King, S. (1983). *Kahuna healing.* Wheaton, IL: The Theosophical Publishing House.

Klinger, E. (1971). *The structure and function of fantasy.* New York: Wiley.

Klinger, E. (1980). Therapy and the flow of thought. In J. E. Shorr, G. E. Sobel, P. Robin, & J. A. Connella (Eds.), *Imagery: Its many dimensions and applications.* New York: Plenum.

Korn, E. R., & Johnson, K. (1983). *Visualization: The uses of imagery in the health professions.* Homewood, IL: Dorsey.

Kosslyn, S. (1980). *Image and mind.* Cambridge: Harvard University Press.

Kripner, S. (1993). Some contributions of native healers to knowledge and the process. *International Journal of Psychosomatics, 40* (1-4), 96-99.

La Barre, W. (1938). *The peyote cult.* New Haven: Yale University Press.

La Barre, W. (1979). Shamanic origins of religion and medicine. *Journal of Psychedelic Drugs, 1-2,* 7-11.

Leuner, H. (1977). Guided affective imagery: An account of its development. *Journal of Mental Imagery, 1,* 73-92.

Leuner, H. (1978). Basic principles and therapeutic efficacy of guided affective imagery. In J. L. Singer & K. S. Pope (Eds.), *The power of human imagination.* New York: Plenum.

Lyons, A. S., & Petrucelli, R. J. (1978). *Medicine: An illustrated history.* New York: Abrams.

McCaffery, M., & Beebe, A. (1989). *Pain: Clinical manual for nursing practice.* Philadelphia: Mosby.

McMahon, C. E. (1976). The role of imagination in the disease process: Pre-Cartesian history. *Psychological Medicine, 6,* 179-184.

McMahon, C. E. & Sheikh, A. A. (1984). Imagination in disease and healing processes: A historical perspective. In A. A. Sheikh (Ed.), *Imagination and healing* (pp. 7-34). Amityville, NY: Baywood.

Meichenbaum, D. (1977). *Cognitive-behavior modification: An integrative approach.* New York: Plenum.

Meichenbaum, D. (1978). Why does using imagery in psychotherapy lead to change? In J. L. Singer & K. S. Pope (Eds.), *The power of human imagination.* New York: Plenum.

Mishra, R. (1973). *Yoga stuvas.* Garden City, NY: Anchor Press.

Mookerjee, A. (1971). *Tantra art.* Paris: Ravi Kumar.

Morrison, J. K. (1980). Emotive-reconstructive therapy: A short-term psychotherapeutic use of mental imagery. In J. E. Shorr, G. E. Sobel, P. Robin, & J. A. Connella (Eds.), *Imagery: Its many dimensions and applications.* New York: Plenum.

Much, N. C., & Sheikh, A. A. (1986). The oneirotherapics. In A. A. Sheikh (Ed.), *Anthology of imagery techniques.* Milwaukee, WI: American Imagery Institute.

Naparstek, B. (1994). *Staying well with guided imagery.* New York: Warner Books.

Noll, R. (1987). The presence of spirit in magic and madness. In S. Nicholson (Ed.), *Shamanism: An expanded view of reality*. Wheaton, Illinois: The Theosophical Publishing House.

Osler, W. (1921). *The evolution of modern medicine*. New Haven: Yale University Press.

Panagiotou, N., & Sheikh, A. A. (1977). The image and the unconscious. *International Journal of Social Psychiatry, 23*, 169-186.

Perls, F. (1970). *Gestalt therapy verbatim*. New York: Bantam.

Pickett, E. (1987-88). Fibroid tumors and response to guided imagery and music: Two case studies. *Imagination, Cognition and Personality, 7*, 165-176.

Pope, K. S. (1977). *The flow of consciousness*. Unpublished doctoral dissertation, Yale University, Cambridge.

Progoff, I. (1970). Waking dream and living myth. In J. Campbell (Ed.), *Myths, dreams and religion*. New York: Dutton.

Reyher, J. (1963). Free imagery, an uncovering procedure. *Journal of Clinical Psychology, 19*, 454-459.

Reyher, J. (1977). Spontaneous visual imagery: Implications for psychoanalysis, psycho-pathology, and psychotherapy. *Journal of Mental Imagery, 2*, 253-274.

Richardson, A. (1969). *Mental imagery*. New York: Springer.

Richardson, A. (1984). Strengthening the theoretical links between imaged stimuli and physiological responses. *Journal of Mental Imagery, 8*, 113-126.

Richardson, A. (1994). *Individual differences in imaging*. Amityville, NY: Baywood.

Rothenberg, J. (Ed.). (1968). *Technicians of the soul*. Garden City, NY: Doubleday.

Samuels, M., & Samuels, N. (1975). *Seeing with the mind's eye*. New York: Random House.

Sawyer, D. (1986). How Jungians work with images. In A. A. Sheikh (Ed.), *Anthology of imagery techniques*. Milwaukee, WI: American Imagery Institute.

Scholem, G. (1961). *Jewish mysticism*. New York: Schocken.

Schultz, K. D. (1984). The use of imagery in alleviating depression. In A. A. Sheikh (Ed.), *Imagination and healing*. Amityville, NY: Baywood.

Schwartz, G. E. (1984). Psychophysiology of imagery and healing: A systems perspective. In A. A. Sheikh (Ed.), *Imagination and healing* (pp. 35-50). Amityville, NY: Baywood.

Sheikh, A. A. (1976). Treatment of insomnia through eidetic imagery: A new technique. *Perceptual and Motor Skills, 43*, 994.

Sheikh, A. A. (1978). Eidetic psychotherapy. In J. L. Singer & K. S. Pope (Eds.), *The power of human imagination*. New York: Plenum.

Sheikh, A. A. (Ed.). (1983). *Imagery: Current theory, research and application*. New York: Wiley.

Sheikh, A. A. (Ed.). (1984). *Imagination and healing*. Amityville, NY: Baywood.

Sheikh, A. A. (Ed.). (1986). *Anthology of imagery techniques*. Milwaukee, WI: American Imagery Institute.

Sheikh, A. A. (Ed). (2002). *Handbook of therapeutic imagery techniques*. Amityville, NY: Baywood.

Sheikh, A. A., & Jordan, C. S. (1981). Eidetic psychotherapy. In R. J. Corsini (Ed.), *Handbook of innovative psychotherapies*. New York: Wiley.

Sheikh, A. A., & Jordan, C. S. (1983). Clinical uses of mental imagery. In A. A. Sheikh (Ed.), *Imagery: Current theory, research, and application*. New York: Wiley.

Sheikh, A. A., & Kunzendorf, R. G. (1984). Imagery, physiology, and psychosomatic illness. *International Review of Mental Imagery, 1*, 95-138.

Sheikh, A. A., Kunzendorf, R. G., & Sheikh, K. S. (1989). Healing images: From ancient wisdom to modern science. In A. A. Sheikh & K. S. Sheikh (Eds.), *Eastern and Western approaches to healing.* New York: Wiley.

Sheikh, A. A., Kunzendorf, R. G., & Sheikh, K. S. (1996). Somatic consequence of consciousness. In M. Velmans (Ed.), *The science of consciousness.* London: Routledge.

Sheikh, A. A., & Panagiotou, N. C. (1975). Use of mental imagery in psychotherapy: A critical review. *Perceptual and Motor Skills, 41,* 555-585.

Sheikh, A. A., & Shaffer, J. T. (Eds.). (1979). *The potential of fantasy and imagination.* New York: Brandon House.

Sheikh, A. A. & Sheikh, K. S. (1996). *Healing East and West.* New York: Wiley.

Sheikh, A. A., Richardson, P., & Moleski, L. M. (1979). Psychosomatics and mental imagery: A brief view. In A. A. Sheikh and J. T. Shaffer (Eds.), *The potential of fantasy and imagination.* New York: Brandon House.

Shorr, J. E. (1978). Clinical use of categories of therapeutic imagery. In J. L. Singer & K. S. Pope (Eds.), *The power of human imagination.* New York: Plenum.

Singer, J. L. (1974). *Imagery and daydream methods in psychotherapy and behavior modification.* New York: Academic Press.

Singer, J. L. (1979). Imagery and affect psychotherapy: Elaborating private scripts and generating contexts. In A. A. Sheikh & J. T. Shaffer (Eds.), *The potential of fantasy and imagination.* New York: Brandon House.

Singer, J. L., & Pope, K. S. (1978). The use of imagery and fantasy techniques in psychotherapy. In J. L. Singer & K. S. Pope (Eds.), *The power of human imagination.* New York: Plenum.

Singer, J. L., & Switzer, E. (1980). *Mind play: The creative uses of imagery.* Englewood Cliffs, NJ: Prentice-Hall.

Stampfl, T., & Lewis, D. (1967). Essentials of therapy: A learning theory-based psychodynamic behavioral therapy. *Journal of Abnormal Psychology, 72,* 496-503.

Stoddard, A. M. (1911). *Life of Paracelsus.* London.

Watkins, M. J. (1976). *Waking dreams.* New York: Harper.

Watson, J. B. (1913). The place of the conditioned reflex in psychology. *Psychological Review, 23,* 89-116.

White, K. D. (1978). Salivation: The significance of imagery in its voluntary control. *Psychophysiology, 15,* 196-203.

Wolpe, J. (1969). *The practice of behavior therapy.* New York: Pergamon.

Yates, F. A. (1966). *The art of memory.* London: Routledge & Kegan Paul.

This chapter is a revised version of part of a previously published paper (Sheikh, Kunzendorf, & Sheikh, 1989). It is included here with permission from John Wiley and Sons, New York.

CHAPTER 2

Physiological Consequences of Imagery and Related Approaches

ANEES A. SHEIKH, ROBERT G. KUNZENDORF,
KATHARINA S. SHEIKH, AND SHEILA M. BAER

> A six-year-old girl . . . having received a bicycle for Christmas, started to ride it immediately, without any difficulty, before the astonished eyes of her parents. When they asked how she had learned to do that, she answered: "I had been imagining it all the time." (Ferrucci, 1982, p. 166)

In the introduction to *The Healing Heart* (Cousins, 1983), Dr. Bernard Lown describes a seriously ill patient: He had suffered a heart attack which had severely damaged the cardiac muscle; he was experiencing chaotic arrhythmia that was hard to control, and his breathing was labored. The patient was being kept alive with oxygen and an intravenous drip of cardiac stimulant. On one of the rounds, Dr. Lown mentioned to the attending staff that the patient's heart had a "wholesome, very loud third sound gallop." This condition indicates that the heart is straining and is on the brink of a failure. However, following this conversation, the patient "miraculously" improved and was discharged from the hospital. When asked by Dr. Lown about his recovery, he responded:

> I was sure the end was near and you and your staff had given up hope. However, Thursday morning when you entered with your troops, something happened that changed everything. You listened to my heart; you seemed pleased by the findings and announced to all those standing about my bed that I had a wholesome gallop. I knew that the doctors, in talking to me, might try to soften things. But I know they wouldn't kid each other. So when I heard you tell your colleagues I had a wholesome gallop, I figured I still had a lot of "kick" to my heart and could not be dying. My spirits were, for the first time, lifted and I knew I would recover.

There is abundant anecdotal evidence demonstrating physiological consequences of conscious mental processes such as imagery, hypnosis, and meditation.

27

Furthermore, an impressive body of empirical research has accumulated over the last two decades which demonstrates quite convincingly that conscious processes, in one form or another, are clearly capable of leading to measurable physiological changes and should be considered significant determinants of disease and health. This chapter first briefly traces the history of thought in the field of psychosomatics and then outlines research dealing with physiological consequences of meditation, imagery, biofeedback, and hypnosis. The concluding section further emphasizes the role that consciousness plays in bringing about extensive physiological changes.

PSYCHOSOMATICS: A BRIEF HISTORICAL REVIEW

Although the term "psychosomatic" was introduced by Heinroth, a German psychiatrist, in 1818, modern psychosomatic medicine came into being in the early 1930s as a result of an integration of two concepts of ancient Greek origin—*psychogenesis* and *holism* (Lipkowski, 1986a, 1986b).

The concept of psychogenesis refers to the belief that psychological factors are capable of causing bodily diseases. Starting with the ancient Greeks, numerous writers have asserted this position. For example, Archer, a 17th-century English physician, said, "The observation that I have made in practice of physik these several years hath confirmed me in this opinion, that the original, or cause, of most mens and womens sickness, disease and death is first, some great discontent which brings a habit of sadness of mind" (1673, p. 121). Similarly, Benjamin Rush (1811), a famous American physician and author of the first American textbook of psychiatry, emphasized that the "actions of the mind" caused many diseases and could be used as therapeutic agents. More recently, Freud and his followers made further contributions to the concept of psychogenesis.

The concept of holism was first introduced by Smuts (1926) but its lineage dates back to ancient Greece. It is derived from the Greek word *holos*, meaning whole. "It refers to the postulate that mind and body constitute an indivisible unity, or whole, and that the study and treatment of the sick need to take into account the whole person rather than isolated parts" (Lipkowski, 1986a, p. 4). For example, Plato, in *Charmides*, subtitled *The Mistake of Physicians*, suggests: "And this is the reason why the cure of many diseases is unknown to the physicians of Hellas, because they are ignorant of the whole which ought to be studied also; for the part can never be well unless the whole is well. It is the greatest mistake in the treatment of disease that there are physicians who treat the body and physicians who treat the mind, since both are inseparable" (quoted in Freyhan, 1976, p. 381).

In 1637, the French philosopher René Descartes proposed the radical view that the body was separate from the mind. The body was regarded as a machine controlled by mechanistic laws, and the mind as an "immaterial substance." Although Descartes had left the possibility of mind-body interaction open, his ideas were profoundly influential in fostering biological determinism in medical theory and research (McMahon & Sheikh, 1989).

However, in spite of Descartes' far-reaching influence, the holistic notions survived and kept appearing in the works of many writers. Two significant 20th-century examples include Canon's (1915) concept of homeostasis which presented a somatic basis for the holistic notion and Adolf Meyer's (1957) psychobiology that asserted that "mind and body were two distinct yet integral aspects of the human organism, a psychobiological unit, as a whole" (Lipkowski, 1986a, p. 5).

In the early 1930s, in reaction to Cartesian dualism and biological reductionism, the concepts of psychogenesis and holism appeared in a reformist movement called psychosomatic medicine. "While core assumptions were of ancient lineage, that movement had a crucial new feature: it initiated a systematic scientific study of the interaction of psychological and biological factors in health and disease" (Lipkowski, 1986a, p. 5).

In 1939, the first issue of the journal *Psychosomatic Medicine* appeared and it formally sanctioned the scientific investigation of psychosomatics in medical thinking and research. This development apparently was overdue; for, within two decades the psychosomatic movement was noticed internationally. By the early 1960s, a dozen journals on this topic appeared in the industrialized countries and membership in professional societies for psychosomatic research has undergone exponential growth (McMahon & Koppes, 1976; McMahon & Sheikh, 1989).

It has become increasingly clear that persons, not cells or organs, have diseases, and that human beings do not merely consist of "self-contained organs carrying out specialized metabolic processes in isolation uninfluenced by external events" (Weiner, 1977, p. 8). Social and psychological variables now appear to play an important role in the predisposition for, and inception and maintenance of, diseases (Gatchel & Blanchard, 1993; Schwab, 1978; Sheikh, Richardson, & Moleski, 1979; Shontz, 1975; Weiner, 1977; Wittkower, 1977). Also, several personality factors (i.e., inability to release emotions) that characterize psychosomatic cases have been noted (Shontz, 1975; Gatchel & Blanchard, 1993).

Many theorists seem to agree that certain stimulus situations, overt or covert, elicit a variety of internal conditions, which if sufficiently intense and prolonged, will lead to structural or somatic alterations. A number of theories have been proposed concerning which structure will undergo alterations (Lachman, 1972; Sheikh, Richardson, & Moleski, 1979).

According to *Constitutional-Vulnerability (Weak-Link) Theories*, stressful stimulation damages the most vulnerable organ: The chain breaks at the weakest link. The elements that render a particular organ more vulnerable are genetic factors, injuries, diseases, and other previous influences. Proponents of *Organ Response Learning Theories* hold that due to a previous connection between emotional stimulation and a reinforced response of an organ, further stressful cues lead to the same organ response. If these stressful situations are frequent, persistent, and sufficiently intense, a malfunction of or damage to that organ may result. Partisans of *Stimulus Situation Theories* contend that certain emotional stimulus situations cause specific physiological reactions and this leads to damage to the organ structure involved. An innate relationship between various patterns of stimulation and those of physiological reaction is often implied. Followers of *Personality-Profile Theories* maintain that various personality structures result in differing reaction tendencies, and thus different individuals are predisposed to different kinds of psychosomatic pathologies. Lastly, *Symptom Symbol Theories* that originated in psychoanalytic conceptions hold that the diseased organ or system has symbolic meaning for the patient (Sheikh, Richardson, & Moleski, 1979).

It should be noted that the proponents of almost all of the foregoing theories have implicitly, if not explicitly, recognized the part played by conscious mental processes in the development of diseases.

MEDITATION AND PHYSIOLOGY

Meditation is perhaps the oldest and the most celebrated way of demonstrating the psychophysiological effects of consciousness (Ramaswami & Sheikh, 1989). A common element of the meditative experience in both Eastern and Western traditions "is an overwhelming and compelling consciousness of the soul's oneness with the ... Divine Ground" (Ramaswami & Sheikh, 1989, p. 435), and many mystics in both traditions are firmly grounded in theism. Meditation is generally thought to consist of four stages: preparation, attention, reception, and higher consciousness (Goleman, 1988; Willis, 1979).

Meditation is obviously a complex subject matter. However, many investigators, for the purpose of research, have defined it as a "stylized mental technique from Vedic or Buddhist [or Sufi] traditions repetitively practiced for the purpose of attaining a subjective experience that is frequently described as very restful, silent, and of heightened alertness, often characterized as blissful" (Jevning, Wallace, & Beideback, 1992, p. 415). After comparing numerous meditation techniques, Benson came to the conclusion that the differences between various techniques are merely "stylistic manners reflecting a core of four universal ingredients" (Lichstein, 1988, p. 33). These four elements in Benson's (1975) *secular* method include: a quiet environment, an object to dwell upon, a passive attitude, and a comfortable position. Benson suggests that the object to concentrate on be a mental device, such as silent repetition of the word *one*, that will "lure one's attention away from worldly concerns" (Lichstein, 1988, p. 33).

While meditation has been practiced for centuries, its scientific study started only a few decades ago. Although a wide variety of meditation techniques exist, most of the available research deals with one specific technique, transcendental meditation (TM). Also, much of this research contains serious methodological flaws. But, in spite of the methodological shortcomings and considerable inconsistency of findings, a review of the literature indicates meditation is not a neutral event in its consequences, that it is different from ordinary rest and sleep, and that it can have definite physiological consequences. Davidson (1976), Delmonte (1985, 1986), Jevning, Wallace, and Beidebach (1992), Lichstein (1988), Ramaswami and Sheikh (1989), Wallace and Benson (1972), West (1987), and Woolfolk (1975) provide excellent reviews of the psychophysiological effects of meditation. It is not within the scope of this chapter to provide a detailed review. For details, the reader should consult the fore-mentioned sources.

In this brief review, various meditation techniques have been lumped together; the aim here is not to compare the effects of different techniques but to see if meditation in general has any physiological consequences.

Cardiopulmonary Responses

Theresa Bross, a French cardiologist who traveled to India in 1935, was perhaps the first to study the physiology of meditation. According to her report, one of the subjects was able to stop his heart (see Jevning et al., 1992; Pelletier & Garfield, 1976). But more than 20 years later, frequently quoted researchers, Wenger, Bagchi, and Anand (1961, 1963), were unable to find consistent changes in heart rate as a function of meditation among yogis. Since then, many studies have demonstrated the conscious control of heart rate, blood pressure, cholesterol levels, angina pectoris, and premature ventricular contraction through meditative experiences (see Barnes, Schneider, Alexander, & Staggers, 1997; Jevning et al., 1992; Lichstein, 1988; Norris, 1989; Ramaswami & Sheikh, 1989; Sudsuang, Chentanez, & Veluvan, 1991; Telles, Nagarathna, & Nagendra, 1998).

In one of the earliest systematic studies on the effects of meditation, Bagchi and Wenger (1957) observed a lowering of the rate of respiration during meditation. Similar results were reported by Wenger, Bagchi, and Anand (1961) and Anand, Chinna, and Singh (1961a). Hirai (1960), Akishige (1968), and Sugi and Akutsu (1968) reported significant reduction in oxygen consumption during meditation. Subsequently, numerous other researchers have reported changes in respiration rate, oxygen consumption, lung volume, and related pulmonary phenomena and, in many cases, the changes are of even higher magnitudes and significance than previously determined (Farrow & Herbert, 1982; Jevning et al., 1992; Kesterson & Clinch, 1989; Lichstein, 1988; Sudsuang et al., 1991; Wallace, 1970; Wallace & Benson, 1972; Wallace, Benson, & Wilson, 1971). Also, in some cases, these changes are accompanied by reports of experiences of pure consciousness.[1]

---

[1] In the TM literature pure consciousness is defined as a state in which the "mind transcends the subtlest level of mental activity and experiences a state of complete mental quiescence in which thoughts are absent and yet consciousness is maintained." These periods are "characterized by the experience of perfect stillness, rest, stability, and order and by a complete absence of mental boundaries" (Farrow & Herbert, 1982, p. 133).

Jevning et al. (1992) think a probable explanation of this discrepancy is "employment of more experienced subjects and, in some cases, use of longer meditation periods, in later research."

Electrodermal Changes

Several reports of the physiological effects of meditation indicate a marked increase of galvanic skin response (GSR) and decreased spontaneous electrodermal response (EDR) (see Jevning et al., 1992; Ramaswami & Sheikh, 1989). Farrow and Herbert (1982) discovered that markedly increased GSR seemed to accompany reports of experiences of pure consciousness provided by the subjects. Orme-Johnson (1973) noted that GSR habituated to aversive auditory stimuli in both meditators and controls, but more quickly in meditators. Researchers also discovered that the GSR of meditators was more stable during meditation than that of resting controls. West (1979) found that meditators had a significant reduction in spontaneous skin conductance responses.

Electroencephalographic Effects

Beginning with Das and Gastaut (1955), numerous other researchers have reported electroencephalographic (EEG) changes during meditation (Akishige, 1968, 1970; Anand, Chinna, & Singh, 1961a; Banquet, 1973; Davidson, 1976; Kasamatsu & Hirai, 1966; Lynch, Paskewitz, & Orne, 1974; Wallace et al., 1971). The most common results include an increase in the occurrence of the alpha wave. The appearance of theta waves has also been reported. In a recent review of physiological effects of transcendental meditation, Jevning et al. (1992) report a number of other EEG changes. These include: high voltage theta burst activity, increased frontal alpha coherence, and fast beta. They note that EEG coherence seems to correlate with subjective experiences of pure consciousness.

Researchers have also noted that external alpha-blocking stimulation, such as strong light, banging noise, or touching with a hot glass tube, did not block the alpha pattern when yogis were in *samadhi*[2], whereas in a nonmeditating state the alpha was blocked (Anand et al., 1961a, 1961b). Kasamatsu and Hirai (1966), in their EEG study, employed 48 Japanese priests and their disciples with meditation experience ranging from one year to more than 20 years. At the beginning of meditation, fast alpha activity was noted. The alpha amplitude then increased; whereas, the alpha frequency decreased. Also, EEG changes among Zen monks seem to positively correlate with subjective reports of deep meditation and the

---

[2] Samadhi is a state of ecstasy, in which the mind is unperturbed by outer distractions or inner turbulence. It also has been called a "sphere of neither perception nor non-perception" where "even the most refined of the pairs of opposites are transcended, even that between the all or nothingness, the all and the void" (Humphreys, 1987, p. 182).

state of transcendence (Kasamatsu & Hirai, 1966; Banquet, 1973). Furthermore, the longer the subjects had spent in Zen training, the more the EEG changed. "There was also a close relationship between degree of EEG changes and the Zen master's ratings of his disciples' mental status" (Ramaswami & Sheikh, 1989, p. 454).

Other Physiological Effects of Meditation

Numerous other effects of meditation have been reported in the literature. These include the decline of adrenocortical activity (Bevan, 1980; Jevning, Wilson, & Davidson, 1978), decreased cortisol secretion (Subrahmanyam & Potkodi, 1980), and increased urinary metabolite serotonin (Bujatti & Riederer, 1976), increased total protein level, and decreased reaction time (Sudsuang et al., 1991), higher levels of melatonin (Coker, 1999; Tooley, Armstrong, Norman, & Sali, 2000), and faster healing of psoriasis lesions (Kabat-Zinn, Wheeler, Light, Skillings, Scharf, Cropley, Hosmer, & Bernard, 1998). Younger biological age[3] has also been reported among long-term meditators in comparison with the general population (Wallace, Dillbeck, Jacobe, & Harrington, 1982). In several clinical studies, it has been noted that meditation can play a significant role in the amelioration of a variety of health problems such as asthma, insomnia, muscular dysfunction, severe migraine and cluster headaches, abuse of nonprescribed drugs, and cancer (Lichstein, 1988; Jevning et al., 1992).

IMAGERY AND PHYSIOLOGY

Recently, mental imagery has become one of the most significant issues in cognitive and health psychology (Sheikh, 1983, 1984, 2001). While interest and research in imagery have mounted, a consensus concerning the nature and function of images is still lacking. However, the question whether images represent a direct encoding of perceptual experiences (Paivio, 1971), an artifact of propositional structuring (Pylyshyn, 1973), or a constructive and reconstructive process (Kosslyn, 1980) has not been of any real concern to the majority of clinicians and experimenters. They assume that everyone experiences mental representations of objects and events, and these representations constitute their subject matter. A definition of imagery such as the one by Richardson (1969, p. 2) is implicit in most of these approaches: "Mental imagery refers to all those quasi-sensory or quasi-perceptual experiences of which we are self-consciously

---

[3] To measure biological age, the authors used Adult Growth Examination developed by Morgan (Morgan & Fevens, 1972) which includes three subtests measuring auditory threshold, near vision, and systolic blood pressure, which are considered the most reliable and easily assessed indicators of biological age.

aware, and which exist for us in the absence of stimulus conditions that are known to produce their genuine sensory or perceptual counterparts."

During the last two decades, a great deal of research has convincingly demonstrated that images can lead to definite somatic consequences (Kunzendorf & Sheikh, 1990; Sheikh & Kunzendorf, 1984; Sheikh, Kunzendorf, & Sheikh, 1989). A brief review of this literature follows.

Imagery and Heart Rate

Studies of heart rate control through imaging had already been reported around the turn of the century (Ribot, 1906; Tuke, 1872). In the last three decades, several researchers obtained heart rate increases to imagined emotional and/or bodily arousal (Bauer & Craighead, 1979; Bell & Schwartz, 1975; Blizard, Cowings, & Miller, 1975; Boulougouris, Rabavilas, & Stefanis, 1977; Carroll, Baker, & Preston, 1979; Carroll, Marzillier, & Merian, 1982; Craig, 1968; Gottschalk, 1974; Grossberg & Wilson, 1968; Jones & Johnson, 1978, 1980; Jordan & Lenington, 1979; Kunzendorf, Francis, Ward, Cohen, Cutler, Walsh, & Berenson, 1996; Lang, Kozak, Miller, Levin, & McLean, 1980; Marks & Huson, 1973; Marks, Marset, Boulougouris, & Huson, 1971; Marzillier, Carroll, & Newland, 1979; Roberts & Weerts, 1982; Schwartz, 1971; Schwartz, Weinberger, & Singer, 1981; Shea, 1985; Wang & Morgan, 1992; Waters & McDonald, 1973). Decreases in heart rate in response to relaxing images have also been reported (Arabian, 1982; Bell & Schwartz, 1975; Furedy & Klajner, 1978; McCanne & Iennarella, 1980; Shea, 1985). Furthermore, a number of studies have indicated a positive correlation between vividness of imagery and control of heart rate (Barbour, 1981; Carroll, Baker, & Preston, 1979; Grossberg & Wilson, 1968; Lang, Kozak, Miller, Levin, & McLean, 1980). Also, biofeedback and imagery have been successfully combined in the treatment of various arrhythmias (Engel, 1979).

Imagery and Blood Pressure

Schwartz, Weinberger, and Singer (1981) and Roberts and Weerts (1982) reported that diastolic blood pressure rises in response to images of anger but not to images of fear, whereas systolic blood pressure is raised both by images of anger and fear. Wang and Morgan (1992) noted an elevation in both systolic and diastolic blood pressure as a result of imagined exercise. In clinical research, long lasting reductions in both systolic and diastolic blood pressure through relaxing images have been recorded (Ahsen, 1978; Crowther, 1983), and in experimental research, imagery-induced increases in blood pressure have correlated positively with greater image-vividness and poorer reality-testing (Kunzendorf et al., 1996).

Imagery and Blood Flow

General blood flow is determined by vasoconstriction and vasodilation. Several studies have indicated that vasomotor activity can be changed by imaging that specific skin regions feel colder or hotter (Dugan & Sheridan, 1976; Kunzendorf, 1981, 1984; McGuirk, Fitzgerald, Friedman, Oakley, & Salmon, 1998; Ohkuma, 1985). The magnitude of these changes seems to be positively correlated with more prevalent visual and tactile images as assessed by scores on Kunzendorf's Prevalence of Imagery Tests (Kunzendorf, 1981).

Since heat images are capable of concentrating blood in localized tissues of the body, they may be a significant factor behind a number of other findings of studies that employed both hypnosis and imagery. These include: increased warmth in feet and hands (Schrieber, Schrieber, & Weeks, 1998); curing of warts through imaging (Spanos, Stenstrom, & Johnston, 1988; Vollmer, 1946); reduced number of migraines (Olness, Hall, Rozniecki, Schmidt, & Theoharides, 1999); enlargement of breast size through repeated imaging of pulsation and warm feelings in the breast area (Willard, 1977); appearance of redness and swelling on skin through touching leaves that were imagined to be poisonous (Ikemi & Nakagawa, 1962); and redness and even blistering of the skin through imaginary burns (Paul, 1963). In contrast, it has been demonstrated that through images of inactivity hemophiliac dental patients (Lucas, 1965), as well as normal dental patients (Chaves, 1980), can reduce external bleeding.

Imagery and Sexual Response

Research shows that erotic images are sufficient to induce penile engorgement in men (Laws & Rubin, 1969; Smith & Over, 1987), and vaginal engorgement in women (Stock & Geer, 1982). It also appears that the degree of engorgement is positively correlated with imaging ability (Smith & Over, 1987; Stock & Geer, 1982). Research also indicates that erotic images frequently arise during sexual relationships and that they improve sexual responding (Hariton & Singer, 1974; Lentz & Zeiss, 1983-1984; Pope, Singer, & Rosenberg, 1984). Moreover, erotic images seem to consistently induce arousal, whereas erotic pictures and X-rated films induce sexual arousal that tends to habituate (Smith & Over, 1987). Whipple, Ogden, and Komisaruk (1992) noted that orgasm from both self-induced imagery and genital self-stimulation led to significant and comparable increases in systolic blood pressure, heart rate, pupil diameter, pain detection threshold, and pain tolerance threshold.

Imagery and Body Chemistry

A few studies have indicated that several changes in body chemistry can be induced through imaging. These include: increase in free fatty acids accompanying anxious dream imagery (Gottschalk, Stone, Gleser, & Iacono,

1966); change in salivary pH by specific taste images (Kunzendorf & Albright, 1981); increase in salivary flow through taste images (Barber, Chauncey, & Winer, 1964); and increase in gastric acid flow through taste images (Luckhardt & Johnston, 1924).

Imagery and Ocular Effects

Experimental research has shown that visual imagery can affect dilation of the pupil (Colman & Paivio 1970; Paivio & Simpson, 1968; Simpson & Climan, 1971), intra-ocular pressure (Kaluza & Strempel, 1995), the electrical activity of the retina (Kunzendorf, 1984; Kunzendorf & Hall, in press; Kunzendorf, Jesses, & Capone, 1994), and the reflex as well as voluntary movements of the eye (Zikmund, 1972; Richardson, 1978). Ruggieri and Alfieri (1992) studied the effects of perceiving and imagining near and far stimuli and discovered that processes of accommodation occur in both real and imagined conditions.

Imagery and Electrodermal Activity

A number of studies have shown that images of emotional and bodily arousal result in increased electrodermal activity both in normal and abnormal subjects (Bauer & Craighead, 1979; Drummond, White, & Ashton, 1978; Gottschalk, 1974; Haney & Euse, 1976; Passchier & Helm-Hylkema, 1981). Also, image-induced galvanic skin response (GSR) seems to be positively correlated with vividness of imagery (Drummond et al., 1978). In an applied investigation, Yaremko and Butler (1975) observed that, compared to 10 pretest shocks, 10 pretest images of electric shock produced faster electrodermal habituation to test shocks.

Imagery and Electromyographs (EMGs)

Arousing images of stressful situations appear to increase frontalis EMG and subjectively experienced tension (Passchier & Helm-Hylkema, 1981); whereas relaxing images reduce these (Thompson & Adams, 1984). In line with William James' (1890) ideo-motor theory of the relationship between imaged activity and real behavior, Lusebrink (1986-1987) discovered that visual images of a pencil produced EMG activity in the right arm and visual images of the letter "P" led to EMG activity in the lip. Similarly, Schwartz, Fair, Greenberg, Freedman, and Klerman (1974) noted that images of sadness and images of happiness, respectively, increased or decreased facial corrugator EMG activity. Also, Quintyn and Cross (1986) observed that images of movement were helpful in disinhibiting the "frozen" body part in clients with Parkinson's disease.

Imagery and the Immune System

It appears that a number of medical disorders result from overreaction or underreaction of the immune system (Goldberg, 1985). Also, it is widely recognized that psychological and psychosocial variables play a significant role in immune-system functioning (Jemmott & Locke, 1984; McClelland, Floor, Davidson, & Saron, 1985; Thackwray-Emmerson, 1988). Among the psychological variables affecting immune responses, mental images have been the focus of numerous researchers as well as clinicians, and their effects have been documented in both healthy subjects and cancer patients.

In healthy subjects, images of "white blood cells attacking germs" increased neutrophil adherence (Schneider, Smith, Minning, Whitcher, & Hermanson, 1991) lymphocyte counts and salivary immunoglobulin A concentration (Hall, Longo, & Dixon, 1981; Jasnoski & Kugler, 1987; Olness, Culbert, & Uden, 1989), whereas images of an unresponsive immune system produced less neutrophil adherence (Schneider et al., 1991) and lower lymphocyte stimulation of immune response (Smith, McKenzie, Marmer, & Steele, 1985). Also, both image-induced increase and decrease in neutrophil adherence are positively correlated with vividness of induced images as judged by the subjects (Schneider et al., 1991). Zachariae, Kristensen, Hokland, Ellegaard, Metze, and Hokland (1990) combined relaxation and guided imagery procedures, instructing the subjects to imagine their immune system becoming very effective, and noted an increase in natural killer cell function in normal healthy subjects. It should be noted that Schneider et al.'s findings concerning neutrophil adherence received support from three recent hypnosis studies (Bogartz, 1990; Hall, Minnes, Tosi, & Olness, 1992; Hall, Papas, Tosi, & Olness, 1996).

Pioneering work in the use of mental imagery with cancer patients was carried out by the Simontons as early as 1978 (Simonton, Mathews-Simonton, & Creighton, 1978; Simonton, Mathews-Simonton, & Sparks, 1980). They clinically tested the effects of imagery and relaxation with 159 patients who were diagnosed to have medically incurable cancer and were expected to die in a year. Of these, 63 were still alive 2 years later. Of the surviving patients, 22.2 percent showed no evidence of cancer, 19.1 percent were in remission, and 31.8 percent were stabilized. Unfortunately, they had no untreated control group, but the findings are quite impressive.

Achterberg and Lawlis (Achterberg, 1984; Achterberg & Lawlis, 1979) and others have extended the Simonton work. In cancer patients, mental images of events such as tumors being absorbed or attacked by white blood cells have been demonstrated to increase the likelihood of remission (Achterberg, 1984, 1985; Gruber, Hall, Hesch, & Dubois, 1988; Norris, 1989; Pickett, 1987-1988). Furthermore, the probability of remission seems to correlate positively with the imaging ability of the patients as assessed by image-CA, a technique developed by Achterberg and Lawlis (1979).

Imagery and Other Physiological Effects

Attempts have also been made to utilize imagery in the treatment of various other medical problems (Gunville, 1991). Recurrent genital herpes (herpes simplex virus, HSV) was effectively treated with an imagery technique involving deep relaxation and imaging viral resistance and lesion-free genital areas (Longo, Clum, & Yaeger, 1988). Epstein (1986) used imagery to treat enlarged prostrate that was accompanied by symptoms of urinary retention and difficulty in initiating the urinary stream. Holden-Lund (1988) successfully used relaxation and guided imagery for wound healing in surgical patients. Other conditions where imagery or related procedures have been tried with some degree of success include: reduction in the number of asthmatic episodes (Castes, Hagel, Palenque, Canelones, Carao, & Lynch, 1999); healing of burn wounds, ulcers, vaginitis, irritable bowel syndrome, and rheumatoid arthritis (Gunville, 1991).

It is true that not all of the studies reported in the section on imagery and physiology are methodologically sound, and a few are merely clinical case studies. Also, negative findings often are not reported in the literature. Consequently one has to be cautious in drawing conclusions. However, overall it seems safe to conclude that imagery has immense potential to bring about a variety of physiological changes and is a significant component in hypnosis, biofeedback, and perhaps meditation. This field of inquiry deserves further attention from competent researchers.

BIOFEEDBACK, IMAGERY, AND PHYSIOLOGY

Perhaps the first experiment employing biological feedback to the subject was carried out around the turn of the century by J. H. Bair (1901); however, formally, this field of study began about 25 years ago. Biofeedback training involves the "continuous monitoring and amplifying of an ongoing biological process of a person, and the feeding back or displaying of this information to a person's . . . conscious awareness. This allows the individual to intentionally self-regulate the physiological activity being monitored by observing the effects of each self-regulation strategy" (Norris, 1989, p. 268). During the last two decades, an enormous amount of experimental and clinical work has been conducted, and numerous physiological processes have thus been regulated or influenced. These include: cardiovascular and cardiopulmonary changes, gastrointestinal motility, brain rhythms, striate muscle activity, blood flow to various parts of the body, blood glucose and insulin levels, and immune system functioning (Norris, 1989). There are many physiological disorders that biofeedback therapists have been able to treat with a considerable degree of success. These include migraine headaches, neurodermatitis, rheumatoid arthritis, asthma, tachycardia, arrhythmia, cardiospasm, hypertension, gastric ulcers, duodenal ulcers, ulcerative colitis, irritable bowel syndrome, inflammatory bowel disease, Raymond's disease, circulatory complications accompanying diabetes, vaginitis, burn wounds, diabetic foot ulcers, and cerebral palsy (Ford, 1982; Green & Green, 1977; Gunville, 1991; Norris, 1986; also see various issues of the journal *Biofeedback and Self-Regulation*).

A critical review of the biofeedback literature reveals that this technique is not equally effective for all subjects (King & Montgomery, 1980), and that individual differences in the effectiveness of biofeedback seem to be due to individual differences in imaging ability (Hirschman & Favaro, 1980; Ikeda & Hirai, 1976; Kunzendorf & Bradbury, 1983). Furthermore, the efficacy of biofeedback appears to be related not only to imaging ability, but also to the use of imagery during biofeedback (LeBouef & Wilson, 1978; Qualls & Sheehan, 1979; Schwartz, 1975; Takahashi, 1984).

Some researchers have explicitly compared the efficacy of biofeedback alone, biofeedback with imaging instructions, and imaging instructions without feedback. It appears that biofeedback with imaging instructions is more effective than biofeedback alone (Herzfeld & Taub, 1980; Ohkuma, 1985) and imaging alone may be more effective than biofeedback alone (Shea, 1985). It seems reasonable to conclude that some of the effects of biofeedback are due to the autonomic effects of imagery.

HYPNOSIS AND PHYSIOLOGY

In recent years, interest in hypnosis as a scientific phenomenon has increased dramatically. Both experimental and clinical work has credited hypnosis with the capability of effecting a wide variety of physiological effects. For example, through hypnosis, allergic reactions have been inhibited, physiological reactions to cold stress have been minimized, labor contractions have been induced and inhibited in some women, some aspects of the narcotic withdrawal syndrome and of narcotic drug effects have been produced in postaddicts, water diuresis has been elicited in some hydrophenic females, ichthyosis has been mitigated, and wheals have been produced in patients with urticaria (see Barber, 1965, 1978, 1984). Increase in gastric acidity, metabolic rate, and heart rate, reduction of blood calcium level, and alteration in spasticity of the bowels have also been noted (Gorton, 1959). Furthermore, attempts at preventing skin reactions produced by plants such as poison ivy (Ikemi & Nakagawa, 1962), at producing localized skin inflammation (Barber, 1970; Johnson & Barber, 1976), at stimulating the remission of warts (Edwin, 1992; Johnson & Barber, 1978; Noll, 1994; Vollmer, 1946), and at stimulating further growth of breasts (Williams, 1974; Willard, 1977) have been successful. Other somatic effects of hypnosis include: changes in hypersensitivity of skin response (Black, 1963; Black, Humphrey, & Niven, 1963), blistering of skin through imaginery burns (Paul, 1963), reduction of external bleeding in hemophiliac dental patients (Lucas, 1965) as well as normal dental patients (Chaves, 1980), immunomodulation (Hall, Longo, &

Dickson, 1981), asthma and hayfever allergic symptoms (Brown & Fromm, 1987; Mason & Black, 1958), dog allergy (Perloff & Spiegelman, 1973), immune-related diseases (Margolis, 1983; Brown & Fromm, 1987), burn wounds (Barber, 1984), involuntary movements associated with Huntington's disease (Moldawsky, 1984), blood flow and bleeding (Barber, 1984), irritable bowel syndrome and peptic ulceration (Whorwell, 1991); wound and fracture healing (Ginandes & Rosenthal, 1999; Patterson, Goldberg, & Ehde, 1996); and treatment of functional infertility (Gravitz, 1995).

It seems that, just like biofeedback and imagery, hypnosis and imagery may also be closely related (Barber, 1978, 1984). It has been pointed out that suggestions employed in hypnosis generally direct the subject to imagine various situations (Honiotes, 1977; Weitzenhoffer & Hilgard, 1962). Hypnotic responsiveness and the ability to be absorbed in activities involving fantasy and imagination seem to be positively correlated (Barber, 1984; Hilgard, 1965; Sheehan, 1972). Sarbin (1976) has described the good hypnotic subject as being very similar to a child engaged in imaginative play and Crawford (1994) has confirmed that hypnosis and imagination are neurophysiologically related. Also, several researchers have concluded that hypnosis basically intensifies the subject's imaginative processes (Barber, Spanos, & Chaves, 1974; Hilgard, 1965; Sarbin & Coe, 1972). Finally, research has shown that autonomic effects of hypnotic suggestion are mediated by mental imagery (Barber, 1984), that individual differences in the effectiveness of hypnosis are attributable to imaging ability of the subjects (Spanos, Senstrom, & Johnston, 1988, Willard, 1977), and that, although hypnotic images produce significant changes in physiological responses, waking images produce equivalent or even greater changes (Ikemi & Nakagawa, 1962; Shea, 1985; Spanos, Senstrom, & Johnston, 1988; Winer, Chauncey, & Barber, 1965). It is interesting to note that the commission appointed by the King of France to investigate Messmer's claims had also concluded that his cures were primarily due to the excitement of the imagination of the patients (Sheikh, Richardson, & Moleski, 1979). Admittedly not all theorists in the field of hypnosis assign a preeminent role to imagery in hypnosis. For further details, the reader is referred to other sources (Lynn & Rhue, 1991).

CONCLUDING REMARKS

The foregoing review makes it abundantly clear that consciousness is not a mere epiphenomenon, a derivative of physiological processes, and in itself of no functional significance. As the Nobel prize-winning physicist Eugene Wigner, reflecting on the connection between consciousness and the physical world, observed, "if mind could not affect the physical world, but was only affected by it, this would be the only known example in modern physics of such a one-way interaction" (Dossey, 1982, p. 208).

It seems obvious that conscious mental activity can bring about far-reaching physiological changes and its role in health and disease has been grossly undervalued in medical communities. Dr. Marcia Angell (1985, p. 1572), in the *New England Journal of Medicine,* sums up the prevalent medical view: ". . . it is time to acknowledge that our belief in disease as a direct reflection of mental state is largely folklore." It is apparent that we have not yet been able to escape the clutches of dualistic thinking. As Patricia Norris (1986) remarks, philosophy gets in the way of reality, and the research of the last three decades has not influenced the everyday practice of medicine. David McClelland describes the situation this way:

> Judging from my own experience, there will be resistance at every level to the notion that psychological variables play a key role in health, illness, and treatment. I have been told flatly by a world famous immunologist, for example, that psychological factors do not affect the immune system, despite, in my estimation, convincing evidence to the contrary. I have found it very difficult to get scientific papers . . . published in medical journals because reviewers have never heard of the variables . . . or simply find it impossible to believe that they could affect physiological processes. We must not assume that it is enough to demonstrate the importance of psychological variables in health areas to our own personal or scientific satisfaction. It will also require much effort to educate the medical and wider community to the role of psychological variables in health. . . . (1985, pp. 465-466)

Although we have been able to confirm the existence of events that the non-interactionist dualism prohibits, we have not been able to come out of its tenacious hold (McMahon, 1986). Perhaps it is so because no viable alternative models of human nature have been presented in any detail. For example, while it is obvious that there is a big leap involved from consciousness to physiology, we have been evading the question of the "how" of physical symptom formation, and so far extremely limited attention has been given to the matter of transition from a purely mental concept, such as consciousness, to very specific somatic alterations (Kunzendorf, 1991; McMahon & Sheikh, 1989). As the eminent physicist Schrödinger (1945) observed regarding the mind-matter issue: "Science has never been able to adumbrate the causal linkage satisfactorily even to its most ardent disciples" (p. 94).

It is commendable that recently a few open-minded scientists are beginning to look beyond the prevalent ideas concerning the relationship of mind and matter, and are trying to formulate new theories that would more adequately account for new observations (Dossey, 1982; Kunzendorf, 1991; McMahon, 1986; Pert, 1987; Sheikh & Sheikh, 1989; Weimer, 1976). In this regard, familiarity with the development of ideas in physics may turn out to be of invaluable significance (McMahon & Sheikh, 1984, 1989).

REFERENCES

Achterberg, J. (1984). Imagery and medicine: Psychophysiological speculations. *Journal of Mental Imagery, 8*, 1-13.

Achterberg, J. (1985). *Imagery in healing.* Boston: Shambhala.

Achterberg, J., & Lawlis, G. F. (1979). A canonical analysis of blood chemistry variables related to psychological measures of cancer patients. *Multivariate Experimental Clinical Research, 4*, 1-10.

Ahsen, A. (1978). Eidetics: Neural experiential growth potential for the treatment of accident traumas, debilitating stress conditions, and chronic emotional blocking. *Journal of Mental Imagery, 2*, 1-22.

Akishige, Y. (Ed.). (1968). Psychological studies on Zen. *Bulletin of Faculty Literature of Kyrushu University, 5 & 11*, Fukuoka, Japan.

Akishige, Y. (Ed.). (1970). *Psychological studies on Zen.* Tokyo: Zen Institute of Komazawa University.

Angell, M. (1985). Disease as a reflection of the psyche. *New England Journal of Medicine, 312*, 1570-1572.

Anand, B. K., Chinna, G. S., & Singh, B. (1961a). Studies on Sri Ramanand Yogi during his stay in an airtight box. *Indian Journal of Medical Research, 49*, 82-89.

Anand, B. K., Chinna, G. S., & Singh, B. (1961b). Some aspects of electroencephalographic studies in yogis. *Electroencephalography and Clinical Neurophysiology, 13*, 452-456.

Arabian, J.M. (1982). Imagery and Pavlovian heart rate decelerative conditioning. *Psychophysiology, 19*, 286-293.

Archer, J. (1673). *Everyman his doctor.* London.

Bagchi, B. K., & Wenger, M. A. (1957). Electrophysiological correlates of some yogi exercises. *Journal of Electroencephalography and Clinical Neurophysiology, 7*, 132-149.

Bair, J. H. (1901). Development of voluntary control. *Psychological Review, 8*, 474-510.

Banquet, J. P. (1973). Spectral analysis of the EEG in meditation. *Electroencephalography and Clinical Neurophysiology, 35*, 143-151.

Barber, T. X. (1961). Physiological effects of "hypnosis." *Psychological Bulletin, 58*, 390-419.

Barber, T. X. (1965). Physiological effects of "hypnotic suggestions": A critical review of recent research (1960-1964). *Psychological Bulletin, 63*, 201-222.

Barber, T. X. (1970). *Suggested ("hypnotic") behavior: The trance paradigm versus an alternative paradigm.* (Medfield Foundation Report 103) Medfield, Mass.: Medfield Foundation.

Barber, T. X. (1978). Hypnosis, suggestions, and psychosomatic phenomena: A new look from the standpoint of recent experimental studies. *American Journal of Clinical Hypnosis, 21*, 13-27.

Barber, T. X. (1984). Changing "unchangeable" bodily processes by (hypnotic) suggestions: A new look at hypnosis, cognitions, imagining, and the mind-body problem. In A. A. Sheikh (Ed.), *Imagination and healing.* Amityville, NY: Baywood.

Barber, T. X., Chauncey, H. H., & Winer, H. A. (1964). Effect of hypnotic and non-hypnotic suggestions on parotid gland response to gustatory stimuli. *Psychosomatic Medicine, 26*, 374-380.

Barber, T. X., Spanos, N. P., & Chaves, J. F. (1974). *Hypnosis, imagination, and human potentialities.* Elmford, NY: Pergamon Press.

Barbour, W. P. (1981). *Vividness of mental imagery and heart rate response to imagined anxiety evoking situations.* Unpublished honours thesis, University of Western Australia.

Barnes, V., Schneider, R., Alexander, C., & Staggers, F. (1997). Stress, stress reduction, and hypertension in African Americans: An updated review. *Journal of the National Medical Association, 89,* 464-476.

Bauer, R. M., & Craighead, W. E. (1979). Psychophysiological responses to the imagination of fearful and neutral situations: The effects of imagery instructions. *Behavior Therapy, 10,* 389-403.

Bell, I. R., & Schwartz, G. E. (1975). Voluntary control and reactivity of human heart rate. *Psychophysiology, 12,* 339-348.

Benson, H. (1975). *The relaxation response.* New York: Morrow.

Bevan, A. J. W. (1980). Endocrine changes in transcendental meditation. *Clinical and Experimental Pharmacology and Physiology, 7,* 75-76.

Black, S. (1963). Inhibition of immediate-type hypersensitivity response by direct suggestion under hypnosis. *British Medical Journal, 6,* 925-929.

Black, S., Humphrey, J. H., & Niven, J. S. (1963). Inhibition of Momtoux reaction by direct suggestion under hypnosis. *British Medical Journal, 6,* 1649-1652.

Blizard, D. A., Cowings, P., & Miller, N. E. (1975). Visceral responses to opposite types of autogenic-training imagery. *Biological Psychology, 3,* 49-55.

Bogartz, W. (1990). The mechanism of hypnotic control of white blood cell count. In R. Van Dyck (Ed.), *Hypnosis: Current theory, research and practice.* Amsterdam: VU University Press.

Boulougouris, J. C., Rabavilas, D. D., & Stefanis, C. (1977). Psychophysiological responses in obsessive-compulsive patients. *Behavior Research and Therapy, 15,* 221-230.

Brown, D. P., & Fromm, E. (1987). *Hypnosis and behavioral medicine.* Hillsdale, NJ: Erlbaum.

Bujatti, M., & Riederer, P. (1976). Serotonin, noradrenaline, and dopamine metabolites in the transcendental meditation technique. *Journal of Neural Transmission, 39,* 257-267.

Cannon, W. B. (1915). *Bodily changes in pain, hunger, fear, and rage.* New York: Appleton.

Carroll, D., Baker, J., & Preston, M. (1979). Individual differences in visual imaging and the voluntary control of heart rate. *British Journal of Psychology, 70,* 39-49.

Carroll, D., Marzillier, J. S., & Merian, S. (1982). Psychophysiological changes accompanying different types of arousing and relaxing imagery. *Psychophysiology, 19,* 75-82.

Castes, M., Hagel, I., Palenque, M., Canelones, P., Carao, A., & Lynch, N. R. (1999). Immunological changes associated with clinical improvement of asthmatic children subjected to psychosocial intervention. *Brain Behavior Immunologies, 13,* 1-13.

Chaves, J. F. (1980, September). *Hypnotic control of surgical bleeding.* Paper presented at Annual Meeting of the American Psychological Association, Montreal.

Colman, F., & Paivio, A. (1970). Pupillary dilation and mediation processes during paired-associate learning. *Canadian Journal of Psychology, 24,* 261-270.

Coker, K. H. (1990) Meditation and prostate cancer: Integrating a mind/body intervention with traditional therapies. *Seminar in Urologic Oncology, 17,* 111-118.

Cousins, N. (1983). *The healing heart.* New York: Norton.

Craig, K. D. (1968). Physiological arousal as a function of imagined, vicarious, and direct stress experience. *Journal of Abnormal Psychology, 73*, 513-520.

Crawford, H. J. (1996). Cerebral brain dynamics of mental imagery: Evidence and issues for hypnosis. In R. G. Kunzendorf, N. P. Spanos, & B. Wallace (Eds.), *Hypnosis and imagination*. Amityville, NY: Baywood.

Crowther, J. H. (1983). Stress management training and relaxation imagery in the treatment of essential hypertension. *Journal of Behavioral Medicine, 6*, 169-187.

Das, H., & Gastaut, H. (1955). Variations de lactivite electrique du cerveau, du couer et des muscles suelettiques an cours de la meditation et de l'extase Yogique. *Electroencephalography and Clinical Neurophysiology* (Suppl. 6), 211-219.

Davidson, J. M. (1976). The physiology of meditation and mystical states of consciousness. *Perspectives in Biology and Medicine, 19*(3), 345-379.

Delmonte, M. M. (1985). Biochemical indices associated with meditation practice: A literature review. *Neuroscience and Biobehavioral Reviews, 9*, 557-561.

Delmonte, M. M. (1986). Meditation as a clinical intervention strategy: A brief review. *International Journal of Psychosomatics, 33*, 9-12.

Dossey, L. (1982). *Space, time, and medicine*. Boulder, CO: Shambhala.

Dossey, L. (1991). *Meaning and medicine*. New York: Bantan.

Drummond, P., White, K., & Ashton, R. (1978). Imagery vividness affects habituation rate. *Psychophysiology, 15*, 193-195.

Dugan, M., & Sheridan, C. (1976). Effects of instructed imagery on temperature of hands. *Perceptual and Motor Skills, 42*, 14.

Edwin, D. M. (1992). Hypnotherapy for warts (Verruca Vulgaris): 41 consecutive cases with 33 cures. *American Journal of Clinical Hypnosis, 35*, 1-10.

Engel, B. T. (1979). Behavioral applications in the treatment of patients with cardiovascular disorders. In J. V. Basmajian (Ed.), *Biofeedback: Principles and practices for clinicians*. Baltimore: Williams and Wilkins.

Epstein, G. (1986). The image in medicine: Notes of a clinician. *Advances, 3*, 22-31.

Farrow, J. T., & Herbert, R. (1982). Breath suspension during tanscendental technique. *Psychosomatic Medicine, 44*, 133-153.

Ferrucci, P. (1982). *What we may be*. Los Angeles: Tancher

Ford, M. R. (1982). Biofeedback treatment for headaches, Raynand's disease, essential hypertension, and irritable bowel syndrome: A review of the long-term follow-up literature. *Biofeedback and Self-Regulation, 7*, 521-536.

Freyhan, F. A. (1976). Is psychosomatic obsolete? A psychiatric appraisal. *Comprehensive Psychiatry, 17*, 381-386.

Furedy, J. J., & Klajner, F. (1978). Imaginational Pavlovian conditioning of large-magnitude cardiac decelerations with tilt as UCS. *Psychophysiology, 15*, 538-548.

Gatchel, R. J., & Blanchard, E. B. (Eds.) (1993). *Psychophysiological disorders*. Washington, D.C.: American Psychological Association.

Ginandes, C. S., & Rosenthal, D. I. (1999). Using hypnosis to accelerate the healing of bone fractures: A randomized controlled pilot study. *Alternative Therapies in Health and Medicine, 5*, 67-70, 72-75.

Goldberg, B. (1985). The treatment of cancer through hypnosis. *Psychology, A Quarterly Journal of Human Behavior, 22*, 36-39.

Goleman, D. (1988) *The meditative mind*, Los Angeles: Tarcher.

Gorton, B. E. (1959). Physiological aspects of hypnosis. In J. M. Schneck (Ed.), *Hypnosis in modern medicine.* Springfield, IL: Charles C. Thomas.

Gottschalk, L. A. (1974). Self-induced visual imagery, affect arousal, and autonomic correlates. *Psychosomatics, 15,* 166-169.

Gottschalk, L. A., Stone, W. N., Gleser, G. C., & Iacono, J. M. (1966). Anxiety levels in dreams: Relation to changes in plasma free fatty acids. *Science, 153,* 654-657.

Gravitz, M. A. (1955). Hypnosis in the treatment of functional infertility. *American Journal of Clinical Hypnosis, 38,* 22-26.

Green, E. E., & Green, A. M. (1977). *Beyond biofeedback.* New York: Delacorte.

Grossberg, J. M., & Wilson, K. M. (1968). Physiological changes accompanying the visualization of fearful and neutral situations. *Journal of Personality and Social Psychology, 10,* 124-133.

Gruber, B. L., Hall, H. R., Hesch, S. P., & Dubois, P. (1988). Immune system and psychological changes in metastatic cancer patients using relaxation and guided imagery: A pilot study. *Scandinavian Journal of Behavior Therapy, 17,* 24-96.

Gunville, T. M. (1991). *Clinical applications of mental imagery: Imagery, physiology and healing.* Unpublished manuscript, Marquette University, Milwaukee, Wisconsin.

Hall, H. R., Longo, S., & Dixon, R. (1981, October). *Hypnosis and the immune system: The effect of hypnosis on T and B cell function.* Paper presented at 33rd Annual Meeting for the Society for Clinical and Experimental Hypnosis, Portland, Oregon.

Hall, H. R., Minnes, L., Tosi, M., & Olness, K. (1992). Voluntary modulation of neutrophil adhesiveness using a cyberphysiological strategy. *International Journal of Neuroscience, 62,* 287-297.

Hall, H., Papas, A., Tosi, M., & Olness, K. (1996). Directional changes in neutrophil adherence following passive resting versus active imagery. *International Journal of Neuroscience, 85,* 185-194.

Haney, J. N., & Euse, F. J. (1976). Skin conductance and heart rate responses to neutral, positive, and negative imagery: Implications for covert behavior therapy procedures. *Behavior Therapy, 7,* 494-503.

Hariton, E. B., & Singer, J. L. (1974). Women's fantasies during sexual intercourse: Normative and theoretical implications. *Journal of Consulting and Clinical Psychology, 42,* 313-322.

Herzfeld, G. M., & Taub, E. (1980). Effect of slide projections and tape-recorded suggestions on thermal biofeedback training. *Biofeedback and Self-Regulation, 5,* 393-405.

Hilgard, E. R. (1965). *Hypnotic susceptibility.* New York: Harcourt, Brace and World.

Hirai, T. (1960). Electroencephalographic Study on the Zen meditation. *Folio Psychiatrica and Neurologica Japanica, 62,* 76-105.

Hirschman, R., & Favaro, L. (1980). Individual differences in imagery vividness and voluntary heart rate control. *Personality and Individual Differences, 1,* 129-133.

Holden-Lund, C. (1988). Effects of relaxation with guided imagery on surgical stress and wound healing. *Research in Nursing and Health, 11,* 235-244.

Honiotes, G .J. (1977). Hypnosis and breast enlargement—A pilot study. *Journal of the International Society for Professional Hypnosis, 6,* 8-12.

Humphreys, C. (1987). *Concentration and meditation.* Longmead, Shaftsbury, Dorset: Element Books.

Ikeda, Y., & Hirai, H. (1976). Voluntary control of electrodrmal activity in relation to imagery and internal perception scores. *Psychophysiology, 13*, 330-333.

Ikemi, Y., & Nakagawa, S. (1962). A psychosomatic study of contagious dermatitis. *Kyushu Journal of Medical Science, 13*, 335-350.

James, W. (1890). *The principles of psychology* (Vol. 2). New York: Henry Holt.

Jasnoski, M. L., & Kugler, J. (1987). Relaxation, imagery, and neuroimmodulation. *Annals of the New York Academy of Sciences, 496*, 722-730.

Jemmott, J. B., & Locke, S. E. (1984). Psychosocial factors, immunologic mediation, and human susceptibility to infectious diseases: How much do we know? *Psychological Bulletin, 95*, 78-108.

Jevning, R., Wallace, R. K., & Beidebach, M. (1992). The physiology of meditation: A review. *Neuroscience and Behavioral Reviews, 16*, 415-424.

Jevning, R., Wilson, A. F., & Davidson, J. M. (1978). Adrenocortical activity during meditation. *Hormones and Behavior, 10*, 54-60.

Johnson, R. F. Q., & Barber, T. X. (1976). Hypnotic suggestions for blister formation: Subjective and physiological effects. *American Journal of Clinical Hypnosis, 18*, 172-181.

Johnson, R. F. Q., & Barber, T. X. (1978). Hypnosis, suggestions, and warts: An experimental investigation implicating the importance of believed-in efficacy. *American Journal of Clinical Hypnosis, 20*, 165-174.

Jones, G. E., & Johnson, H. J. (1978). Physiological responding during self-generated imagery of contextually complete stimuli. *Psychophysiology, 15*, 439-446.

Jones, G. E., & Johnson, H. J. (1980). Heart rate and somatic concomitents of mental imagery. *Psychophysiology, 17*, 339-347.

Jordan, C. S., & Lenington, K. T. (1979). Physiological correlates of eidetic imagery and induced anxiety. *Journal of Mental Imagery, 3*, 31-42.

Kabat-Zinn, J., Wheeler, E., Light, T., Skillings, A., Scharf, M. J., Cropley, T. G., Hosmer, D., & Bernard, J. D. (1998). Influence of a mindfulness meditation-based stress reduction intervention on rats of skin clearing in patients with severe psoriasis undergoing phototherapy (UVB) and photochemotherapy (PUVA). *Psychosomatic Medicine, 60*, 625-632.

Kaluza, G., & Strempel, I. (1995). Effects of self-relaxation methods and visual imagery in IOP in patients with open-angle glaucoma. *Opthalmoligica, 209*, 122-128.

Kasamatsu, A., & Hirai, T. (1966). An electroencephalographic study of the Zen meditation (zazen). *Folio Psychiatria and Neurological Japanica, 20*, 315-336.

Kesterson, J., & Clinch, N. F. (1989). Metabolic rate, respiratory exchange ratio and apnea during meditation. *American Journal of Physiology, 256*, 632-638.

King, N. J., & Montgomery, R. B. (1980). Biofeedback-induced control of human peripheral temperature: A critical review. *Psychological Bulletin, 88*, 738-752.

Kosslyn, S. (1980). *Image and mind.* Cambridge, MA: Harvard University Press.

Kunzendorf, R. G. (1981). Individual differences in imagery and autonomic control. *Journal of Mental Imagery, 5*, 47-60.

Kunzendorf, R. G. (1984). Centrifugal effects of eidetic imaging on flash electroretinograms and autonomic responses. *Journal of Mental Imagery, 8*, 67-76.

Kunzendorf, R. G. (1991). The causal efficacy of consciousness in general, imagery in particular: A materialistic perspective. In R. G. Kunzendorf (Ed.), *Mental imagery.* New York: Plenum.

Kunzendorf, R. G., & Albright, L. M. (1981). *Voluntary imaging abilities and voluntary control of salivary pH: A litmus paper test for gustatory and visual images.* Unpublished.

Kunzendorf, R. G., & Bradbury, J. L. (1983). Better liars have better imaginations. *Psychological Reports, 52,* 634.

Kunzendorf, R. G., Francis, L., Ward, J., Cohen, R., Cutler, J., Walsh, J., & Berenson, S. (1996). Effect of negative imaging on heart rate and blood pressure, as a function of image vividness and image "realness." *Imagination, Cognition and Personality, 16,* 139-159.

Kunzendorf, R. G., & Hall, S. (2001). Electroretinographic after-effects of visual imaging: Individual differences in imagery vividness and reality testing. *Journal of Mental Imagery, 25,* 79-92.

Kunzendorf, R. G., Jesses, M., & Capone, D. (1997). Conscious images as "centrally excited sensations." *Journal of Mental Imagery, 21,* 155-166.

Kunzendorf, R. G., & Sheikh, A. A. (1990). *The psychophysiology of mental imagery: Theory, research, and application.* Amityville, NY: Baywood.

Lachman, S. J. (1972). *Psychosomatic disorders: A behavioristic interpretation.* New York: Wiley.

Lang, P. J., Kozak, M. J., Miller, G. A., Levin, D. N., & McLean, A. (1980). Emotional imagery: Conceptual structure and pattern of somato-visceral response. *Psychophysiology, 17,* 179-192.

Laws, D. R., & Rubin, H. B. (1969). Instructional control of an autonomic sexual response. *Journal of Applied Behavior Analysis, 2,* 93-99.

LeBouef, A., & Wilson, C. (1978). The importance of imagery in maintenance of feedback-assisted relaxation over extinction trials. *Perceptual and Motor Skills, 47,* 824-826.

Lentz, S. L., & Zeiss, A. M. (1983-1984). Fantasy and sexual arousal in college women: An empirical investigation. *Imagination, Cognition and Personality, 3,* 185-202.

Lichstein, K. L. (1988). *Clinical relaxation strategies.* New York: Wiley.

Lipkowski, Z. J. (1986a). Psychosomatic medicine: Past and present. Part I. Historical background. *Canadian Journal of Psychiatry, 31,* 2-7.

Lipkowski, Z. J. (1986b). Psychosomatic medicine: Past and present. Part II. Current state. *Canadian Journal of Psychiatry, 31,* 8-13.

Longo, D. J., Clum, G. A., & Yaeger, N. J. (1988). Psychosocial treatment for recurrent genital herpes. *Journal of Consulting and Clinical Psychology, 56,* 61-66.

Lucas, O. (1965). Dental extractions in the hemophiliac: Control of the emotional factors by hypnosis. *American Journal of Clinical Hypnosis, 7,* 301-307.

Luckhardt, A. B., & Johnston, R. L. (1924). Studies in gastric secretions: I, The psychic secretion of gastric juice under hypnosis. *American Journal of Physiology, 70,* 174-182.

Lusebrink, V. B. (1986-1987). Visual imagery: Its psychophysiological components and levels of information processing. *Imagination, Cognition and Personality, 6,* 205-218.

Lynch, J. J., Paskewitz, D. A., & Orne, M. T. (1974). Some factors in the feedback control of human alpha rhythm. *Psychosomatic Medicine, 36*(5), 399-410.

Lynn, S. J., & Rhue, J. W. (1991). *Theories of hypnosis: Current models and perspectives.* New York: Guilford Press.

Margolis, C. G. (1983). Hypnotic imagery with cancer patients. *American Journal of Clinical Hypnosis, 25,* 128-134.

Marks, I., & Huson, J. (1973). Physiological aspects of neutral and phobic imagery: Further observations. *British Journal of Psychiatry, 122,* 567-572.

Marks, I., Marset, P., Boulougouris, J., & Huson, J. (1971). Physiological accompaniments of neutral and phobic imagery. *Psychological Medicine, 1,* 299-307.

Marzillier, J. S., Carroll, D., & Newland, J. R. (1979). Self-report and physiological changes accompanying repeated imaging of a phobic scene. *Behavior Research and Therapy, 17,* 71-77.

Mason, A. A., & Black, S. (1958). Allergic skin responses abolished under treatment of asthma and hayfever by hypnosis. *Lancet, 1,* 877-880.

McCanne, T. R., & Iennarella, R. S. (1980). Cognitive and somatic events associated with discriminative changes in heart rate. *Psychophysiology, 17,* 18-28.

McClelland, D. C. (1985). Health psychology mandate. *American Behavioral Scientist, 28,* 451-467.

McClelland, D. C., Floor, E., Davidson, R .J., & Saron, C. (1985). Stressed power motivation, sympathetic activation, immune function, and illness. *Advances, 2,* 43-51.

McGuirk, J., Fitzgerald, D., Friedman, P. S., Oakley, D., & Salmon, P. (1998). The effect of guided imagery in a hypnotic context on forearm blood flow. *Contemporary Hypnosis, 15,* 101-108.

McMahon, C. E. (1986). *Where medicine fails.* New York: Trado-Medic Books.

McMahon, C. E., & Koppes, S. (1976). The development of psychosomatic medicine: An analysis of growth of professional societies. *Psychosomatics, 17,* 185-187.

McMahon, C. E., & Sheikh, A. A. (1984). Imagination in disease and healing processes: A historical perspective. In A. A. Sheikh (Ed.), *Imagination and healing.* Amityville, NY: Baywood.

McMahon, C. E., & Sheikh, A. A. (1989). Psychosomatic illness: A new look. In A. A. Sheikh and K. S. Sheikh (Eds.), *Eastern and Western approahes to healing.* New York: Wiley.

Meyer, A. (1957). *Psychobiology: A science of man.* Springfield, IL: Charles C. Thomas.

Moldawsky, R. J. (1984). Hypnosis as an adjunctive treatment in Huntington's disease. *American Journal of Clinical Hypnosis, 26,* 229-231.

Morgan, R. F., & Fevens, S. K. (1972). Reliability of the adult growth examination: A standardized test of individual aging. *Perceptual and Motor Skills, 34,* 415-419.

Noll, R. (1994). Hypnotherapy for warts in children and adolescents. *Journal of Developmental and Behavioral Pediatrics, 15,* 170-173.

Norris, P. (1986). Biofeedback, voluntary control and human potential. *Biofeedback and Self-Regulation, 11,* 1-20.

Norris, P. (1989). Current conceptual trends in biofeedback and self regulation. In A. A. Sheikh & K. S. Sheikh (Eds.), *Eastern and Western approaches to healing.* New York: Wiley.

Ohkuma, Y. (1985). Effects of evoking imagery on the control of peripheral skin temperature. *Japanese Journal of Psychology, 54,* 88-94.

Olness, K., Culbert, T., & Uden, D. (1989). Self-regulation of salivary immunoglobulin A by children. *Pediatrics, 83,* 66-71.

Olness, K., Hall, H., Rozniecki, J. H., Schmidt, W., & Theoharides, T. C. (1999). Mast cell activation in children with migraine before and after training in self-regulation. *Headache, 39,* 101-107.

Orme-Johnson, D. W. (1973). Autonomic stability and transcendental meditation. *Psychosomatic Medicine, 35*(4), 341-349.

Paivio, A. (1971). *Imagery and verbal processes.* New York: Holt, Rinehart and Winston.

Paivio, A., & Simpson, H. M. (1968). Magnitude and latency of the pupillary response during an imagery task as a function of stimulus abstractness and imagery ability. *Psychonomic Science, 12,* 45-46.

Passchier, J., & Helm-Hylkema, H. (1981). The effect of stress imagery on arousal and res implications for biofeedback of the frontalis muscles. *Biofeedback and Self-Regulation, 6,* 295-303.

Patterson, D. R., Goldberg, M. L., & Ehde, D. M. (1996). Hypnosis in the treatment of patients with severe burns. *American Journal of Clinical Hypnosis, 38,* 200-213.

Paul, G. L. (1963). The production of blisters by hypnotic suggestion: Another look. *Psychosomatic Medicine, 25,* 233-244.

Pelletier, K. R., & Garfield, C. (1976). *Consciousness East and West.* New York: Harper and Row.

Perloff, M. M., & Spiegelman, T. (1973). Hypnosis in the treatment of a child's allergy to dogs. *American Hypnosis, 15,* 269-272.

Pickett, E. (1987-1988). Fibroid tumors and response to guided imagery and music: Two case studies. *Imagination, Cognition and Personality, 7,* 165-176.

Pope, K. S., Singer, J. L., & Rosenberg, L. C. (1984). Sex, fantasy and imagination: Scientific research and clinical applications. In A. A. Sheikh (Ed.), *Imagination and healing.* Amityville, NY: Baywood.

Pylyshyn, Z. W. (1973). What the mind's eye tells the mind's brain: A critique of mental imagery. *Psychological Bulletin, 80,* 1-24.

Qualls, P. J., & Sheehan, P. W. (1979). Capacity for absorption and relaxation during electromyograph biofeedback and no-feedback conditions. *Journal of Abnormal Psychology, 88,* 652-662.

Quintyn, M., & Cross, E. (1986). Factors affecting the ability to initiate movement in Parkinson's disease. *Physical and Occupational Therapy in Geriatrics, 4,* 51-60.

Ramaswami, S., & Sheikh, A. A. (1989). Meditation east and west. In A. A. Sheikh & K. S. Sheikh (Eds.), *Eastern and Western approaches to healing.* New York: Wiley.

Ribot, T. (1906). *Essay on the creative imagination* (A. H. N. Baron, Trans.). Chicago: Open Court. (Reprinted in New York by Arno Press, 1973.)

Richardson, A. (1969). *Mental imagery.* New York: Springer.

Richardson. A. (1978). Subject, task, and tester variables associated with initial eye movement responses. *Journal of Mental Imagery, 2,* 85-100.

Roberts, R. J., & Weerts, T. C. (1982). Cardiovascular responding during anger and fear imagery. *Psychological Reports, 50,* 219-230.

Ruggieri, V., & Alfieri, G. (1992). The eyes in imagery and perceptual processes: First remarks. *Perception and Motor Skills, 75,* 287-290.

Rush, B. (1811). *Sixteen introductory lectures.* Philadelphia: Bradford and Innskeep.

Sarbin, T. R. (1976). *The Quixotic principle: Believed-in imaginings.* Santa Cruz, CA: Department of Psychology, University of California.

Sarbin, T. R., & Coe, W. C. (1972). *Hypnosis: A social psychological analysis of influence communication.* New York: Holt, Rinehard and Winston.

Schneider, J., Smith, C. W., Minning, C., Whitcher, S., & Hermanson, J. (1991). Guided imagery and immune system function in normal subjects: A summary of research findings. In R. G. Kunzendorf (Ed.), *Mental imagery.* New York: Plenum.

Schreiber, E. H., Schreiber, K. N., & Weeks, A. S. (1998). A study of hypnosis with Raynaud's disease. *Australian Journal of Clinical and Experimental Hypnosis, 26,* 165-171.

Schrödinger, E. (1945). *What is life?* Cambridge: Cambridge University.

Schwab, J. J. (1978). *Sociocultural roots of mental illness.* New York: Plenum.

Schwartz, G. E. (1971). Cardiac responses to self-induced thoughts. *Psychophysiology, 8,* 462-467.

Schwartz, G. E. (1975). Biofeedback, self-regulation, and the patterning of physiological processes. *American Scientist, 63,* 314-324.

Schwartz, G. E., Fair, P. L., Greenberg, P. S., Freedman, M., & Klerman, J. L. (1974). Facial electromyography in assessment of emotion. *Psychophysiology, 11,* 237.

Schwartz, G. E., Weinberger, D. A., & Singer, J. A. (1981). Cardiovascular differentiation of happiness, sadness, anger, and fear following imagery and exercise. *Psychosomatic Medicine, 43,* 343-364.

Shea, J. D. (1985). Effects of absorption and instructions on heart rate control. *Journal of Mental Imagery, 9,* 87-100.

Sheehan, P. W. (1972). Hypnosis and the manifestations of "imagination." In E. Fromm & R. E. Shor (Eds.), *Hypnosis: Research development and perspectives.* Chicago: Aldine-Atherton.

Sheikh, A. A. (Ed.). (1983). *Imagery: Current theory, research and application.* New York: Wiley.

Sheikh, A. A. (Ed.). (1984). *Imagination and healing,* Amityville, NY: Baywood.

Sheikh, A. A. (Ed.). (2001). *Handbook of therapeutic imagery techniques.* Amityville, NY: Baywood.

Sheikh, A. A., & Kunzendorf, R. G. (1984). Imagery, physiology, and psychosomatic illness. *International Review of Mental Imagery, 1,* 94-138.

Sheikh, A. A., Kunzendorf, R. G., & Sheikh, K. S. (1989). Healing mages: From ancient wisdom to modern science. In A. A. Sheikh & K. S. Sheikh (Eds.), *Eastern and Western approaches to healing.* New York: Wiley.

Sheikh, A. A., Kunzendorf, R. G., & Sheikh, K. S. (1996). Somatic consequences of consciousness. In M. Velmans (Ed.), *The science of consciousness.* London: Routledge.

Sheikh, A. A., Richardson, P., & Moleski, L. M. (1979). Psychosomatics and mental imagery: A brief view. In A. A. Sheikh & J. T. Shaffer (Eds.), *The potential of fantasy and imagination.* New York: Brandon House.

Sheikh, A. A., & Sheikh, K. S. (Eds.). (1989). *Eastern and Western approaches to healing.* New York: Wiley.

Shontz, F. C. (1975). *The psychological aspects of illness and disability.* New York: Macmillan.

Simonton, O. C., Matthews-Simonton, S., & Creighton, J. (1978). *Getting well again: A step-by-step, self-help guide to overcoming cancer for patients and their families.* Los Angeles: J. P. Tarcher.

Simonton, O. C., Matthews-Simonton, S., & Sparks, T. F. (1980). Psychological intervention in the treatment of cancer. *Psychosomatics, 21,* 226-227.

Simpson, H. M., & Climan, M. H. (1971). Pupillary and electromyographic changes during an imagery task. *Psychophysiology, 8,* 483-490.

Smith, D., & Over, R. (1987). Does fantasy-induced sexual arousal habituate? *Behaviour Research and Therapy, 25,* 477-485.

Smith, G. R., McKenzie, J. M., Marmer, D. J., & Steele, R. W. (1985). Psychologic modulation of the human immune response to varicella zoster. *Archives of Internal Medicine, 145,* 2110-2112.

Smuts, J. C. (1926). *Holism and evolution.* New York: Macmillan.

Spanos, N. P., Senstrom, R. J., & Johnston, J. C. (1988). Hypnosis, placebo and suggestion in the treatment of warts. *Psychosomatic Medicine, 50,* 245-260.

Stock, W. E., & Geer, J. H. (1982). A study of fantasy-based sexual arousal in women. *Archives of Sexual Behavior, 11,* 33-47.

Subrahmanyam, S., & Potkodi, D. (1980). Neurohumoral correlates of transcendental meditation. *Journal of Biomedicine, 1,* 73-88.

Sudsuang, R., Chentanez, V., & Veluvan, K. (1991). Effect of Buddhist meditation on serum cortisol and total protein levels, blood pressure, pulse rate, lung volume and reaction time. *Physiology and Behavior, 50,* 543-548.

Sugi, Y., & Akutsu, K. (1968). Studies on respiration and energy metabolism during sitting in zazen. *Research Journal of Physical Education, 12,* 190.

Takahashi, H. (1984). Experimental study on self-control of heart rate: Experiment for a biofeedback treatment of anxiety state. *Journal of Mental Health, 31,* 109-125.

Telles, S., Nagarathna, R., & Nagendra, H. R. (1998). Autonomic changes while mentally repeating two syllables—One meaningful and the other neutral. *Indian Journal of Physiology and Pharmacology, 42,* 57-63.

Thackwray-Emmerson, D. (1988). Stress and disease: An examination of psycho-physiological effects and alternative treatment approaches. *Counseling Psychology Quarterly, 1,* 413-420.

Thompson, J. K., & Adams, H. E. (1984). Psychophysiological characteristics of headache patients. *Pain,* 41-52.

Tooley, G. A., Armstrong, S. M., Norman, T. R., & Sali, A. (2000). Acute increases in nighttime plasma melatonin levels following a period of meditation. *Biological Psychology, 53,* 69-78.

Tuke, D. H. (1872). *Illustrations of the influence of the mind upon the body in health and disease: Designed to elucidate the action of the imagination,* London: J. and A. Churchill.

Vollmer, H. (1946). Treatment of warts by suggestion. *Psychosomatic Medicine, 8,* 138-142.

Wallace, R. K. (1970). Physiological effects of transcendental meditation. *Science, 167,* 1251-1254.

Wallace, R. K., Benson, H., & Wilson, A. F. (1971). A wakeful hypometabolic physiologic state. *American Journal of Physiology, 221,* 795-799.

Wallace, R. K., & Benson, H. (1972). The physiology of meditation. *Scientific American, 262,* 84-90.

Wallace, R. K., Dillbeck, M. C., Jacobe, E., & Harrington, B. (1982). The effects of the transcendental meditation and TM-Sidhi program on the aging process. *International Journal of Neuroscience, 16,* 53-58.

Wang, Y., & Morgan, W. P. (1992). The effect of imagery perspectives on the psychophysiological responses to imagined exercise. *Behavioral Brain Research, 52*, 167-174.

Waters, W. F., & McDonald, D. G. (1973). Autonomic response to auditory, visual and imagined stimuli in a systematic desensitization context. *Behaviour Research and Therapy, 11*, 577-585.

Weimer, W. B. (1976). Manifestations of mind. Some conceptual and empirical issues. In. G. Globus, G. Maxwell, & J. Savodnik (Eds.), *Consciousness and the brain.* New York: Plenum.

Weiner, H. (1977). *Psychobiology and human disease,* New York: Elsevier.

Weitzenhoffer, H. M., & Hilgard, E. R. (1962). *Stanford Hypnotic Susceptibility Scale, Form C.* Palo Alto, CA: Consulting Psychologist Press.

Wenger, M. A., Bagchi, B. K., & Anand, B. K. (1961). Experiments in India on voluntary control of the heart and pulse. *Circulation, 24*, 1319-1325.

Wenger, M. A., Bagchi, B. K., & Anand, B. K. (1963). Voluntary heart and pulse control by yoga methods. *International Journal of Parapsychology, 5*, 25-41.

West, M. A. (1979). Physiological effects of meditations: A longitudinal study. *British Journal of Social and Clinical Psychology, 18*, 219.

West, M. A. (1987). *The psychology of meditation.* Oxford: Clarendon Press.

Whipple, B., Ogden, G., & Komisaruk, B. R. (1992). Physiological correlates of imagery-induced orgasm in women. *Archives of Sexual Behavior, 21*, 121-123.

Whorwell, P. J. (1991). Use of hypnotherapy in gastrointestinal disease. *British Journal of Hospital Medicine, 45*, 27-29.

Williams, J. E. (1974). Stimulation of breast growth by hypnosis. *Journal of Sex Research, 10*, 316-326.

Willard, R. D. (1977). Breast enlargement through visual imagery and hypnosis. *American Hypnosis, 19*, 195-200.

Willis, R. J. (1979). Meditation to fit the person: Psychology and the meditative way. *Journal of Religion and Health, 18*(2), 93-119.

Winer, R. A., Chauncey, H. H., & Barber, T. X. (1965). The influence of verbal or symbolic stimuli on salivary gland secretion. *Annals of the New York Academy of Sciences, 131*, 874-883.

Wittkower, E. D. (Ed.). (1977). *Psychosomatic medicine: Its clinical applications.* Hagerstown, MD: Harper and Row.

Woolfolk, R. L. (1975). Psychophysiological correlates of meditation. *Archives of General Psychiatry, 32*, 1326-1333.

Yaremko, R. M., & Butler, M. C. (1975). Imaginal experience and attention of the galvanic skin response to shock. *Bulletin of the Psychonomic Society, 5*, 317-318.

Zachariae, R., Kristensen, J. S., Hokland, P., Ellegaard, J., Metze, E., & Hokland, M. (1990). The effect of psychological intervention in the form of relaxation and guided imagery on cellular immune function in normal healthy subjects: An overview. *Psychotherapy and Psychosomatics, 54*, 32-39.

Zikmund, V. (1972). Physiological correlates of visual imagery. In P. Sheehan (Ed.), *The function and nature of imagery.* New York: Academic Press.

This chapter is a revised version of a previously published paper (Sheikh, Kunzendorf, & Sheikh, 1996). It is included here with permission from Routledge, London, England.

CHAPTER 3

How Could Images Heal Anything?[1]

MAX VELMANS

A CONUNDRUM

Question: Is it possible for consciousness to do something to or about something that it is not conscious of?

If the answer is NO. We are not aware of the activity of our own brains. So we conclude that consciousness as such does not influence brain activity.

If the answer is YES. We are not aware of the activity of our own brains. So consciousness must influence brain activity unconsciously. So we conclude that consciousness as such does not influence brain activity.

Yet consciousness is central to human being. Without it our existence would be like nothing. So the notion that consciousness does nothing makes no sense. (Velmans, 2000)

THE PROBLEM OF MENTAL CAUSATION

Psychosomatic medicine assumes that the conscious mind can affect the body, and this is supported by evidence that the use of imagery, hypnosis, biofeedback, and other "mental interventions" can be therapeutic in a variety of medical conditions. However, there is no accepted theory of mind/body interaction and this has had a detrimental effect on the acceptance of mental causation in many areas of clinical practice (McMahon & Sheikh, 1989). Biomedical accounts typically translate the effects of mind into the effects of brain functioning, for example, explaining mind/body interactions in terms of the interconnections and reciprocal control of cortical, neuroendocrine, autonomic, and immune systems. While such accounts are instructive, they are implicitly reductionist, and beg the question of how *conscious experiences* could have bodily effects. On the other hand, non-reductionist accounts have to cope with three

---

[1] This chapter selects from and develops some of the ideas presented in Chapter 11 of Velmans (2000) *Understanding Consciousness*, Routledge/Psychology Press.

problems: 1) The physical world appears causally closed, which would seem to leave no room for conscious intervention. 2) One is not conscious of one's own brain/body processing, so how could there be conscious control of such processing? 3) Conscious experiences appear to come too late to causally affect the processes to which they most obviously relate (see below). The present chapter suggests a way of understanding mental causation that resolves these problems. It also suggests that "conscious mental control" needs to be partly understood in terms of the voluntary operations of the *preconscious* mind.

DIFFERENT WAYS IN WHICH BODY/BRAIN AND MIND/CONSCIOUSNESS MIGHT INTERACT

There are four distinct ways in which body/brain and mind/consciousness might, in principle, enter into causal relationships. There might be physical causes of physical states, physical causes of mental states, mental causes of mental states, and mental causes of physical states. Establishing which forms of causation are effective in *practice* has clear implications for understanding the aetiology and proper treatment of illness and disease.

Within conventional medicine, physical→physical causation is taken for granted. Consequently, the proper treatment for physical disorders is assumed to be some form of physical intervention. Psychiatry takes the efficacy of physical→mental causation for granted, along with the assumption that the proper treatment for psychological disorders may involve psychoactive drugs, neurosurgery, and so on. Many forms of psychotherapy take mental→mental causation for granted, and assume that psychological disorders can be alleviated by means of "talking cures," guided imagery, hypnosis, and other forms of mental intervention. Psychosomatic medicine assumes that mental→physical causation can be effective ("psychogenesis"). Consequently, under some circumstances, a physical disorder (for example, hysterical paralysis) may require a mental (psychotherapeutic) intervention. Given the extensive evidence for *all* these causal interactions (cf. readings in Velmans, 1996a), how are we to make sense of them?

CLINICAL EVIDENCE FOR THE CAUSAL EFFICACY OF MENTAL STATES

The problems posed by mental→physical causation are particularly acute as reductionist, materialistic science generally takes it for granted that the operation of physical systems can be entirely explained in physical terms. Yet there is a large body of evidence that states of mind can affect not only subsequent states of the mind but also states of the body. For example, Barber (1984), Sheikh, Kunzendorf, and Sheikh (1996), and many readings in Sheikh (2002—this volume) review evidence that the use of imagery, hypnosis, and biofeedback may be therapeutic in a variety of medical conditions.

Particularly puzzling is the evidence that under certain conditions, a range of *autonomic* bodily functions, including heart rate, blood pressure, vasomotor activity, blood glucose levels, pupil dilation, electrodermal activity, and immune system functioning, can be influenced by conscious states. In some cases these effects are striking. Baars and McGovern (1996), for example, report that

> The global influence of consciousness is dramatized by the remarkable phenomenon of biofeedback training. There is firm evidence that *any* single neuron or *any* population of neurons can come to be voluntarily controlled by giving conscious feedback of their neural firing rates. A small needle electrode in the base of the thumb can tap into a single motor unit—a muscle fibre controlled by one motor neuron coming from the spinal cord, and a sensory fiber going back to it. When the signal from the muscle fibre is amplified and played back as a click through a loudspeaker, the subject can learn to control his or her single motor unit—one among millions—in about ten minutes. Some subjects have learned to play drumrolls on their single motor units after about thirty minutes of practice! However, if the biofeedback signal is not conscious, learning does not occur. Subliminal feedback, distraction from the feedback signal, or feedback via a habituating stimulus—all these cases prevent control being acquired. Since this kind of learning only works for *conscious* biofeedback signals, it suggests again that consciousness creates global access to all parts of the nervous system. (p. 75)

The most well accepted evidence for the effect of states of mind on medical outcome is undoubtedly the "placebo effect"—well known to every medical practitioner and researcher. Simply receiving treatment, and having confidence in the therapy or therapist has itself been found to be therapeutic in many clinical situations (Skrabanek & McCormick, 1989; Wall, 1996). As with other instances of apparent mind/body interaction, there are conflicting interpretations of the causal processes involved. For example, Skrabanek and McCormick (1989) claim that placebos can affect illness (how people feel) but not disease (organic disorders). That is, they accept the possibility of mental→mental causation but not of mental→physical causation.

However, Wall (1996) cites evidence that placebo treatments may produce organic changes. Hashish, Finman, and Harvey (1988), for example, found that use of an impressive ultrasound machine reduced not only pain, but also jaw tightness and swelling after the extraction of wisdom teeth whether or not the machine was set to produce ultrasound. Wall also reviews evidence that placebos can remove the sensation of pain accompanying well-defined organic disorders, and not just the feelings of discomfort, anxiety, and so on which may accompany it.

As McMahon and Sheikh (1989) note, the absence of an acceptable theory of mind/body interaction within philosophy and science has had a detrimental effect on the acceptance of mental causation in many areas of clinical theory and practice. Conversely, the extensive evidence for mental causation within some clinical settings forms part of the database that any adequate theory of mind/consciousness–body/brain relationships needs to explain.

SOME USEFUL ACCOUNTS OF MENTAL CAUSATION

The effects of imagery on brain, body, and other conscious experience is often explained in terms of *refocusing and redirection of attention*, linked where plausible to the operation of known biological mechanisms. For example, in their pain control induction program, Syrjala and Abrams (1996) explain the effectiveness of imagery to patients in terms of the gate-control theory of pain:

> Even though the pain message starts in your leg, you won't feel pain unless your brain gets the pain message. The pain message moves along nerves from where the injury is located to the brain. These nerves enter the spinal cord, where they connect to other nerves, which send information up the spinal cord to the brain. The connections in the spinal cord and brain act like gates. These gates help you to not have to pay attention to all the messages in your body all the time. For example, right now as you are listening, you do not notice the feelings in your legs, although those feelings are there if you choose to notice them. If you are walking, you might notice feelings in your legs but not in your mouth. One way we block the gates to pain is with medications. Or we can block the gates by filling them with other messages. You do this if you hit your elbow and then rub it hard. The rubbing fills the gate with other messages, and you feel less pain. You've done the same thing if you ever had a headache and you get busy doing something that takes a lot of concentration. You forget about the headache because the gates are full of other messages. Imagery is one way to fill the gate. You can choose to feel the pain if you need to, but any time you like you can fill the gate with certain thoughts and images. Our goal is to find the best gate fillers for you. (p. 243)

While this account is nicely judged in terms of its practical value to patients, it does not give much detail about the actual mechanisms involved. Nor is it intended to be a general account of mental causation, for example in cases that seem to require a more sophisticated understanding of the intricate, reciprocal balance of mind/brain/body relationships. The evidence that involuntary processes can sometimes be brought under voluntary control, for example, appears to blur the classical boundary between voluntary and autonomic nervous system functions, and extends the potential scope of top-down processing in the brain. And the evidence that imagery can sometimes have bodily effects that resemble the effects of the imaged situations themselves suggest that the conventional, clear distinction between "psychological reality" and "physical reality" may not be so clear in the way that these are *responded to* by body and brain. As Kenneth Pelletier (1993) puts it:

> Asthmatics sneeze at plastic flowers. People with a terminal illness stay alive until after a significant event, apparently willing themselves to live until a

graduation ceremony, a birthday milestone, or a religious holiday. A bout of rage precipitates a sudden, fatal heart attack. Specially trained people can voluntarily control such "involuntary" bodily functions as the electrical activity of the brain, heart rate, bleeding, and even the body's response to infection. Mind and body are inextricably linked, and their second-by-second interaction exerts a profound influence upon health and illness, life and death. Attitudes, beliefs, and emotional states ranging from love and compassion to fear and anger can trigger chain reactions that affect blood chemistry, heart rate, and the activity of every cell and organ system in the body—from the stomach and gastrointestinal tract to the immune system. All of that is now indisputable fact. However, there is still great debate over the extent to which the mind can influence the body and the precise nature of that linkage. (p. 19)

One productive route to a deeper understanding of such linkages is the traditional biomedical one, involving a fuller understanding of the interconnections and reciprocal control between cortical, neuroendocrine, autonomic, and immune systems. These have been extensively investigated within psychoneuroimmunology. Following a detailed review of this research, Watkins (1997) concludes that

It is apparent that the immune system can no longer be thought of as autoregulatory. Virtually every aspect of immune function can be modulated by the autonomic nervous system and centrally produced neuropeptides. These efferent neuroimmunomodulatory pathways are themselves modulated by afferent inputs from the immune system, the cortex and the limbic emotional centers. Thus the brain and the immune sytem communicate in a complex bidirectional flow of cytokines, steroids, and neuropeptides, sharing information and regulating each other's function. This enables the two systems to respond in an integrated manner to environmental challenges, be they immunological or behavioral, and thereby maintain homeostatic balance. (p. 15)

SO WHY DOES MENTAL CAUSATION REMAIN A PROBLEM?

Such innovative findings and their practical consequences for the development of "mind-body medicine" demand careful investigation. It is important to note however that such explanatory accounts routinely translate *mind*-body interactions into *brain*-body interactions. Unless one is prepared to accept that mind and consciousness are *nothing more* than brain processes,[2] this finesses the classical mind/body problems that are *already* posed by *normal* voluntary, "mental" control. How imagery might affect autonomic or immune system

[2] I present a detailed case against such materialist reductionism in Velmans (2000) chapters 3, 4, and 5.

functioning is mysterious, but how a conscious wish to lift a finger makes that finger move is equally mysterious. Why? There are many reasons, but I will focus on just three.

Problem 1. The physical world appears causally closed.

As noted previously, it is widely accepted in science that the operation of physical systems can be entirely explained in physical terms. For example, if one examines the human brain from an external third-person perspective one can, in principle, trace the effects of input stimuli on the central nervous system all the way from input to output, without finding any "gaps" in the chain of causation that consciousness might fill. Indeed, the *neural correlates* of consciousness would fill any "gaps" that might potentially be filled by consciousness in the activities of brain. In any case, if one inspects the operation of the brain from the outside, no subjective experience can be observed at work. Nor does one need to appeal to the existence of subjective experience to account for the neural activity that one *can* observe. The same is true if one thinks of the brain as a functioning system described in information processing terms rather than neural terms. Once the processing within a system required to perform a given function is sufficiently well specified in procedural terms, one does not have to add an "inner conscious life" to make the system work. In principle, the same function, operating to the same specification, could be performed by a non-conscious machine.[3]

Problem 2. One is not conscious of one's own brain/body processing. So how could there be conscious control of such processing?

How "conscious" is conscious, voluntary control? It is surprising how few people bother to ask.[4] One might be aware of the fact *that* relaxing imagery can lower heart rate, but one has no awareness of *how* it does so, nor, in biofeedback, does one have any awareness of how consciousness might control the firing of a single motor neurone. One isn't even conscious of *how* to control the articulatory system in everyday "conscious speech"! Speech production is one of the most complex tasks humans are able to perform. Yet, one has no awareness

---

[3] Note that being physically closed does not preclude "downward causation." Higher order brain states or functions may for example constrain lower order brain states and functions, for example in the way that computer software constrains and controls the switching in the hardware of the machine. The software, like the higher order functioning of the brain, is best described in functional terms (e.g., as an information processing system), but this does not alter the fact that the software is entirely embodied in the physical hardware and exercises its causal effects through its embodiment in that hardware.

[4] See the initial discussion of this issue in Velmans (1991).

whatsoever of the motor commands issued from the central nervous system that travel down efferent fibers to innervate the muscles, nor of the complex motor programming that enables muscular coordination and control. In speech, for example, the tongue may make as many as 12 adjustments of shape per second— adjustments which need to be precisely coordinated with other rapid, dynamic changes within the articulatory system. According to Lenneberg (1967), within one minute of discourse as many as 10 to 15 thousand neuromuscular events occur. Yet only the *results* of this activity (the overt speech) normally enters consciousness.

Preconscious speech control might of course be the result of *prior* conscious activity, for example, planning *what* to say might be conscious, particularly if one is expressing some new idea or expressing some old idea in a novel way. Speech production is commonly thought to involve hierarchically arranged, semantic, syntactic, and motor control systems in which communicative intentions are translated into overt speech in a largely top-down fashion. Planning *what* to say and translating nonverbal conceptual content into linguistic forms requires effort. But to what extent is such planning conscious? Let us see.

A number of theorists have observed that periods of conceptual, semantic, and syntactic planning are characterized by gaps in the otherwise relatively continuous stream of speech (Boomer, 1970; Goldman-Eisler, 1968). The neurologist John Hughlings Jackson, for example, suggested that the amount of planning required depends on whether the speech is "new" speech or "old" speech. Old speech (well-known phrases, etc.) requires little planning and is relatively continuous. New speech (saying things in a new way) requires planning and is characterized by hesitation pauses. Fodor, Bever, and Garrett (1974) point out that breathing pauses also occur (gaps in the speech stream caused by the intake of breath). However, breathing pauses do not generally coincide with hesitation pauses.

Breathing pauses nearly always occur at the beginnings and ends of major linguistic constituents (such as clauses and sentences). So these appear to be coordinated with the syntactic organization of such constituents into a clausal or sentential structure. Such organization is largely automatic and preconscious. By contrast, hesitation pauses tend to occur within clauses and sentences and appear to be associated with the formulation of ideas, deciding which words best express one's meaning, and so on. If this analysis is correct, conscious planning of *what* to say should be evident during hesitation pauses—and a little examination of what one experiences during a hesitation pause should settle the matter. Try it. During a hesitation pause one might experience a certain sense of effort (perhaps the effort to put something in an appropriate way). But nothing is revealed of the *processes* which formulate ideas, translate these into a form suitable for expression in language, search for and retrieve words from memory, or assess which words are most appropriate. In short, no more is revealed of conceptual or semantic planning in hesitation pauses than is revealed of syntactic planning in breathing pauses. The fact that a process demands processing *effort* does not ensure that it is *conscious*. Indeed, there is a sense in which one is only conscious of what one wants to say *after one has said it!*

It is particularly surprising that the same may be said of *conscious verbal thoughts*. That is, the same situation applies if one formulates one's thoughts into "covert speech" through the use of phonemic imagery, prior to its overt expression. Once one *has* a conscious verbal thought, manifested in experience in the form of phonemic imagery, the complex cognitive processes required to generate that thought, including the processing required to encode it into phonemic imagery *have already operated*. In short, covert speech and overt speech have a similar relation to the planning processes that produce them. In neither case are the complex antecedent processes available to introspection. It should be clear that this applies equally to the processes that generate the detailed spatial arrangement, colors, shapes, sizes, movements, and accompanying sounds and smells of an imaged visual scene.

Problem 3. Conscious experiences appear to come too late to causally affect the processes to which they most obviously relate.

In the production of overt speech and covert speech (verbal thoughts) the conscious experience that we normally associate with such processing *follows* the processing to which it relates. Given this, in what *sense* are these "conscious processes" conscious? The same question can be asked of that most basic of conscious voluntary processes, *conscious volition itself.*

It has been known for some time that voluntary acts are preceded by a slow negative shift in electrical potential (recorded at the scalp) known as the "readiness potential," and that this shift can precede the act by up to one second or more (Kornhuber & Deeke, 1965). In itself, this says nothing about the relation of the readiness potential to the *experienced wish* to perform an act. To address this, Libet (1985) asked subjects to note the instant they experienced a wish to perform a specified act (a simple flexion of the wrist or fingers) by relating the onset of the experienced wish to the spatial position of a revolving spot on a cathode ray oscilloscope, which swept the periphery of the face like the sweep-second hand of a clock. Recorded in this way, the readiness potential preceded the voluntary act by around 550 milliseconds, and preceded the experienced wish (to flex the wrist or fingers) by around 350 milliseconds (for spontaneous acts involving no preplanning). This suggests that, like the act itself, the experienced wish (to flex one's wrist) may be one output from the (prior) cerebral processes that actually select a given response. If so, "conscious volition" may be no more necessary for such a (preconscious) choice than the consciousness of ones own speech is necessary for its production.[5] And the same is likely to apply to more complex voluntary acts, such as the voluntary control of autonomic functions through imagery and biofeedback discussed previously.[6]

THE CURRENT THEORETICAL IMPASSE

As noted, there is extensive experimental and clinical evidence that conscious experiences can affect brain/body processes, and the importance of conscious experience is rightly taken for granted in everyday life. In one sense this can be explained by a more sophisticated biomedical understanding of mind/brain/body relationships. But in a deeper sense, current attempts to understand the role of conscious experience face an impasse. How can experiences have a causal influence on a physical world that is causally closed? How can one consciously control something that one is not conscious of? And how can experiences affect processes that *precede* them? Dualist-interactionist accounts of the consciousness-brain relationship, in which an autonomously existing consciousness influences the brain, do not even recognize these "how" problems let alone address them. Materialist reductionists attempt to finesse such problems by challenging the accuracy, causal efficacy, and even the existence of conscious experiences. This evades the need to address the "how" questions, but denies the validity of the clinical evidence and defies common sense. I have given a detailed critique of the many variants of dualism and reductionism elsewhere and will not repeat this here.[7] In what follows I suggest a way through the impasse that is neither dualist nor reductionist.[8]

---

[5] As Libet observed, the experienced wish *follows* the readiness potential, but *precedes* the motor act itself (by around 200 msec)—time enough to consciously *veto* the wish before executing the act. In a manner reminiscent of the interplay between the libidinous desires arising from Freud's unconscious *id* and the control exercised by the conscious *ego,* Libet suggested that the *initiation* of voluntary act and the accompanying wish are developed preconsciously, but consciousness can then act as a form of censor which decides whether or not to carry out the act. While this is an interesting possibility, it does invite an obvious question. If the wish to perform an act is developed preconsciously, why doesn't the decision to censor the act have its own preconscious antecedents? Libet (1996) argues that it *might* not need to do so as voluntary control imposes a change on a wish that is already conscious. Yet, it seems very odd that a wish *to do* something has preconscious antecedents while a wish *not to do* something does not. As it happens, there is evidence that bears directly on this issue. Karrer, Warren, and Ruth (1978) and Kanttinen and Lyytinen (1993), for example, found that *refraining* from irrelevant movements is associated with a slow *positive-going* readiness potential.

[6] This could be tested using Libet's procedures, by examining the relation of the readiness potential to an experienced wish to control a given bodily function via imagery or biofeedback.

[7] See Velmans (2000) chapters 2, 3, 4, and 5.

[8] In the space available I can only give a rough idea of how one might resolve these problems. A far more detailed and carefully defended treatment is given in Velmans (2000) chapter 11.

ONTOLOGICAL MONISM COMBINED WITH EPISTEMOLOGICAL DUALISM

How can one reconcile the evidence that conscious experiences are causally effective with the principle that the physical world is causally closed? One simple way is to accept that for each individual there is *one* "mental life" but *two* ways of knowing it: first-person knowledge and third-person knowledge. From a first-person perspective conscious experiences appear causally effective. From a third-person perspective the same causal sequences can be explained in neural terms. It is not the case that the view from one per- spective is right and the other wrong. These perspectives are complementary. The differences between how things appear from a first- versus a third-person perspective has to do with differences in the *observational arrangements* (the means by which a subject and an external observer access the subject's mental processes).

Let's see how this might work in practice. Suppose you have a calming image of lying in a green field on a summer's day, and you can feel the difference this makes in producing a relaxed state, slowing your breathing, removing the tension in your body, and so on. You give a causal account of what is going on, based on what you experience. From my external observer's perspective, I can also observe what is going on—but what I observe is a little different. I can measure the effects on your breathing and muscle tension, but no matter how closely I inspect your brain, I cannot observe your experienced image. The closest I can get to it are its neural correlates in the visual system, association areas, and so on.[9] Nevertheless, if I could observe all the neurophysiological events operating in your brain to produce your relaxed bodily state, it would be a complete, physical account of what is going on. So, now you have a first-person account of what is going on that makes sense to you and I have a third-person account of what is going on that makes sense to me. How do these relate? To understand this we need to examine the relation of your visual image to its neural correlates with care.

The Neural Correlates of Conscious Experience

Although we know little about the physical nature of the neural correlates of conscious experiences, there are three plausible, functional constraints imposed by the phenomenology of consciousness itself. Normal human conscious experi- ences are representational (phenomenal consciousness is always *of* something).

---

[9] The neural correlates of a given experience accompany or *co-occur* with given experiences, and are by definition as close as one get to those experiences from an external observer's perspective. This differentiates them from the antecedent causes (such as the operation of selective attention, binding, etc.) which may be thought of as the necessary and sufficient *prior* conditions for given experiences in the human brain.

Given this, it is plausible to assume that the physical correlates of such experiences are representational states. A representational state must also represent *something*. For a given physical state to be the correlate of a given experience, it is plausible to assume that it represents the *same* thing. Finally, for a physical state to be the correlate of a given experience, it is reasonable to suppose that it has the same "grain." That is, for every discriminable attribute of experience there will be a distinct, correlated, physical state. As each experience and its physical correlate represents the same thing, it follows that each experience and its physical correlate encodes the same information about that thing. That is, they are representations with the same *information structure*.[10]

In short, your experience and the neural correlates I observe relate to each other in a very precise way. What you experience takes the form of visual or other imagery accompanied by feelings about lying on the grass on a summer day. What I observe is the same information (about the visual scene) encoded in the physical correlates of what you experience in your brain. The information structure of what you and I observe is identical, although it is displayed or "formatted" in very different ways. From your point of view, the only information you have about your own state of mind is the imagery and accompanying feelings that you experience. From my point of view, the only information you have (about your own state of mind) is the information I can see encoded in your brain. The way your information (about your own state) is displayed appears to be very different to you and me for the reason that the "observational arrangements" by which we access that information are entirely different. From my external, third-person perspective I can only access the information encoded in your neural correlates by means of my visual or other exteroceptive systems, aided by appropriate equipment. Because you *embody* the information encoded in your neural correlates and it is already at the interface of your consciousness and brain, it displays "naturally" in the form of the visual scene and feelings that you experience.

But what is your mind *really* like? From my "external observer's perspective," can I assume that what you experience is really nothing more than the physical correlates that I can observe? From my external perspective, do I know what is going on in your mind/brain/consciousness better than you do? No. I know something about your mental states that you do not know (their physical

---

[10] Note that having an identical referent and information structure does not mean that experiences are *nothing more than* their neural correlates (as eliminativists and reductionists assume). A filmed version of the play "Hamlet," recorded on videotape, for example, may have the same sequential information structure as the same play displayed in the form of successive, moving pictures on a TV screen. But it is obvious that the information on the videotape is not ontologically identical to the information displayed on the screen. In this instance, the same information is embodied in two different ways (patterns of magnetic variation on tape versus patterns of brightness and hue in individual pixels on screen) and it is displayed or "formatted" in two different ways (only the latter display is in visible form).

embodiment). But you know something about them that I do not know (their manifestation in experience). Such first- and third-person information is *complementary*. We need your first-person story and my third-person story for a complete account of what is going on. If so, the nature of the mind is revealed as much by how it appears from one perspective as the other. It is not *either* physical *or* conscious experience, it is at once physical *and* conscious experience (depending on the observational arrangements). For lack of a better term we may describe this nature as *psychophysical*.[11,12] If we combine this with the representational features above, we can say that mind is a psychophysical process that encodes information, developing over time.

AN INITIAL WAY TO MAKE SENSE OF THE CAUSAL INTERACTIONS BETWEEN CONSCIOUSNESS AND BRAIN

This brief analysis of how first- and third-person accounts relate to each other can be used to make sense of the different *forms* of causal interaction that are taken for granted in everyday life or suggested in the clinical and scientific literature. Physical→physical causal sequences describe events from an entirely third-person perspective (they are "pure third-person" accounts). Mental→mental causal sequences describe events entirely from a first-person perspective (they are "pure first-person" accounts). Physical→mental and mental→physical causal

---

[11]The struggle to find a model or even a form of words that somehow captures the dual-aspect nature of mind is reminiscent for example of wave-particle complementarity in quantum mechanics— although this analogy is far from exact. Light either appears to behave as electromagnetic waves or as photon particles depending on the observation arrangements. And it does not make sense to claim that electromagnetic waves really *are* particles (or vice versa). A complete understanding of light requires both complementary descriptions—with consequent struggles to find an appropriate way of charac- terizing the nature of light which encompasses both descriptions ("wave-packets," "electron clouds," and so on). This has not prevented physics from developing very precise accounts of light viewed *either* as waves *or* as particles, together with precise formulae for relating wave-like properties (such as electromagnetic frequency) to particle-like ones (such as photon energy). If first- and third-person accounts of consciousness and its physical correlates are complementary and mutually irreducible, an analogous "psychological complementarity principle" might be required to understand the nature of mind. A more detailed discussion of how psychological complementarity relates to physical complementarity is given in Velmans (2000) chapter 11, note 19.

[12]At the macrocosmic level, the relation of electricity to magnetism also provides a clear parallel to the form of dual-aspect theory I have in mind. If one moves a wire through a magnetic field this produces an electrical current in the wire. Conversely, if one passes an electrical current through a wire this produces a surrounding magnetic field. But it does not make sense to suggest that the current in the wire is nothing more than the surrounding magnetic field, or vice-versa (reductionism). Nor is it accurate to suggest that electricity and magnetism are energies of entirely different kinds that happen to interact (dualist-interactionism). Rather these are two manifestations (or "dual-aspects") of *electro-magnetism*, a more fundamental energy that grounds and unifies both, described with elegance by Maxwell's Laws.

sequences are *mixed-perspective* accounts employing *perspectival switching* (Velmans, 1996b).

Physical→mental causal sequences start with events viewed from a third-person perspective and switch to how things appear from a first-person perspective. For example, a causal account of visual perception starts with a third-person description of the physical stimulus and the visual system but then switches to a first-person account of what the subject experiences. Mental→physical causal sequences switch the other way. From your subjective point of view, for example, the imagery that you experience is causing your heart rate to slow down and your body to relax (effects that I can measure). If I could identify the exact neural correlates of what you experience, it might be possible for me to give an entirely third-person account of this sequence of events (in terms of higher order neural representations having top-down effects on other brain and body states). But the mixed-perspective account actually gives you a more immediately useful description of what is going on in terms of the things that you can do (maintain that state of mind, deepen it, alter it, and so on).

In principle, complementary first- and third-person sources of information can be found whenever body or mind/brain states are represented in some way in subjective experience. A patient might for example have insight into the nature of a psychological problem (via feelings and thoughts), that a clinician might investigate by observing his/her brain or behavior. In medical diagnosis, a patient might have access to some malfunction via interoceptors, producing symptoms such as pain and discomfort, whereas a doctor might be able to identify the cause via his/her exteroceptors (eyes, ears, and so on) supplemented by medical instrumentation. As with conscious states and their neural correlates, the clinician has access to the physical embodiment of such conditions, while the patient has access to how such conditions are experienced. In these situations, neither the third-person information available to the clinician nor the first-person information available to the patient is *automatically* privileged or "objective" in the sense of being "observer-free." The clinician merely reports what he/she observes or infers about what is going on (using available means) and the patient does likewise. Such first- and third-person accounts of the subject's mental life or body states are complementary, and mutually irreducible. *Taken together*, they provide a global, psychophysical picture of the condition under scrutiny.

CONSCIOUS EXPERIENCES PROVIDE GLOBAL REPRESENTATIONS OF WHAT IS GOING ON

The above, I hope, gives an initial indication of how one can reconcile the evidence that conscious experiences appear causally effective with the principle that the physical world is causally closed. But there are two further, equally perplexing problems. How can the contents of consciousness affect brain and body states when one is not conscious of the biological processes that govern those states? And how can conscious experiences be causally effective if they come too late to affect the processes to which they most obviously relate?

I suggest that to make sense of these puzzles, one has to begin by accepting the facts rather than sweeping them under some obscuring theoretical carpet. Why do experiences come too late to affect the processes to which they most closely relate? For the simple reason that experiences are *representations*, and representations of an event or process can only be formed *after that event or process has taken place*! Barring illusions and hallucinations, one can only see an event or object in the external world if it already exists and one can only feel a state in one's own body if one's body is already in that state. In the same way, one can only experience a state of one's own mind/brain if it already exists, or has already taken place. As shown above, once one has a conscious thought (manifest in inner speech) the cognitive processes which have created that thought, along with the processes responsible for translating that thought into phonemic imagery (inner speech) have already operated. Just as perceived events in the world or body represent current states in the world or body, an experienced thought consciously represents the current state of one's own cognitive system. Likewise, a visually imaged peaceful world and one's conscious feelings about it represent a current, voluntarily produced representational state (and responses to it) within one's own cognitive and conative systems.

Why don't we have more detailed experience of the processes which produce such conscious experiences, or of the detailed workings of our own bodies, minds and brains? Because for normal purposes we don't need them! Our primary need is to interact successfully with the external world and with each other—and for that, the processes by which we arrive at representations of ourselves in the world, or which govern the many internal adaptive adjustments we have to make are best left on "automatic." This is exemplified by the well-accepted transition of skills from being conscious to being nonconscious as they become well learned (as in reading or driving a car). The global representations that we have of ourselves in the world nevertheless provide a useful, reasonable accurate representation of what is going on.[13]

HOW TO MAKE SENSE OF THE CAUSAL ROLE OF THE CONTENTS OF CONSCIOUSNESS

As noted above, normal experiences are *of* something, i.e., they represent entities, events, and processes in the external world, the body and the mind/brain

---

[13] It is reasonable to suppose that the detail of conscious representation has been tailored by evolutionary pressures to be useful for everyday human activities (although these remain global, approximate, and species-specific). To obtain a more intricate knowledge of the external world, body, or mind/brain we usually need the assistance of scientific instruments. A much fuller analysis of these points is given in Velmans (2000) chapter 7.

itself. In everyday life, we also behave as "naïve realists." That is, we take the events we experience to *be* the events that are actually taking place, although sciences such as physics, biology, and psychology might represent the same events in very different ways. For everyday purposes, the assumption that the world just *is* as we experience it to be serves us well. When playing billiards, for example, it is safe to assume that the balls are smooth, spherical, colored, and cause each other to move by mechanical impact. One only has to judge the precise angle at which the white ball hits the red ball to pocket the red. A quantum mechanical description of the microstructure of the balls or of the forces they exert on each other won't improve one's game.

That said, the experienced world is not the world *in itself*—and it is not our experience *of* the balls that governs the movement of the balls themselves. Balls as-experienced and their perceived interactions are global *representations* of autonomously existing entities and their interactions, and conscious representations (of what is happening) can only be formed *after* the occurrence of the events they represent. The same may be said of the events and processes that we experience to occur in our own bodies or minds/brains. When we withdraw a hand quickly from a hot iron, we experience the pain (in the hand) to cause what we do, but the reflex action actually takes place before the experience of pain has time to form. This can also happen with voluntary movements. Suppose, for example, that you are required to press a button as soon as you feel a tactile stimulus applied to your skin. A typical reaction time is 100 ms or so. It takes only a few milliseconds for the skin stimulus to reach the cortical surface, but Libet, Wright, Feinstein, and Pearl (1979) found that awareness of the stimulus takes at least 200 ms to develop. If so, the reaction must take place preconsciously, although we *experience* ourselves as responding *after* we feel something touching the skin. Just as the interactions among experienced billiard balls represent causal sequences in the external world, but are not the events themselves, experienced interactions between our sensations, thoughts, images, and actions represent causal sequences within our bodies and brains, but are not the events themselves. The mind/brain requires time to form a conscious representation of a pain or of something touching the skin and of the subsequent response. Although the conscious representations accurately place the cause (the stimulus) before the effect (the response), once the representations are formed, both the stimulus and the response have already taken place.

A similar pattern applies to other inner experiences. The thoughts, images, and feelings that appear in our awareness are both *generated by* processes in our bodies and mind/brains and *represent* the current states of those processes. Thoughts and images represent the ongoing state of play of our cognitive systems; feelings represent our internal (positive and negative) reactions to and judgments about events (see, e.g., Mangan, 1993).

In sum, conscious representations of inner body and external events are not the events themselves, but they generally represent those events and their causal interactions sufficiently well to allow a fairly accurate understanding of what is happening in our lives. Although they are only *representations* of events and their causal interactions, for everyday purposes we can take them to *be* those events and their causal interactions. When we play billiards we can line up a shot without the assistance of physics. Although our knowledge of our own inner states is not incorrigible, when we experience our verbal thoughts expressed in covert or overt speech, we usually know all we need to know about what we currently think—without the assistance of cognitive psychology. When we image ourselves in green grass on a summer's day and feel relaxed, we are usually right to assume that the mental state that is represented in our imagery has produced a real bodily effect, even though we don't understand how such imagined scenarios are constructed by preconscious mental processes or exercise top-down control in the mind/brain/body system. And when we experience ourselves to have acted out of love or fear, we usually have an adequate understanding of our motivation—although a neuropsychologist might find it useful to give a third-person account of this in terms of its origins in the brain's limbic system. It is not the case that a lower level (microscopic) representation is always better than a macroscopic one (in the case of billiard balls). Nor are third-person accounts always better than first-person ones (in describing our thoughts, images, and emotions). The value of a given representation, description, or explanation can only be assessed in the light of the purposes for which it is to be used.

WHO'S IN CONTROL?

The difference between voluntary and involuntary bodily functions is accepted wisdom, enshrined in the voluntary/autonomic nervous system distinction in medical texts. As we have seen previously, some processes that are normally involuntary can also become partly voluntary once they are represented in consciousness. But if we don't have a detailed conscious awareness of the workings of our own bodies and brains and if consciousness comes too late to affect the processes to which it most closely relates, how can this be? Consider again the dilemma posed by Libet et al.'s (1979) experiments on the role of conscious volition described previously. If the brain prepares to carry out a given action around 350 milliseconds before the conscious wish to act appears, then how could that action be "conscious" and how could it be "voluntary"? Doesn't the preceding readiness potential indicate that the action is determined preconsciously and automatically by processing in the mind/brain?

Let us consider the "conscious" aspect first. The decision to act is taken preconsciously but it becomes conscious at the moment that it manifests *as* a wish to do something in conscious experience. The wish then becomes conscious in the same way that your perception of this WORD is conscious. Like the wish, once you become conscious of this WORD, the physical, syntactic, and semantic analyses required to recognize it have already taken place. Nonetheless, once you become conscious of the wish or the WORD, the mental/brain processes make a transition from a preconscious to a conscious state—and it is only when this happens that you consciously realize what is going on.[14]

But how could an act that is executed *preconsciously* be "voluntary"? Voluntary actions imply the possibility of choice, albeit choice based on available external and internal information, current needs and goals. Voluntary actions are also potentially flexible and capable of being novel. In the psychological literature these properties are traditionally associated with controlled rather than automatic processing or with focal-attentive rather than pre-attentive or non-attended processing.[15] Unlike automatic or pre-attentive processing, both controlled processing (in the execution of acts) and focal-attentive processing (in the analysis of input) are thought to be "conscious."[16] None of the above argues against such traditional wisdom. In Libet's experiments the conscious experience appears around 350 milliseconds after the onset of preconscious processes that are indexed by the readiness potential. This says something about the timing of the conscious experience in relation to the processes that generate it and about its role once it appears. However, it does not argue against the voluntary nature of that preconscious processing. On the contrary, the fact that the act consciously feels as if it is voluntary and controlled suggests that the processes which have generated that experience *are* voluntary and controlled, as conscious experiences generally provide reasonably accurate representations of what is going on (see above).[17] This applies equally to the voluntary nature of more complex, mental processing such as the self-regulating, self-modifying operations of our own psychophysical minds evidenced by the effects of conscious imagery, meditation, and biofeedback.

So *who*'s in control? Who chooses, has thoughts, generates images and so on? We habitually think of ourselves as being our *conscious selves*. But it should be clear from the above that the different facets of our experienced, conscious selves are generated by and represent aspects of our own preconscious minds. That is, we are *both* the pre-conscious generating processes *and* the conscious results. Viewed from a third-person perspective our own preconscious mental processes

[14] I do not have space to develop this theme in more detail here. In Velmans (2000) chapters 10, 11, and 12 I develop a broader "reflexive monist" philosophy in which the function of consciousness is to "real-ise" the world. That is, once an entity, event or process enters consciousness it becomes *subjectively* real.

[15] Such functional differences are beyond the scope of the present chapter. However they have been extensively investigated, e.g., in studies of selective attention, controlled versus automatic processing, and so on (see e.g., Kihlstrom, 1996; Velmans, 1991).

[16] In Velmans (1991) I argue that there are three distinct senses in which a process may be said to be conscious. It can be conscious a) in the sense that one is conscious *of* it, b) in the sense that it results in a conscious experience, and c) in the sense that consciousness causally affects that process. Conscious volition is conscious in senses a) and b) but not c) (see also Velmans, 2000, chapter 9).

[17] This contrasts for example with the experienced involuntary feeling associated with a muscle twitch or the uncontrolled movements found in Parkinson's disease.

look like neurochemical and associated physical activities in our brains. Viewed introspectively, from a first-person perspective, our preconscious mind seems like a personal, but "empty space" from which thoughts, images, and feelings spontaneously arise. *We* are as much one thing as the other—and this requires a shift in our sensed "center of gravity" to one where our consciously experienced self becomes just the visible "tip" of our own embedding, preconscious mind.

REFERENCES

Baars, B. J., & McGovern, K. (1996). Cognitive views of consciousness: What are the facts? How can we explain them? In M. Velmans (Ed.), *The science of consciousness: Psychological, neuropsychological, and clinical reviews*. London: Routledge.

Barber, T. X. (1984) Changing "unchangeable" bodily processes by (hypnotic) suggestions: A new look at hypnosis, cognitions, imagining, and the mind-body problem. In A. A. Sheikh (Ed.), *Imagination and healing*. Amityville, NY: Baywood.

Boomer, D. S. (1970). Review of F. Goldman-Eisler *Psycholinguistics: Experiments in spontaneous speech. Lingua, 25,* 152-164.

Fodor, J. A., Bever, T. G., & Garrett, M. F. (1974). *The psychology of language*. New York: McGraw-Hill.

Goldman-Eisler, F. (1968). *Psycholinguistics: Experiments in spontaneous speech*. New York: Academic Press.

Hashish, I., Finman, C., & Harvey, W. (1988). Reduction of postoperative pain and swelling by ultrasound: A placebo effect. *Pain, 83,* 303-311.

Kanttinen, N., & Lyytinen, H. (1993). Brain slow waves preceding time-locked visuo-motor performance. *Journal of Sport Sciences* 11, 257-266.

Karrer, R., Warren, C., & Ruth, R. (1978). Slow potentials of the brain preceding cued and non-cued movement: Effects of development and retardation. In D. A. Otto (Ed.), *Multidisciplinary perspectives in event-related potential research*. Washington D.C.: U.S. Government Printing Office.

Kihlstrom, J. F. (1996). Perception without awareness of what is perceived, learning without awareness of what is learned. In M. Velmans (Ed.), *The science of consciousness: Psychological, neuropsychological, and clinical reviews*. London: Routledge.

Kornhuber, H. H., & Deecke, L. (1965). Hirnpotentialänderungen bei willkürbewegungen und passiven bewegungen des menchen: Bereitschaftspotential und reafferente potentiale. *Pflügers Archiv für die Gesampte Physiologie des Menschen und Tiere, 284,* 1-17.

Lenneberg, E. H. (1967). *Biological foundations of language*. New York: Wiley.

Libet, B. (1985). Unconscious cerebral initiative and the role of conscious will in voluntary action. *Behavioral and Brain Sciences, 8,* 529-566.

Libet, B. (1996). Neural processes in the production of conscious experience. In M. Velmans (Ed.), *The science of consciousness: Psychological, neuropsychological, and clinical reviews*. London: Routledge.

Libet, B., Wright Jr., E. W., Feinstein, B., & Pearl, D. K. (1979). Subjective referral of the timing for a conscious experience: A functional role for the somatosensory specific projection system in man. *Brain, 102,* 193-224.

Mangan, B. (1993). Taking phenomenology seriously: The "fringe" and its implications for cognitive research. *Consciousness and Cognition, 2*(2), 89-108.

McMahon, C. E., & Sheikh, A. (1989). Psychosomatic illness: A new look. In A. Sheikh & K. Sheikh (Eds.), *Eastern and Western approaches to healing.* New York: Wiley-Interscience.

Pelletier, K. R. (1993). Between mind and body: Stress, emotions, and health. In D. Goleman & J. Gurin (Eds.), *Mind body medicine: How to use your mind for better health.* New York: Consumer Reports Books.

Sheikh, A. A., Kunzendorf, R. G., & Sheikh, K. S. (1996). Somatic consequences of consciousness. In M. Velmans (Ed.), *The science of consciousness: Psychological, neuropsychological, and clinical reviews.* London: Routledge.

Sheikh, A. A. (Ed.). (2002). *Healing images: The role of imagination in health.* Amityville, NY: Baywood.

Skrabanek, P., & McCormick, J. (1989). *Follies and fallacies in medicine.* Glasgow: The Tarragon Press.

Syrjala, K. A., & Abrams, J. R. (1996). Hypnosis and imagery in the treatment of pain. In R. J. Catchel & D. C. Turk (Eds.), *Psychological approaches to pain management: A practitioner's handbook.* New York: The Guilford Press.

Velmans, M. (1991). Is human information processing conscious? *Behavioral and Brain Sciences, 14*(4), 651-726.

Velmans, M. (Ed). (1996a). *The science of consciousness: Psychological, neuropsychological and clinical reviews.* London: Routledge.

Velmans, M. (1996b). Consciousness and the "causal paradox." *Behavioral and Brain Sciences, 19*(3), 537-542.

Velmans, M. (2000). *Understanding consciousness.* London: Routledge/Psychology Press.

Wall, P. D. (1996). The placebo effect. In M. Velmans (Ed.), *The science of consciousness: Psychological, neuropsychological and clinical reviews.* London: Routledge.

Watkins, A. (1997). Mind-body pathways. In A. Watkins (Ed.), *Mind-body medicine: A clinician's guide to psychoneuroimmunology.* New York: Churchill Livingstone.

CHAPTER 4

Imagery, Cerebral Laterality, and the Healing Process: A Cautionary Note

SVEN VAN DE WETERING, DANIEL M. BERNSTEIN, AND ROBERT G. LEY

Something I owe to the soil that grew,
More to the life that fed,
But most to Allah
Who gave me two separate sides of my head.

I would go without shirts or shoes,
Friends, tobacco, or bread,
Sooner than for an instant
Lose either side of my head.

Rudyard Kipling (1928)

What does mental imagery have to do with the healing process? In 1983, we proposed a model to explain the action of imagery on healing (Ley & Freeman, 1983). We argued for a series of links connecting inescapable stress with hopelessness, catecholamine depletion, depression, oversecretion of corticosteroids, and immune dysfunction. We further argued that imagery could inhibit these undesirable processes, both by weakening the link between stress and hopelessness and by stimulating the right hemisphere of the brain, thus improving emotional function.

The model we proposed was provisional, intended to help explain a complex network of phenomena, but somewhat speculative. The intervening years have produced masses of research relevant to that early model, and in many ways have not been kind to it. Some of our proposed linkages have been amply corroborated by subsequent findings, such as that between excess corticosteroid secretion and immune dysfunction. Some have been corroborated, but our interpretation of them has been called into question, largely because what we regarded as unidirectional linkages now appear to be bidirectional. The link between depression and immune dysfunction falls into this category, as does the link between lateralized cerebral activation and depression. Finally, some links have been seriously called into question; both the catecholamine depletion theory of depression and the idea that imagery is largely confined to the right cerebral hemisphere fall in this category.

Because of these developments, our original model, considered as a whole, no longer looks very helpful in making sense of phenomena relating to stress, imagery, cerebral laterality, depression, and health. The goal of this chapter is to examine some of those new developments and how they affect our understanding of the relevant phenomena. Our untenable old model will not be replaced by a new model, but rather by a tentative series of assertions about linkages which will not lend themselves readily to being assembled into a coherent picture. In the end, we find no cause to reject the use of imagery in treating depression or aiding healing, but also no strong theoretical or empirical grounds for endorsing it.

LATERALITY, IMAGERY, AND BRAIN ORGANIZATION

The Concept of Laterality

The brain is a marvelous piece of symmetry. How much of this symmetry, though, extends to brain function? Much work in the past century has aimed at unveiling functional differences in the two cerebral hemispheres. Early observations by Broca and Wernicke over a century ago led to two important conclusions. First, the left hemisphere is more vital than the right for various aspects of language. Second, different regions within the left hemisphere are responsible for different aspects of language (production vs. comprehension). The logic underlying both notions is that particular brain regions serve particular functions. Although this idea appears perfectly reasonable, the brain may be organized in such a way that any given behavior or function is executed simultaneously and conjointly in multiple brain regions (Sergent, 1990).

Despite the brain's beautiful complexity and our present lack of complete understanding of even the simplest of cognitive functions (Effron, 1990), researchers have attempted to explain behaviors as diverse as tennis playing (Gallwey, 1974), seating arrangements in classrooms (Gur, Sackheim, & Gur, 1976), and purchase decisions (Heath, 1999) on the basis of hemispheric functional differences. The following briefly examines research on cerebral asymmetry in preparation for more specific discussion of the links among laterality, imagery, and the healing process.

The "Basics" of Laterality. "The two [cerebral] hemispheres control vastly different aspects of thought and action. Each half has its own specialization and thus its own limitations and advantages. The left brain is dominant for language and speech. The right excels at visual-motor tasks. The language of these findings has become part of our culture: writers refer to themselves as left-brained, visual artists as right-brained" (Gazzaniga, 1998, p. 3).

How much of human behavior can be so clearly dichotomized as occurring in either one or the other cerebral hemisphere? Do the two cerebral hemispheres really subserve "vastly" different cognitive functions? The past 35 years of laterality research have produced a dizzying array of data, only some of which is consistent. Nevertheless, some findings are well established. It is known that, for the most part, each hemisphere controls sensory input on the opposite side of the body. For example, sounds, images, and sensations on the left side of the body are transmitted largely to the right hemisphere and vice versa. Although no right hemisphere cognitive ability is as firmly established as the left hemisphere's dominance for speech and language (and even this is not as clear as was once thought), several behaviors seem to rely on the right hemisphere. These include music perception (Gates & Bradshaw, 1977), face recognition (Geffen, Bradshaw, & Wallace, 1971), emotional expression (Ley & Bryden, 1979), perception of degraded visual stimuli (Bryden & Allard, 1976), distribution of attention across space (Hellige, 1993) and perception of global aspects of visual stimuli (Robertson & Lamb, 1991).

Despite its intuitive and lasting appeal as an area of scientific investigation, laterality research has been marred by myriad methodological and logical shortcomings. Wood, Flower, and Naylor (1991) stress the importance of external environment and task demands in laterality research. Effron (1990) mentions that the differences found within a hemisphere are typically much greater than those found between hemispheres. Moreover, the robust differences in performance on certain cognitive tasks (e.g., dichotic listening, which involves the simultaneous presentation of different words to each ear) reflect stable performance in only 40 percent of subjects. Effron also argues cogently for more attention to be paid to subcortical structures which have been largely ignored in laterality research. Perhaps Effron's most damning criticism is one that strikes the very foundation of much of laterality research: "The concept of 'specialization' is used merely as a short-hand way of re-stating the existence of a correlation between the site of a brain lesion and some type of cognitive deficit" (p. 27).

It is important to view the relative hemisphere advantages for verbal, as opposed to visual-spatial tasks, as reflecting the different cognitive "styles" of each hemisphere. If one considers the logic driving most laterality research, one might be led to falsely infer that the different hemispheres evolved to perform fairly specific functions. However, it is unlikely that the brain evolved to process words in the left hemisphere and to detect music in the right hemisphere. Rather, each hemisphere is most likely structured to efficiently process a variety of environmental stimuli.

Imagery: Definition and Relation to the Right Hemisphere. Imagery has been broadly defined as "conscious reproductions of previously experienced events" (Trojano & Grossi, 1994, p. 213). Alternatively, images have been described as propositional constructs that are more accurately represented as symbolic, conceptual descriptions (Pylyshyn, 1978) than as "pictures in the head."

Originally, visual imagery was thought to be related to right hemisphere activation (Springer & Deutsch, 1981). By analyzing single cases of brain damaged patients who lacked visual imagery, Farah (1984) challenged this view as overly simplistic, and instead proposed a computational account of visual imagery in which damage to the posterior left hemisphere results in impaired imagery generation. This view was based on earlier work by Kosslyn (1980). Computational models assume that any given mental process (in this case, imagery) is reducible to discrete component processes (e.g., image generation, inspection, and transformation of images) that are likely executed in different brain regions and possibly different hemispheres. Computational models have come to dominate much of visual imagery research as well as most other research in cognitive psychology.

Sergent (1990) carefully re-examined Farah's (1984) analysis, as well as other studies in the literature on split-brain patients, group studies of brain damaged patients, and behavioral studies of normal subjects. From her review, Sergent found little evidence to support the notion that either hemisphere controls image generation. Instead, Sergent argues for reciprocal and simultaneous contributions from both hemispheres in the generation of mental imagery.

More recent reviews of imagery generation (Loverock & Modigliani, 1995; Tippet, 1992; Trojano & Grossi, 1994) tend to accord more involvement to the left hemisphere than to the right. Shuren, Greer, and Heilman (1996) use a straightforward imagery procedure designed to evoke hemisphere asymmetry. Right-handed subjects asked to imagine simple, common objects like a paper cup or a mountain were more likely to image the right side of the object, indicating more left hemisphere involvement in image generation. Recent work using imaging techniques such as positron emission tomography (PET) and functional magnetic resonance imaging (fMRI) has revealed conflicting data. While some have shown bilateral hemisphere activation during image generation (e.g., Mellet, Tzourio, Denis, & Mazoyer, 1998), others report more left hemisphere involvement (D'Esposito, Detre, Aguirre et al., 1997).

With respect to visual perception and visual imagery, Brown and Kosslyn (1993) have argued that the right hemisphere is better than the left at encoding coordinate metric spatial relations involving distances (vs. categorical spatial relations that involve categories like "above" or "inside") and at representing specific instances of visual forms (vs. more abstract categories of visual forms). Michimata (1997) has recently demonstrated that this hemisphere difference in processing imaged spatial relations is largely task dependent, and that "there is no 'dominant' hemisphere in general imagery processing" (p. 381).

The same logic that compelled some researchers (cf. Farah, 1984; Kosslyn, 1987) to abandon the global divisions of hemispheric specialization for a computational description of neural specialization might also be applied to computational approaches. The level of analysis has merely been refined, leaving the logic of localization of function largely intact. Thus, while imagery used to be considered a right hemisphere controlled process, now most researchers would agree that the two hemispheres operate in tandem on different aspects of the imagery process (e.g., image generation vs. inspection). There are likely few "pure" specializations of function found anywhere in the brain. That is, every operation and process may involve multiple networks, simultaneously interacting to perform a given function. Thus, the components of imagery and perception may be no more localizable than the gross-level functions of imagery and perception. The logical extension of this argument is that each of the components of imagery (e.g., image generation and inspection) is reducible to yet further subcomponents (ad infinitum?) and that each of these subcomponents will be processed in different hemispheric subsystems. This and other problems with the computational approach have led some theorists to propose that the computational approach to many problems in cognitive science should be supplemented or replaced by a dynamical approach (van Gelder, 1998).

Emotion: Depression and the Right Hemisphere. Although, as can be seen above, there is no obvious hemispheric dominance for imagery processing, there does appear to be a right hemisphere specialization for the perception, experience and expression of emotion (Coffey, 1987). Recent conceptualizations tend to ascribe a communicative nature to emotion, whereby emotion explains to ourselves and to others our intentions and actions (Oatley & Jenkins, 1992).

Heller (1993; Heller, Nitschke, & Miller, 1998) uses Russel's (1980) circumplex model of emotion to explain differences in emotional experience. According to the model, all emotion can be represented by arousal (low to high) and valence (unpleasant to pleasant). Heller believes that emotional valence is subserved by the frontal lobes and that arousal is associated with right parieto-temporal regions.

"The experience of emotion is not lateralized to one or the other hemisphere: Rather, it involves dynamic processes that include interactions between anterior and posterior regions of both hemispheres, as well as between cortical and subcortical structures of the brain" (Heller et al., 1998, pp. 26-27). Despite this caveat, Heller et al. present a model of hemispheric asymmetry that might be used to explain differences in depression and anxiety. According to this model, depression is associated with decreased right posterior activation while anxiety is linked to increased right posterior activation. Heller et al. break anxiety down into anxious apprehension (worry) and anxious arousal (panic). The former is believed to be related to increased left hemisphere activation while the latter is related to increased right hemisphere activation. Unfortunately, as Heller (1993) points out, anxiety and depression often co-occur and are very difficult to disentangle (cf., Pine, Kentgen, Bruder, Leite, Bearman, Ma, & Klein, 2000).

Coffey (1987) argues that the right hemisphere is linked to negative affect while the left hemisphere is related to positive affect. In support of this notion, Schiff and Lamon (1989) have been able to induce positive or negative emotions in subjects simply by having subjects contract their facial muscles to the left or right side, respectively. What is perhaps most impressive about this phenomenon is that subjects do not appear to be cognizant of the effects. Thus, facial expression itself may influence emotion by activating the right and left hemispheres.

There is also evidence that the perception and expression of emotion is lateralized. Recent evidence has revealed that faces with negative expressions are more easily processed by the right hemisphere, while faces with positive expressions are more easily processed by the left hemisphere (Jansari, Tranel, & Adolphs, 2000). Kakolewski, Crowsen, Sewell, and Cromwell (1999) provide data in which positive words (e.g., "vibrant") are more easily processed by the left hemisphere. However, they found no evidence that negative words (e.g., "failure") favored right hemispheric processing.

Another theory of the lateralization of emotion relates hemispheric lateralization of positive (left hemisphere) and negative (right hemisphere) emotions to approach and withdrawal responses, respectively (Davidson, 1995; Kinsbourne, 1978). Davidson proposes that either decreased left frontal activation or damage to left frontal regions of brain may be associated with depression. He points to a variety of EEG studies in support of this position. Bruder (1995) reviews ERP evidence in support of the notion that depression is linked to both left frontal and right posterior inactivation. Schiff and Bassel (1996) provide further support for a model of left frontal inactivation in depression. They found that right hemispheric activation facilitated finger extension (a withdrawal response), whereas left hemispheric activation facilitated finger flexion (an approach response). Further support for the lateralization of withdrawal and approach responses has recently been provided by Yecker, Borod, Brozgold, Martin, Alport, and Welkowitz (1999), who compared the facial emotional expressions of controls, schizophrenics, and patients with unipolar depression.

Depression has also been linked to increases in pain sensitivity (Pauli, Wiedermann, & Nickola, 1999; Romano & Turner, 1985) and somatization (Min & Lee, 1997) on the left side of the body. Moreover, depression has been related to increases in left conjugate lateral eye movements and increased left-hand skin conductance, suggestive of right hemisphere hyperexcitability (Lenhart & Katkin, 1986).

Finally, Bulman-Fleming and Bryden (1994) have shown in a single dichotic listening task the simultaneous occurrence of a left hemisphere superiority for verbal material and a right hemisphere superiority for affective material. Subjects were asked to listen for a particular word presented in one ear spoken in a particular tone of voice presented in the other ear.

From the above discussion, we may conclude that the right hemisphere plays a vital role in the processing of emotion. Although several theories exist that are not entirely compatible, there does appear to be enough evidence to confidently assert a relationship between emotion and the right hemisphere. At present, depression seems to be related to either right hemispheric hyperactivity or left hemispheric hypoactivity or both. However, the direction of this relationship may be either unidirectional (e.g., right hemisphere activation causes depression or depression causes right hemisphere activation) or bidirectional.

We suspect that laterality research on emotion will likely follow a similar path to that followed by imagery research: the global construct of emotion will have to be broken down into its components. Indeed, Borod (1993) has already called for a componential approach to the study of emotion involving perception, expression, physiology, arousal and activation, and subjective experience. These components will largely be found to favor either the left or the right hemisphere. However, as we argue above, this fractionation has no logical end. The more we learn about the components of emotion, the finer will be its subdivisions. Few, if any, researchers would argue that emotion is a unitary construct. Thus, it remains to be seen how finely we can split emotion and still feel confident that we are studying emotion.

THE EFFECTS OF STRESS, DEPRESSION, AND NEGATIVE AFFECT ON ILLNESS AND HEALING

When we proposed our 1983 model, the field of psychoneuro-immunology was still in its infancy. We devoted considerable energy to demonstrating that a person's psychological state could have an influence on his/her physical health. By the late 1990s, this assertion was no longer controversial. Although we will devote some space to showing that there are links between psychological and physical functioning, it now seems just as important to inject a note of caution into the discussion, and state that, while some effect of emotions on health have been established, the magnitude of this effect is usually modest, and the mechanisms by which, for example, a good mood improves health are not well understood.

Perhaps the most widely reported findings in this area concern the effect of stress on immune functioning. Being psychologically stressed seems to decrease people's ability to resist illness and heal from wounds.

One frequently studied example of this phenomenon is in the area of stress and upper respiratory infections (URI, also known as the common cold). Evans and Edgerton (1991) found in a naturalistic study in which subjects kept diaries of life events that subjects had experienced more hassles and fewer "uplifts" in the last few days before catching a cold, particularly on the day four days before onset of the cold. In a subsequent study, Evans and Edgerton (1992) report that cold onset was related to self-reports of previously experiencing hostile depression. Unfortunately, Stone, Porter, and Neale (1993) were unable to replicate these results, despite using a similar methodology. Turner Cobb and Steptoe (1996) have found evidence that life stress can increase susceptibility to colds, but that this effect was moderated by psychosocial resources.

In a review of the literature on stress and infectious disease in humans, Cohen and Williamson (1991) point out that even if findings of correlations between stress and susceptibility to acute infectious illness are accepted as reliable, there is no proof that this link is mediated by direct physiological effects of psychological stress. At least two other mechanisms are possible. One of these is that psychological stress could lead to a change of behaviors that may increase exposure to pathogens. For example, a psychologically distressed person may engage in more support-seeking behaviors, including bodily contact with large numbers of people, which may increase exposure to infectious agents. The other possibility is that psychological distress may increase reporting of symptoms because of oversensitivity to bodily cues, with a resulting tendency to label innocuous sensations as symptoms and to label symptom clusters as illnesses.

Cohen, Tyrrell, and Smith (1991) dealt with one of these problems by controlling for exposure to pathogens. Exposure to a cold virus was controlled by administering the viruses to subjects in nose drops and then quarantining the subjects for two days prior to and seven days subsequent to administration of the virus. Under these circumstances, it was possible to demonstrate a modest but reliable effect of self-reported stress over the past year on people's susceptibility to colds, and to further show that the relationship is roughly linear, i.e., the greater the stress, the greater the likelihood of catching a cold.

Studies of wound healing have helped deal with the second problem, that of differential reporting of symptoms. The progress of wound healing can be precisely assessed by means of photographs and reaction to hydrogen peroxide. Both the stress of caring for a demented relative (Kiecolt-Glaser, Marucha, Malarkey, Mercado, & Glaser, 1995) and the stress of preparing for university examinations (Marucha, Kiecolt-Glaser, & Favagehi, 1998) have been shown to slow healing of standardized wounds inflicted by the experimenters.

Another way to circumvent issues surrounding the ambiguity of the mediating link between stress and health is to use laboratory measures of immune system efficacy as a dependent measure in such studies. Many studies assess the concentration of various types of immune cells in the bloodstream, the activity of Natural Killer (NK) cells, or the proliferative response of lymphocytes to stimuli (called mitogens) that mimic the effect of antigens. In a review of such studies, O'Leary (1990) finds that the results often contradict each other. This is likely due to the fact that the body has at least two major endocrine systems, the sympathetic adrenal-medullary (SAM) system, which releases catecholamines into the bloodstream, and the hypothalamic-pituitary-adrenocortical (HPAC) system, which releases corticosteroids. The effect of catecholamines is generally to take lymphocytes out of storage and put them into the circulatory system. This is often interpreted as enhanced immune function, but because it only involves reallocation of existing resources, this may not actually represent an improvement in ability to fight infection. Corticosteroids, on the other hand, tend to suppress most aspects of immune functioning. The net result of this is that different forms of stress will have different effects on immunity, depending on the degree to which they activate each of these two systems.

"Stress" is a slippery concept, incorporating as it does both the idea of external circumstances and of psychological psychological reactions to those circumstances. Depression, anxiety, and negative affect, being more clearly internal phenomena, are also frequently studied in psychoneuroimmunology. In a meta-analysis of studies of depression and immunity, Herbert and Cohen (1994) found that there was sufficient evidence to warrant firm claims that depressive illness was associated with significant negative changes in a number of measures of cellular immunity. It has also been found that trait negative affect is associated with greater severity of symptoms of colds (Cohen, Doyle, Skoner, Fireman, Gwaltney, & Newsom, 1995), though it is plausible that this increased severity can be traced to biases in complaining about symptoms rather than to impaired immune function. Attempts have also been made to demonstrate the converse, that optimism and positive mood decrease illness. Segerstrom, Taylor, Kemeny, and Fahey (1998), for example, were able to show an association between optimism and more robust immune functioning in the face of stress.

Psychosocial Intervention

If we accept that long-term stress and negative emotion have a negative impact on health and immune system functioning, and that positive mood may have a positive impact, then it seems logical to ask whether psychosocial interventions can be used to positively affect the health of people who are chronically ill or distressed. On the whole, studies that have attempted to measure the effects of such interventions have shown encouraging results (Kiecolt-Glaser & Glaser, 1995). This sort of intervention has been particularly widely studied in cancer patients. For example, Spiegel, Bloom, Kraemer, and Gottheil (1989) found that supportive group therapy and hypnosis for pain significantly increased the mean survival time for patients with metastatic breast cancer. Another study involving patients with melanoma was able to demonstrate not only long-term improvements in survival rates and decreases in relapse rates as a result of psychological support and stress management training (Fawzy, Fawzy, Hyun, Elashoff, Guthrie, Fahey, & Morton, 1993), but also relatively short-term improvements in a number of measures of immune functioning as a result of this psychosocial manipulation (Fawzy, Kemeny, Fawzy, Elashoff, Morton, Cousins, & Fahey, 1990).

AIDS is another form of a chronic health problem that has been extensively studied in this regard. AIDS is particularly interesting from the point of view of psychoneuroimmunology, both because AIDS is a disease of the immune system and because the stigma associated with AIDS infection is such that mere labeling as an AIDS victim constitutes a significant source of psychosocial stress. Notification that one is HIV positive has been shown to result in a number of decrements in immune functioning independent of the actual damage caused by the infection (Antoni, Baggett, Ironson, LaPerriere, August, Klimas, Schneiderman, & Fletcher, 1991; LaPerriere, Fleischer, Antoni, Klimas, Ironson, & Schneiderman, 1991). These decrements can be reduced or even eliminated by psychosocial manipulations such as training in cognitive-behavioral stress management techniques (Antoni et al., 1991) or enrolment in an aerobic exercise training program (LaPerriere et al., 1991).

Imagery and Healing

Imagery continues to be widely used in healing contexts, as it was at the time of our 1983 model. Nevertheless, the use of imagery continues to encounter skepticism, due largely to the absence of well controlled studies demonstrating its efficacy (Hall, Anderson, & O'Grady, 1994). This is due less to oversight than to the inherent difficulty of adequately controlling such studies. In particular, imagery manipulations tend to be tailored to the patient, and are therefore difficult to subject to the sort of tight experimental control that is usually desired for such studies.

To the extent that imagery does have a positive effect, it likely does so through its ability to reduce anxiety and decrease the perceived stressfulness of challenging life events (Fiore, 1988; Hammer, 1996; Jordan & Lenington, 1979; Sapp, 1994). Thus, we can reaffirm our statement of 1983 that imagery can serve as a coping mechanism, which weakens the tendency for an environmental stressor to produce a strain within the organism.

DIFFICULTIES IN INTERPRETATION OF PSYCHONEUROIMMUNOLOGICAL FINDINGS

The findings that have been sketched in the previous two sections are often interpreted as demonstrating that feeling good is good for the immune system and therefore for one's physical health, whereas feeling bad is bad for the immune system and therefore for one's health. As a rule of thumb, this is probably a good one, but it is important to be aware of some limitations and subtleties that may cloud the simplicity of this generalization.

One of the most obvious caveats is that boosting the numbers of immune cells in the bloodstream is not the same as improving immune function; instead, it should probably be thought of as mobilizing stored resources (O'Leary, 1990). This can have a positive effect on health if there is in fact a threat to health present that can be combated with immune cells; for example, there is an obvious functional reason for the body's mobilization of leukocytes in response to catecholamines, namely that catecholamines are usually secreted from the adrenal gland in response to an external threat. External threats, at least during the time period when the immune system did most of its evolving, were usually associated with risk of wounds, which were in turn in danger of becoming infected. This risk of infection was and is minimized by mobilizing leukocytes before any wound is inflicted. Nevertheless, the adaptiveness of this mechanism in the case of threat of wounds does not mean that this response is valuable in all circumstances; presumably, the body stores leukocytes for a reason, and is likely to be negatively affected by having them mobilized when that mobilization serves no defensive purpose.

A second subtlety that is easy to miss is that psychosocial therapies that make many people happier and more resistant to disease are not universally helpful. Individual differences in response to therapy are easy to miss in studies where individuals are members of a statistical aggregate. One example of the differential effects of therapy on different people can be found in a study by Christensen, Edwards, Wiebe, Benotsch, McKelvey, Andrews, and Lubaroff (1996). These investigators were interested in the effects of self-disclosure on immunity, because previous work had shown self-disclosure to be beneficial to many people's health. They found that self-disclosure caused a short-term rise in natural killer cell (NK) cytotoxicity in all participants, but that this effect was much stronger in participants high on the trait of cynical hostility. The likely interpretation for this is that self-disclosure was much more acutely stressful for cynically hostile people than for others, resulting in large catecholamine-induced increases in NK cytotoxicity. The long term therapeutic implications of this moderating effect are uncertain, because of the major discontinuities between short-term and long-term psychoneuroimmunological effects (Christensen et al., 1996; Delahunty, Dougall, Craig, Jenkins, & Baum, 1997; Solomon, Segerstrom, Grohr, Kemeny, & Fahey, 1997).

Finally, great caution is needed when making assertions about the direction of causation. Much popular writing about psychoneuroimmunology gives the impression that the only direction of causation worthy of notice is from psychological states to immune function. Nevertheless, there are writers who point out that the converse may also happen: changes in immune functioning may have psychological consequences. In fact, some writers go so far as to describe the immune system as a "diffuse sense organ," one of whose principal roles is to provide information about threats to health from the brain (Maier & Watkins, 1998). This information is valuable, because a group of behaviors, sometimes called the "sick response," plays an important role in combating disease (Hart,

1988; Kent, Bluthe, Kelley, & Dantzer, 1992; Maier & Watkins, 1998). Much of this response is probably a behavioral support for fever, which inhibits reproduction of many pathogens (Hart, 1988). Nevertheless, some of these aspects of the sick response, such as reductions in motivation, activity, and appetite, mimic the symptoms of depression quite closely (Hart 1988; Maier & Watkins, 1998; Yirmiya, 1996). Such behavioral responses appear to be induced by cytokines, which are chemicals produced by various immune cells when they are busy fighting infection (Kent, Bluthe, Kelley, & Dantzer, 1992; Maier & Watkins, 1998). Thus, the widely cited findings of a link between depression and changes in the immune system (Herbert & Cohen, 1994) should not be cited as conclusive evidence that depression causes immune changes; the converse may be at least as true.

Stress and Depression

Until recently, it was widely held that inescapable stress could lead to depletion of certain neurotransmitters, and that this neurotransmitter depletion in turn leads to depression. Norepinephrine and dopamine played an important part in our 1983 model. Since that time serotonin has emerged as a neurotransmitter whose scarcity is frequently invoked to explain depression, thanks to the recent successes of the selective serotonin reuptake inhibitors in treating depression. Nevertheless, some recent researchers have expressed skepticism over the importance of neurotransmitter depletion in explaining depression (Delgado, Moreno, Potter, & Gelenberg, 1998; Holsboer, 2000). They argue that the much touted efficacy of antidepressants that increase the quantities of these neurotransmitters in the brain actually works against the idea of neurotransmitter depletion as a cause for depression. This is because these drugs increase neuro-transmitter levels immediately, but have an effect on depression only after a number of weeks. Thus, antidepressants work not because they restore depleted neurotransmitter levels, but rather because of some indirect change induced by these changed neurotransmitter levels. A further problem with neurotransmitter depletion is that it has been notoriously difficult to consistently demonstrate that depressed people do in fact have depressed levels of norepinephrine or serotonin (Holsboer, 2000).

A very different idea that we also invoked in 1983 is the learned helplessness theory of depression, which still constitutes an active research program. This theory states that depression is the result of a (perceived) inability to control important environmental factors (Overmier & LoLordo, 1998). The effects of uncontrollable stress on depression-like symptoms is well documented in both rodents and humans, as is the effect of human attributions of helplessness on depression. If we no longer believe that neurotransmitter depletion mediates this effect, do we have to give up the possibility of a physiological mechanism altogether?

The idea of a link between helplessness and physiology can be rescued if we look at cross-sensitization between immune and non-immune stressors (Tilders & Schmidt, 1999). The basic idea is that both immune stressors (e.g., invading microorganisms, injection with cytokines) and non-immune stressors (e.g., being attacked by a predator or a boss) lead to a general stress response that includes activation of the hypothalamus-pituitary-adrenal (HPA) axis and release of corticosteroids. The activation of the HPA axis leads to sensitization to further stressors that lasts on the order of 1-2 weeks, leading to even greater activation of the HPA axis if another stressor is encountered. Thus, if an infection is followed by one or more ill-timed major stressors, this can lead to dysregulation of the HPA axis, such as is seen in depression. Furthermore, such dysregulation may be accompanied by the release of cytokines and consequent activation of the sick response, which, as has already been discussed, corresponds closely to the symptoms of depression (Tilders & Schmidt, 1999).

Given this causal pathway, the use of imagery and other coping mechanisms can still be valuable in preventing depression, inasmuch as such coping techniques decrease the perceived stressfulness of events. Such a reduction in perceived stressfulness would also reduce HPA activation and sensitization to stressors, such that the cascade of events that may lead to depression is less likely to be set into motion.

Laterality and Immunity

In 1983, we speculated that activation of the right hemisphere might improve immune function by preventing catecholamine depletion in the left hemisphere. Since that time, one article has appeared in the literature that has a bearing on the issue of lateral activation and immune function (Kang, Davidson, Coe, Wheeler, Tomarken, & Ershler, 1991). Kang and colleagues examined immune parameters of two small groups of subjects, which had been selected for their extreme, stable pattern of either right or left frontal EEG activity. There were no significant group differences on measures of recent history of infectious illness or measures of current anxiety, depression, or stress. Nevertheless, the group with high right frontal activation did show lower NK cytotoxicity than members of the left frontal activation group, though the groups did not differ on other immune measures such as lymphocyte proliferation responses or ratios of T-cell subsets. Kang et al. (1991) are hesitant in the interpretation of their findings, but suggest that stable high levels of activation of the right frontal cortex are instrumental in predisposing individuals to depression, even in cases such as the present one, where little current depression was observed. This right frontal activation is also directly responsible for lowering NK cytotoxicity rather than being mediated by overt depression.

This finding and its interpretation would appear to contradict our 1983 model. If stable patterns of right frontal activation lead to a suppression of immune functioning, then presumably interventions intended to increase right frontal activation should not be expected to improve immune function. Nevertheless, we must inject a note of caution here. As has been discussed above, there is good evidence that interactions between brain and immune system are reciprocal (Maier & Watkins, 1998); in fact, certain forms of immune challenge may lead to depression, rather than be a result of it. There is no pressing reason to think that intense right frontal activation causes reduction in NK cytotoxicity rather than the reverse direction of causality; nor is there any reason to rule out some as yet unidentified third factor.

CONCLUSIONS

The evidence for links among laterality, emotional well-being, and immune function has accumulated over the past 19 years, but with this accumulation of evidence has come an emerging realization that these links constitute a tremendously complex web, rather than a few straightforward, unidirectional causal chains. Awareness of this complexity is intellectually invigorating, but also inclines us to be increasingly reluctant to endorse any simple models of the interaction among these components of the human organism.

At present, it appears that only one of the two pathways that we postulated to explain the positive role of imagery in healing can still be sustained. To the extent that imagery-based techniques can be used to increase relaxation, induce a sense of control, or reduce anxiety, they are valuable in reducing the stressfulness of life events. Given the amply documented role of stress in precipitating depression, reducing immune function, and inhibiting healing, this is no small service to the cause of promoting physical and psychological health, and the use of imagery in healing settings can be endorsed for that reason. On the other hand, there is relatively little reason to believe that the use of imagery results in a global stimulation of the right cerebral hemisphere compared to the left, and even if such stimulation were to occur, it is not certain that it would have a beneficial effect. Therefore, attempts to link imagery to healing via cerebral laterality are premature, if not simply ill-advised.

REFERENCES

Antoni, M. H., Baggett, L., Ironson, G., LaPerriere, A., August, S., Klimas, N., Schneiderman, N., & Fletcher, M. A. (1991). Cognitive-behavioral stress management intervention buffers distress responses and immunologic changes following notification of HIV-1 seropositivity. *Journal of Consulting and Clinical Psychology, 59,* 906-915.

Borod, J. C. (1993). Emotion and the brain—Anatomy and theory: An introduction to the special section. *Neuropsychology, 7,* 427-432.

Brown, H. D., & Kosslyn, S. M. (1993). Cerebral lateralization. *Current Opinion in Neurobiology, 3,* 183-186.

Bruder, G. E. (1995). Cerebral laterality and psychopathology: Perceptual and event-related potential asymmetries in affective and schizophrenic disorders. In R. J. Davidson & K. Hugdahl (Eds.), *Brain asymmetry* (pp. 661-691). Cambridge, MA: MIT Press.

Bryden, M. P., & Allard, F. (1976). Visual hemifield differences depend upon typeface. *Brain and Language, 3,* 191-200.

Bulman-Fleming, M. B., & Bryden, M. P. (1994). Simultaneous verbal and affective laterality effects. *Neuropschologia, 32,* 787-797.

Cherry, B. J., & Hellige, J. B. (1999). Hemispheric asymmetries in vigilance and cerebral arousal mechanisms in younger and older adults. *Neuropsychology, 13,* 111-120.

Christensen, A. J., Edwards, D. L., Wiebe, J. S., Benotsch, E. G., McKelvey, L., Andrews, M., & Lubaroff, D. M. (1996). Effect of verbal self-disclosure on natural killer cell activity: Moderating influence of cynical hostility. *Psychosomatic Medicine, 58,* 150-155.

Coffey, C. E. (1987). Cerebral laterality and emotion: The neurology of depression. *Comprehensive Psychiatry, 28,* 197-219.

Cohen, S., Doyle, W. J., Skoner, D. P., Fireman, P., Gwaltney, J. M., & Newsom, J. T. (1995). State and trait negative affect as predictors of objective and subjective symptoms of respiratory viral infections. *Journal of Personality and Social Psychology, 68,* 159-169.

Cohen, S., Tyrrell, D. A. J., & Smith, A. P. (1991). Psychological stress and susceptibility to the common cold. *New England Journal of Medicine, 325,* 606-612.

Cohen, S., & Williamson, G. M. (1991). Stress and infectious disease in humans. *Psychological Bulletin, 109,* 5-24.

Davidson, R. J. (1995). Cerebral asymmetry, emotion and affective style. In R. J. Davidson & K. Hugdahl (Eds.), *Brain asymmetry* (pp. 362-387). Cambridge, MA: MIT Press.

Delahunty, D. L., Dougall, A. L., Craig, K. J., Jenkins, F. J., & Baum, A. (1997). Chronic stress and natural killer cell activity after exposure to traumatic death. *Psychosomatic Medicine, 59,* 467-476.

Delgado, P. D., Moreno, F. A., Potter, R., & Gelenberg, A. J. (1998). Norepinephrine and serotonin in antidepressant action: Evidence from neurotransmitter depletion studies. In M. Briley & S. Montgomery (Eds.), *Antidepressant therapy at the dawn of the third millennium* (pp. 141-161). London: Martin Dunitz.

D'Espositio, M., Detre, J. A., Aguirre, G. K., et al. (1997). A functional MRI study of mental image generation. *Neuropsychologia, 35,* 725-730.

Effron, R. (1990). *The decline and fall of hemispheric specialization.* Hillsdale, NJ: Lawrence Erlbaum.

Evans, P. D., & Edgerton, N. (1991). Life events and mood as predictors of the common cold. *British Journal of Medical Psychology, 64,* 35-44.

Evans, P. D., & Edgerton, N. (1992). Mood states and minor illness. *British Journal of Medical Psychology, 65,* 177-186.

Farah, M. J. (1984). The neurological basis of mental imagery: A componential analysis. *Cognition, 18,* 245-271.

Fawzy, F. I., Fawzy, N. W., Hyun, C. S., Elashoff, R., Guthrie, D., Fahey, J. L., & Morton, D. L. (1993). Malignant melanoma. Effects of an early structured psychiatric intervention, coping, and affective state on recurrence and survival 6 years later. *Archives of General Psychiatry, 50,* 681-689.

Fawzy, F. I., Kemeny, M. E., Fawzy, N. W., Elashoff, R., Morton, D. L., Cousins, M., & Fahey, J. L. (1990). A structured psychiatric intervention for cancer patients: II. Changes over time in immunological measures. *Archives of General Psychiatry, 47,* 729-735.

Fiore, N. A. (1988). The inner healer: Imagery for coping with cancer and its therapy. *Journal of Mental Imagery, 12,* 79-82.

Gallwey, W. T. (1974). *The inner game.* New York: Random House.

Gates, A., & Bradshaw, J. L. (1977). The role of the cerebral hemispheres in music. *Brain and Language, 4,* 403-431.

Gazzaniga, M. S. (1998). The split brain revisited. *Scientific American* (Special Report).

Geffen, G., Bradshaw, J., & Wallace, G. (1971). Interhemispheric effects on reaction time to verbal and nonverbal stimuli. *Journal of Experimental Psychology, 87,* 415-422.

Gur, R. C., Sackheim, H. S., & Gur, H. E. (1976). Classroom seating and psychopathology: Some initial data. *Journal of Abnormal Psychology, 85,* 122-124.

Hall, N. R. S., Anderson, J. A., & O'Grady, M. P. (1994). Stress and immunity in humans: Modifying variables. In R. Glaser & J. K. Kiecolt-Glaser (Eds.), *Handbook of human stress and immunity* (pp. 183-215). San Diego: Academic Press.

Hammer, S. E. (1996). The effects of guided imagery through music on state and trait anxiety. *Journal of Music Therapy, 33,* 47-70.

Hart, B. L. (1988). Biological basis of sick behavior in animals. *Neuroscience and Biobehavioral Reviews, 12,* 123-137.

Heath, R. (1999). "Just popping down to the shops for a packet of image statements": A new theory of how consumers perceive brands. *Journal of the Market Research Society, 41,* 153-169.

Heller, W. (1993). Neuropsychological mechanisms of individual differences in emotion, personality, and arousal. *Neuropsychology, 7,* 476-489.

Heller, W., Nitschke, J. B., & Miller, G. A. (1998). Lateralization in emotion and emotional disorders. *Current Directions in Psychological Science, 7,* 26-32.

Hellige, J. B. (1993). *Hemispheric asymmetry: What's right and what's left.* Cambridge, MA: Harvard University Press.

Herbert, T. B., & Cohen, S. (1994). Depression and Immunity: A meta-analytic review. *Psychological Bulletin, 113,* 472-486.

Holsboer, F. (2000). Current theories of the pathophysiology of mood disorders. In U. Halbreich & S. A. Montgomery (Eds.), *Pharmacotherapy for mood, anxiety, and cognitive disorders* (pp. 13-35). Washington: American Psychiatric Press.

Jansari, A., Tranel, D., & Adolphs, R. (2000). A valence-specific lateral bias for discriminating emotional facial expressions in free field. *Cognition and Emotion, 14,* 341-353.

Jordan, C. S., & Lenington, K. T. (1979). Physiological correlates of eidetic imagery and induced anxiety. *Journal of Mental Imagery, 3,* 31-42.

Kakolewski, K. E., Crowsen, J. J., Sewell, K. W., & Cromwell, R. L. (1999). Laterality, word valence, and visual attention: A comparison of depressed and non-depressed individuals. *International Journal of Psychophysiology, 34,* 283-292.

Kang, D.-H., Davidson, R. J., Coe, C. L., Wheeler, R. E., Tomarken, A. J., & Ershler, W. B. (1991). Frontal brain assymetry and immune function. *Behavioral Neuroscience, 105,* 860-869.

Kennedy, S., Kiecolt-Glaser, J. K., & Glaser, R. (1988). Immunological consequences of acute chronic stressors: Mediating role of interpersonal relationships. *British Journal of Medical Psychology, 61,* 77-85.

Kent, S., Bluthe, R. M., Kelley, K. W., & Dantzer, R. (1992). Sickness behavior as a new target for drug development. *Trends in Pharmacological Sciences, 13,* 24-28.

Kiecolt-Glaser, J. K., & Glaser, R. (1995). Psychoneuroimmunology and health consequences: Data and shared mechanisms. *Psychosomatic Medicine, 57,* 269-274.

Kiecolt-Glaser, J. K., Marucha, P. T., Malarkey, W. B. Mercado, A. M., & Glaser, R. (1995). Slowing of wound healing by psychological stress. *The Lancet, 346,* 1194-1196.

Kinsbourne, M. (1978). The biological determinants of functional bisymmetry and asymmetry. In M. Kinsbourne (Ed.), *Asymmetrical functions of the brain.* New York: Cambridge University Press.

Kipling, R. (1928). *Kim.* New York: Modern Library.

Kosslyn, S. (1980). *Image and mind.* Cambridge, MA: Harvard University Press.

LaPerriere, A., Fletcher, M. A., Antoni, M. H., Klimas, N. G., Ironson, G., & Schneiderman, N. (1991). Aerobic exercise training in an AIDS risk group. *International Journal of Sports Medicine, 12,* S53-S57.

Lenhart, R. E., & Katkin, E. S. (1986). Psychophysiological evidence for cerebral laterality effects in a high-risk sample of students with subsyndromal bipolar depressive disorder. *American Journal of Psychiatry, 143,* 602-607.

Ley, R. G., & Bryden, M. P. (1979). Hemispheric differences in processing emotion and faces. *Brain and Language, 7,* 127-138.

Ley, R. G., & Freeman, R. J. (1983). Imagery, cerebral laterality and the healing process. In A. A. Sheikh (Ed.), *Healing images: The role of imagination in the healing process* (pp. 51-68). New York: Baywood.

Loverock, D. S., & Modigliani, V. (1995). Visual imagery and the brain: A review. *Journal of Mental Imagery, 19,* 91-132.

Maier, S. F., & Watkins, L. R. (1998). Cytokines for psychologists: Implications of bidirectional immune to brain communication for understanding behavior, mood, and cognition. *Psychological Review, 105,* 83-107.

Marucha, P. T., Kiecolt-Glaser, J. K., & Favagehi, M. (1998). Mucosal wound healing is impaired by examination stress. *Psychosomatic Medicine, 60,* 362-365.

Mellet, E., Tzourio, N., Denis, M., & Mazoyer, B. (1998). Cortical anatomy of mental imagery of concrete nouns based on their dictionary definition. *Neuroreport, 9,* 803-808.

Michimata, C. (1997). Hemishperic processing of categorical and coordinate spatial relations in vision and visual imagery. *Brain and Cognition, 33,* 370-387.

Min, S., & Lee, B. O. (1997). Laterality and somatization. *Psychosomatic Medicine, 59,* 236-240.

Oatley, K., & Jenkins, J. M. (1992). Human emotions: Function and dysfunction. *Annual Review of Psychology, 43,* 55-85.

O'Leary, A. (1990). Stress, emotion, and human immune function. *Psychological Bulletin, 108,* 363-382.

Overmier, J. B., & LoLordo, V. M. (1998). Learned helplessness. In W. O'Donohue (Ed.), *Learning and behavior therapy* (pp. 352-373). Boston: Allyn and Bacon.

Pauli, P., Wiedermann, G., & Nickola, M. (1999). Pain sensitivity, cerebral laterality, and negative affect. *Pain, 80,* 359-364.

Pine, D. S., Kentgen, L. M., Bruder, G. E., Leite, P., Bearman, K., Ma, Y., & Klein, R. G. (2000). Cerebral laterality in adolescent major depression. *Psychiatry Research, 93,* 135-144.

Pylyshyn, Z.W. (1978). What the mind's eye tells the mind's brain: A critique of mental imagery. *Psychological Bulletin, 80,* 1-24.

Robertson, L., & Lamb, M. (1991). Neuropsychological contributions to part/whole organization. *Cognitive Psychology, 23,* 299-330.

Romano, J. M., & Turner, J. A. (1985). Chronic pain and depression: Does the evidence support a relationship? *Psychological Bulletin, 97,* 18-34.

Russel, J. A. (1980). A circumplex model of affect. *Journal of Personality and Social Psychology, 39,* 1161-1178.

Sapp, M. (1994). The effects of guided imagery on reducing worry and emotionality components of test anxiety. *Journal of Mental Imagery, 18,* 165-180.

Schiff, B. B., & Bassel, C. (1996). Effects of asymmetrical hemispheric activation on approach and withdrawal responses. *Neuropsychology, 10,* 557-564.

Schiff, B. B., & Lamon, M. (1989). Inducing emotion by unilateral contraction of vacial muscles: A new look at hemispheric specialization and the experience of emotion. *Neuropsychologia, 27,* 923-935.

Segerstrom, S. C., Taylor, S. E., Kemeny, M. E., & Fahey, J. L. (1998). Optimism is associated with mood, coping, and immune change in response to stress. *Journal of Personality and Social Psychology, 74,* 1646-1655.

Sergent, J. (1990). The neuropsychology of visual image generation: data, method, and theory. *Brain and Cognition, 13,* 98-129.

Shuren, J. E., Greer, D., & Heilman, K. M. (1996). The use of hemi-imagery for studying brain asymmetries in image generation. *Neuropsychologia, 34,* 491-492.

Solomon, G. F., Segerstrom, S. G., Grohr, P., Kemeny, M., & Fahey, J. (1997). Shaking up immunity: Psychological and immunological changes after a natural disaster. *Psychosomatic Medicine, 59,* 114-127.

Spiegel, D., Bloom, J. R., Kraemer, H. C., & Gottheil, E. (1989). Effect of psychosocial treatment on survival of patients with metastatic breast cancer. *Lancet, II,* 888-891.

Springer, S., & Deutsch, G. (1981). *Left brain, right brain.* San Francisco, CA: Freeman.

Stone, A. A., Porter, L. S., & Neale, J. M. (1993). Daily events and mood prior to the onset of respiratory illness episodes: A non-replication of the 3-5 day 'desirability dip.' *British Journal of Medical Psychology, 66,* 383-393.

Tilders, F. J. H., & Schmidt, E. D. (1999). Cross-sensitization between immune and non-immune stressors. In R. Dantzer, E. E. Wollmann, & R. Yirmiya (Eds.), *Cytokines, stress, and depression* (pp. 179-192). New York: Kluwer Academic/ Plenum.

Tippet, L. J. (1992). The generation of mental images: A review of neuropsychological research and theory. *Psychological Bulletin, 112,* 415-432.

Trojano, L., & Grossi, D. (1994). A critical review of mental imagery defects. *Brain and Cognition, 24,* 213-243.

Turner Cobb, J. M., & Steptoe, A. (1996). Psychosocial stress and susceptibility to upper respiratory tract illness in an adult population sample. *Psychosomatic Medicine, 58,* 404-412.

van Gelder, T. (1998). The dynamical hypothesis in cognitive science. *Behavioral and Brain Sciences, 21,* 615-665.

Wittling, W. (1995). Brain asymmetry in the control of autonomic-physiologic activity. In R. J. Davidson & K. Hugdahl (Eds.), *Brain asymmetry* (pp. 304-357). Cambridge, MA: MIT Press.

Wood, F. B., Flowers, D. L., & Naylor, C. E. (1991). Cerebral laterality in functional neuroimaging. In F. L. Kitterle (Ed.), *Cerebral laterality: Theory and research* (pp. 103-116). Hillsdale, NJ: Lawrence Erlbaum.

Yecker, S., Borod, J. C., Brozgold, A., Martin, C., Alpert, M., & Welkowitz, J. (1999). Lateralization of facial emotional expression in schizophrenic and depressed patients. *Journal of Neuropsychiatry and Clinical Neuroscience, 11,* 370-379.

Yirmiya, R. (1996). Endotoxin produces a depressive-like episode in rats. *Brain Research, 711,* 163-174.

CHAPTER 5

Imagery, Love, and Health: How Dynamical Energy Systems Theory Can Integrate Conventional and Complementary Medicine

GARY E. SCHWARTZ AND LINDA G. RUSSEK

> He knew how to listen so others could talk,
> he knew how to talk so others could listen,
> so love and the best medicine could win the battle.
>> Henry I. Russek, M.D., 1921-1990[1]

INTRODUCTION AND OVERVIEW—FROM BIOFEEDBACK AND EMOTION TO ENERGY MEDICINE AND LOVE

Can an expanded vision of love and caring, viewed from the perspective of a synthesis of modern systems theory with the physics of energy and information, provide a common thread that 1) fosters the integration of conventional and complementary medicine, and 2) stimulates an "info-energy" vision for understanding the role imagery in the healing process?

The history of our current research in complementary and alternative medicine (e.g., Schwartz & Russek, 1999) was inspired by principles derived from general and living systems theory (Miller, 1978; Von Bertallanfy, 1968). The early work began with biofeedback and health (reviewed in Schwartz, 1977), and was expanded to include emotion and health (reviewed in Schwartz, 1986) and repression and health (reviewed in Schwartz, 1990). A recent addition has

---

[1]Credo of Dr. Henry I. Russek, Director of the New York Meetings of the American College of Cardiology for 25 years. This chapter is dedicated to his memory and to his values as a clinician, scientist, and humanitarian.

been love and health (e.g., Russek & Schwartz, 1996a) and energy and health (reviewed in Russek & Schwartz, 1996b; Schwartz & Russek, 1997a; Schwartz & Russek, 1999).

As will become clear, focusing on love and energy, using a dynamical energy systems perspective, is paradigm expanding for both conventional and complementary medicine. The purpose of this chapter is to summarize some of the implications of a dynamical energy systems approach (Russek & Schwartz, 1996b; Schwartz & Russek, 1997a) for conventional and complementary medicine. As will become clear, when systems theory is joined with the concepts of energy and information, our vision of imagery, health, and healing expands dramatically.

This chapter begins with a review of the fundamentals of systems theory and the concepts of information and energy. Five hypotheses derived from dynamical energy systems theory (Russek & Schwartz, 1996b) are illustrated, using the heart, the largest generator of electromagnetic energy in the body, as a model system. Procedures for measuring cardiac synchronized energy patterns are explained, and novel experimental predictions are illustrated (for example, that cardiac synchronized energy patterns may interact between people and play an important role in certain therapies). Therapeutic touch is briefly described from the perspective of dynamical energy systems theory. Some challenging implications for potential new fields, such as energy clinical psychology and energy psychotherapy, are outlined.

Implications of a dynamical energy systems approach for memory are then described. The logic of how all dynamical systems inherently store information and energy (termed the systemic memory hypothesis—Schwartz & Russek, 1997a,b) is explained, and implications for therapy involving other organs besides the brain are considered. Finally, new research and theory on love and health (Russek & Schwartz, 1996a; 1997a,b) are reviewed and interpreted from a dynamical energy systems perspective.

As the chapter unfolds, the implications for imagery and healing become increasingly novel and controversial. This is unavoidable. Puthoff, a physicist, described the logic of dynamical energy systems theory and energy cardiology as "inexorably" leading to certain conclusions (see Russek & Schwartz, 1996b). Though some of the hypotheses developed in this chapter challenge our classical theories about human interaction and health, they do inexorably follow from established principles in systems theory and modern physics. A challenge for the emerging integrative medicine is to consider dynamical energy systems theory and to evaluate how it expands our vision of mind, spirit, and health (Schwartz & Russek, 1997c; Schwartz & Russek, 1999).

Systems Theory, Information, and Energy

The root meaning of the word "system," which derives from the Greek *synhisanai* ("to place together"), is the concept of an *integrated whole whose essential properties arise from the relationships between its parts.*

Systems theory, including general systems theory (von Bertalanffy, 1968) and general living systems theory (Miller, 1978), was developed as a conceptual tool to organize and integrate knowledge within and across disciplines, from the physical and biological sciences to the behavioral and social sciences (Schwartz, 1982, 1984, 1987, 1989).

According to Miller (1978):

> A system is a *set* of *interacting units* with *relationships* among them. The word "set" implies that the units have some *common* properties. These common properties are essential if the units are to interact or have relationships. *The state of each unit is constrained by, conditioned by, or dependent on the state of the other units.* The units are *coupled.* Moreover, there is at least one measure of the sum of its units which is *larger than the sum* of that measure of its units. [italics added].

It can be said that the "heart" of systems theory is the notion of dynamic interaction. When two or more components are connected in a system, the components do not simply "act" upon each other, they "interact" with each other. Feedback loops therefore have complex, often non-linear, emergent effects. Complexity theory, chaos theory, and self-organization theory (reviewed in Capra, 1996; Kauffman, 1993) are current examples reflecting the evolution of our understanding of this fundamental principle.

According to Miller (1978), information in systems refers to the abstract concept of patterns (literally, to give form). Information may be simply descriptive (physical structure and mathematical order), it may reflect complex meanings and knowledge, or it may convey deep wisdom (Rubik, 1995). Paraphrasing Miller, living systems can be defined as *dynamic organizations of intelligent information expressed in energy and matter* (Russek & Schwartz, 1996b). Energy is defined as the capacity to do work. Organized energy is informational energy. Hence, when we speak, for example, of the heart generating electromagnetic energy, we are also speaking of information (generated by the heart and the brain) that is carried by the energy that affects matter.

Energy is one of the most mundane yet mysterious concepts in modern physics. Though the measurement of energy may be defined precisely, its interpretation is abstract and is difficult to comprehend (even by seasoned physicists).

Becker and Selden (1988) illustrate this point beautifully:

> Electromagnetism can be discussed in two ways—in terms of fields and in terms of radiation. A field is "something" that exists in space around an object that produces it. We know there's a field around a permanent magnet because it can make an iron particle jump through space to the magnet. Obviously there's an invisible entity that exerts a force on the iron, but as to just what it consists of—don't ask! No one knows. A different but analogous something—an electric field—extends outward from electrically charged objects.

We believe that this difficulty of interpretation may be one reason why the concept of energy has yet to make its way into the mainstream of modern psychology and medicine. Systems theory reminds us that what we measure is the *functioning of systems*. Energy and force are *concepts* we invent to make sense of the *observation* that iron particles do, in fact, jump through space to a permanent magnet, and we use this observation to explain how, for example, the heart can be observed to contract when an electromagnet is placed near the chest (Ragan, Wang, & Eisenberg, 1995).

The Dynamical Energy Systems Approach and Energy Cardiology

We have recently derived five general hypotheses from systems theory, applied them to the concept of energy (termed the dynamical energy systems approach), and then specifically applied them to the heart as a prototypic energy generating system (termed energy cardiology) (Russek & Schwartz, 1996b). Table 1 illustrates five dynamical energy systems hypotheses and their application to energy cardiology.

Table 1 lists two parallel sets of hypotheses. The first set—the dynamical energy systems hypotheses—is drawn from general systems theory, and conceived in terms of energy. The second set—the energy cardiology hypotheses—applies the first set to biological systems, as illustrated by the heart and cardiovascular system.

The hypotheses, necessarily abbreviated here for the sake of space, are organized from the least to the most controversial.

Hypothesis 1. The body is a dynamic organization of intelligent information expressed in energy as well as matter.

Hypothesis 2. Energy helps regulate and coordinate the body interactively.

Hypothesis 3. Energy is generated in parallel (organized energy patterns).

Hypothesis 4. Energy operates dynamically between people, as well as within people.

Hypothesis 5. Consciousness modulates energy—and so the body— and is modulated by energy. Hence, imagery modulates energy, and vice versa.

These five dynamical energy systems hypotheses can be applied to any organ system or combination of organ systems. In Russek and Schwartz (1996b), our focus was on the heart, which can be viewed as a generator of a broad spectra of types and frequencies of energies occurring over time. We could as well have focused on the brain, typically taken to be the prime generator of bodily processes.

Table 1. Five Dynamical Energy Systems Hypotheses and Their Expression in Energy Cardiology (from Russek & Schwartz, 1996b)

Dynamical energy systems hypotheses	Energy cardiology hypotheses
1. Systems are expressions of organized energy and emit energy.	1. The heart is a dynamical energy generating system.
2. Energy activates and regulates systems interactively.	2. Energy from the heart may regulate organs and cells throughout the body interactively.
3. Different energies (types and frequencies) are emitted simultaneously, including at the quantum level.	3. The heart generates patterns of energy. The cardiac energy pattern includes electrical, magnetic sound, pressure, temperature.
4. Energy is transmitted between systems dynamically and interactively.	4. Cardiac energy patterns may have interaction effects interpersonally and environmentally as well as intrapersonally.
5. Levels of consciousness may modulate patterns of energy in health and illness, and conversely, patterns of energy may modulate levels of consciousness.	5. Levels of consciousness may modulate cardiac energy patterns in health and illness, and conversely, cardiac energy patterns may modulate levels of consciousness.

However, we wanted to show the new insights that can be derived from a dynamical energy systems approach to the body.

When the biophysical consequences of organized energy are considered, far reaching implications for the role of the heart in health and healing emerge. For example, since the electromagnetic energy from the heart literally reaches every cell within the body, the heart (in concert with the brain) may be the major organizer and integrator of coordinated cellular functioning in the body. Moreover, since electromagnetic energy and information from the heart is not contained within the skin (it leaves the body roughly at the speed of light), cardiac energy patterns may interact *between* people (even at a distance). It is possible that cardiac energy patterns communicated between people may be involved in both conventional and alternative therapies.

A central mystery in modern biology is how a system that contains literally trillions of highly specialized cells can ever function as an organized whole. The metaphor of a symphonic orchestra is useful here. If the body was thought to be an orchestra containing trillions of separate instruments, from "piccolos" (generating high frequency patterns) to "tubas" (generating low frequency patterns), how could these individual instruments ever play their unique melodies as a symphonic whole? The need for a "conductor" becomes self-evident. We believe that the heart may serve a fundamental synchronizing function since its energy and information reaches every cell within the body (including the brain). Using this metaphor, the heart becomes the "conductor," and the brain provides the "score."

The Energy to Do This Need Not Be Strong. Consider: very tiny electromagnetic signals have been shown to influence cellular functioning (reviewed in Becker, 1990 and in many articles in the journal *Bioelectro-magnetics)*. Moreover, serious scientists are entertaining the possibility that biological cells can "rectify and signal average" weak electric fields through "stochastic resonance" (see Astumian, Weaver, & Adair, 1995). Though space precludes reviewing this research here, it is important to note that these new findings and models indicate that bioelectromagnetic effects often show an *inverted U shaped function*—weak signals can produce resonance whereas strong signals may not.

Of course, all systems have boundaries that protect them from external matter and energy, and therefore information as well. As Miller (1978) writes, "an important function of boundary processes is fending off matter-energy excess stresses." Since the human body contains trillions of highly specialized cells designed to perform specific tasks, it makes sense that cells should not be excessively regulated by the heart (or any other organ or cell). It is conceivable that cells of the body (including the brain) have mechanisms that prevent them from being over-controlled by the heart (or any other energy generating system).

However, depending upon the state of the cell at a given moment, it may be more or less sensitive to the energy generated by the heart. A dynamical energy systems approach to heart-cell interactions requires that we consider each cell as a semi-independent unit (in effect, a subsystem) that responds dynamically and interactively with other semi-independent units, including the heart and, as we propose in Hypothesis 5, consciousness.

Energy and Heart/Brain Relationships

Of all the organs within the body, the heart is preeminent in terms of the centrality of its location, the richness of its connections to all the cells within the body, and particularly relevant here, the intensity of its energy transmission. This energy aspect of the heart does not receive much attention. But just as the heart not only pumps patterns of biochemical nutrients to every cell within the body through the circulation, it also "pumps" patterns of energy and information to every cell within the body through the circulation as well.

For example, it is well known that the electrical potential generated by the heart, identified by the electrocardiogram, can be recorded from *any site on the body* because of "volume conduction," a mechanism that is well known in physics and biology and is not, in and of itself, controversial (Malmivuo & Plonsey, 1995).

A natural example of volume conduction is the simultaneous recording of fetal and maternal cardiac electrical fields (potentials) *from the same pair of ECG electrodes* placed on the abdomen (Wakai, Wang, & Martin, 1994). For the first nine months of life, the developing fetus is literally "bathed" in cardiac energy generated by the mother, and the mother, in turn, is similarly bathed in the emerging cardiac energy of the developing fetus. Historically, the mother's electrocardiogram has been considered to be an annoying recording "artifact" that seriously confounds the measurement of the fetus's electrocardiogram rather than reflecting the actual "sharing" of cardiac energy and information that may have, heretofore, unrecognized yet important biophysical consequences for the fetus, the mother, and the mother-fetus relationship.

It turns out that of all the internal organs, the heart is by far the largest generator of magnetic energy. Superconducting quantum interference devices that measure magnetic fields outside the body have shown that the heart generates over 50,000 femtoteslas (a measure of intensity of magnetic field), compared to less than 10 femtoteslas recorded from the brain (Clarke, 1994), which makes the heart's magnetic field 5,000 times greater than the brain's. For this reason, when researchers try to record the magnetic field of the brain (the magneto-encephalogram) they discover that it is "contaminated" by the magnetic field of the heart (the magnetocardiogram). The magnetic field of the heart travels through the brain and mixes with the brain's magnetic field.

As is well known in radio and television transmission, information can be transmitted on top of waves of energy (i.e., carrier waves) that also have specific timing functions. Further, different radio or television stations—each a different frequency band—carry different kinds of information. It is conceivable that each of the various energies in the pattern of cardiac energy may contain different information.

For example, frequency patterns in addition to the patterns comprising the electromagnetic activity of the heart can be carried and observed in the electro-cardiogram, ranging from very low frequencies (.01 to 30 Hertz) to high frequencies (thousands of Hertz)—"noise" that is "riding" on top of the electro-cardiogram. In traditional cardiologic measurement, however, these additional patterns are deliberately "removed" and disregarded.

Additional energy and information is routinely removed, for example, by careful electrode placement. If electrodes are placed on the chest across the heart (with an appropriate ground), the primary signal *observed* is the electrical activity arising from the heart. With this electrocardiogram electrode placement, the electrical activity of the brain, for example, which is also volume conducted throughout the cardiovascular system, is very small (because much of the EEG is subtracted using ECG leads) and is typically treated as "noise" to be ignored.

Conversely, if electrodes are placed on the scalp across the brain (for example, scalp to linked ears), the primary signal *observed* is the electrical activity arising from the brain. With this electroencephalogram electrode placement, the electrical activity of the heart is relatively small (because much of the ECG is subtracted using EEG leads referenced to linked ears) and is typically treated as "noise" to be ignored.

However, if one electrode is placed on the scalp, and the other electrode is placed below the heart on the chest, what will be observed is the *electro-cardiogram combined with the electroencephalogram*—one will literally see brain waves riding, so to speak, on top of cardiac waves. With this scalp-chest (brain/heart) electrode placement, the true mixing of brain and cardiac electrical signals becomes self-evident.

Just as the blood contains a *mixture* of both molecules (for example, hormones) and cells (for example, red and white blood cells), it also contains a *mixture* of types (for example, electrical and thermal) and frequencies of energies. The dynamical energy systems approach encourages us to attempt to measure the wholistic (mixed) nature of multiple types and frequencies of energies within and between organs such as the heart and the brain.

Why is this worth doing? To discover what the "noise" is conveying. For example, the electromagnetic signal coming from the heart may be a carrier wave for additional information that is not only diagnostic of cardiac function and disease but also indicative of the functioning of other biological systems.

Simply stated, the ECG and the EEG mix with each other and travel to every organ and cell within the body (and by extension, beyond the body). When the heart is used as a "trigger," and the EEG is averaged using event related potential procedures, the R spike of the ECG can be clearly observed in the EEG. Moreover, there is a clear topographic pattern of the ECG observed in the EEG.

In Russek and Schwartz (1994), we recorded averaged cardiac synchronized energy patterns from 20 male subjects during a 2 minute eyes closed resting baseline. The data were collected as part of a 42-year follow-up to the Harvard Mastery of Stress study (Funkenstein, King, & Drolette, 1957; Russek, King, Russek, & Russek, 1990). Nineteen channels of EEG (referenced to linked ears) and the ECG (arm to arm placement) were recorded at 128 Hz using a Lexicor Neurosearch 24 System.

Cardiac synchronized energy patterns were obtained using special purpose software written to calculate averaged waveforms per trial per subject per site. Using the raw EEG and ECG data files, the program calculated averaged ECG and EEG waveforms synchronized either with the subject's own ECG (*intra*personal cardiac synchronized energy patterns) or another person's ECG (*inter*personal cardiac synchronized energy patterns).

When the subject's own ECG was used as the trigger, significant evidence of the subject's ECG in the subject's EEG was found, primarily in the posterior regions. When the experimenter's ECG was used as the trigger, significant evidence of the experimenter's ECG in the subject's EEG was found, primarily in anterior regions, in subjects who rated themselves in college as having been raised by loving parents. These subjects were also significantly healthier in late adulthood than subjects who rated their parents low in loving.

We will return to the question of the relationship of perceptions and images of love and caring to health later in the chapter. The important point to appreciate here is that energy from the heart (the ECG) can be recorded from the brain (the EEG) not only within an individual, but between individuals as well. It follows that interpersonal interaction, therefore, involves energetic interaction. Even behavior per se (the movement of muscles and fluids) creates electrostatic energy effects that can be registered from a distance (for example, on a copper wall at a distance from the subject—Green, Parks, Guyer, Fahrion, & Coyne, 1991).

Physiology and behavior, then, can generate electromagnetic fields that can be transmitted between individuals.

Is it possible that electromagnetic resonance between individuals may play a role in interpersonal interactions, and therefore may play a role in psychotherapy, body therapies, and therapies that explicitly are derived from dynamical energy systems concepts as explicated in Hypotheses 1-5 (Table 1). Some examples using the heart as a model dynamical energy system are described below.

It is possible that biobehavioral factors that are well known to contribute to health, including exercise, relaxation, and social support (Russek & Russek, 1980), work in part because of heretofore unrecognized energetic consequences of the phenomena. Exercise, relaxation, and social support may all function to improve patterned energy flow within the body, thereby improving the cardiac energy patterns and hence the functioning of the heart, the cardiovascular system, and the body as a whole. Concerning social support, it is possible that good therapist-patient relationships improve cardiac energy flow within the body and so promote healing through empathy and caring (part of the so-called placebo effect) as much as by treatment. Also, many alternative medicine techniques, including acupuncture, meditation, massage, Tai Chi, homeopathy, and therapeutic touch, typically provide a strong caring relationship between therapists and patients, which in turn may make an important contribution in restoring energetic equilibrium to the body by enhancing the generation, transmission, and/or registration of cardiac energy patterns.

Therapeutic touch, a set of procedures involving both contact (physical touch) and "non-contact" touch (that is, placing the hands a few inches above the body), has been reported to reduce stress, improve cardiovascular and immune function, and foster healing (Krieger, 1990). If Hypotheses 1 to 5 in Table 1 are correct, it would be intriguing to consider the possibility (and potential consequences) of cardiac energy patterns emitted from the hands of nurses and other therapists (in terms of synchronized patterns of cardiac electrical potentials, magnetism, sound, pressure, and temperature).

The hands may be a powerful transmitter of cardiac energy patterns. The hands are rich with blood flow, and sweat is a wonderful conductor. By applying the cardiac synchronized energy patterns methodology to both the therapist and patient simultaneously, one could scientifically determine the role, if any, that cardiac energy patterns play in mediating non-contact therapeutic healing effects. If positive results are obtained, it then may become possible to determine methods for optimizing the transmission of this energy from therapist to patient as well as the preferred distance for energy transmission from the therapist's hands to the patient's body.

A related implication concerns assessing the sensitivity of therapists (including psychotherapists) to energy generated by patients and, vice versa, the capacity of therapists to transmit energy to patients. The cardiac synchronized energy patterns paradigm could be applied systematically to assessing 1) how sensitive a given therapist is to the cardiac energy pattern emitted by a given patient, and 2) how effective a given therapist is in transmitting her or his cardiac energy patterns to the patient. In short, the cardiac synchronized energy patterns paradigm provides a new, objective procedure for quantifying the therapist-patient relationship, and the role of imagery in this relationship.

Energy cardiology has implications for understanding the potential power of interpersonal interactions, not only between two individuals such as therapist and patient, but also between groups of individual engaged in meditation, chanting, singing, and dancing. When two or more people move and breathe in synchrony, it is possible that increases in cardiac synchrony may also occur. Summation if not synergy of cardiac energy (and related energy due to synchronized electrostatic effects of movement) may affect the health and functioning of individuals within the group as well as the health and functioning of the group as a whole. Respiratory synchronized energy patterns can be computed. Moreover, respiratory synchronized energy patterns can be calculated at various phases in the respiratory cycle (for example, cardiac synchronized energy patterns can be calculated separately during inspiration, the peak inspiration, expiration, and the pause). As will be explained in the last section, from a dynamical energy systems perspective, the capacity for interpersonal synchronization is a hallmark of love and caring, not only between humans, but between all systems as well.

Memory and Holism in Dynamical Systems:
The Systemic Memory Hypothesis

It is typically assumed that memory involves the storage and retrieval of information in the brain, and that neurons are the only cells capable of storing information. However, a profound implication that can be derived from dynamical energy systems theory is that all dynamical systems inherently store information as memory to varying degrees.

When the logic of interaction is carefully analyzed, especially interactions that occur recurrently (i.e., circular feedback), the logic leads to the conclusion that a complex version of the history of the recurrent feedback interactions are stored within the inherent circulation of information and energy in systems. The emergence of a system, therefore, involves the storage of systemic memory, and as will become clear, systemic memory is memory of the whole. Since the logic of recurrent (circular feedback) interaction is systemic and general, it can be applied to any system at any level.

According to Webster (1977), one of the original definitions of circulation was *a series in which the same order is preserved, and things return to the same state.* When the concept of circulation is reinterpreted in terms of dynamically changing, recurrent feedback interactions, things are not predicted to return precisely to the same state. Instead, the order that is predicted to be preserved is the *evolution (accumulation) of the dynamical interactions among the parts.*

The hypothesis of systemic memory was anticipated in 1890 by William James. He proposed that "When two elementary brain-processes have been active together or in immediate succession, one of them, on re-occurring, tends to propagate its excitement into the other" (James, 1890).

When the word "subsystems" is substituted for "brain-processes," the systemic memory hypothesis is anticipated. "When two subsystems have been active together or in immediate succession, one of them, on re-accruing, tends to propagate its excitement into the other."

The hypothesis of systemic memory is implicit in writings of Warren McCulloch. Not only did he propose in 1951 the idea of "reverberatory memory," he pointed out "The reverberating activity patterned after something that happened retains the form of the happening but loses track of when it happened. Thus it shows that there was some time at which such and such occurred. The 'such and such' is the idea wrenched out of time" (McCulloch, 1951). He went on to say, "It is an eternal idea in a transitory memory wherein the form exists only so long as the reverberation endures. When that ceases, the form is no longer anywhere."

McCulloch did not extend his logic to physical and biological systems other than neurons. Had he done so, he would have discovered that "reverberation" (circulating interaction) in systems is the rule, not the exception, and that according to modern quantum dynamics, reverberation persists, even at absolute zero temperature and in a vacuum.

The modern concept of recurrent feedback loops in neural networks (e.g., Lisberger & Sejnowski, 1992) is actually a special case of systemic feedback cycles—circulating recurrent feedback interactions—in all systems at all levels. However, the fact that the logic used to explain recurrent feedback loops in neural networks can be equally applied to recurrent feedback networks in all dynamical systems at all levels is not widely appreciated. Moreover, the insight that circulating recurrent feedback interactions provide an explanation for holism in all dynamical systems has not been previously explicated.

We use the term memory here to refer to the storage of information and energy in systems. In everyday experience, episodic (explicit) memory can be recalled consciously. However, substantial research in psychology documents that the storage of information can occur in the absence of awareness (reviewed in Schacter, 1996). Typically these implicit memories cannot be recalled consciously. The use of the term memory in computer science (e.g., hard disk memory) and electrical engineering (e.g., DC battery memory) refers to the storage of information and energy. From a systems perspective, the phenomenon of explicit memory may be a special case of implicit memory.

We can illustrate the fundamental logic of how recurrent feedback interactions create systemic (holistic) memory using the example from classical physics of two tuning forks that come into resonance. Once the fundamental logic of this simple system is understood, the deep complexity of its application to complex systems will be self-evident (see Schwartz & Russek, 1999).

The interaction between tuning forks A and B (or between any As and Bs—e.g., photons, subatomic particles, atoms, molecules, cells, organs, organisms, groups of organisms, etc.) contains a profound implication. As A and B interact with each other, they literally create a memory of their interaction over time through the circulation of their information and energy. *In fact, this memory is part of the expression of their interactions as a whole, and is a natural requirement for them to interact.* The memory is the relationship. The relationship information is systemic information, and systemic information is an expression of the whole. Moreover, it follows that the information of the whole of a system is stored within each of the parts comprising the system to varying degrees.

We illustrate this conclusion by considering memory from the point of view of tuning fork A. At time 0, before A is struck, A is spontaneously vibrating as predicted by quantum dynamics (e.g., its atoms and subatomic particles are vibrating and moving in complex, interacting, resonating ways). When A is struck at time 1, it vibrates with a frequency "a1." The frequency "a1" moves (at the speed of sound) to tuning fork B at time 2. B begins to vibrate at time 2, which is some complex (linear and non-linear) product of "a1" (we will, for the sake of simplicity, assume for the moment that "a1" has not changed much as it travels to B) and B's state at time 2. We will call this complex interactive product "a1b2."

As B vibrates, the sound now returns to A at time 3. The sound that returns to A at time 3 is a complex interactive product of "a1b2" plus whatever interference occurs with the continued sound coming from A at time 3 (a3). This gives us "a1b2a3" that returns to A at time 3.

Now, let us hypothesize that A is influenced by this return sound at time 3 to some degree, and starts to interact with A's vibration at time 3. Not only will A's vibration have changed spontaneously by time 4 (e.g., it might be decreasing—the simplest case), *but it will have further changed by the "a1b2a3" feedback interaction returning to it.* The resulting sound will be a4 modulated by "a1b2a3," or "a1b2a3a4."

In other words, in one complete "cycle" of A–B interaction, the sound coming from A at time 4 contains the *complex history (both linear and non-linear) of the A–B interaction (their relationship) over the cycle.* We see an "image" of a1, modulated by b2, interacting back with a3, reaching A, so that A at time 4 includes the *complex history of the first A-B interaction in its next interaction.* Meanwhile, from the perspective of B, a somewhat parallel set of interactions is also occurring.

Each cycle includes the previous information, hence the history (memory) continues to grow. *As long as the units are connected (e.g., the two forks are interacting through the air), the memory trace circulating between them will be retained, albeit modified as time goes on.* All things being equal, the memory trace will "grow" with time through the continued circulation of the recurrent feedback interactions (even if the intensity of the recurrent feedback interactions decrease, which is the case for the simple two tuning fork example).

The logic and simple mathematics of the two tuning fork example are obviously grossly oversimplified. We have chosen only four time points, and have described the interaction only from the perspective of tuning fork A. However, the essence of the logic should be self-evident. Any time two (A + B) or more (A + B + n) things interact, information concerning their history accumulates. Recurrent feedback interactions are systemic—theoretically they occur between electrons, protons, and neutrons, between the two strands of DNA, or between the brain and the heart, to name just a few. From a systems perspective, *at whatever levels the systems are interacting, the interactive history of the energy and information should be contained in a complex way.* Hence, this mechanism suggests that memory will occur to varying degrees in all dynamical systems. It is a general model of stored systemic (relationship) information. *It is the inherent capacity of a system to circulate interactive information and energy that enables a system to have a holistic history and therefore be whole.*

It logically follows that the more rapidly recurrent feedback interactions occur in a given system, the more rapidly a stabile holistic history should emerge. For example, atoms vibrate billions of times a second. Therefore, although it would be predicted that it should take a finite amount of time for a molecular holistic history to form when hydrogen and oxygen come together as H_2O, the time it actually takes may be a few nanoseconds.

According to systems theory, systems are always interconnected to various degrees in various ways. Hence, energy (and the information riding with the energy) is continually being exchanged and circulated to various degrees in various ways. As a result, the memories should continue naturally.

When tuning forks A and B resonate, they become a two tuning fork system. Each tuning fork functions as a subsystem in the two tuning fork system (or we can say each tuning fork is a system in the two tuning fork suprasystem—the principle is the same). The two tuning forks become a whole.

Tuning forks A and B each contain molecules. Molecules are subsystems within each tuning fork system (or we can say each molecule is a system within a single tuning fork suprasystem—the principle is the same). Hence, it follows that resonance not only can occur *between* tuning forks A and B, resonance can occur *within* tuning forks A and B. In fact, tuning forks A and B cannot vibrate as individual tuning forks unless their molecules can vibrate (resonate) interactive within each tuning fork as a whole. In other words, the logic of what happens *between* tuning forks A and B applies to what happens *within* tuning forks A and B as well.

Recurrent resonance, therefore, not only occurs *between* physical systems (e.g., between tuning forks A and B), but also occurs *within* physical systems (e.g., within tuning fork A and within tuning fork B) as well. For this reason, the logic that leads to the hypothesis that recurrent interaction creates memory *between* tuning forks A and B, also requires that we entertain the hypothesis that recurrent feedback interaction simultaneously creates memory *within* tuning fork A and within tuning fork B as well, and this intra-tuning fork memory is sustained, even after tuning forks A and B have been separated. The same logic requires that we entertain the hypothesis that once hydrogen and oxygen have interacted recurrently as H_2O, if hydrogen and oxygen are subsequently separated, some version of their history as H_2O will be retained within the hydrogen and oxygen, expressed potentially in terms of their individual, dimensional complexities.

Modern quantum physics indicates that even at the temperature of absolute zero, matter vibrates, and hence, resonates. Quantum mechanical fluctuation energy of the atoms in matter has been measured by measuring the vibrations in a crystal as the temperature of the crystal is lowered. The experimental data agree with the predictions of the equations of quantum mechanics suggesting that quantum mechanical zero-temperature vibrational fluctuations of atoms in matter is a general property of matter. For example, residual quantum mechanical vibrational energy is used to explain why liquid helium does not freeze even when it is cooled to within micro degrees of absolute zero temperature (reviewed in Forward, 1996). For the sake of completeness, it should be noted that modern quantum physics also suggests that a vacuum can sustain an infinity of electromagnetic vibrations (the quantum mechanical electromagnetic fluctuations of the vacuum). Hence, interactive recurrent resonance not only occurs within matter, but it would be predicted to occur within a vacuum as well (Milonni, 1994).

By definition, systems can potentially store only what they are capable of responding to (and hence processing), and they will process this information in their own ways. It follows that the nature of information stored between subatomic particles, for example, will be of a different order than the nature of information stored between neurons. Also, the more reliable and flexible the components of the system (and hence, the more complex the system), the more reliable and flexible should be the storage (and complexity) of the information.

Of course, outlining the logic that memory is intrinsically created and stored in systems does not imply that this information, once stored, can be accessed and retrieved (at least in human consciousness). Everyday experience and substantial empirical research reminds us that our ability to recognize information is typically far greater than our ability to recall information (Schacter, 1996). Clearly, failure to observe recall does not necessarily imply that memory has not occurred. Forgetting, therefore, does not necessarily imply that memory has been erased—the process may involve an alteration in retrieval. The deep question of retrieving memory, once stored in systems, remains a central challenge for future science. The solution may require a deep understanding of recurrent resonance as a systemic recurrent pattern recognition process.

A controversial implication of the hypothesis of systemic memory is the prediction that information, once received, is retained in some form forever, so long as the system remains intact and recurrent feedback interactions (cycling) continue. Not only will the information continue, but it potentially will evolve over time. In fact, in a deep sense, it may be virtually impossible to erase information in an intact system completely. Only in the case of presumed complete entropy would it be predicted that systemic memory should be eliminated completely. Theoretically, if the experiment is sensitive enough, evidence for savings or other subtle measures of change in functioning or behavior of a system should be demonstrable in all systems as a function of the evolution of the hypothesized memory process.

In summary, the wholeness of a system may derive from its capacity not only to interact, but to interact recurrently, and to circulate (and therefore mix and accumulate) this information and energy within the system. Though neurons are especially gifted in storing sensory and psychological information (because neurons are so highly interconnected, creating profoundly complex recurrent feedback interactive networks), it may be time to evolve our intellectual heritage and re-envision the brain as being a marvelous special case of a ubiquitous systemic (holistic) memory process in nature. It is our belief that in the process of researching the phenomenon of recurrent feedback interaction in nature, science will gain a deeper understanding of the essence of holism and evolution, and in the process, will enable us to understand certain heretofore unexplained observations that strain our current models of how memory works.

Imagery, involving memory, may also be a ubiquitous systemic (holistic) process.

Memory and the Heart:
The Challenge of Cardiac Transplants

A common phrase is that we learn things "by heart," and that we know things "by heart." Is this simply a misplaced metaphor, or is there some deep significance to this particular choice of words? If all cells store information, if the heart is especially involved because of the centrality of its location and connections, and if the heart is especially involved in emotion, then memories (in particular, implicit emotional memories) may literally involve the heart in addition to the brain (Russek & Schwartz, 1996b).

If the heart of one person is transplanted into another (something that does not happen naturally in nature), the history of the donor (as witnessed and stored by the heart) will be potentially available to the recipient. Since the recipient's body typically treats the donor's heart as foreign matter to be rejected, drugs are required to suppress this natural reaction. Is it possible that the rejection response is not simply the rejection of the matter comprising the heart, but the rejection of stored energy and information contained in the heart as well?

It would take a special recipient, indeed, to possibly retrieve the hypothesized information stored in the donor's heart. However, sporadic reports have surfaced suggesting that strange changes in recipient's perceptions and preferences sometimes occurs (e.g., Siegel, 1995). The critical question is, do the recipient's new perceptions and preferences correspond to the donor's known preferences?

Consider the challenging experiences of a former dancer, Claire Sylvia, who received a heart/lung transplant in Boston. Hers was the first successful heart/lung transplant in New England. According to Sylvia and Novack (1997), Sylvia remembered that six weeks after her transplant, when she was allowed to drive again she had driven "straight to the nearest Kentucky Fried Chicken, a place she'd never been before, and this former dancer and fit, thin person had ordered chicken nuggets." She later learned that the 18-year-old person whose heart and lungs now lived inside her had a fondness for fried chicken nuggets. Moreover, at the time of the young man's death, uneaten chicken nuggets were found stuffed inside the pocket of his leather jacket.

Claims such as these are typically treated as nonsense—that is, they do not make any sense—from a strictly non-systemic materialistic perspective. They are explained away as coincidences, misperceptions, self-deceptions, or magical thinking. However, when systems are viewed not only as matter systems, but as information and energy systems as well, strange claims such as these from select transplant patients begin to make sense, whether we are comfortable with these claims or not.

As William James put it, "If you wish to upset the law that all crows are black . . . it is enough if you prove one single crow to be white." It is possible that Claire Sylvia may be the "white crow." Claire Sylvia may be a special case because she is artistic, a skilled dancer, in touch with her body and emotions, open minded and spiritual. Maybe her experiences do not simply reflect her creative consciousness, but reflect actual information retrieval from the essential organs she has inherited. Whether this information is truly episodic and cognitive in nature (e.g., explicit cognitive memory), or is more stylistic and emotional/motivational in nature (e.g., implicit emotional memory), is a completely open question that can and should be addressed in future research.

How should modern clinical psychology approach the treatment of such a person? Should we interpret her psychological changes post surgery only as symptoms of the medication, the stress of the surgery, and/or a sign of her preexisting psychopathology? Or, should we also take an energy clinical psychology approach, and entertain the possibility that she is meaningfully interacting with stored information in the donor's heart? A dynamical energy systems approach encourages us to be open to such a possibility (several more cases have been reported by Pearsall, 1998).

Perceptions of Love and Long-Term Health

"That love promotes health surprises few people, yet the scientific study of love and physical health is in its infancy" begins Green and Shellenberger (1996) in their review of research on "the healing energy of love." Green and Shellenberger suggest that because love has "many facets and is manifested in many ways, it was banned from Western science, which insisted on observable and simple independent variables." Because love is complex, and may have effects that operate biophysically, psychosocially, and spiritually (Dossey, 1996; Green & Shellenberger, 1996; Levin, 1996; Russek & Schwartz, 1996b) the study of the relationship of love and health is extraordinarily difficult.

We recently discovered that 1) simple independent variables can be created to measure the perception of love, and 2) these measures can serve as powerful prospective predictors of long-term health and illness (Russek & Schwartz, 1997a).

Justification for measuring the perception of love and caring can be found in the social support literature. The perception of social support has been reported to be a significant predictor of future health (Shumaker & Czajkowski, 1994). Carefully controlled prospective studies document that the extent to which individuals achieve health is directly related to the extent to which they perceive their relationships to be strong and supportive (Welin, Tibblin, Svardsudd, Tibblin, Ander-Perciva, Larsson, & Wilhelmsen, 1985; Ruberman, Weinblatt, Goldberg, & Chaudhary, 1984; Seeman, Berkman, Kohout, LaCroix, Glynn, & Blazer, 1993). In a review of population-based research on mortality risk over the past 20 years, Berkman (1995) found that people who are isolated are at increased risk from a number of causes. More recent studies, furthermore, indicate that social support is significantly related to survival post myocardial infarction (Williams et al., 1992).

Social support reflects loving and caring relationships in people's lives, and this fact may be assessed directly. The results of two major studies suggest that simple ratings of "feeling loved" may be as effective, if not more effective, in assessing social support and predicting future health than more comprehensive instruments that quantify network size, structure, and function. In a five year prospective study of ten thousand Israeli men, Medalie and Golbourt (1976) found that the question, "Does your wife show you her love?" was the best predictor of the outcome measure of angina pectoris. Correspondingly, Seeman and Syme (1987) reported, in a sample of 119 men and 40 women undergoing coronary angiography, that simple ratings of "feeling loved" exerted an independent and direct effect on coronary atherosclerosis that was not confounded or mediated by any of the standard risk factors.

In the first 20 years of life, parents are often identified as the most important and meaningful providers of social support and love. The attachment literature (Bowlby, 1969; Parkes, Stevenson-Hinde & Marris, 1991) highlights the powerful role that parental love and caring plays in shaping the biological as well as psychosocial health of infants, children and adolescents. Presently, however, the extent to which the positive perception of parental love and caring predicts health status later in life remains unknown. We use the term caring, in addition to the term love, because caring is a many faceted term that includes positive perceptions of love, understanding, empathy, and justice, as well as other positive and responsible parental role attributes.

To examine the relationship between perceptions of parental love and caring and health later in life, Russek and Schwartz (1997a) analyzed data from Harvard undergraduates who participated in the Harvard Mastery of Stress Study (Funkenstein, King, & Drolette, 1957) in the early 1950s and were followed up 35 years later, when the subjects were in their mid 50s (Russek et al., 1990). As part of a very large battery of psychological tests administered in college, the subjects were asked, directly and simply, to rate their mothers and their fathers separately in terms of how "loving," "just," "fair," "clever," "hardworking," and "strong" they were, using the numbers 1 to 9. The results indicated that subjects who gave their parents lower ratings on the average of these perceived parental caring items while in college, were identified, in mid-life, as suffering from significantly more illnesses such as coronary artery disease, hypertension, duodenal ulcer, and alcoholism. This effect was independent of subject's age, family history of illness, smoking behavior, and the death and /or divorce of parents.

Prospective analyses revealed that 87 percent of subjects who rated both their mothers and fathers low on parental love and caring had diagnosed diseases in mid-life, whereas only 25 percent of subjects who rated both their mothers and fathers high on parental love and caring had diagnosed diseases in mid-life (Russek & Schwartz, 1997a). Similar findings were obtained for narrative descriptions of parental love and caring (Russek & Schwartz, 1996a) and multiple choice questions of perceptions of parental warmth and closeness (Russek & Schwartz, 1997b).

Future research is clearly needed to determine the physical, biological, psychological, social and/or spiritual mechanisms that may mediate how parental love and caring contributes to health and illness over the life span. Possible sets of factors influenced by parental love and caring include 1) nutrition, stress, and loving energy before and after birth, 2) healthy and unhealthy behaviors developed during childhood (e.g., sleep, exercise, use of drugs), 3) coping styles such as anxiety, anger, hostility, depression, negative affectivity, optimism, and self-esteem, 4) choice and stability of work, marriage, family relationships and friendships, 5) the presence/social support of parents in one's adult life, and 6) spiritual values and practices. *The perception of parental love and caring may be a powerful predictor of future health because parental love and caring involves and integrates so many potential mechanisms.*

Levels of Love and Caring Energy: The Systemic Love Hypothesis

When a dynamical energy systems approach is applied to love and caring, some far reaching implications emerge (Russek & Schwartz, 1996b), termed the systemic love hypothesis. The hypothesis that love is a fundamental organizing force in nature can be seen in the ancient ideas of chi energy and is explicit or implicit in both eastern and western spiritual philosophies (Kraft, 1983). Scientists who adopted a vitalist position implicitly adopted the vision that some sort of fundamental organizing force was necessary to explain the evolution of order in nature (see Capra, 1996). Though vitalism fell out of favor and was replaced with molecular biology, deep questions about the origin and evolution of order remained. Modern systems theorists employ concepts from self-organization, chaos and complexity theory (modern extensions of systems theory) to attempt to explain the origin and evolution of living systems (reviewed in Capra, 1996).

However, implicit in the logic of circular (recurrent) feedback interactions is the requirement that 1) parts can connect in a circular arrangement, and remain connected in a circular arrangement, to function as a system, and 2) energy and information (as well as matter) can be circulated within a system (Schwartz & Russek, 1997a,b). Physics and chemistry invented concepts such as "attractive" forces and "affinity" to explain how atomic and molecular systems emerge and become whole. The concepts of attraction and affinity are required to explain how circular systems are created that can circulate information, energy, and matter. Simply stated, the concept of a system requires the assumption that some sort of circulating force exists, and some systems theorists have labeled this the force of love (Kraft, 1983). In fact, Isaac Newton, who invented the concept of gravity and described its mathematics, saw gravity as a physical expression of the universal force of love (the love of God). Gravity was envisioned to be the fundamental attractive force that interconnected everything and enabled the universe to function as a grand system.

A simple analysis of the way the term love is used in everyday language reinforces the idea that the concepts of attraction and affinity are fundamental to the concept of love. It is commonly said "I love my mother, I love my spouse, I love my daughter, I love my dog, I love my house, I love music, I love salmon, I love the Grand Canyon, I love science. Obviously, the meaning of "I love my spouse" is very different than "I love salmon"—the former includes the concept of loving (implying the giving of love, nurturing, protection, etc.), the latter typically does not. However, both imply a strong attraction and affinity. Through attraction and affinity comes the potential for attachment and bonding.

When it is hypothesized that every system requires attractive forces that enable circular feedback interactions to occur (and that these attractive forces can be termed a basic level of love), it logically follows that as systems become more complex, and show new emergent properties, the expression of these loving forces may become more complex and emergent as well. Theoretically, the more complex the system, the more complex is the system's capability to experience and express love. It is meaningful that the human species, the most complex biological system known to mankind, has the extraordinary capability to love virtually everything in nature. Love as an emergent process goes far beyond simple attraction and affinity—emergent higher levels of love (especially in humans) include the expression of interest and appreciation, empathic understanding and caring wisdom, altruism and compassion, purpose and meaning.

When species are born, they are clearly open to levels of love, beginning with (but not limited to) basic physical energy (e.g., warmth), sensory stimulation (e.g., touch), and chemical sustenance (e.g., milk). The growing infant naturally seeks love and affection, and finds everything in life interesting and exciting. In the wild, organisms not only learn to love, they also learn to fear. They develop appropriate cautions in order to survive into adulthood. As humans grow into adulthood, they too do not only learn to love, they also learn to fear. As mentioned above, the perception of parental love and caring appears to be a strong predictor of long term physical health (Russek & Schwartz, 1996a; 1997a,b).

Moreover, it is well recognized in the psychotherapy literature that the perceived personal warmth of the therapist, and her or his ability to engage in empathic understanding, is an important predictor of successful therapy.

A person's love history (a person's systemic memories of love), profoundly shapes her or his capacity to thrive and prosper. If the essence of love, and the very existence of systems, involves energy, it logically follows from dynamical energy systems theory that caring energy has effects on human functioning and health (Russek & Schwartz, 1996b). It is important to remember that physical movements per se of living systems cause electrostatic field effects that can be measured at a distance (Green et al., 1991).

Is it possible that personal warmth and empathy have an energetic component, and that this energetic component should be added to our theories of caring and health? Is it possible that the expression of anger, as communicated by angry words and angry gestures, involves dynamical energy patterns that literally assault the energy systems of people? Is it possible that unwanted sexual words and sexual gestures, even if they are "non-contact," may literally involve a kind of energetic rape? Do the energetic needs of patients literally contribute to the phenomenon of burn-out in health professionals? From a dynamical energy systems perspective, controversial hypotheses such as these are logically plausible and scientifically testable (Russek & Schwartz, 1996b).

If trends in modern science continue, the integration of the physical, biological, behavioral, and social sciences will expand. As explicated in this chapter, topics of relevance to conventional and complementary medicine may in the future involve more intimate connections with fundamental physics and biophysics in addition to biology and neuroscience. The integration of biophysical concepts of energy with psychology and mind-body medicine may be a new frontier, sparking the evolution of new fields such as energy clinical psychology and energy psychotherapy in the context of integrative medicine.

Healing Images and Energy Clinical Psychology: A New Frontier?

As most human beings have experienced firsthand, a subset of our images propel us to action. Images can motivate, encourage, and inspire. Images of love and caring can foster feelings of safety, security, peace, warmth, and hope.

If the dynamical energy systems perspective outlined in this chapter has utility, it has the potential to widen our vision of imagery and the role of images in healing. Images may be viewed someday as dynamic integrative info-energy systems that can foster connection and holism, and therefore health and healing.

If the current chapter motivates, encourages, and even potentially inspires researchers and clinicians who are interested in imagery to develop a new, biophysical image of imagery process itself, then it will have served its goal.

REFERENCES

Astumian, R. D., Weaver, J. C., & Adair, R. K. (1995). Rectification and signal averaging of weak electric fields by biological cells. *Proceedings of the National Academy of Sciences, 92,* 3740-3743.

Becker, R. O (1990). *Cross currents.* New York: Jeremy P. Tarcher/Perigee.

Becker, R. O., & Selden, G. (1988). *The body electric.* New York: Quill, William Morrow.

Berkman, L. F. (1995). The role of social relations in health promotion. *Psychosomatic Medicine, 57,* 245-254.

Bowlby, J. (1969) *Attachment and loss Vol I: Attachment.* New York: Basic Books.

Capra, F. (1996). *The web of life: A new scientific understanding of living systems.* New York: Anchor Books.

Clarke, J. (1994, August). SQUIDs. *Scientific American,* 46-53.

Dossey, L. (1996). What's love got to do with it? *Alternative Therapies in Health and Medicine, 2,* 8-15.

Forward, R. (1996). Mass modification definition study. *Journal of Scientific Exploration, 10,* 325-254.

Funkenstein, D., King, S. H., & Drolette, M. (1957). *Mastery of stress.* Cambridge, MA: Harvard University Press.

Green, E. E., Parks, P. A, Guyer, P. M., Fahrion, L. S., & Coyne, L. (1991). Anomalous electrostatic phenomena in exceptional subjects. *Subtle Energies, 2,* 69-94.

Green, J., & Shellenberger, R. (1996). The healing energy of love. *Alternative Therapies in Health and Medicine, 2,* 46-56.

James, W. (1890). *Psychology (Briefer Course).* New York: Holt.

Kauffman, S. A. (1993). *The origins of order.* New York: Oxford University Press.

Kraft, R. W. (1983). *A reason to hope: A synthesis of Teilhard de Chardin's vision and systems thinking.* Seaside, CA: Intersystems.

Krieger, D. (1990). Therapeutic touch: Two decades of research, teaching and clinical practice. *NSNA/Imprint, 37,* 83-88.

Levin, J. S. (1996). How prayer heals: A theoretical model. *Alternative Therapies in Health and Medicine, 2,* 66-73.

Lisberger, S. G., & Sejnowski, T. J. (1992). Motor learning in a recurrent network model based on the vistibulo-ocular reflex. *Nature, 360,* 159-161.

Malmivuo, J., & Plonsey, R. (1995). *Bioelectromagnetism.* New York: Oxford University Press.

McCulloch, W. S. (1951). Why the mind is in the head. In L. A. Jeffress (Ed.), *Cerebral mechanisms in behavior.* New York: John Wiley.

Medalie, J. H., & Goldbourt, U. (1976). Angina pectoris among 10,000 men: Psychosocial and other risk factors. *American Journal of Medicine, 60,* 910-921.

Miller, J. G. (1978). *Living systems.* New York: McGraw-Hill.

Milonni, P. W. (1994). *The quantum vacuum: An introduction to quantum electronics.* New York: Academic Press.

Orear J. (1962). *Fundamental physics.* New York: John Wiley & Sons.

Parkes, C. M., Stevenson-Hinde, J., & Marris, P. (Eds.), (1991). *Attachment across the life cycle.* London: Tavistock/Routledge.

Pearsall, P. (1998). *The heart's code.* New York: Broadway Books.

Ragan, P. A., Wang, W., & Eisenberg, S. R. (1995). Magnetically induced currents in the canine heart: A finite element study. *IEEE Transactions on Biomedical Engineering, 42,* 1110-1115.

Rubik, B. (1995). Energy medicine and the unifying concept of information. *Alternative Therapies in Health and Medicine, 1,* 34-39.

Ruberman, W., Weinblatt, E., Goldberg, J. D., & Chaudhary, B. S. (1984). Psychosocial influences on mortality after myocardial infarction. *New England Journal of Medicine, 311,* 552-559.

Russek, H. I., & Russek, L. G. (1980). Emotion and the heart. In G. H. Bourne (Ed.), *Hearts and heart-like organs: Volume II.* New York: Academic Press.

Russek, L. G., King, S. H., Russek, S. J., & Russek, H. I. (1990). The Harvard Mastery of Stress Study 35-year follow-up: Prognostic significance of patterns of psychophysiological arousal and adaptatron. *Psychosomatic Medicine, 52,* 271-285.

Russek, L. G., & Schwartz, G. E. (1997a). Perceptions of parental caring predict health status in mid-life: A 35 year follow-up of the Harvard Mastery of Stress Study. *Psychosomatic Medicine, 59,* 144-149.

Russek, L. G., & Schwartz, G. E. (1996a). Narrative descriptions of parental love and caring predict health status in mid-life: A 35 year follow-up of the Harvard Mastery of Stress Study. *Alternative Therapies in Health and Medicine, 2*(6), 55-62.

Russek, L. G., & Schwartz, G. E. (1996b). Energy cardiology: A dynamical energy systems approach for integrating conventional and alternative medicine. *Advances: The Journal of Mind-Body Health, 12*(4), 4-24.

Russek, L. G., & Schwartz, G. E. (1997b). Feelings of parental caring predict health status in mid-life: A 35 year follow-up of the Harvard Mastery of Stress Study. *Journal of Behavioral Medicine, 20*(1), 1-13.

Schacter, D. L. (1996). *Searching for memory.* New York: Basic Books.

Shumaker, S. A., & Czajkowski, S. M. (Eds.). (1994). *Social. support and cardiovascular disease.* New York: Plenum Press.

Schwartz, G. E. (1977). Psychosomatic disorders and biofeedback: A psychobiological model of disregulation. In J. D. Maser & M. E. P. Seligman (Eds.), *Psychopathology: Experimental models.* San Francisco: W. H. Freeman.

Schwartz G. E. (1982). Cardiovascular psychophysiology: A systems perspective. In J. T. Cacioppo & R. E. Petty (Eds.), *Perspectives in cardiovascular psychophysiology.* New York: Guilford Press.

Schwartz, G. E. (1984). Psychobiology of health: A new synthesis. In B. L. Hammonds & C. J. Scheirer (Eds.), *Psychology and health: The master lecture series. Volume 3.* Washington, D.C.: American Psychological Association.

Schwartz, G. E. (1986). Emotion and psychophysiological organization: A systems approach. In M. G. H. Coles, E. Donchin, & S. Porges (Eds.), *Psychophysiology.* New York: Guilford Press.

Schwartz, G. E. (1987). Personality and the unification of psychology and modern physics: A systems approach. In J. Aronoff, A. I. Robin, & R. A. Zucker (Eds.), *The emergence of personality.* New York: Springer.

Schwartz, G. E. (1989). Disregulation theory and psychosomatic disease: A systems approach. In S. Cheren (Ed.), *Psychosomatic medicine: Theory, research and practice.* New York: International University Press.

Schwartz, G. E. (1990). Psychobiology of repression and health: A systems approach. In J. E. Singer (Ed.), *Repression and dissociation.* Chicago: The University of Chicago Press.

Schwartz, G. E., & Russek, L. G. (1997a). Dynamical energy systems and modern physics: Fostering the science and spirit of complementary and alternative medicine. *Alternative Therapies in Health and Medicine, 3*(3),46-56.

Schwartz, G. E., & Russek, L. G. (1997b). Do all dynamical systems have memory? Implications of the systemic memory hypothesis for science and society. In K. Pribram & J. S. King (Eds.), *Brain and values: Behavioral neurodynamics V.* Hillsdale, NJ: Erlbaum.

Schwartz, G. E., & Russek, L. G. (1997c). The challenge of one medicine: Theories of health and "eight world hypotheses." *Advances, 3*(13), 7-23.

Schwartz, G. E. R., & Russek, L. G. (1999). *The living energy universe: A fundamental discovery that transforms science and medicine.* Charlottesvile, VA: Hampton Roads.

Seeman, T. E., & Syme, L. (1987). Social networks and coronary artery disease: A comparison of the structure and function of social relations as predictors of disease. *Psychosomatic Medicine, 49,* 341-354.

Seeman, T. E., Berkman L. F., Kohout, F., LaCroix, A. Z., Glynn, R. J., & Blazer, D. G. (1993). Intercommunity variations in the association between social ties and mortality in the elderly: A comparative analysis of three communities. *Annals of Epidemiology, 3,* 325-335.

Siegel, B. S. (1995). Exploring what can't be explained. *Advances: The Journal of Mind-Body Health, 11,* 2-3.

Sylvia, C., with Novack, W. (1997). *A change of heart.* New York: Little, Brown.

von Bertalanffy, L. (1968). *General system theory.* New York: Braziller.

Wakai, R. T., Wang, M., & Martin, C. B. (1994, March). Spatiotemporal properties of the fetal magnetocardiogram. *American Journal of Obstetrics and Gynecology,* 770-776.

Webster, N. (1977). *Webster's new twentieth century dictionary of the English language. Unabridged, 2nd Edition.* New York: Collins World.

Welin, L., Tibblin, G., Svardsudd, K., Tibblin, B., Ander-Perciva, S., Larsson, B., & Wilhelmsen, L. (1985). Prospective study of social influences on mortality: The study of men born in 1913 and 1923. *Lancet, 1,* 915-918.

Williams, R. B., Barefoot, J. C., Califf, R. M., et al. (1992). Prognostic importance of social and economic resources among medically treated patients with angiographically documented coronary artery disease. *Journal of the American Medical Association, 267,* 520-524.

CHAPTER 6

Music, Imagery, and Healing

PAT MOFFITT COOK

The universe is a tonal harmony of many sounds—many lives interacting and vibrating together as they fill the great silence. Music's rhythm and melodies echo the eternal harmonies of the heavens. In this way music is a mirror of holy resonance: it opens transparencies in us, enlarging our horizons and helping us to feel what is beautiful and inspiring . . . it attunes us to powerful waves of life energy and to the unfathomable Source of all Good. (Hal Lingerman, cited in Brigham, 1994, p. 289)

And we must learn that to know a man is not to know his name but to know his melody. (Unknown Oriental Philosopher)

Music combined with imagery provides a conduit through which we can access images, feelings, and memories that support the healing process (Bonny & Savary, 1990; Rider, 1997; Warming, 1992). Human beings respond universally to the power of musical language, its harmonic, rhythmic, and melodic elements, without having to formally learn it (Blacking, 1990; Rider 1997). This phenomenon, believed to be intuitively understood by ancient and traditional healers, continues to motivate contemporary health care professionals to use music for stress reduction (Rosch, 2000), and pain control (Taylor, 1997), to induce altered states of consciousness and to evoke emotional catharsis for healing (Grof, 1985). A growing number of music and sound therapists now compliment Western medical interventions in the hospital and hospice settings (Crowe, 2000; Schroeder-Sheker, 1997). Music also promotes and intensifies spiritual experiences (Bush, 1995; Rider, 1997), and in some cultures it plays a significant role in the death and dying process (Gaynor, 1999; Schroeder-Sheker, 1997).

In this chapter, the ancient and cross-cultural uses of music and imagery are traced and a recent, heightened interest, in the West, in music and healing is noted. Also bases for the therapeutic efficacy of music are examined in detail and a number of methods that employ music and imagery are discussed. Finally a list of suggested music for imagery and healing is provided.

115

MUSIC AND IMAGERY IN ANCIENT, EASTERN, AND INDIGENOUS TRADITIONS

Healing with music and music-evoked imagery is part of an ancient therapy still practiced in many parts of the world by holy men and women, shamans, and indigenous healers. Throughout the ages, selected tones, song melodies, harmonic structures, and rhythmic patterns were discovered by healers and used as sonic remedies (Cook, 1997a). Physicians in ancient Greece prescribed music-making and singing (Bush, 1995; Rosch, 2000). Indigenous healers directed sound as energy toward (or into) a patient, negotiated with disease-causing entities, cooled fevers (Cook, 1997b), induced trance states and evoked powerful images useful in the healing process. Rouget (1985) and Friedson (1996) have done extensive research on this subject with non-Western cultures.

Among the Hindus in India, "the central act of worship is hearing the *mantra* or sacred sound with one's own ears and chanting the mantra with ones own voice" (Coward & Goa, 1996, p. 4). This sacred act is believed to tune a person with divine vibration, which eventually purifies, heals, and transforms. The Parama-Samhita says, "It is by mantra that God is drawn to you. It is by mantra that he is released" (Beck, 1995, p. 1). The Hindu notion of *Nada-Brahman,* God as divine sound, and of Nada-Yoga, the yoga of sacred sound, are an ancient science that is still practiced today. Through Nada-Yoga, practitioners achieve spiritual release, *moksa* (Beck, 1995). This belief forms the foundation of an ancient science and practice of healing with sound.

The ancient Indian sages studied this carefully and discerned foundational vibrations, which are expressed in the Sanskrit alphabet, in which each letter represents a particular vibration. "These foundational vibrations interact with centers of resonance which are called chakras" (Soule, 1995, p. 16). Soule teaches his meditation students that meditating, chanting, and visualizing the chakras and/or symbols associated with them, bring stability to the body, breath, mind, and emotions. Houston (1997) suggests that the person chanting is put back into a state of harmonic resonance from which he/she may have deviated. This resonance can be manipulated and generated outwardly to patients who are mentally or physically ill, affecting them in positive ways. Vibration is also referred to as energy. When practitioners intone sacred seed syllables, *bijas,* or sing a healing song, they place their body, mind, and soul in a desired state of vibration. "The energy patterns it sets into motion, naturally gives access to states of consciousness not available through the ordinary experience of senses" (Houston, 1997, p. 20).

Early Greek physicians used instrumental music to cure melancholy, aggression, and psychic disturbances. Pythagoras prescribed daily singing as a cathartic to cleanse emotions of worry, sorrow, and fear. Musican-physicians composed melodies to cure passions of the psyche, as well as depression and anger (Rosch,

2000). In Rome, special modal music was played as a cure for snakebites. Special songs and chants were played in curative temples in Greece, inspiring patients to wellness by altering their emotions and creating a sense of harmony (Crowe, 2000).

Medical anthropologists, ethnomusicologists, and other scholars have documented how music accompanies a wide variety of musical healing rituals led by shamans (Gouk, 2000). Community singing in many indigenous cultures provides a medium to dissolve tension and maintain a balanced society. For example, among the Raramuri (Tarahumara of Northern Mexico), the *Owiruame* (medicine man) sings to drive sadness away; for, they believe that sadness is the cause of illness (Cook, 1997a).

Central American Kuna song healer Maestro Demosdenes Ramirez sings the *Nia Ikar,* the medicine song (story) for mental illness. His patients lie beside him in a hammock and listen to song verses that retell the epic battle against one of four devils. The song evokes vivid imagery. The patients come face-to-face with their illness. Both patients and healer relive the dramatic story of their ancestor's fight against mental illness (known as the devil). The devil is overcome on the fourth day when the empowered *nuchus* (medicine dolls) capture him, burn him, and bury his ashes deep in the earth. The patients go home cured and rejoin their family and community (Cook, 1997a).

Songs invite benevolent deities to aid in healing sessions. Babaji, a Hindu *ojah* (village healer), sings to the goddess Shitala (Cool One, the goddess associated with smallpox and fevers) to help relieve a patient who is suffering from delusional fevers caused by smallpox. When Shitala's image possesses the healer's heart and he holds her in his minds eye, he transfers her divine power to the person who is suffering. Soon the fever breaks and the patient's temperature cools (Cook, 1997b).

A Peruvian patient with malignant brain tumors ingests *ayahuasca,* a psychotropic hallucinogenic. His mind and emotions attach themselves to a flowing flute melody followed by an intoxicating guided-imagery-journey sung by the *ayahuascero* (shaman). The sound of shaking rattles penetrates the patient's mind and slows his breathing and heart rate. At this point the *ayahuascero* performs non-invasive surgical operations with rattles and ceremonial rods. The image of the rods probing, pulling, and extracting the infirmities takes the sickness away. "The sickness can come out when we use our imaginations well," said Don Agustin (Cook, 1997a, pp. 23-27).

These examples point out that music combined with imagery is used to intercept the course of mental and physical illnesses by the ancient and traditional healers. The music forms a multi-layered canvas that invites both patient and healer to paint images upon it—cultural myths, symbols of illness and wellness, and powerful remedies—drawn from imaginal realms. The healer resounds sonic remedies, and at the same time, he improvises musically and intuitively based upon the spontaneous revelations that emerge from the patients' psycho-spiritual and psychosocial experiences of pain and suffering. It is evident that the practitioners in these systems do not separate the mind, body, and spirit; for, they believe that the human being is a tripartite unity. Music by its very nature encourages and helps to reveal and stimulate this relationship. It supports "the unification of breath, rhythm, and tone of the human body. . . . It patterns and reinforces the powers of listening, attention and memory (emotions) for people of every culture" (Campbell, 1991, p. 243). It is noteworthy that ancient and traditional music therapy practices share common approaches and are considered precursors to contemporary music-centered therapies.

RECENT WESTERN INTEREST IN MUSIC AND HEALING

The therapeutic efficacy of music now commands recognition in Western medicine, alternative health care, and special education. A substantial body of historical information has provided background for contemporary research and for new applications of music-centered therapies. "Today modern technologies allow us to analyze, produce, and reproduce musical processes much more precisely than ever before" (Rosch,[1] 2000, p. 10). As a result, a wide range of music disciplines are available for different patient populations and for individuals interested in sound and music tools for health-maintenance at home.[2]

Clinical studies in music therapy and music in medicine have measured changes in mood and emotional responses to musical elements, such as pitch, rhythm, and melody (Maranto, 1992; Radocy & Boyle, 1997; Rider, 1997). Researchers have assessed the effects of stimulating and sedative music on anxiety and arousal (Radocy & Boyle, 1997) and have demonstrated how elements in music affect physiological changes in blood pressure, heart rate, body temperature, and brain wave states. They have examined the effects of music as a psychotherapeutic agent for improving self-concept and promoting self-expression (Aigen, 1998). Bonny's research indicated that guided imagery and music helped listeners access archetypal roots and experience transpersonal realms (Bush, 1995).

Interdisciplinary research in the health sciences continues to help refine music and imagery modalities. Music-centered therapists now can better assess client responses during music-enhanced imagery sessions. Music and imagery techniques alone or in combination with other medical interventions can address mood-related performance, psychosomatic illnesses, and immune responsiveness. In music-evoked or music-enhanced imagery techniques the listener experiences visual, auditory, olfactory, noetic, and body imagery as well as emotions, thoughts, and memories (Wrangsjo & Korlin, 1995).

---

[1] Paul J. Rosch, M.D. is editor-in-chief of the Newsletter of the American Institute for Stress in Yonkers, New York.
[2] Three good resources for further investigation into music tools for home use are Campbell (1992, 1997), Leeds (2001), and Bush (1995).

Bonny theorizes that quieting music combined with imagery specifically relieves pain by producing the pain-relieving peptides that affect brain responses. Rider (1997) says that a patient learns to develop mental images of pain, "a red-hot, bubbling mass for example, when music that matches the image," either by its mood or musical properties, is played (Pinkerton, 1996, p. 17).

Music is a temporal art. Its sounds are organized cumulatively through time in rhythm. Its effects are experienced from within and without, and it has the power to stimulate the intellect and emotions (Tusler, 1991).

WHAT CONSTITUTES THE THERAPEUTIC POWER OF MUSIC?

This section will define musical elements and explain how they help make music therapeutic.

Pitch

The highness or lowness of a sound, pitch, is determined by the frequency of vibrations, the number of vibrations per second. Pitch is any periodic frequency between 20 and 20,000 Hz (normal human hearing range). A pitched note can be used to help listeners focus on general (lower, middle, upper) or specific (i.e., forehead, heart, shoulder) areas in the body. A resonating tuning fork or a vowel sound toned by a therapist can be directed at tight muscles and pressure points on the body. This form of "sound acupressure" on body meridians is said to break up stagnant energy and to stimulate the flow of energy or *chi*.[3]

Mid- to high-pitched sustained notes played on Tibetan *tinkshas* (hand bells) and singing bowls (metal bowls that produce rich overtones) are used in Eastern and Western meditation practices to help focus one's attention on a single point. With the eyes closed, images can arise from the subconscious, bubble up, present themselves to the listener, and move on.

High-pitched, fast-tempo instrumental music, as opposed to low, can stimulate a more alert state in listeners. Tomatis, the French physician and specialist in otolaryngology, uses filtered music through an electronic device to treat auditory disorders. He discovered that high-frequency sounds supply more concentrated nervous influx and thus increase the effect of charging the brain. Tomatis researched the use of high-frequency sounds for the purpose of increasing energy levels, of restoring the ears' ability to process auditory information, and of helping to motivate the unmotivated (Leeds, 2001; Madaule, 1994; Radocy & Boyle, 1997).

---

[3] Wind Records produces and distributes Chinese healing music performed by the Shanghai orchestra. Their recording entitled "Cancer" as well as other recordings are based on sound acupressure.

Bonny designed a series of surgery tapes called "Music Rx. for Hospitals" (1979). For recovery room music, she utilized "Spring," a movement in Vivaldi's "Four Seasons." Bonny's research indicated that patients who listened to classical music performed on higher-pitched instruments (i.e., violins and flutes), came to a conscious state more easily and quickly than those patients who did not listen to music in the recovery room.

Visual images, thoughts, and body sensations change with music performed in different registers (bass, baritone, alto, and soprano). Therapists use imagery scripts that suggest that listeners imagine colors and shapes that seem to resonate with pitch registers.

Siberian composer Mourashkin discovered that he could write and record musical compositions that brought him relief from severe and chronic pain caused by a traumatic car accident. Rhythmically energetic music laced with interesting high-pitched random sounds captured Mourashkin's attention, drawing his focus away from his acute pain. Mourashkin's album "Points of Light" is used in the United States today for pain control, anxiety, and stress reduction. His recordings are part of a series called "bio-energetic" music (Mourashkin, 1997).

The lower-pitched instruments more easily resonate with the body. Low-pitched large percussion, brass, or stringed instruments penetrate physical tension. Low to mid-range melodies that are rich in overtones connect strongly with the physical body, such as David Darling's cello piece, "Only One Wish," on his album "Eight String Religion" or any of the six Bach cello suites.

Interval

The distance from one pitch to another or intervals are classified as perfect consonances (unisons, perfect fourths, perfect fifths, and octaves), imperfect consonances (major and minor thirds and sixths), and dissonances (seconds, sevenths, and all diminished and augmented intervals). Interval ratios determine how two or more notes played simultaneously sound. In theory, the number of possible musical intervals is unlimited. But for musical evocation, the simpler acoustic intervals are most often used. "They appear so natural that without external help it is vocally almost impossible to get away from them" (Danielou, 1995, p. 12).

Consonant sounds are most accurately detected by the human ear and reproduced by the voice. The ear hears and decodes consonant properties of interval ratios far better than dissonant ones. Thus, in part, tuning systems for musical instruments grow out of human perception and ability to process sound information and the desire to accompany the voice and ear. Consonant harmony requires less work for listeners (Danielou, 1995). This phenomenon is important in selecting music for healing. In general, consonant music creates an atmosphere of safety, familiarity, and organization. For example, Bill Douglas's choral arrangement of "Deep Peace," a well-known Celtic poem, suggests and mirrors harmonious relationships with the external and internal world. This same musical mirror can amplify and exaggerate psychological and physiological disharmonies in a listener in the midst of such sonic organization and balance.

Dissonant music (in the West more than the East) generates feelings of tension, chaos, and conflict. Dissonance suggests conflict, stretches and stresses time, and anticipates release. Harmonic tension stimulates energy, serves as a catalyst for stirring emotions, and is used to match mental confusion, negative moods, and experiences of physical pain (Danielou, 1995). Dissonant music is used in music-evoked imagery sessions to encourage problem solving.

Melody

It is a series of tones of different pitches arranged in a rhythmic pattern. The melody is also thought of as the tune or theme. Melody is perhaps the most expressive element in music, possibly because melodies were first created by the human voice.[4]

Our experience has taught us that melody tends to invite inner dialogue. Melody leads the way and takes listeners on a journey into a personal story. It becomes the voice of the listener. If the melody is bold and confident, so can the inner voice be. If the melody wanders, feeling unsure of itself, a similar feeling can overcome the listener. A melancholy tune evokes sadness and can enhance imagery associated with grief and loss. If the melody is harmonized in a minor key, it can elicit regret or remorse. It can bring up memories and feelings of the past. Melody is easily stored in our memories. In music-enhanced imagery sessions, a minor or major melody sung by a woman or man, or played by an instrument in a specific register, can evoke the voice of a mother, father, child, or partner. The timbre of the instrument creating the melody can express unevenness, anger, rawness, and attitude.

Familiar music can be chosen to help an ill person visualize himself/herself in earlier times of wellness. Research indicates that the brain records and responds to familiar tonal material (Taylor, 1997). Melody can be utilized in therapy to connect listeners with people, places, and eras.

Volume and Intensity

This refers to how loud or soft a sound or music piece is performed or played (decibels, amplitude of vibrations). Loud volume drowns out other environmental sounds and often a person's thoughts. Low volume helps quiet listeners and accompanies reflective moments or efforts to fall asleep. Soft music can feel inviting, mysterious, while loud music is strong and sometimes imposing.

---

[4] For further reading on melodic foundations, review chapter six in Radocy and Boyle (1997).

Grof, the originator of "Holotropic Breath Work," combines the consciousness-altering effect of breath with evocative music, which is played very loudly. This psychotherapeutic process evokes personal, archetypal, and transpersonal visual imagery and can lead to therapeutic effect through spontaneous body movements (Grof, 1985).

During an interview for the *Noetic Sciences* video entitled "Of Sound, Mind and Body," music therapist Barbara Crowe explained that, when a loud repetitive sound is presented to the ear, the sound travels via the auditory nerve and enters at the lowest level of the brain. Then the sound stimulus enters and arouses a structure called the Reticular Activating System (RAS). RAS is an alert system for the cortex. It assigns meaning to incoming sensory information. A loud repetitive drumbeat, for example, causes the RAS to send out a constant signal to the cortex. This signal masks the sensory input from other senses, decreasing activity in the left brain. This allows other forms of cognition and problem solving to emerge from the right brain, the seat of our mythology. We can use this to access deeply buried psychological materials, and, in Jungian terms, archetypal symbols and images, in a psychiatric setting. It has also been discovered that because of music's ability to affect the arousal functions of the RAS system, the brain focuses on an incoming music stimulus instead of pain. In other words, the music distracts patients from pain sensations (Taylor, 1997).

Rhythm

This is the organization of pitch or musical tones in time. Rhythm includes beat, pulse, meter, tempo, as well as long- and short-note values. Rhythm has to do with all musical timing. It is a common factor in all cultures and remains the most important factor in musical organization.

There are many ways in which rhythm affects us. When we hear rhythm, we begin to entrain to it (Leeds, 1997). This affects our cardiorespiratory rhythm. This rhythm is a result of "complicated interactions between several populations of respiratory neurons located in the lower brain stem" (Koepchen, Spintge, & Droh, 1992, p. 47). Therefore, music entrains our heart rate, blood pressure, and muscle movement. This bidirectional process is the very reason rhythm is one of the most effective musical elements in sound and music therapy. Our biological rhythms will entrain to a presented external tempo or musical beat, thus controlling biological and mental functions through the central nervous system (Koepchen, Spintge, & Droh, 1992).

Rhythm is a complex phenomenon. It is much more than pulse, periodicity, or movement. Different rhythms control and influence our state of consciousness and physiology. For this reason, music's rhythmic element can be used as therapy for relieving stress and anxiety and inducing sleep.

Shamans enter trance states associated with healing on the sound of a shaking rattle or the steady beat of a drum. They experience visions and gather diagnostic information for those who are sick (Achterberg, 1992; Kalweit, 1992) of the past and the present, and they continue to travel to other realms on the beat of a drum or repetitive shaking of a rattle.

On the Suquamish Indian reservation in Poulsbo, Washington, Steve Old Coyote leads sweat lodges weekly for young members of the reservation. He teaches songs and drumming to the youth. "It keeps our young people out of trouble," Steve said. "The music we make in the sweat lodge encourages them to talk about their problems. We share our dreams and visions about the future. Our song meetings support teenagers who are dealing with alcoholism and drug addiction. The beat of the peyote rattle and water drum matches our heart beat. It connects us and heals us for the time being" (Cook, 1997a, p. 83).

Spintge and Droh (1992) have conducted research on the effect of neuro-vegetative rhythmicity on stress and relaxation. Music therapist and composer Janalea Hoffman (1995) composes and produces musical recordings based solely on the relationship between the body rhythms and musical tempo for the purpose of regulating heart rate. Hoffman says that "the listener's heart responds to the external stimulus of the slow, steady beat of the music and her/his heart rate begins to synchronize.[5] Hoffman's rhythmic music synchronizes a heart beating at 70 or 80 times per minute to slower tempos, gradually decreasing the rate to 60 and 50 beats per minute. Her tapes for Parkinson patients and children include music-enhanced guided imagery scripts.

Strong, percussionist and sound healer, recorded "Calming Rhythms" for use with autistic children and by individuals who are coping with high anxiety and aggression. The drumming sounds from his compact disc make use of shifting gravity, where the stress of the beat takes place. This prevents habituation and boredom and engages the mind in the music. Therefore listeners listen longer and can shift the attention to the music instead of to feelings of anxiety, for example.

Psychotherapist and author of *The Healing Power of the Drum,* Friedman, conducts drumming workshops in hospitals for adults and children with cancer to help them feel more energy, life inside themselves. Thaut has investigated the effect of rhythmic music or a simple drum pattern on motor coordination of Parkinson patients. He reports that a significant number of patients have walked 50 percent faster at the end of studies than at the beginning (Leeds, 2001).

Rhythm provides a structure and a sense of security. It organizes time and space. Music therapist Nancy Houghton described one of her clients during a sound therapy training at the Open Ear Center in Washington: "Charles, struggling with a stroke-induced shuffle-walk, sensed the metered cadence of a march I played. He recalled his military days, he saw himself able to walk, and then blended his gait with the beat."

[5] Dutch scientist Christian Huygens discovered in 1665 that two pendulum clocks placed side by side would entrain, synchronize (Hoffman, 1995).

Rhythm and tempo are capable of revving us up or calming us down. Assiogoli called rhythm "the primordial and fundamental element of music" (Friedman, 2000, p. 40). Most researchers in this field will agree that rhythm is the element which has the most intense and immediate influence on human beings because it affects directly both the body and the mind.

Timbre

It is the tone color or quality of the sound an instrument produces. Each instrument has a unique timbre as a result of its harmonic content. The harp sounds different than a bell, for example, even when the same pitch is played. The size and shape of an instrument and the way it is played create its unique timbre. This is the reason our ears can discriminate between instruments.

A timbre can enhance a mood, become the attitude of a listener in a guided-imagery session. In a music and imagery session, instruments with different timbres in musical composition are played to evoke attitudes, feelings of strength, or compassion. In their book *Music and Your Mind,* Bonny and Savary (1990) present a researched music repertoire and the mood each selection may elicit from a listener. Timbre reveals the nature of the individual voice of an instrument. It intensifies perceptions of color and creates musical texture.

Duration

It is the length of time any one element is sustained. The duration an instrument sustains a note or a harmony produces responses that are useful in music and imagery sessions. Short tones are thought to suggest movement. On the other hand, long-held notes or chords can cause anticipation, a sense of suspension, or the opposite, relief from movement. Long-held tones can induce a meditative state in some listeners, and for others they may cause them to "space out" or lose interest in the music and imagery process.

Orchestration and Texture

They refer to the arrangement of instruments in a musical score. The combinations of musical instruments and their unique timbres and rhythms create texture. Musical orchestration and the texture it creates affect the size of the sound container. A score can call for solo instruments or full orchestras. An orchestra creates a large container. This can be daunting for someone who needs containment and safety. If a listener lacks confidence or requires a more intimate container, a solo instrument, a duet, or a quartet would be more suitable. Different orchestrations and textures are more suitable for different moments in a thera-peutic process (Bonny & Savary, 1990).

MUSIC, IMAGERY, AND HEALING

"Music creates a continuity and connection in the various states of consciousness, and when used therapeutically, creates a continuous carrying wave that helps the subject move through difficult sequences and impasses" (Grof, 1985, p. 386). Campbell delineates six elements which he considers "essential for the successful process of integration of music, imagery and healing" (Campbell, 1991, p. 245-252).

1. *Music modifies the environment.* Music may be specifically selected for its ambient effect, to calm a frantic emergency room, to stimulate movement and mood in a geriatric setting, or to organize the study habits of students.
2. *Music modifies our relationship to time and space.* Classical or baroque music can serve to order our movements and thoughts and to enhance our learning process. Impressionistic or new age music may serve to stretch our perception of time and reality, allowing space for imagery and release.
3. *Effective visualization incorporates both the concrete and the metaphorical.* Music may allow one to flow from a position of impasse into more fluid thinking. An individual stuck in a concrete thought process may move into forming more creative associations through properly chosen music.
4. *Imagery incorporates the emotional along with the visual.* For thought to be a true image, sensory qualities must be introduced. Music operates on a multi-modal level in which we hear and feel our world. Music facilitates the creation of pathways between the inner and outer worlds, stimulating healing of the psyche and the physical being.
5. *Music can effect physical and mental curation, which is known as physio-audiation.* Therapist-led or client-created imaging can lead to the reduction of stress, increased concentration, and other desirable effects. Music aids in repatterning the mind and may lead to emotional, physical, mental, or spiritual benefits.
6. *For effective healing, integration and grounding must occur.* Campbell states, "For grounding, select music that is solid, that has a beat. Music for integration needs to impart the feeling of safety—of connectedness to self and to the environment" (Campbell, 1991, p. 251).

The Bonny Method of Guided Imagery and Music (GIM)

GIM is a psychotherapeutic one-on-one process with a "guide" (facilitator) who assists a "traveler" (client) on a music journey into a dreamlike associative state. The facilitator encourages the traveler to respond verbally with any impressions, images, and thoughts that come to mind while listening to Western classical music. She/he records these impressions on paper or with a tape recorder for review and discussion with the client after each session.

During a GIM session, clients listen in a relaxed state and either lie down or recline in a chair. A music and imagery session can last from 30 minutes to an hour. The process evokes imagery from "metaphoric levels of the psyche while uncovering feelings and facilitating release" (Bush, 1995, p. xi). "The music is selected to pace clients through different states of emotional awareness and remembrance so as to reach a peak experience; then the client is gradually returned to a safe, quiet and relaxed state" (Campbell, 1991, p. 250). The guide then helps the traveler to integrate his/her imagery experience through discussion or artwork.

The Bonny Method was developed by Helen L. Bonny. She began her work at the Maryland Psychiatric Research Center in the late 1960s, with Walter Pahnke and Stanislov Grof. Bonny found that by combining relaxation and imagery techniques with carefully selected music programs "she could produce therapeutic results with alcoholic and psychiatric patients which had been previously attainable only through the use of drugs" (Jarvis, 1988, p. 69).

GIM has proven itself an effective therapeutic strategy for the following reasons. 1) Music is a nonverbal medium that contains emotional suggestions. 2) Music affects the center of the brain and the limbic system and controls emotional responses (pain and pleasure) and involuntary processes (blood pressure, body temperature). 3) Music activates stored tonal memory, which can then evoke images and memories from the past. 4) Music stimulates peptides and causes the release of endorphins. 5) "Listening to music while identifying with evoked mental images induces a state of synchronization of the music, feelings and images, breath, and pulse rate. When this entrainment occurs, it increases the joint effect on the body/mind for healing" (Bush, 1995, p. 25).

Pickett works with the GIM technique to heal delayed Post Traumatic Stress Disorder. She reported this case study in the *Association for Music and Imagery Journal* (1995): The course of W's treatment spanned over 12 music sessions.

> This 28-year-old business man sought relief from his fear of losing emotional control or physically hurting someone. His goals were to uncover unimaginable hidden feelings caused by childhood sexual abuse by a Catholic priest in third grade and to recover memories before his adoption at age 9. Together with Pickett, he sought to heal the child and the grown man. Then he felt he would be able to gain control and adapt solutions to his emotional stresses and fears now.
>
> The music sessions enabled him to image himself in those childhood years. Successive sessions with appropriate music brought up rage, feelings of abandonment, and a grieving period. These initial sessions helped him finish the work he needed to do with his biological father. He made internal peace with both his mother and father and the priest. His progress motivated him to join a weekly therapy group.
>
> In 12 sessions, the client accepted his anger and as a result gained more control over himself and his feelings. He stopped drinking, enjoyed a renewed interest in his sexual life, and became more productive at work. "He experienced a healing of his own internal self-representation of trauma" (Pickett, 1995, p. 99). The music provided a canvas, a container to support and promote this process as W. resolved the hurt and angry feelings. His solutions arose

spontaneously in his imaginative process and in tandem with the classical music selected for him." (Pickett, 1995, p. 99)

GIM is being used with a large variety of patient populations in the United States and Europe.[6]

Cross-Cultural Music and Other Music with Imagery Techniques

In our experience, clients often respond better to relatively unfamiliar cross-cultural music than to familiar Western music (Cook, 2000). The following case history illustrates this point.

Josef (pseudonym), a German professor teaching at an American University, participated in a "Cross-cultural Music in Healing" weekend workshop at the Open Ear Center, and he then asked me, a GIM facilitator, for a series of private music and imagery sessions. His work also included home sound exercises.

Josef was divorced and estranged from his two teenage daughters. He was soft-spoken and had a noticeable tremor in his left hand. He filled his teacup only half way to avoid spilling. He felt that his life was empty. He had lost his self-confidence and spent a tremendous amount of energy suppressing a lifetime of anger.

Josef's first session indicated that the melodic and consonant harmonies of Western classical music were not sufficient to empower him or to connect him with his authentic voice, which he so desperately needed. He was too familiar with this music repertoire and the sounds of Western classical instruments. It was more productive, in his case, to use music with which he had little association.

For Josef's second session, I guided him through an East Indian breathing technique and suggested several body positions that felt natural to him, if the need arose to move. The music selection that day began with Boris Mourashkin's "Points of light" followed by an Australian didjeridu recording, and the Tibetan Buddhist chants of the Gyoto Monks. The didjeridu stimulated sensations in his bones. "I can feel my bones vibrating; the music is inside me," Josef reported.

Just minutes into the Tibetan chanting, Josef clasped his chest and struggled to speak. He gritted his teeth, holding back long-held emotion-filled words. The resonant deep-penetrating voices of the monks gave Josef courage to speak. He spontaneously spewed impressions as they emerged from his psyche. For the next 15 minutes he wept, stuttered, and shouted painful memories of childhood, dominated by images of his father. "My father refused to become a Nazi soldier," he said. "They black-listed him so he couldn't find work. He became depressed and an alcoholic. He often beat me. I was so afraid of him."

---

[6] For further investigation of the Bonny Method of Guided Imagery, review Bonny and Savary (1990), Bush (1995), and *The Journal of the Association for Music and Imagery*, volume 1-4.

In later sessions, Josef forgave his father and visualized embracing him. Josef found strength in the voices of the Tibetan monks. I prescribed a daily breathing and sound meditation for Josef to do at home. Lying down for 15 to 30 minutes, he rested a Tibetan singing bowl on his abdomen, struck it, and allowed the vibration to penetrate his abdomen. Immediately afterward, he sat upright in a chair and intoned the "OOO" sound for 10 to 20 minutes. The release, he said, brought him so much internal freedom that he telephoned his estranged daughters and asked them to meet him upon his return to Germany.

The day before his departure, he came by to say goodbye. He requested a full cup of tea. "Pat look," he said, picking up his cup in his left hand. The tremor was gone. Two years later a letter arrived with a photo of Josef with his two daughters and a new wife. He wrote that he was happy and life felt full again. He continues to work with his singing bowl, toning and listening to his collection of Tibetan Buddhist chanting.

In his book *Sounds of Healing,* Gaynor (1999, p. 16), an oncologist, describes how "chanting, listening to music, playing bells and hand cymbals, wind gongs, drums, whistles, etc., and toning can positively affect our minds as well as our physiology." Gaynor and other sound healing practitioners accept the principle underlying all sound healing modalities, that "there is a tendency toward harmony in nature, which researchers confirmed is indeed a universal rule" (Gaynor, 1999, p. 16).

Gaynor integrates crystal singing bowls into his medical practice. One of his patients, George, who was having a recurrence of lymphoma, was instructed by Gaynor to practice a sound meditation using his voice, a crystal singing bowl, and specific images of himself healthy, before his diagnosis. One night while practicing, George let out a low moan that originated in his abdomen. He asked Gaynor if he thought that it was a coincidence that that was where his lymphoma had started and then recurred. Gaynor did not consider it a coincidence. Like many other case histories Gaynor mentions, both doctors and patients feel that they may not have fended off another recurrence without the conscious use of vibration and imagery for deep healing (Gaynor, 1999).

The Power of the Human Voice

One of the primary instruments in sound healing and music therapy is the human voice. The voice is our center of creativity and empowerment. It is perhaps our greatest personal healing instrument. Stimulating internal sensations by making nonverbal sounds (moaning, wailing, keening) or humming, toning, chanting, or singing can affect mood, breathing, heart rate, and physical balance.

Toning the EEE sound, rich in higher overtone frequencies, can help dissipate a headache. Facilitators instruct people to combine tone with color or tone with a visual image. An individual is sometimes instructed to visualize the head pain and use the vowel sound to match its intensity. Campbell says, when you are tired, toning "EEE" is invigorating. He suggests that using a higher pitch is energizing.

To resonate your whole body, intone "OOO." Choose the most natural pitch for your voice and tone the vowel (Campbell, 1987). Fill your body with the color of OOO to help you increase your ability to resonate more. Sound therapists, like the Indian sages and practitioners of Nada-Yoga, claim that toning a specific vowel sound can resonate different parts of your body and helps you focus on that area. From any physical resonating location, a sensation, a story, or an emotion can emerge, freeing memories and healing old wounds. It promotes the realization that a person is over-stimulated or cannot feel parts of himself/herself. "How long have I been numb here?" a man asked at a Campbell workshop.

Even if someone is not performing a daily practice of toning, these experiences often take place during sessions with a sound therapist. Techniques such as vocal scanning, overtone chanting, toning, humming, and singing in a group can produce an experience or resonance and movement of energy in the body and mind. A depressive mood can be uplifted. The vibration causes individuals to twitch, shake, release emotion, laugh, or enter into deep meditative states. Practitioners and patients report visual impressions entering their mind's eye when they tone.

A sound therapy prescription can be toning specific vowel sounds or chanting bija mantras for a period of time to facilitate a return of resonance to the voice and body. Visualizing color and "seeing" parts of the body facilitates connecting to physical areas.

The Tomatis Method and Auditory Stimulation Programs

Methods of auditory stimulation use filtered music to accentuate and deliver, through earphones, a range of frequencies that stimulate auditory processing networks in the brain. Preliminary listening tests measure a person's ability to perceive and process air- and bone-conducted sound frequencies between 125 and 8000 hertz without distortion. For physical, social, or psychological reasons, listening can become distorted, obscured, impaired, or shut down. This important fact helps practitioners understand that not all persons hear or listen to music in the same way. Some individuals cannot process frequencies, music, or voices as others do. People can choose not to listen to music presented in a therapy session. In many cases individuals cannot process voices even though they hear well.

"Listening involves far more than the passive physical act of picking up sounds at random," says psychologist and listening therapist Paul Madaule. "It requires the ability to actively attune the ear to a particular sound signal, with both the intention and the desire to understand and communicate" (Madaule, 1994, p. 9).

The aim of the Tomatis Method is to reeducate the ear via an auditory training device called the Electronic Ear. The device presents sounds via music (Mozart and Gregorian Chant) that have been modified (filtered) so that they can be boosted to the higher frequency range (Gilmore, Madaule, & Thompson, 1989). Auditory processing difficulties and listening problems can complicate or cause

Attention Deficit Disorder (ADD), depression, poor communication and social skills, and speech problems. Poor listeners often have poor auditory memories and have difficulties in receptive and expressive language skills. The program is also used with autistic children and brain-injured patients.

Tomatis-based programs are gaining wide international acceptance. Among organizations adopting Tomatis' theories and techniques are the Berard Method: Auditory Integration Training, Listening Fitness Training Program, Open Ear Listening and Learning Program, and The Listening Program.

"Encounters in a person's life can detrimentally affect the desire to listen, and thus communicate," says Madaule. At birth we have the desire to listen, says Tomatis. A difficult birth, separation from a parent, physical health problems at an early age, severe or frequent ear infections, or a traumatic event shut down our desire to listen and participate.

Candidates enrolled in any of the above programs undergo up to 100 hours of auditory training. The programs combine other therapies with auditory training programs. These include counseling, voice work, art therapy, and occupational therapy. Functional, emotional, and relational issues are dealt with through daily social activities, creative writing, painting, and drawing, while listening to filtered music (Leeds, 2001; Leeds & Wise, 2000; Madaule, 1994). A case history follows:

> Alex was 9 years old when he took part in a Tomatis Program in a San Diego learning center. The family had already sought help from a number of other therapies. He was failing in school, was on probation for poor behavior, and lacked language and social skills. His pediatrician had prescribed three medications for ADD, aggressive behavior, and sleep problems.
>
> When Alex was 5 he barely survived a car accident. He was thrown through the windshield and flung onto the pavement 20 yards in front of the car. Flesh was scraped off the left side of his face, and he suffered injuries to his forehead. It took five surgeries to reconstruct his face. The trauma from the accident and surgeries caused Alex to withdraw from the world. By the age of 7, he was labeled ADD, had the reputation of a bully and misfit at school and at home.
>
> When I tested Alex, he looked like a normal 9-year-old. Though faded, three scars had earned him the name of "scarface" among peers.
>
> The surgeries had been a success, but Alex did not see it that way. He imagined himself as ugly and rejected. He made little eye contact and even less conversation. Weeks before starting the auditory stimulation program, his pediatrician had decided to wean Alex from dexidrine and ritalin with close observation.
>
> For the first 4 days in the program, Alex kept to himself, guarded his territory, and remained unfriendly. During this time he received auditory stimulation, and was instructed to paint daily. On the fifth and sixth days he exhibited more interest in the other children in the room.
>
> Seven days into the program, Alex began to awaken as a result of the sound stimulation. He was conversational with teachers' aides and spent more time than usual completing his required daily painting.

Alex drew a large oval head on an 11-inch by 17-inch sheet of art paper. He painted it red, like dripping blood. He divided the head with a track of black stitches. Then he lettered his name at the top. Alex smiled when he handed his "art" to me at the end of the listening period. He described the face of his worst enemy in words.

Alex told his mother that he felt happy. She reported that he was compliant all day and went to bed without the usual struggle. He was affectionate and for the first time initiated authentic contact with her. The next morning he complimented one of his classmates on his "awesome" new tennis shoes. The boy returned the compliment by inviting Alex to play monopoly with him and two other classmates. Alex reached out and met with success.

Over 2 nonconsecutive months, Alex listened to modified music with headsets for 2 hours each day, read positive stories, or hummed into a microphone with filtered music in the background. He painted on art paper, images that arose each day as the frequency stimulation shifted. He painted with brighter colors, in more detail, and often included other children with him in his pictures. His negative self-image changed to a positive one. He was constructing a new self-image, taking a chance and was attracting friends. His grades rose from Ds and Cs to Bs and As, and his teachers sent home positive comments about his behavior. A year later, Alex was medication free and was doing well socially and academically.

Clients who participate in the Tomatis Method programs, Open Ear Listening Program, and Listening Fitness Programs are required to write daily comments about their listening experience. These include thoughts, feelings, and kinesthetic responses to the sound stimulation. Most clients report better posture, more active dreaming at night, awareness of colors, sounds, and smells, and a desire to paint or draw with vibrant colors. These dreams and drawings are many times "spring-boards" in counseling sessions.

Robert Monroe

In 1950 Robert Monroe began investigating the connection between electronically produced audio patterns and brain wave rhythms. He used "pulsed audio stimuli to create an electrical frequency following response (FFR) in the brain, evoking psychological and mental states in direct relationship to the original audio wave forms" (Monroe Institute, 1995a, p. 3). In 1975 Monroe patented a sound technology called "Hemi-Sync." It combines sound frequencies, embedded at very low volume in an audio program of music and guided imagery. These embedded binaural beats stimulate a "whole-brain state," one in which both hemispheres are synchronized. This technology is used to induce concentration, alertness, positive imaging, release, relaxation, and sleep.

The whole-brain state aids the individual to be receptive to new information and can lead to higher levels of performance. A person entering a whole-brain state, via sound and music, becomes more receptive to therapeutic imagery scripts.

Monroe realized that if individuals could simulate and sustain this hemispheric synchronization for longer periods, they could train themselves to reproduce these states at will, and thus gain access to innate abilities to heal, via healing types of imagery.

Since the 1970s, numerous Hemi-Sync recorded series have been developed that support different patient populations and facilitate self-help programs. These include pain control, concentration, surgical support series, energy walk, and the positive immune program. Each program blends slow-moving simple harmonious music and imagery narrations. Research results confirmed that individuals could free themselves of negative cognition, solve problems, improve learning capacity, increase relaxation, and induce sleep.

With the use of a Hemi-Sync tape series called "Positive Immune Program," HIV-infected patients learned to boost innate immunity, augment energy levels, and produce positive emotional and physical states. Many individuals using the eight-tape program are able to "fall asleep by intent and to use sleep for restorative purposes, reduce stress, and increase relaxation" (Monroe, 1995a, p. 4). A half-hour listening period is prescribed each day and can be repeated when necessary. The guided imagery script and suggestions facilitate the listener's ability to experience a range of imagery from different colors and the visual and kinesthetic experience of them to a journey through the T-cells in the body. Affirmations and "resonant tuning" (toning with other voices on each tape) are included from time to time to encourage a patient and shift negative to positive cognition and reduce internal dialog.

Methods of perception are suggested to direct a listener toward therapeutic goals. He/she may experience physical sensations of rising and falling, rocking or tingling, vibrations, twitches, or pressure. Visual imagery is directed by a woman's voice on each tape, always supported by music and binaural beats. This helps in visualizing parts of the body and moving through them more easily (visually, kinesthetically, or auditorily).

For example, in tape #3 entitled "Living Body Map," the facilitator asks the listeners to see or feel themselves as pure energy, as a nonphysical map—the body is outlined by sparkling, white light. Then the listeners practice changing the white light to red, representing their circulatory system; blue, the nervous system; yellow, organs and the glandular system; and orange, muscle and bone structures.

Auditory perception manifests as voices, buzzing sounds, tones, and auditory impressions from emerging visualizations. Patients learn auditory and visual cues that strengthen their ability to experience positive images, sensations, and states of relaxation. The images become guides, and are perceived by listeners based on their ability to call them forth. On tape #7, a woman's voice directs patients to communicate with an individual cell that serves as a representative for all the helper cells. It is called a "Journey Through the T-Cells." Following this powerful imaging experience and training, patients can achieve three outcomes: 1) a sense of personal control; 2) states of relaxation, restorative sleep, and a positive immune response; and 3) emotional balance during difficult periods.

Health care practitioners throughout the United States recommend the Hemi-Sync "Surgical Support Series" for selected patients preparing for surgery or surviving a traumatic injury. The tapes offer a blend of music, embedded sound signals producing the whole-brain state, guided imagery and "exercises that reinforce the minds ability to escalate the physical, mental and emotional components of the total healing process" (Monroe, 1995b, p. 2). The tapes assist in the maintenance of a positive attitude and in the promotion of states of relaxation. Effectiveness is not dependent on whether the patient is conscious or unconscious. Reported outcomes have included less anesthesia for surgery, stable blood pressure, quick return to consciousness in the recovery room, less need for pain medication, feelings of empowerment, and the belief in positive outcomes from their surgery.

Music stimulates physiological changes by affecting brainwave states. Through measuring electrical impulses in the brain, neuroscientists have measured four bioelectric brainwave states, the beta, alpha, theta, and delta states. These states can be influenced by sound pulses within a musical composition, by a solo instrument, or by electronically generated pulses that match the frequencies of each of the brain states. The brain is stimulated to match the pulse of the music or entrain itself to their rhythm, a phenomenon known as "acoustic brainwave entrainment" (Cook & Thompson, 1999).

Brain waves are produced by the electrical activity of the brain cells. They can be measured with the electroencephalograph (EEG). The frequencies of these electrical waves are measured in cycles per second, or hertz (Hz). Brain waves change frequencies based on neural activity in the brain. They are closely tied to changes in mind or consciousness. Brainwave measurement shows that our states of mind fall into four general classes: beta (30-13 Hz), alpha (13-8 Hz), theta (8-3.5 Hz), and delta (3.5-0.5 Hz) (Cook & Thompson, 1999).

A music and imagery session can be enhanced by selecting music that enhances a specific brainwave state. For example, sound and music that entrain beta brainwaves arouse listeners, stimulate linear thinking, and enhance productivity. The mind is focused and active in beta. Beta brainwaves are also associated with anxiety. Alpha brainwaves produce a quiet, inner, and reflective mental state. The alpha state is easily accompanied by therapeutic imagery scripts and relaxation techniques. Theta brainwaves are found in waking and sleeping states. In sleep they are associated with dreaming. In waking states, deep insight and creativity are possible. Intense visualization, mental images, and emotional resolutions or insights are possible. Theta can be used in music-centered therapy sessions to help clients change core self-defeating behaviors. The delta brainwave state is associated with deep sleep, with the lowest metabolic rate, the lowest blood pressure, the lowest body temperature, and the slowest heart rate. It is a state of recuperation and physical healing (Cook & Thompson, 1999).

CONCLUDING REMARKS

Music combined with imagery facilitates healing. Music becomes an empty canvas on which to paint mental images. "Imagery from the right brain emerges in clusters of life-related metaphors, each encoded with significant symbolism" (Bush, 1995, p. 31). Musical elements have the ability to shift our state of consciousness to cause our critical faculties to recede.

Music-evoked imagery sessions allow us to override censorship. Once we relinquish control, images appear spontaneously. In an altered state of consciousness, experiences emerge from the unconscious. In a therapy session, this can lead to the completion of unresolved issues and the reintegration of disconnected and dissonant parts of ourselves. Music-enhanced imagery allows the mind to present material that helps reframe negative experiences and thinking into healthy connections and insights. Music has the ability to evoke and enhance visual imagery; therefore, it has developed into a vehicle, a medical technology for controlling voluntary and involuntary processes ranging from stress-management to facilitating self-transformation.

Interdisciplinary research in acoustics, music psychology, psycho-immunology, and psychology is providing new perspectives reinforced by empirical data that support the evolution of music in healing. Music with imagery provides a conduit through which we can access images, feelings, and memories that support the healing process. We respond universally to the power of a musical language and its harmonic, rhythmic, and melodic elements without having to learn it.

Therapists and sound healers access an individual's musical preferences, tolerances, cultural background, and overall sensitivity prior to prescribing music-enhanced or evoked imagery. Depending on the nature of the therapeutic intention, music may be chosen to mirror feelings, called the "iso" principle, or to oppose and challenge them. The therapist evaluates what the desired effect of the music session will be: to nudge the listener off a stuck position, to create an open, safe place to access disturbing memories, to cradle and support feelings of belonging, or to induce relaxation and a regulated heart and breath rate.

In a one-on-one process between a facilitator and client, imagery emerges while listening to music in a specific body position, or while being guided through a therapeutic visualization script. The challenge for the sound or music therapist in this case is to work with client-reported imagery as it is taking place to facilitate appropriate movement toward a therapeutic goal and to assess the type of imagery the client is reporting. This process can be likened to practices of indigenous healers, who evoke imagery through singing, drumming, and movement, while encouraging their patients to sing back their problems and report their visions, auditory images, hallucinations, and dreams.

The conscious use of music is a valuable service to both patient and health care professionals. Music and imagery assists the patient and their caregivers when anxiety, fear, confusion, denial, loneliness, boredom, depression, and pain become obstacles to finding physical, psychological, and spiritual wellness. Music has the ability to stimulate or contain varied experiences and support the patient in the healing process.

MUSIC SUGGESTIONS FOR IMAGERY AND HEALING

When choosing music to accompany imaging, it is important to set a specific length of time, ranging between 5 and 30 minutes. It is important to have a tablet and pen at hand to record any thoughts or images that may arise while listening. These images can be written down while listening or immediately afterwards.

For those who enjoy painting and sketching, it may be fruitful to have art materials nearby. Also, exercises should be done in a safe and comfortable environment, away from disturbances.

To prepare for a music and imagery experience, it is helpful to take a moment to focus on breathing, to take several deep breaths, and to relax.

Music for Relaxation and Imagery

Advanced Brain Technologies	Music for Relaxation
Albinon	Adagio
Arcangelos Chamber Ensemble	Hearts of Calm
J. S. Bach	Lute Suites
Don Campbell	The Mozart Effect, II
	Music for Healing the Body
Pat Cook and Jeffrey Thompson	Brainwave Symphony, "Alpha"
David Darling	Musical Massage, balance
Bill Douglas	Deep Peace
Janalea Hoffman	Therapeutic Drumming
Vyass Houston	Songs to Shiva (sacred songs)
Vyass Houston	Gayatri Mantra: The Sound of Light
David Ison	The Musical Body Tape Series
Daniel Kobialka	When You Wish Upon A Star
Monroe Institute	Deep 10 Relaxation
Joseph Nagler	Rejuvenation
Oruc Guvenc & Tumata	Rivers of One: The Rast Makam
	(Traditional Sufi Healing Music)
Pachelbel	Canon in D
Stan Richardson	Shakuhachi Meditation Music
Will Seachnasaigh	Dreamings: Aboriginal Healing Didjeridu

Music for Concentration and Learning

These musical selections can be played in the background while studying or writing.

Tommaso Albinoni	Oboe concerto in B-flat
Arcangelos Chamber Ensemble	Music for Concentration
J. S. Bach	Prelude and Fugue in G major
Don Campbell	Mozart Effect I, Strengthen the Mind. III Unlock the Creative Spirit
Gregorian Chant	Any recording available
Hayden	Cello Concerto in C, Moderato
Mendelssohn	Octet
Monroe Institute	Einstein's Dream
Monroe Institute	Baroque Garden
Monroe Institute	Concentration
Mozart	Concerto no. 5 in A major for violin Symphony in D major
Vivaldi	Five Concerti for Flute

Music to Match and Calm Anxiety

Arcangelos Chamber Ensemble	Relaxation
Bhaskar Chandavarkar	The Elements, Fire
Corelli	Concerti Grossi
Philip Glass	Pruit Igoe, from Koyaanisqatsi
Hebrew Traditional	Hatikvoh
Holst	Mars, The Bringer of War
Boris Mouraskin	Points of Light
Jeff Strong	Calming Rhythms
Vivaldi	Mandolin Concertos
Glen Velez	Rhythms of the Chakras

Music Sets for Multiple Use in Imagery and Healing

Cook and Thompson	Brainwave Symphony
Thompson	Brainwave Suite
East Indian Composers	The Elements
Don Campbell	The Mozart Effect
Don Campbell	The Mozart Effect for Children
Relaxation Company	Music for Health and Balance Series
Monroe Institute	Positive Immune Series
Monroe Institute	Surgical Support Series
Andrew Weil	Sound Body and Sound Mind

David Ison   Musical Body Series
Relaxation Company   The Yoga of Sound

REFERENCES

Achterberg, J. (1992). Drumming, shamanic work and healing: An interview by Don Campbell. In D. Campbell (Ed.), *Music and miracles*. Wheaton: Quest Books.

Aigen, K. (1998). *Paths of development in Nordoff-Robbins music therapy*. Gilsum: Barcelona Publishers.

Beck, G. L. (1995). *Sonic theology*. Delhi: Motilal Banarsidass Publishers.

Blacking, J. (1990). *How musical is man?* Seattle: University of Washington Press.

Bonny, H. L. (1978). *GIM Monograph 1: Facilitating GIM sessions*. Baltimore: ICM Books.

Bonny, H. L. (1979). *Music Rx for surgery* (Pamphlet). Baltimore: ICM Books.

Bonny, H. L., & Savary, L. (1990). *Music & your mind: Listening with a new consciousness*. Barrytown: Station Hill Press.

Brigham, D. D. (1994). *Imagery for getting well*. New York: Norton.

Bush, C. A. (1995). *Healing imagery and music*. Portland: Rudra Press.

Campbell, D. G. (1987). *The roar of silence*. Wheaton: Quest Books.

Campbell, D. G. (1991). *Music: Physician for times to come*. Wheaton: Quest Books,

Campbell, D. G. (1992). *Music and miracles*. Wheaton: Quest Books.

Campbell, D. G. (1997). *The Mozart effect*. New York: Avon Books.

Cook, P. M. (1997a). *Shaman Jhankri and Nele: Music healers of indigenous cultures*. Rosyln: Ellipsis Arts.

Cook, P. M. (1997b). Sacred music therapy in north India. In M. P. Baumann & L. Fujie (Eds.), *Music and healing in transcultural perspectives*. Bamberg: The University of Bamberg.

Cook, P. M., & Thompson, J. (1999). *Brainwave symphony booklet* (with compact discs). Rosyln: Relaxation Company.

Cook, P. M. (2000). Crosscultural music in healing. *Open Ear Journal, 28*(1), 193.

Coward, H., & Goa, D. (1996). *Mantra: Hearing the divine in India*. New York: Columbia University Press.

Crowe, B. (2000). The profession of music therapy in the United States. *Open Ear Journal, 28*(1), 170-173.

Danielou, A. (1995). *Music and the power of sound: The influence of tuning and intervals on consciousness*. Rochester: Inner Traditions.

Friedman, R. L. (2000). *The healing power of the drum*. Reno: White Cliffs Media.

Friedson, S. (1996). *Dancing prophets: Musical experience in Tumbuka healing*. Chicago: Chicago Press.

Gaynor, M. L. (1999). *Sounds of healing*. New York: Broadway Books.

Gilmor, T. M., Madaule, P., & Thompson, B. (1989). *The Tomatis method*. Toronto: The Listening Centre Press.

Gouk, P. (2000). *Musical healing in cultural contexts*. Aldershot: Ashgate.

Grof, S. (1985). *Beyond the brain: Birth, death and transcendence in psychotherapy*. New York: State University of New York Press.

Hoffman, J. (1995). *Rhythmic medicine: Music with a purpose*. Leawood: Jamillan Press.

Houston, V. (1997). Sanskrit: Planetary language of sonic healing. *Open Ear Journal,* *21*(2), 19-21.

Jarvis, J. (1988). Guided imagery and music (GIM) as a primary psychotherapeutic approach. *Music Therapy Perspectives, 5,* 69-72.

Kalweit, H. (1992). *Shamans, healers and medicine men.* Boston: Shambala.

Koepchen, H. P., Spintge, R., & Droh, R. (1992). Physiological rhythmicity and music in medicine. In R. Sprintge & R. Droh (Eds.), *MusicMedicine.* St. Louis: MMB, Inc.

Leeds, J. (1997). *Sonic alchemy: Conversations with leading sound practitioners.* Sausalito: InnerSong Press.

Leeds, J. (2001). *The power of sound: How to manage your personal soundscape for a vital, productive and healthy life.* Rochester: Healing Arts Press.

Leeds, J. & Wise, A. (2000). The making of sound body, sound mind. *Open Ear Journal,* *28*(1), 183-184.

Madaule, P. (1994). *When listening comes alive: A guide to effective learning and communication.* Norval: Moulin Publishers.

Monroe Institute. (1995a). *Positive immune booklet.* Faber: Interstate Industries, Inc.

Monroe Institute. (1995b). *Surgical support series booklet.* Faber: Interstate Industries, Inc.

Maranto, C. D. (1992). Music in the treatment of immune-related disorders. In R. Spintge & R. Droh (Eds.), *Musicmedicine.* St. Louis: MMB, Inc.

Mourashkin, B. (1997). Bio-energetic music. *Open Ear Journal, 20*(1), 2-8.

Pickett, E. (1995). Guided imagery and music: A technique for healing trauma. *Journal of the Association for Music & Imagery, 4,* 93-101.

Pinkerton, J. (1996). *The sound of healing.* Brooklyn: Alliance.

Radocy, R. E., & Boyle, J. D. (1997). *Psychological foundations of musical behavior.* Springfield: Charles C Thomas Publisher, LTD.

Rider, M. (1997). *The rhythmic language of health and disease.* St. Louis: MMB, Inc.

Rosch, P. J. (2000). The stress reduction effects of music. *Open Ear Journal, 28*(1), 8-11.

Rouget, G. (1985). *Music and trance: A theory of the relations between music and possession.* Chicago: University of Chicago Press.

Soule, D. (1995). The sound in inner resonance. *Open Ear Journal, 12*(4), 6-9.

Spintge, R., & Droh, R. (Eds.). (1992). *Musicmedicine.* St. Louis, MMB, Inc.

Schroeder-Shekar, T. (1997). Music for the dying. In J. Leeds (Ed.), *Sonic alchemy.* Sausalito: InnerSong Press.

Taylor, D. B. (1997). *Biomedical foundations of music as therapy.* St. Louis: MMB Music, Inc.

Tusler, R. L. (1991). *Music: Catalyst for healing.* Alkmaar, The Netherlands: Drukkeriji Krijgsman.

Warming, P. (1992). Psyche and sound. In D. Campbell (Ed.), *Music: Physician for times to come* (pp. 230-241). Wheaton, IL: Quest Books.

Wrangsjo, B., & Korlin, D. (1995). Guided imagery and music as a psychotherapeutic method in psychiatry. *Journal of the Association for Music & Imagery, 4,* 79-80.

Clinical Applications

CHAPTER 7

Healing Images: Connecting with Inner Wisdom

SHEILA M. BAER, AMY C. HOFFMANN,
AND ANEES A. SHEIKH

> When I asked Dr. [Albert] Schweitzer how he accounted for the fact that anyone could possibly expect to become well after having been treated by a witch doctor, he said that I was asking him to divulge a secret that doctors have carried around inside them ever since Hippocrates.
>
> "But I'll tell you anyway," he said, his face still illuminated by that half-smile. "The witch doctor succeeds for the same reason that all of us succeed. Each patient carries his own doctor inside of him. They come to us not knowing that truth. We are at our best when we give the doctor who resides within each patient a chance to go to work." (Cousins, 1980, pp. 68-69)

According to the above quote, the physician that is perhaps the most effective healer is not in an office but within the psyche of the individual. In the face of complex illness, knowledge of exactly what is out of order and how to regain order is maintained within the individual as unconscious material. This is not a new concept; many religions and spiritual traditions have posited the existence of an inner wisdom that guides and heals:

> Open yourself to the Tao, trust your natural responses and everything
>   will fall into place. (Taoism)
> The kingdom of heaven is within you. (Christianity)
> Look within, thou art the Buddha. (Buddhism)
> He who knows himself, knows God. (Islam)
> Atman (individual consciousness) and Brahman (universal
>   consciousness) are one. (Hinduism)

Furthermore, it has been asserted that this inner wisdom is inherent not only in humans, but in all beings and things in nature:

> Such a principle makes even more sense when we look around us and see that healing is a universal property of all creation. Life everywhere naturally tends toward wholeness and growth. Animals and plants are able to heal themselves

without the help of a doctor. Whole ecosystems heal themselves. Take, for example, a field in which trees have been cut. It will go through a slow process of regeneration—first with grasses, then with brush, and finally the return of trees. Even stars are capable of healing themselves as evidenced by Nova explosions. (Mein, 1989, p. 7)

Thus, the view may be taken that the nature of all things is health, which is maintained by an inherent wisdom of the right operation of all things. In order to regain health, one simply needs to tap into this unconscious store of inner wisdom to view the true origin of the problem and the manner in which it may be resolved.

Imagery has been used extensively as a means of accessing the unconscious for various reasons. Through imagery people have had experiences that defy the understanding of modern allopathic medicine. Examples of spontaneous healing, remission of chronic health problems (both physical and mental), and accounts of enlightenment and insight in the literature suggest an innate healing ability. Although this healing ability appears to manifest spontaneously, it may also be accessed through direct attempts to connect with the unconscious and the inner wisdom therein. Perhaps imagery, through its connection with the unconscious, is the royal road to this wisdom.

This chapter will provide the reader with an understanding of the healing power of imagery through its connection with inner wisdom. The chapter begins with a brief introduction to the paradigm shift from dualism to holism, followed by a discussion of the various ways in which our bodies possess an innate inner wisdom that may be accessed in the service of healing. Next, research supporting imagery as an alternative method of healing is reviewed. The underlying basis for the effectiveness of imagery in connecting with inner wisdom is discussed from two perspectives—the similarities between imaginal and sensorial perceptual processing and the depth of understanding accessed by imagery as opposed to verbal or linguistic processes. Finally, a variety of imagery techniques that utilize inner wisdom for the development of insight, healing, and transcendence will be presented.

THE PARADIGM SHIFT

Modern allopathic medicine is largely based on the Cartesian dualistic model. Under this prevailing paradigm it has been possible to study health and disease within the physical body without interference, yielding a detailed under-standing of anatomy and physiology. The body is seen as a separate entity from the mind and/or spirit, that may be affected negatively by the presence of a material causal pathogen, such as a bacterium or virus. Thus, dualism has focused on curing disease through elimination of the causal pathogen or disease/distress state (Chez & Jonas, 1997). Within this paradigm many advances in both medical and psychological treatment have been made.

As science explores the body, it adds details that reinforce this sense of wonder. For example, the heart beats a hundred thousand times every 24 hours and pumps 6,300 gallons of blood a day through 96,000 miles of blood vessels. To replenish this blood, 3 million new red blood cells are created every second. When one realizes that these are only a few of the thousands of operations continually going on in our body, one has to be filled with a sense of awe. The fact that over 70 trillion cells, each containing ten thousand more molecules than the Milky Way has stars, work in a coordinated fashion is, indeed, a miracle. (Mein, 1989, pp. 11-12)

As the above indicates, the processes of the human body are incomprehensibly vast; any paradigm that automatically or arbitrarily limits interaction between two or more subcomponents is bound to be lacking. In fact, despite the numerous benefits of the dualistic paradigm, it has fallen short of providing sufficient explanation for many processes of the human body. A systems-based, holistic framework, however, conceptualizes mental processes and physical states as interwoven and having significant effects upon each other, thereby increasing its explanatory power. However, this approach also raises important new issues regarding curing disease versus healing a person.

Within a holistic model, the view of mind and body has been expanded to acknowledge that our mental state can affect our physical state, and vice versa. Evidence exists to show that the negative emotions we experience may lead to or exacerbate certain physiological health problems (Carlson, 1998; Cobb & Rose, 1973; Cohen, 1953; Drugan, Basile, Ha, & Ferland, 1994; Gatchel, Baum, & Krantz, 1989; Jensen, Genefke, & Hyldebrandt, 1982; Kiecolt-Glaser, Marucha, Malarkey, Mercado, & Glaser, 1995; Locke & Colligan, 1986; Manuck, Kaplan, & Clarkson, 1983; Manuck, Kaplan, & Matthews, 1986; Sapolsky, 1986; Sapolsky, Krey, & McEwen, 1986; Theorell et al., 1992; Uno, Tarara, Else, Suleman, & Sapolsky, 1989; Weiss, 1969; Wood, Sheps, Elveback, & Schirder, 1984), as well as impair natural healing processes (Achterberg, 1984; Achterberg & Lawlis, 1979; Burns, 2000; File, 1996; Gilbert, Stunkard, Jensen, Detwiler, & Martinko, 1996; Kiecolt-Glaser, Page, Marucha, MacCallum, & Glaser, 1998; Petrie, Booth, & Pennebaker, 1998; Posluszny, 1999; Roberts & Weerts, 1982; Susman, Dorn, Inoff-Germain, Nottelmann, & Chrousos, 1997).

The evidence for the veridicality of the new paradigm raises questions regarding past definitions of health and disease. Health is defined as "the condition of being sound in body, mind, or spirit, especially freedom from physical disease or pain; a flourishing condition; well being" (Merriam-Webster, 1995), and as "a state of complete physical, mental and social well-being, and not just the absence of disease and infirmity" (World Health Organization, 1964). Disease is defined as "a condition of the living animal or plant body or one of its parts that impairs normal functioning" (Merriam-Webster, 1995). These definitions suggest a tripartite view of health, ranging from a state of flourishing well-being, to the absence of disease, to non-impaired functioning (and a similar view of disease, ranging from impaired functioning, to the presence of disease, to a lack of flourishing well-being).

A key tenet of mind-body medicine is that health is not the mere absence of disease; it is the dynamic integration of our environment, body, mind, and spirit (Chopra, 2000). Therefore, an essential difference between medical models that uphold dualism versus those that uphold a mind-body-spirit unity (nondualistic models) is the emphasis in treatment on curing versus healing the diseased state. One may be healed without being cured of the pathogenic state; one may suffer physically from chronic or terminal illness but nevertheless maintain a sense of dignity and inner peace throughout. Similarly, a person may be cured of a disease without being healed, and elimination of a pathogen does not necessarily eliminate feelings of fragmentation or imbalance.

To conclude, the shift away from Cartesian dualism toward an integrated view of the mind, body, and spirit has led to a revision of beliefs regarding the nature of symptoms, whether they are of a physical or psychological nature, and the causal mechanisms of disease. If the body and mind are not separate, but function as an integrated whole, then the ultimate health of the individual depends on the achievement of a balanced state within the body-mind rather than the absence of a pathogen. This balance depends not only on a physical being that is self-healing and self-regulating, but also on a mind that possesses natural wisdom concerning the proper balance and the mechanisms to assess and maintain it.

EVIDENCE AND EXAMPLES OF INNER WISDOM

Examples suggestive of an innate, inner wisdom that continually guides the individual toward flourishing well-being abound; these are particularly evident within the physiological systems of the body. The delicate balance maintained by the body's homeostatic processes; the coordinated activity, speed, and strength of the immune system; and the nature of spontaneous healing and the placebo effect, are all testaments to the astounding wisdom within. Since much of this work is conducted automatically, without the conscious awareness of the individual, it has generally been assumed that this wisdom resides within the unconscious. Thus, the individual functions not only as the healer and the one being healed, but also as the healing process itself. It is this view of the unconscious, as a unifying and regulating force working to achieve wholeness in the individual, that has led to the use of unconscious material for healing—both physical and psychological. Jaffe (1980) describes a similar process occurring within psychotherapy:

> The major premise of psychotherapy is that the wisdom to confront, under-
> stand, and resolve . . . dilemmas lies within each person. In the psycho-
> therapeutic process, the patient moves from his initial expectation that
> discovery will come from the outside (specifically his therapist) toward the
> ultimate discovery that the answers exist within the hidden corners of his
> own psyche. (pp. 228-229)

At the point when this awareness reaches consciousness, the patient often makes huge leaps toward recovery of his psychological health. As the patient begins to take more responsibility for his own and others' well-being, a snowball effect begins, in which competence and mastery increase, efficacy and coping are enhanced, and feelings of powerlessness, vulnerability, or despair diminish. Thus, just as the physiological system has the ability to regulate its inner environment and to heal itself when injured or invaded, the mental/emotional system has the ability to accommodate as well. While internal and external stresses may threaten to impair normal mental or emotional functioning, the ability to adapt or cope reduces their negative effects, thus playing a large role in promoting and maintaining mental health. This process may be considerably more effortful (i.e., conscious) than physiological self-regulation, although there is evidence to suggest the existence of an internal mechanism (i.e., inner wisdom) that automatically adapts or regulates responses to distressing events (Lambert & Bergin, 1994).

The most obvious evidence for inner wisdom and the body's innate capacity to heal itself is the immune system. It can destroy foreign and potentially health-threatening invaders, such as bacteria and viruses, and can also assist in wound healing. We are constantly bombarded with pathogens and insults from the environment, yet we become ill relatively infrequently. The large majority of pathogens we encounter in the environment fail to have a negative impact internally due to certain mechanisms of the body; chief among these are the autonomic nervous system (ANS) and the immune system. Together, these systems protect us from threats to our safety by increasing our ability to fight or flee from danger in the external environment via activation of the sympathetic division of the ANS, and by controlling and eliminating internal threats of disease via immune cell activation. Additionally, the parasympathetic division of the ANS controls functions that occur during a relaxed state, having a counteracting effect on the excitatory effects of the sympathetic division of the ANS, which, if prolonged, can be deleterious to health. These processes serve to maintain health by increasing the body's supply of stored energy, decreasing the body's heart rate, and increasing activity of the digestive system.

Inner wisdom is not limited to the immune system, however. Mein (1989) describes additional health-promoting processes, such as wound repair, that rely upon an inner sense of knowing for maintenance of a stable physiological organism:

> This amazing capacity to balance on the tightrope of health extends beyond our immune systems. Whether walking on the beach on a warm August day or on a cold January morning, our body's temperature is maintained at 98.6 degrees Fahrenheit. Similarly, almost regardless of what we eat, our blood makeup stays constant. It is this inner wisdom that allows us to recover from illnesses and other assaults on our well-being.
>
> A simple example of this innate healing ability that we often take for granted is wound repair. The entire sequence of events—from the wound

bleeding to cleanse itself to the blood clotting to form a scab to the redness and warmth signaling that the white blood cells have arrived to remove the debris and defend against infection—is a thing of beauty. This process has been so perfected that healing usually occurs without loss of sensation or movement to the area of the cut. (p. 4)

The human body contains numerous systems that work in concert to maintain a homeostatic norm that is stress and illness-free. One such system, the neuropeptide network, has been researched extensively by Candace Pert and her colleagues over the last 15 years. Neuropeptides are amino acid-based chemicals that have been found to lie at the heart of numerous experiences in people, including the experience of emotions within the brain and the rest of the body and emotions' effects on immunity (Pert, 1986, 1997). Initially, the limbic system was found to be enriched with receptors for the first neuropeptides identified, opiates, as well as for most of the other neuropeptides that were identified. Based on the role of the limbic system as the emotional center, the high concentration of opiate neuropeptide receptors in the limbic system, and the distribution pattern of the receptors in emotion-regulating areas of the brain (as well as their role as communicators), neuropeptides were hypothesized to be the chemical substrate of emotions (Pert, 1986, 1997; Pert, Ruff, Weber, & Herkenham, 1985).

Further research about neuropeptides and their function within the body as emotional information transmitters led to the discovery of the presence of receptors for the same neuropeptides elsewhere in the body, at nodal points (Pert, 1997). These nodal points are anatomically located in areas of the body that tend to receive a great deal of emotional modulation, such as the dorsal horn of the spinal cord (Pert, 1986). In addition, a mode of transmission that did not involve linear synaptic transmission seemed to be occurring. Rather, information transmission appeared to be directly linked to the specificity of the receptors. Hence, these substances were attaching to their receptors on various organs and having an effect within the body.

The groundbreaking discovery of receptors on traveling immune cells was the first step toward altering the traditional view that emotions arise solely in the brain. Research by Pert and colleagues (1985) identified receptors for nearly every neuropeptide, or "chemical of emotion," on human monocytes, a type of immune cell. In addition, not only do immune cells contain the receptors for neuropeptides, but they have also been found to manufacture the chemicals themselves. This was demonstrated through findings that immunocytes, or immune cells, store, synthesize, and secrete neuropeptides. Since neuropeptides are direct products of DNA without any enzyme regulation, there is little chance that the brain could be modulating their production (Pert, Dreher, & Ruff, 1998).

All of this neuropeptide activity occurs continuously in the body without conscious involvement of the person. The body and mind are aspects of a bi-directional communication system that maintains and regulates emotions as well as immunity through its own inner wisdom. Thus, Pert et al. (1998) have asserted that the bodymind can no longer be characterized as a hierarchical, hard-wired system with connections that descend down from the brain into the body. Rather, it needs to be conceptualized as an expansive network of free-flowing information transmitted by chemicals that can enter at any nodal points.

The placebo effect is another phenomenon that suggests the existence of a mind-body system in which inner wisdom regulates the process of healing. It has been invoked to account for spontaneous healing and pain relief, as well as physiological effects in direct opposition to a drug that has been administered (Rossman, 1987). Robert Delap, head of one of the Food and Drug Administration's Offices of Drug Evaluation, said: "Expectation is a powerful thing. The more you believe you're going to benefit from a treatment, the more likely it is that you will experience a benefit" (cited in Nordenberg, 2000, p. 14).

Herbert Benson, founder of the Harvard Mind/Body Medical Institute, refers to the placebo effect as *remembered wellness* (Benson, 1996). Much of his early research was driven by criticisms that his *relaxation response* was "nothing but a placebo effect" (Benson, 1996, p. 27), reflecting the predominant view of the medical community that the placebo effect was simply an irritating anomaly, undeserving of scientific scrutiny.

The *remembered wellness* model of healing promoted by Benson (1996) involves three interrelated aspects of healing: self-care, medications, and medical procedures. Self-care is described as the critical component which may elevate one's state of health from *absence of disease* to *flourishing wellness*, though all three aspects of healing are thought to be enhanced by remembered wellness. Benson conceptualizes remembered wellness as a product of beliefs and expectancies generated by the patient, the caregiver, and the relationship between the patient and the caregiver. These beliefs and expectancies, often triggered by healing rituals, have been found to generate a profound physiological response that affects the body's ability to heal. Unfortunately, the flip side of this mechanism is the power of belief to define oneself as "sick" or "weak." Patients may just as unwittingly create self-fulfilling prophecies, leading to an increased likelihood of illness, through identification with the label "sick."

Benson (1996) also recognizes the powerful healing that often results from spiritual beliefs and the capacity to live in accord with nature; this is the underlying basis for his suggestion that humans may be "wired for God" (1996, p. 198). Benson's experience with the impact of beliefs on health suggested to him that the most powerful belief, evidenced in rituals of worship and prayer to a higher power, may be a primal motive or survival instinct. Faith or belief in some greater meaning provides a mechanism for incorporating the certain knowledge of one's own mortality in a manner that promotes survival, similar to other innate or instinctual responses that have developed over time. This instinct involves finding significant meaning in one's life, through religious, spiritual, or other beliefs. This inspires us and helps us transcend the meaninglessness of our existence, generating a kind of hope inaccessible by reason alone. Since this faith transcends reality and experience to generate hope and expectancy, it evokes *remembered wellness*—the "neurosignature messages of healing that mobilize the body's resources and reactions" (Benson, 1996, p. 203).

The problem, according to Benson, is that we often fail to allow the inherent wisdom of the mind-body to emerge, either because we do not know how to access it or because we are conditioned to *act* rather than to wait for answers to present themselves. "Remembering" a state of health is the key, according to Benson, not learning something new. Critical in promoting one's health is to know you are the expert on what hurts or heals you, to trust your inner instincts, and to honor your beliefs and emotions:

> It is the client who knows what hurts, what directions to go, what problems are crucial, what experiences have been deeply buried. It began to occur to me that unless I had a need to demonstrate my own cleverness and learning, I would do better to rely upon the client for the direction of movement in the process. (Rogers, 1961, pp. 11-12)

IMAGERY AS A METHOD OF HEALING

Alternative methods of healing that rely on the power of the mind appear to be breaking through the barriers into mainstream medical practice as fast as new evidence supporting the changing paradigm is discovered. The National Institute of Health (NIH), one of the world's foremost biomedical research institutions, comprises 25 separate centers, including the National Center for Complimentary and Alternative Medicine (NCCAM) established in 1998. NCCAM was established by Congressional mandate for the purpose of facilitating the evaluation of alternative medical therapies in order to determine their effectiveness. Primarily a research and training organization, NCCAM is supported by the federal government; the FY2000 budget of $68.7 million testifies to the growing importance of alternative medicines and healing practices in the United States (NCCAM, 2000).

According to NCCAM,

> most traditional medical systems make use of the interconnectedness of the mind and body and the power of each to affect the other. During the past 30 years, a growing scientific movement has focused on the mind's capacity to affect the body. The clinical aspect of this enterprise is called mind-body medicine. Mind and body are so integrally related that it makes little sense to refer to therapies as having impact just on the mind or the body. Interest in the mind's role in the cause and course of cancer has been substantially stimulated by the discovery of the complex interactions between the mind and the neurological and immune systems, the subject of the rapidly expanding discipline of psychoneuroimmunology. (2000)

Within NCCAM, seven classifications of complimentary and alternative medicine (CAM) have been established. Within each of these classifications, specific practices are designated along a continuum with respect to degree of acceptance within conventional medicine. Those practices designated as "behavioral medicine" are among the most widely accepted and practiced, and those designated as "CAM" are among the least accepted and practiced. Imagery is classified by NCCAM as *Mind-Body Medicine: Mind-Body Methods*, and is designated as *behavioral medicine*, indicating a relatively large degree of acceptance and use within the conventional medical establishment. Other methods in this category include psychotherapy, meditation, hypnosis, biofeedback, and support groups.

NCCAM describes imagery as

> both a mental process (as in imagining) and a wide variety of procedures used in therapy to encourage changes in attitudes, behavior, or physiological reactions. As a mental process, it is often defined as "any thought representing sensory quality." It includes, as well as the visual, all the senses—aural, tactile, olfactory, proprioceptive, and kinesthetic. Imagery has been successfully tested as a strategy for alleviating nausea and vomiting associated with chemotherapy in cancer patients, to relieve stress, and to facilitate weight gain in cancer patients. It has been successfully used and tested for pain control in a variety of settings; as adjunctive therapy for several diseases, including diabetes, and with geriatric patients to enhance immunity. Imagery is usually combined with other behavioral approaches. It is best known in the treatment of cancer as a means to help patients mobilize their immune systems, but it also is used as part of a multidisciplinary approach to cardiac rehabilitation and in many settings that specialize in treating chronic pain. (2000)

Results of clinical trials at several large university and teaching hospitals and clinics provide ample evidence for the effectiveness of imagery and self-hypnotic relaxation in healing (see Dreher, 1998, for a review). Recent studies indicating support for the efficacy of imaginal techniques have been conducted at these centers: College of Physicians and Surgeons, Columbia University (Ashton et al., 1997); UCLA School of Medicine (Fawzy et al., 1993); Maine Medical Center, Central Maine Medical Center, and Eastern Maine Medical Center (Fillon, 2000); Harvard Medical School (Ginandes & Rosenthal, 1999; Irvin, Domar, Clark, Zuttermeister, & Friedman, 1996; Lang et al., 2000); Medical College of Wisconsin (Hudetz, Hudetz, & Klayman, 2000); University of Akron (Kolcaba & Fox, 1999); University College, London (Manyande et al., 1995); Medical College of Ohio (McGrady, Bush, & Grubb, 1997); Mount Sinai School of Medicine, NY (Pan, Morrison, Ness, Fugh-Berman, & Leipzig, 2000); University of Texas-Houston School of Public Health (Richardson et al., 1997); Department of Family Practice, University of Texas Health Science Center, San Antonio (Shrock, Palmer, & Taylor, 1999); Center for Stress Management and Research, Monash University, Victoria, Australia (Sharpley, 1994); Children's Hospital of Denver

(Smart, 1997); University of Arizona, Tucson (Song, Schwartz, & Russek, 1998); Stanford University (Tiller, McCraty, & Atkinson, 1996); University of Wisconsin-Green Bay (Wichowski & Kubsch, 1999); University of Akron (Wynd, 1992a); and Cleveland Clinic Foundation (Tusek, Church, Strong, Grass, & Fazio, 1997; Wynd, 1992b).

Imagery as a Tool for Accessing Inner Wisdom

Imagery has been shown to be a highly effective tool for accessing inner wisdom, primarily due to a unique ability to access deeper modes of understanding than those accessed through more linear verbal reasoning and expression. The technique of imagery has been used successfully in psychotherapy for several years. Additionally, research has begun to show strikingly consistent similarities between imaginal and sensorial perceptual processing. Dadds, Cutmore, Novbjerg, and Redd (1997) reviewed research linking neurological processes involved in imagery with those involved in perceptual responses. Their review indicates that imagery resembles actual perception, produces psychophysiological responses, and is associated with relevant behavioral responses.

Imagery Resembles Sensory Perception. Strong evidence for the notion that the formation of a mental image resembles the actual perception of the corresponding external stimuli has been reviewed by Finke (1985) and Kosslyn (1988, 1994). It appears that humans generate a mental image of a stimulus by activating and integrating stored perceptual information; thus, when creating an image of an apple, information related to the visual characteristics of apples (red, round, with a stem) is made available to the visual system, which then "constructs" an apple as if the person were actually perceiving it (Kosslyn, 1988).

Three main lines of evidence support this proposition. First, vision and visual imagery share a common neural basis. Studies using measures of localized cerebral blood flow, electrocephalography (EEG), and event-related potentials (ERP) have shown that localized areas of the brain involved in visual processing are selectively activated during visual imagery tasks (Farah, 1988; Kosslyn, 1988).

Second, substantial evidence indicates that perception and imagery share common functional properties (Kosslyn, 1988, 1994). Segal and Fusella (1970) showed that holding a mental image interferes with perception tasks that rely on the same sensory mode, but not tasks involving different sensory modes. For example, instructing participants to visualize an apple impairs visual perception more than it impairs auditory perception, and vice versa for an auditory image. Other studies by Kosslyn (1994) indicate that the resolution possible between two closely spaced dots is similar whether a participant is working with imagery or physical stimuli. A similar finding occurs for the resolution possible for vertical and horizontal lines versus obliquely parallel lines (Kosslyn, 1987).

Third, extensive evidence from clinical neuropsychology shows that damage to visual areas of the brain causes parallel dysfunction in both sensory and imaginal systems. Patients with damage to the right parietal lobe who have difficulty scanning their left visual field also have problems scanning the left side of a mental image (Bisiach & Luzzatti, 1978; Farah, 1988). Particularly strong evidence comes from studies of color perception, which have repeatedly shown that acquired deficits in the perception of color are associated with similar deficits in color imagery (see Farah, 1988, for a review).

Thus, there is strong evidence that the generation, manipulation, and scanning of mental images is functionally similar to the processes involved in perceiving the external world, and that image formation uses neural sensory processing mechanisms in abstract information processing about absent or imagined stimuli.

Imagery Produces Psychophysiological Responses. A substantial body of literature indicates that when humans engage in mental imagery involving certain kinds of noxious or salient stimuli (e.g., violence, phobic stimuli, and aversive stimuli such as toxic foods), reliable changes in physiology and subjective arousal occur (King, 1973; Lichstein & Lipshitz, 1982; Marzillier, Carroll, & Newland, 1979; Pitman, Orr, Forgue, de Jong, & Claiborn, 1987). Similarly, mental imagery of relaxing scenes is reliably associated with decreases in physiological arousal (Carroll, Marzillier, & Merian, 1982; Lang, 1979), making imagery-induced relaxation a standard intervention for a number of medical disorders that are aggravated by psychophysiological factors (e.g., insomnia, headache). One of the most rigorous demonstrations that mental contents can directly influence a physiological response was undertaken by Barber, Chauncey, and Winer (1964). Participants were asked to drink either water or a citric acid solution prior to measuring salivation. Participants who imagined that the water was sour showed increased salivation, and those who imagined that the citric acid was water showed decreased salivation. Numerous studies have demonstrated the power of imagery to produce physiological changes across a wide variety of systems, including changes in heart rate, blood pressure, skin and body temperature, breathing rate, blood glucose, pupillary dilation, vasodilation for blood flow to the brain and muscles, gastrointestinal activity, gastric-acid secretion, and blister formation. In fact, imagery has been suggested as possibly the only practical method of controlling several autonomic responses (Miller, 1972).

Imagery is Associated with Behavioral Responses. There is also substantial evidence for a link between imagery and behavioral responses. As early as the 1930s, Jacobson demonstrated that muscular movement corresponds with the content of mental imagery; for example, vertical eye movement was observed when participants were asked to imagine themselves looking at the Eiffel Tower (Jacobson, 1932). Similarly, Lusebrink and McGuigan (1989) showed that when participants with high imagery skills imagined words beginning with "p" or "b" they produced corresponding lip movement, and when they imagined objects such as a pencil they produced movement in the preferred writing arm. These findings provide further evidence that people process mental images in much the same manner as actual physical stimuli.

As this review indicates, a variety of innovative methods of studying imagery have been designed. Kosslyn's (1987, 1988) method—imposing tasks that require the use of imagery for their solution—has been particularly useful. It not only provides a methodology by which various characteristics of image formation may be quantified, but it also reduces reliance on participants' subjective descriptions and self-reports. Overall, then, evidence based on localization of neural function, psychophysiological responses, and behavioral indices suggests that when participants report that they are generating, scanning, or manipulating a mental image, they are actually doing so.

Imagery is Involved in the Development and Treatment of Psychological Disorders. The notion that conscious and unconscious mental images may be involved in the development and maintenance of traumatic reactions is not new; this has been a central theme in psychodynamic theory since Freud first suggested it. Ericksonian hypnotherapy also asserts that unconscious images (e.g., internal maps of the world or schema), rather than sensory experience alone, are major determinants of people's actions (Lankton & Lankton, 1983). Unconscious or internal images also play a central role in contemporary theories of posttraumatic stress disorder (PTSD; Brett & Ostroff, 1985). Imagery also provides the underlying basis for a variety of treatment approaches, including behaviorally-oriented exposure treatments and experiential therapy.

Images appear to represent goal objects (McMahon, 1973), acting as motivators for future behavior (Mowrer, 1977; Sarbin & Coe, 1972). According to Shephard (1978) and Tower and Singer (1981), individuals often act more on the basis of imagined than actual consequences. Images seem to provide a unique representation consisting of the integration of perception, motivation, subjective meaning, and realistic abstract thought (Shorr, 1980). Meaning and emotional responses to objects appear to be contained in images rather than in verbal representations (Arieti, 1976; Bugelski, 1970; Forisha, 1979); images appear to have a greater affinity for emotionally laden associations than the more linear verbal processing mode (Sheikh & Panagiotou, 1975). In addition, imagery has unique capabilities regarding past events—not only does imagery allow one to maintain contact with phenomenological experiences from the past (Singer, 1979), but preverbal experiences may be accessible only through imagery (Sheikh & Panagiotou, 1975). Singer (1974) notes that spontaneous images often emerge in therapeutic settings when exploration through verbal means becomes blocked; imagery appears to "outwit" the defenses that are causing the blockage. According to Horowitz (1970), this is possible because imagery provides a medium by which unconscious material may enter consciousness, bypassing the more critical mechanisms of verbal expression.

In summary, the similarity of neurological and experiential characteristics to sensory processing, as well as the more unique integrated or holistic effects of visual as opposed to linguistic processing, provide the bases for imagery's effectiveness in clinical and therapeutic settings, and thus in accessing inner wisdom.

IMAGERY TECHNIQUES TO CONNECT WITH INNER WISDOM

Several imagery techniques for connecting with inner wisdom are described in the following sections, including imagery and relaxation, the inner advisor, dialogue with symptoms, a rose opening, and temple of silence.

Imagery and Relaxation

Relaxation, that peaceful state in which mental anxiety and muscle tension are at a minimum, is the essential common denominator of all forms of healing imagery. Relaxation actually serves two very important functions with respect to healing imagery and connecting with inner wisdom. First, relaxation has numerous beneficial side effects of its own, such as reducing the breathing rate, heart rate, and other signs of autonomic arousal. Prolonged practice with relaxation, like meditation, has been shown to reduce blood pressure, to alleviate psychological or emotional difficulties involving anxiety, fear, anger, and depression, and to enhance the body's natural healing powers (Fanning, 1994). Second, by eliminating the distractions of the outer world, relaxation provides the peaceful environment necessary for imaginal and intuitive thinking to emerge. In fact, relaxation may lead to a special state of awareness that facilitates access to inner wisdom. The following section outlines the important role of relaxation as a component of healing imagery, describes the most common methods of achieving total body-mind relaxation, and focuses on various healing images used to elicit or enhance relaxation.

Relaxation helps to still the active and demanding external world, allowing attention to be drawn slowly inward to the realm of imaginal experience: "Imagery comes very well and very richly during highly relaxed states" (Gendlin, 1981, p. 71). According to Singer (1974, p. 226) relaxation is "conducive to the occurrence or awareness of imaging and ongoing daydreams." Relaxation helps allay chronic fear and anxiety, and effectively interrupts the nearly constant inner chatter within the mind, both of which interfere with intuitive functioning and inhibit access to inner wisdom. Thus, relaxation is much more than a physiological process, it is psychological as well:

> Beyond physically relaxing, we need to clear our minds of all the busy-ness, the "mental noise"—analyzing, worrying, judging, remembering, looking ahead, comparing, associating, and scanning the environment—that

we normally do. It is only when the mind has quieted down that the weaker signal of our intuitive voice can be heard. (Naparstek, 1997, p. 54)

There are numerous methods of relaxation, but most include a mental device to block distracting thoughts (e.g., a focus), a passive and accepting attitude, a quiet environment, a comfortable position, and a set of behavioral techniques which have been previously conditioned to induce relaxation, such as deep abdominal breathing and peaceful images (Benson, 1976; McCaffery & Beebe, 1989). Nearly all relaxation and imagery exercises begin with the suggestion to "close your eyes and relax." For experienced users, this is typically sufficient to set in motion the physiological changes in muscle relaxation and breathing that lead to total body-mind relaxation.

The two most commonly mentioned aspects of relaxation are a loosening of physical tension and proper breathing. Beginners often learn to reduce physical tension through a procedure called *progressive muscle relaxation* (PMR), first described in 1929 by physician Edmund Jacobson in his book *Progressive Relaxation*. The procedure, simple to learn and to perform, consists of alternately tensing and relaxing different muscles throughout the body, while fully experiencing the different sensations associated with the two states. The second basic component of relaxation, proper breathing, is essential in order to provide an adequate supply of oxygen to the bloodstream and to enhance a deeper sense of relaxation. The basic PMR procedure, along with a variety of shortcuts for more experienced users, will be described in the following sections, followed by a review of both basic and specialized breathing techniques.

Basic PMR Technique. The basic PMR technique alternates between tensing muscles for about 5 seconds, and relaxing muscles for about 15 seconds; two sets of tensing/relaxing are generally performed for each muscle group. In addition, many people find it helpful to repeat a silent affirmation, such as the following from Fanning (1994, p. 36): *I'm letting go of the tension/ I'm throwing the tension away/ I feel calm and rested/ Let the tension melt away.*

Begin in a comfortable position, either lying down or sitting, with arms and legs uncrossed, and eyes closed. Clench your right fist for about 5 seconds, squeezing harder and harder, feeling the tension and tightness increase as you clench even harder—focus all your attention on the feeling of tightness in your fist. Now relax your fist for about 15 seconds—again, focus all your attention on the sensation of looseness in your fist. Pay special attention to the difference in sensation between tensing and loosening. Do this twice for your right fist, then repeat for your left fist, and then do both fists together. Next, bend your elbows and tense your biceps, holding the tension for about 5 seconds. Straighten your arms as you relax; perform twice with each arm.

Next, move your attention up to your head, scalp, forehead, and face. Beginning with your forehead, wrinkle your brow as tightly as you are able, and then relax—feel the smoothing of your brow as the tension disappears. Move on to your face, alternately tensing and relaxing your eyes, cheeks, jaw, tongue, and lips. Now focus on your neck; press your head back as far as possible and feel the tightness; gently roll your head to the right, and to the left, and then let your head drop down in front so your chin is resting on your chest. Feel the tension at each point and the corresponding lack of tension as you relax. Now move down to your shoulders—raise them as high as you can and hold. As your shoulders drop, feel the relaxation spreading from your head through your neck to your shoulders, arms, and hands.

Shift your attention to your torso; breathe in as deeply and slowly as you can, and hold for a couple of seconds, noting the tension in your chest. As you exhale, relax your chest, feeling the sensation of looseness. Repeat this step several times, releasing more and more tension with each exhalation. Now place your hand on your stomach, breathing in deeply so that your hand rises with each breath. Feel the relaxation continue to spread with each breath. Move down to your back, and arch your back, feeling the tightness in your lower back, and relax (do not arch your back if you have back problems, simply focus on relaxing those muscles).

Move down to your lower body, tightening the muscles in your buttocks and thighs, then to your calves and feet. Point your toes toward the floor as tightly as you can, feeling the tension in your feet and calves, then flex your toes upward, feeling the tight pull on your shins as you stretch those muscles.

Finally, allow your attention to focus on your entire body—feel the relaxation spreading from your feet and ankles up through your calves, thighs, and buttocks, to your stomach, back, and chest, out to each arm, hand, and finger, now up through your shoulders to your neck, face, and scalp. Do a final scan of your entire body, searching for any remaining pockets of tension, and repeat the tension/relaxation routine as necessary.

If you practice this procedure for about 15 minutes twice daily, in a week or two you should be able to achieve total body-mind relaxation fairly easily. At this point, you may want to experiment with your own procedures, or try one of the several shortcut procedures designed to induce relaxation quickly.

Shortcut Relaxation Procedure. You may want to try tensing and relaxing your muscles in combinations of major muscle groups simultaneously. Begin with your hands and arms, tightening your fists and biceps; then move on to your face, neck, and shoulders. Next, tense your back and chest together by arching your back, taking in a deep breath, and tightening your stomach; then relax. Finally, move down to your buttocks, thighs, calves, and feet, tensing your leg muscles and pointing your toes down, then up.

Once you have become adept at shortcuts, or quick induction of relaxation, you may require only a simple body scan to determine where the tension in your body is and to release it. You should then be able to enter a state of total body-mind relaxation relatively quickly, at will.

Basic Breathing Techniques. How you breathe is crucial to your emotional and physical state. Proper breathing can help lead you to relaxation, while improper or shallow breathing, filling only the top portion of your lungs, may lead to an increase in anxiety and tension. Proper breathing is deep and slow, with the breath filling the lower portion of your lungs first, and then filling the upper portion.

Assume a comfortable position, close your eyes, and place your hand over your stomach; focus on filling the space beneath your hand. When your lungs are filling from the bottom your stomach will rise first, followed by your chest. As you exhale, your stomach should fall back down first, followed by your chest, as your lungs empty from the bottom up. Repeat this at a steady pace, holding each in-breath and out-breath for a couple of seconds before moving on; maintain your focus on a smooth and steady rhythm of breathing, so that your stomach and chest are rising and falling in the patterns suggested above.

Two specialized breathing exercises, one designed for cleansing the other for enhancing energy, are described next.

Cleansing Breath. This is an adaptation of an ancient eastern breath exercise designed to enhance physical, mental, and spiritual development. Begin as before, breathing in deeply and slowly to a natural rhythm. As you inhale, imagine your breath as white steam or fog, and see yourself inhaling this pure white cleansing cloud through the heels of your feet. See the cloud enter your body through the heels of your feet, and sweep up one side of your body, picking up debris and toxins along the way. As your lungs become full, imagine the cloud has reached your head, still cleansing and purifying. As you exhale, visualize the cleansing cloud sweeping down the other half of your body, collecting additional impurities as it passes, finally exiting through your toes. As your lungs empty, the cloud leaves the body and disintegrates into the air around it, along with all the negative particles and toxins removed from your body. Repeat this exercise as many times as necessary to feel cleansed and purified; with each pass of the cleansing breath, see your body growing brighter, lighter, and more pure.

Energizing Breath. This breathing exercise is designed to impart a sense of power, vibrancy, enthusiasm, and glowing health. It is similar to the cleansing breath, although the images are designed to energize rather than cleanse.

Begin as before, in a comfortable position, with your eyes closed. Visualize the air you inhale as white light, filling your lungs and chest. As you exhale, see the white light expand, filling every niche in your body with energizing white light. Repeat this exercise several times; imagine more energy entering with each inhalation. You may want to experiment with different techniques or combinations of colors, intensities, even vibrations, to find the best method for you.

Relaxation Images. This final section lists a variety of relaxing images from Fanning (1994) that may be used to evoke or deepen relaxation. Because images are highly subjective, no single image will have the same effect on any two people, and you may want to use your own spontaneous images.

Twisted ropes, untwisting and going slack
Ice or butter melting
Harsh red light changing to soft blue or white light
Musical discords changing to harmonious chords
Peaceful forest glade or meadow
Blankets being piled high to make you warm and heavy
Warm sunlight
Beach scene with warm sand, surf noise, soaring gulls
Your limbs being gently covered with warm, heavy sand
Rocking in a hammock or cradle
Crumpled paper being smoothed out
Waves subsiding to ripples, ripples to glassy smoothness
A warm bath
A gentle massage

The remaining sections of this chapter will present several healing imagery techniques for connecting with inner wisdom.

The Inner Advisor

What I call coming to terms with the unconscious, the alchemists call medi-tation [Ruland says of this]: "Meditation, the name of an internal talk of one person with another who is invisible, as in the invocation of the Deity, or communion with one's self, or with one's good angel." (Jung, 1963, p. 497)

Carl Jung specified in the above quote the action of connecting with some inner being who embodies the unconscious in the service of healing and/or development. The process by which contact with this inner wisdom is made has been touted by practitioners of Jungian psychoanalysis as active imagination, so-called because the ego plays an active role in dropping into a fantasy state and working with images that arise during this state in the service of growth (Hannah, 1976). This process has been described as the very essence of psychological transformation (Dallett, 1984); it is not specific to one particular method, but can be present in various spontaneous activities, such as drawing mandalas, building sand castles, experiencing visual images, and communicating with unconscious figures (Watkins, 1976). In addition, all images experienced through the process of active imagination are viewed as symbolic manifestations of the unconscious and its contents (Watkins, 1976). Jung (1963) describes the actual process of active imagination as follows:

Take the unconscious in one of its handiest forms, say a spontaneous dream, a fantasy, an irrational mood, an affect, or something of the kind, and operate with it. Give it your special attention, concentrate on it, and observe its alterations objectively. Spare no effort to devote yourself to this task, follow the subsequent transformations of the spontaneous fantasy attentively and carefully. Above all, don't let anything from the outside, that does not belong, get into it, for the fantasy image has "everything it needs." (p. 79)

Thus, active imagination allows unconscious elements of thought to come to the fore in visual form through their association with parallel elements. For this reason, it is believed that Jung felt that active fantasy was one of the highest forms of psychic activity, in that both conscious and unconscious are allowed to flow together as a united common product in the service of healing and development through utilization of the transcendent function (Hannah, 1976).

Jung was the first Western practitioner to use techniques utilizing the process of active imagination to contact inner wisdom, the high Self, or the inner physician, etc. Specifically, Jung was the first practitioner who attempted contact with an internal image of inner wisdom and used this image and its alterations to serve the personal development of the client. Jung felt that merely observing how a fragment of fantasy develops while holding ego consciousness at bay yields information on the unconscious processes of the psyche at work in the individual (Stein, 1984). This process and its concomitant results are theoretically identical to the practice of the Inner Advisor technique. In fact, Oyle (1975) drew directly from the practice of active imagination when he first began working with the inner advisor technique. Since Oyle (1975), numerous other researchers and practitioners of imagery techniques have expanded upon Jung's original ideas of using inner wisdom in the service of healing. These will be described in sections to come.

The inner advisor technique, sometimes also called *inner dialogue* (Ferrucci, 1983), is so named due to an assumption that through the imagery experience, the individual dialogues with an inner advisor who is a symbolic emanation of inner wisdom, the inner physician, or the high Self (Shore, 1993). Various people have created and used inner advisor imagery scripts to facilitate this dialogue in the service of healing and gaining insight (Bresler & Trubo, 1979; Emery, 1999; Ferrucci, 1983; Houston, 1982; Jaffe, 1980; Rossman, 1987; Samuels & Bennett, 1978). The inner advisor is most frequently viewed as a liaison or ambassador between the conscious and the unconscious (Shore, 1993). The process of change, therefore, is understood to occur because the body is a self-regulating mechanism under the control of the psyche or unconscious (Shore, 1993). This technique, according to Ferrucci (1983), avails itself of hidden truth within the person, typically hidden in the realm of the unconscious. Through accessing the contents of the unconscious through an evolved superconscious aspect of oneself, insight may be gained and healing may be facilitated.

Although physiological or psychological symptom reduction may occur due to a dialogue between the inner advisor and the symptoms, it is not the sole benefit (Shore, 1993). Symptoms are not seen as residing solely within the body. Rather, the presenting problem and corresponding symptoms are actually seen as a message from the unconscious that perceives itself to have been driven into opposition or conflict. Through the use of imagery, the client takes a conscious attitude of listening to and cooperating with the unconscious, thus changing the nature of the presenting problem (Shore, 1993; Rossman, 1987). Thus, it can be stated that the goal of therapy using the inner advisor technique is increased communication with the unconscious.

There are currently many different views regarding the meaning, significance, and contents of the inner advisor. Archetypal images from analytical psychology that share a strong resemblance to the inner advisor are the crone, the wise old man, the wild woman (Estes, 1995; Robertson, 1987, 1995; Signell, 1990), and the Self (Signell, 1990; Singer, 1994). In particular, the Self is a body of wholeness in connection to the conscious and unconscious. Thus, it allows for the development and maintenance of wholeness through being able to relate to the world consciously while drawing on the wisdom of the unconscious. When viewed as an advisor image, perhaps as a wise old man or woman, people are allowed to tap into its healing and illuminating energy (Ferrucci, 1983).

In attempting to understand the nature of the inner advisor, more recent theories have sought to create an equivalence between the unconscious, the right hemisphere of the brain, and the intuition of the individual (Bresler & Trubo, 1979). In specific, one of these theories posits a relationship between the inner advisor and the unconscious, where the inner advisor acts as a liaison between the rational, conscious mind and the information held within the unconscious (Rossman, 1987). An additional recent conceptualization for the inner advisor is that of an inner doctor who resides in the unconscious and "will become your alter ego, advisor, or helper" (Samuels & Bennett, 1978, p. 6). Finally, other conceptualizations have described the inner advisor as a made-up form who can tap into unconscious information and bring it back in usable form (Jaffe, 1980), as the embodiment of the superconscious Self of the individual (Ferrucci, 1983), and as the intuitive healer within (Emery, 1999).

The common aspect among all of these views is that the inner advisor has access to the unconscious. By accessing the wisdom of the unconscious, clients can gain a new perspective on their symptoms or presenting problems and often experience relief by utilizing a new way of thinking about what is happening within them. Through maintenance of a regular dialogue with the inner advisor, people are enabled to rely on the wisdom of their own Self rather than following pressures outside of their highest essence (Ferrucci, 1983).

Therapeutic use of the inner advisor begins by inviting the client to relax and imagine a special place of safety, peace, and comfort, where contact with an inner advisor figure can occur, and, hopefully, some information relating to the presenting problem can be obtained (Shore, 1993). The meeting between the client and the advisor may take place in one session, immediately following induction into relaxation, or it may need to be preceded by several relaxation sessions and imagery-building inductions (Shore, 1993). The success of the inner advisor technique lies in the client's belief that it works, as well as in the client's ability to obtain and work with relatively vivid images (Shore, 1993). Therefore, progression through all of the phases of an inner advisor imagery session should be done at the client's pace rather than based on an agenda of the therapist (Shore, 1993).

Although different therapists may use variations on these phases, the general progression of an inner advisor imagery session is as follows. The first phase involves guiding, in which the technique is introduced and explained to the client. Phase two involves inducting the client into general relaxation. Any relaxation induction that the therapist and client find effective may be used, and there is no time limit on the length of the relaxation induction. Once relaxation has been achieved to the satisfaction of both the client and the therapist, the therapist initiates phase three by asking the client to go to a special place in his/her "mind's eye" or imagination. This place should evoke feelings of peace, safety, and comfort for the client; it can be an actual location or a place that is imagined (Shore, 1993). When the client tells the therapist that he/she is at the special place, the therapist asks a series of questions to allow the client to fully experience the imagery with different sensory modalities (Shore, 1993). This phase should continue until the therapist has determined the vividness of the client's imagery, the predominant sensory modality being used by the client, and the affective state of the client in relation to this imagery (Shore, 1993).

Once the special place has been explored, the therapist moves the client into the next phase: the client is asked to find a spot in the image where he/she can pause and rest for a few moments (Shore, 1993). When the client reports having found this spot, he/she is instructed to look around and to report on the first living creature that he/she sees (or hears, smells, etc.) (Shore, 1993). Enhancement of the imagery of the creature progresses in the same manner as for the special place (Shore, 1993). It is assumed that the creature contacted represents an inner advisor figure. At this time the therapist guides the client through a dialogue with the advisor. Initial questions include obtaining the name of the advisor and often involve striking a deal with the advisor; the advisor may agree to dialogue with the client if the client fulfills conditions set forth by the advisor (Shore, 1993).

Fulfillment of the agreement made by the client constitutes the next part of the session (Shore, 1993). This may also require ascertaining the primary communication method of the advisor, which may be gestures or noises rather than direct verbal communication (Shore, 1993). Upon completion of contacting the advisor, obtaining the name, and meeting conditions for dialoguing, the therapist may begin to facilitate a dialogue between the advisor and the client using the prearranged, open-ended questions concerning the presenting problem of the client (Shore, 1993). The therapist continues to guide the question and answer session by deciding the order in which questions should be asked, and, depending on the answers received, which questions should be asked as follow-ups (Shore,

1993). The therapist should also record the advisor's answers, since the client often does not remember important details or points made by the advisor and may need to be reminded when he/she returns to waking consciousness (Shore, 1993). Dialoguing proceeds between the client and the advisor until there is a transition in the dialogue. At this time, the therapist invites the client to ask if the advisor has any concluding remarks (Shore, 1993). Once the advisor concludes the dialogue, the client is then instructed to thank the advisor for dialoguing with him/her, and for anything in particular that the client has gained (Shore, 1993). The therapist also instructs the client to ask the advisor if the advisor wishes the client to do anything before they meet again, and if the advisor is willing to meet with the client again (Shore, 1993). If the advisor agrees to meet again, a mutually agreed upon time and place for that meeting is set (Shore, 1993). The client then says goodbye and is gently brought back to full, waking consciousness by the therapist (Shore, 1993).

The final phase of treatment involves consultation between the therapist and the client about the experience of contacting the inner advisor, and any possible gains. The therapist also answers any questions that the client may have (Shore, 1993). This discussion may deal with what, if anything, the client will do differently in the coming week as a result of having spoken with the advisor, or with the client's feelings about the advice from the advisor (Shore, 1993). The therapist also encourages the client to honor the future meeting with the advisor, or, if the meeting cannot be honored, to contact the advisor to explain the change and reschedule (Shore, 1993).

One prominent feature of this technique that is shared by many other techniques that contact inner wisdom is the utilization of the unconscious to achieve insight about current concerns or conditions. Through using the inner advisor, a symbolization of inner wisdom that has access to all of the information of the unconscious, a person is able to gain insight not previously available and to use this in the service of personal growth.

Dialogue with Symptoms

Engaging in a dialogue with one's symptoms is another method of accessing inner wisdom. In this technique, the individual focuses directly on the source of the problem—the symptom itself—using receptive imagery to promote understanding of the symptom's purpose and what is required in order for healing to begin. The following section explores the notion of symptoms as messages, and describes the most common meanings and functions of symptoms. This is followed by a description of various techniques for entering into an imaginal dialogue with symptoms or illness, in order to contact one's inner wisdom and natural healing abilities.

Pain, a primary symptom, conveys the message that something is wrong, encouraging the body to take action in order to prevent further injury. From an evolutionary perspective, it is one of the most powerful ways to insure the survival of an organism in a dangerous world. However, pain may also be a symptom generated by one's inner wisdom, frequently as a message concerning the process of change (Bresler, 1992).

Symptoms may also reflect one of several additional unconscious processes. LeCron (in Edelstein, 1981) suggested seven common unconscious reasons for the development of symptoms. 1) The symptom may be a symbolic physical expression of feelings the individual is otherwise unable to express. This is often called "organ language"—a broken heart, a pain in the neck, not being able to stomach something, getting cold feet, feeling weak in the knees, putting something behind you, and so on. 2) The symptom may be the result of the unconscious acceptance of a negative idea or image implanted earlier in life, such as "you're a bad girl, and no one worthwhile could ever love you." The images we form of ourselves in our earliest years are frequently the basis for unconscious patterns later in life. 3) Symptoms may be the result of an unconscious need for self-punishment; this is often the result of the negative childhood messages described above. Alternatively, the symptom may be an unconscious attempt to atone for a traumatic event for which the individual feels responsible. 4) The symptom may result from highly emotional and traumatic experiences from the past that have been generalized; these experiences are often the basis of phobias. 5) The symptom may provide certain benefits, or solve a particular problem. This aspect was further explored by Simonton, Matthews-Simonton, and Creighton (1978), who compiled a list of the five most common benefits of illness listed by cancer patients. These benefits included: having permission to avoid dealing with problems; receiving attention, care, and nurturing from others; having the opportunity to regroup psychologically; finding motivation for personal growth or for modifying undesirable habits; and not having to meet the high expectations of others (or themselves). 6) The symptom may be the result of an unconscious identification with an important, beloved person in one's life. The "anniversary illness," a well-known phenomenon in medicine, occurs when people fall ill on the anniversary date of a loved one's death, frequently exhibiting similar symptoms to those experienced by the deceased. 7) Finally, the symptom may be a manifestation of an inner conflict. There may be an unmet need or desire that is forbidden by family, friends, society, or one's own inner judgment; the symptom may either prevent the individual from carrying out the forbidden action, or it may allow him to fulfill the desire symbolically.

One unfortunate aspect of our rushed and often thoughtless modern times is that people are less and less inclined to be in touch with their bodies; people are generally unaware of how well their body is functioning, or whether it requires special attention or care. Jaffe (1980) recommends two techniques which may be useful in enhancing awareness of the body's current state of health.

The first technique involves exploring how your body tends to respond to stressful events. First, draw a timeline across the bottom of a large sheet of paper, with marks for each five-year period. Above the line mark important health events in your life, such as serious illnesses, recurrent health problems, and accidents; above that, note the important events and changes in your life during those periods. Notice if there seems to be a relationship between negative health events and stressful changes in your life. Your purpose is to discover what your unconscious response may have been to a difficult situation, so that you can play a more conscious role in your recovery.

The second technique recommended by Jaffe (1980) for ascertaining your body's current state of being involves deep relaxation and imagery. Once you are relaxed, allow your imagination to create an image of yourself in perfect health. Examine this image in all its detail, then ask yourself how the image seems different from the present you—what can the healthy image do that you cannot? This exercise is especially helpful in becoming aware of the differences between your current state of health and the desired state, and may point out areas that demand particular attention.

Using Imagery to Explore Specific Symptoms. At times it may be more helpful to explore the nature and meaning of a specific symptom. A simple and direct technique is to engage in a dialogue with your symptom. Simply relax, focus your attention on the symptom, and allow an image representing the symptom to come to mind. Have a conversation with your symptom—ask why it is there, and what it wants or needs from you.

Oyle (1975) suggests the following technique: Sit quietly in a comfortable and safe place. If you are indoors, a door will open; if you are outdoors, someone will appear on a path. When the figure appears, ask it "Are you the one who created my symptoms?" If the figure affirms, ask it to clarify the nature of the symptom's message. The most common message of symptoms is that we need to attend to some previously ignored aspect of our lives. The phrase "the wisdom of the body," coined by Walter Cannon, expresses the inherent tendency of the body to take responsibility for managing itself; this includes issuing warnings to the conscious mind, via symptoms, when some type of effort or change is required to restore health and balance.

When you use imagery to explore your symptoms, focus on your symptoms as you experience them. If you have back and leg pain diagnosed as a herniated disc, focus on the symptom of pain, not on the disc itself, as the object of your imaginal dialogue. Healing often begins with the initiation of this dialogue, in which the biological wisdom, neglected for so long, is finally reclaimed.

There may be times when you question the response offered by your symptom. If you doubt the information you have been given, or for some other reason feel uneasy, you may want to test the information. There are several questions you may wish to ask: What specifically is required in order for healing to occur? How will you know when the healing is coming true? Is there any way to objectively track your progress? Are there any risks involved in fulfilling the symptom's request or following its advice? You may also wish to determine whether there are ways of minimizing potential risks, and you may even want to consider whether the potential risks are worth the possible gain.

Many people become aware of negative feelings toward their symptoms or toward the image representing their symptoms. These are frequently the emotional result of accumulated pain, fear, and difficulties caused by the symptom in the past. However, should this occur, it is important to begin a dialogue with your symptom. If you express your feelings to the image and allow it to respond, this may be the beginning of an enhanced understanding and sense of cooperation. Take the stance of a good negotiator: find out what the symptom wants and needs, what it will settle for, and what it has to offer in exchange. This is the essence of the symptom dialogue technique, and an open attitude, free of judgment, will facilitate this dialogue.

According to Remen, "If you have a chronic illness, you already have a relationship with it. That relationship is often not the best it could be and may be characterized by mistrust, hostility, and fear. Dialoging with the symptom or with an image that represents it opens up lines of communication that may have been closed, and may lead to an improvement in the relationship. This improvement is often experienced as a decrease in pain, anxiety, or depression, and in some cases, as improvement in the illness itself" (see Rossman, 2000; this excerpt is taken from the introduction to an audiotape recorded by Remen as part of Rossman's *Healing Yourself* tape series, available on Rossman's Web site).

You may not be able to come to an immediate agreement with your symptom. As with any negotiation, extensive exchange and consideration may need to take place before a bargain is struck. Make sure any agreement is mutually acceptable—one-sided pacts do not work. If you do make a bargain with your symptoms, make sure you keep your agreement, and watch carefully for improvement in your health.

A technique called *symptom substitution* allows the symptom or pain to be relocated to a different area of the body, where it will be less disturbing or disruptive. For example, you may learn to experience your headaches in your little finger instead of in your head. In using this technique, you are not asking for the removal of pain, or to mask the message it may be trying to communicate; rather, you simply ask the pain to relocate to a less troublesome area of your body until you have been able to identify what message it is trying to send you (Bresler, 1992).

As you progress, you may become increasingly aware of additional information you had not recognized during the imagery itself. You may even notice this information emerging over a period of several days following your healing dialogue, and in a variety of different ways (e.g., through friends, television, books, and so forth). Jung cautioned that once a connection with the unconscious has been established, symbols and messages will spontaneously pop into your consciousness, appearing at times to be coming from some external source rather than from within. It is vital to assimilate these disparate aspects of your inner self which had previously been rejected or cast off. You may also find that repeating the dialogue process in a few days will allow you to explore the relationship between you and your symptoms at an even deeper level, culminating in a dialogue marked by forgiveness and growth, in which you find yourself able to care for and honor your symptom as a part of your inner self.

If you are new to working with imagery in this way, keep in mind that there is a difference between medical diagnosis and the personal meaning of your illness, and that each is a valuable aspect of your total health care. Dialoguing with your symptoms to find out what personal meaning they hold for you does not negate the necessity of obtaining adequate medical attention for symptoms and illness. However, relying on your own inner wisdom will provide you with a unique way of participating more deeply, and taking increased responsibility for your own healing.

A Rose Opening

Healing is often visualized as an unfolding process of the psyche. Within this unfolding, contact with a higher level of consciousness, namely the super-conscious, typically precedes the evolution of the person to a higher level of awareness. Experiences of contact with the superconscious, or transpersonal experiences, have been reported to occur both spontaneously and as the result of imagery practice (Ferrucci, 1983). According to Ferrucci (1983), accounts from people who have accessed this higher level of consciousness are widely varied and may include any of the following:

An insight
The sudden solution of a difficult problem
Seeing one's life in perspective and having a clear sense of purpose
A transfigured vision of external reality
The apprehension of some truth concerning the nature of the universe
A sense of unity with all beings and of sharing everyone's destiny
Illumination
An extraordinary inner silence
Waves of luminous joy
Liberation
Cosmic humor
A deep feeling of gratefulness
An exhilarating sense of dance
Resonating with the essence of beings and things we come in contact with
Loving all persons in one person
Feeling oneself to be the channel for a wider, stronger force to flow through
Ecstasy
An intimation of profound mystery and wonder

The delight of beauty
Creative inspiration
A sense of boundless compassion
Transcendence of time and space as we know them

In addition, the rhythm of the experiences may vary greatly, sometimes coming on suddenly and sharply and other times gradually increasing and unfolding (Ferrucci, 1983). Despite these variations, some form of contact with a timeless essence or being appears to be present in all experiences (Ferrucci, 1983).

Many theories attempt to explain the nature of these experiences. According to Ferrucci (1983) some of the most plausible explanations relate to human evolution. Biological evolution, as proposed by Darwin, is thought to be only one facet of the total evolution of human consciousness (Ferrucci, 1983). Maslow (1970) felt that peak experiences and meta-needs were the highest level of human evolution. He argued that these should be viewed as inherent aspects of human biology, not separate from the entire human condition.

Regardless of the reason for their existence, Ferrucci (1983) proposed that these experiences have the potential to lead to personal transformation and healing. People who have experienced the superconscious through transpersonal experiences do not deny the reality of its existence (Ferrucci, 1983). The Transpersonal Self, contacted during these experiences, rises above the ordinary state of the personality and all of its incompleteness and busy-ness (Ferrucci, 1983). As during the process of mindfulness, as defined by Kabat-Zinn (1990), the person is allowed to transcend all of the subjective falseness of the personality that leads to distress and to view the truth that exists in pure experience. Through this unadulterated perspective each event is viewed from a new perspective and new connections are brought to light. The shedding of the subjective falseness of experience that is generated by the personality reduces habitual distress reactions, thereby facilitating healing.

Various techniques aid in establishing contact with the superconscious through facilitation of a transcendent experience. Techniques that utilize symbols to facilitate this process include the inner advisor, described previously, and the exercise of imagining the blossoming of a rose (Ferrucci, 1983; Moleski, Ishii, & Sheikh, 2001). This technique was created by Assagioli (1971) and involves first imagining a rosebush in detail: roots, stems, leaves, and one rosebud on top. The rosebud is completely enclosed in its sepals. After clearly developing this image, the person is instructed to begin imagining the opening of the rosebud, sepals first. The closed petals are revealed and are imagined in detail. Once the petals are clear in the person's mind, they, too, begin to open slowly. While this is occurring, the person is instructed to become aware of something deep within that is also opening up and coming to light. As this rose is visualized, the person is guided to feel that the rhythm of the rose is the person's rhythm, the opening is the person's opening. He/she watches the rose opening up in its entirety, revealing all its beauty. He/she smells its perfume and absorbs it into his/her being. Next, the person is instructed to gaze into the very center of the rose, where its life is most intense. He/she is instructed to allow an image to spontaneously emanate from that center, without force or thought, that represents that which is most beautiful, most meaningful, most creative, that wants to come to light in his/her life right at that moment. The person is instructed to stay with that image and absorb its quality. Finally, the person is instructed to be receptive to any messages that emanate from this image.

This technique shares many similarities with some of the above-mentioned techniques. Similar to the inner advisor technique, it uses symbols to facilitate growth and healing through the imagery experience (Moleski, Ishii, & Sheikh, 2001). Specific to this technique is the viewing of the process of unfolding into superconsciousness and identifying the process that is occurring in an image with a process that is concurrently occurring within the psyche of the person. There is no contact of symptoms within this method, nor is there any acknowledgement that symptoms hold messages about areas in need of change. The rose opening imagery enhances the perspective of *moving toward wholeness* without any attention to symptoms. The individual is able to see the core nature, or essence, of being, as inherently perfect. In addition, intuition of the superconscious is accessed within the silence of the transpersonal experience (Ferrucci, 1983).

As in the case of the inner advisor technique, healing is not a primary focus of this method; rather, it is seen as a secondary gain in insight and enlightenment. Within the inner advisor technique, symptoms may be acknowledged within the dialogue between the person and the advisor, which may lead to understanding of the imbalance that underlies symptomatology. Symptom dialogue more explicitly uses symptoms to determine areas of the person's psyche in need of attention. In the rose-unfolding imagery, the process of unfolding is the focus.

Temple of Silence

This last technique, referred to as the Temple of Silence, has as its primary goal *inner silence*, which has immense therapeutic value. Inner silence is essentially an extension of relaxation; although the effects are often much deeper than those achieved with relaxation alone. When one is immersed in inner silence, subjective conflict seems to disappear, scattering becomes unity, and energy is saved and restored rather than thoughtlessly tossed about. This type of silence has been likened to the "steady flame of a candle in still air, or to the sea when it is so calm and clear that one can see the bottom undistorted" (Ferrucci, 1983, p. 217). True inner silence allows our inner healing capacity to emerge without fear of the controlling influence of the mind, noise, information, and action; thus, our inner wisdom, and a spontaneous harmony of being, may also feel free to emerge.

However, true inner silence is difficult to achieve. It occurs only when the mind has become focused on a chosen object; as the mind becomes unified in its focus, the object itself begins to fade, and the individual is left with a silent, calm, and still mind.

The Temple of Silence technique of connecting with inner wisdom is a visualization exercise designed to evoke true inner silence. The script that follows is from Ferrucci (1983):

> Imagine a hill covered with greenery. A path leads to the top, where you can see the Temple of Silence. Give that temple the shape of your highest consciousness: noble, harmonious, and radiant.
>
> It is a spring morning, sunny and pleasantly warm. Notice how you are dressed. Become conscious of your body ascending the path, and feel the contact of your feet with the ground. Feel the breeze on your cheeks. Look about you at the trees and the bushes, the grass, and the wildflowers as you go up.
>
> You are now approaching the top of the hill. Ageless stillness pervades the atmosphere of the Temple of Silence. No word has ever been uttered here. You are close to its big wooden portals: see your hands on them and feel the wood. Before opening the doors, know that when you do so, you will be surrounded by silence.
>
> You enter the temple. You feel the atmosphere of stillness and peace all around you. Now you walk forward into the silence, looking about you as you go. You see a big luminous dome. Its luminosity not only comes from the rays of the sun, but also seems to spring from within and to be concentrated on an area of radiance just in front of you.
>
> You enter this luminous silence and feel absorbed by it. Beams of beneficent, warm, powerful light are enveloping you. Let this luminous silence pervade you. Feel it flowing through your veins and permeating every cell in your body.
>
> Remain in this silence for two or three minutes, recollected and alert. During this time, *listen* to the silence. Silence is a living quality, not just the mere absence of sounds.
>
> Slowly leave the area of radiance; walk back through the temple and out to the portals. Outside, open yourself to the impact of the spring, feel its gentle breeze once more upon your cheek, and listen to the singing of the birds. (pp. 219-220)

According to Ferrucci (1983), this special type of inner silence creates a channel for superconscious energy, and allows for the flow of symbolic messages, whose meaning is not always perfectly clear. However, the more valuable aspect of this inner silence is that it awakens an expansive and transcendent superconscious intuition. Compared with ordinary intuition, superconscious intuition reveals the "big picture." It conveys the mystical notion that everything makes sense or is as it should be, along with a felt sense of unity, oneness, inner connectedness with all things and eternity.

Connecting with one's inner wisdom through the Temple of Silence offers the potential for a powerful experience of healing. This essential contact with the more subtle aspects of your inner nature can have a profound effect on all aspects of the inner being, including mental, emotional, physical, and spiritual forms of being. At its peak, although rarely, true inner silence may even evoke *illumination*. Ferrucci (1983, p. 225) describes illumination as the "complete view of the world," and as intuition's "glimpse of the world in which the Self lives." The Temple of Silence technique, by accessing inner silence, superconscious intuition, and even illumination, may be an essential and transformational mystical experience, leading to the experience of the power of inner wisdom.

CONCLUSION

While many spiritual traditions emphasize the inner core of wisdom within the individual, many also insist that access to this inner core is reserved for the few deemed worthy of transcendence or direct communication from God. The techniques of healing imagery explored in this chapter, however, are accessible to all persons desiring to contact that inner core of wisdom and healing. The use of imagery as a means of accessing this innate inner wisdom, and of stimulating understanding and our innate healing mechanisms, amplifies the understanding of body, mind, and spirit as interconnected.

In an attempt to explain why psychological traits and states should be so fully intertwined with biological systems of healing, some scientists have proposed that the immune system is engaged in a broad process of self-determination, in which the psychological, neurological, and immunological subsystems share a common goal of establishing and maintaining self-identity (Booth & Ashbridge, 1993). The unifying principle underlying this process, referred to as *teleological coherence*, is thought to represent the interconnectedness that maintains harmony both within and outside the organism, to distinguish "self" from "nonself," and to uphold organismic integrity.

However, innumerable questions still exist concerning both teleological coherence and the body-mind system in general. How are we to explain the body's inherent ability to heal itself, and the aspect of nonconscious processing that represents inner wisdom? How are these processes, as purposeful and coherent as they seem to be, susceptible to conscious intervention?

While we lack complete answers for these questions, we do have some insight into the more basic processes. Although the operation of this system generally occurs outside the level of consciousness, interventions based on imaginal abilities can bring these unconscious mental processes into awareness. Interventions designed to facilitate emotional expression are an example of the ability of conscious awareness and intent to enhance autonomic, unconscious processes, resulting in improved health. Thus, the forms of mind-body medicine that awaken our unconscious healing potential are those that arouse emotion and generate spirit, which might be defined in terms once used by Rollo May (1981, p. 220):

"Spirit is that which gives vivacity, energy, liveliness, courage, and ardor to life," and spirit is the true nature of the universe.

REFERENCES

Achterberg, J. (1984). Imagery and medicine: Psychophysiological speculations. *Journal of Mental Imagery, 8,* 1-13.

Achterberg, J., & Lawlis, G. F. (1979). A canonical analysis of blood chemistry variables related to psychological measures of cancer patients. *Multivariate Experimental Clinical Research, 4,* 1-10.

Arieti, S. (1976). *Creativity: The magic synthesis.* New York: Basic Books.

Ashton, C., Whitworth, G. C., Seldomridge, J. A., Shapiro, P. A., Weinberg, A. D., Michler, R. E., Smith, C. R., Rose, E. A., Fisher, S., & Oz, M. C. (1997). Self-hypnosis reduces anxiety following coronary artery bypass surgery. A prospective, randomized trial. *Journal of Cardiovascular Surgery, 38,* 69-75.

Assagioli, R. (1971). *Psychosynthesis.* New York: Viking.

Barber, T. X., Chauncey, H. H., & Winer, R. A. (1964). Effects of hypnotic and non-hypnotic suggestions on parotid gland response to gustatory stimuli. *Psychosomatic Medicine, 26,* 374-380.

Benson, H. (1976). *The relaxation response.* New York: Avon.

Benson, H. B. (1996). *Timeless healing: The power and biology of belief.* New York: Scribner.

Bisiach, E., & Luzzatti, C. (1978). Unilateral neglect of representational space. *Cortex, 14,* 129-133.

Booth, R. J., & Ashbridge, K. R. (1993). A fresh look at the relationship between the psyche and immune system: Teleological coherence and harmony of purpose. *Advances, 9,* 4-23.

Bresler, D. E. (1992). Health promotion and chronic pain: Challenges and choices. In A. Kaplun (Ed.), *Health promotion and chronic illness: Discovering a new quality of health* (pp. 139-151). Cologne: The Federal Centre for Health Education and the Regional Office for Europe of the World Health Organization.

Bresler, D., & Trubo, R. (1979). *Free yourself from pain.* New York: Simon and Schuster.

Brett, E. A., & Ostroff, R. (1985). Imagery and posttraumatic stress disorder: An overview. *American Journal of Psychiatry, 142,* 417-424.

Bugelski, B. R. (1970). Words and things and images. *American Psychologist, 25,* 1002-1012.

Burns, J. W. (2000). Regression predicts outcome following multidisciplinary treatment of chronic pain. *Health Psychology, 19,* 75-84.

Carlson, N. R. (1998). *Physiology of behavior.* Needham Heights, MA: Allyn and Bacon.

Carroll, D., Marzillier, J. S., & Merian, S. (1982). Psychophysiological arousal accompanying different types of arousing and relaxing imagery. *Psychophysiology, 19,* 75-82.

Chez, R. A., & Jonas, W. B. (1997). The challenge of complementary and alternative medicine. *American Journal of Obstetrics and Gynecology, 177,* 1156-1161.

Chopra, D. (2000). http://www.chopra.com/aboutmindbody.htm.

Cobb, S., & Rose, R. M. (1973). Hypertension, peptic ulcer, and diabetes in air traffic controllers. *Journal of the American Medical Association, 224,* 489-492.

Cohen, E. A. (1953). *Human behavior in the concentration camp.* New York: W. W. Norton.

Cousins, N. (1980). *Anatomy of an illness.* New York: W. W. Norton.

Dadds, M. R., Cutmore, T. R. H., Novbjerg, D. H., & Redd, W. H. (1997). Imagery in human classical conditioning. *Psychological Bulletin, 122,* 89-103.

Dallett, J. (1984). Active imagination in practice. In M. Stein (Ed.), *Jungian analysis.* London: William Heinemann.

Dreher, H. (1998). Mind-body interventions for surgery: Evidence and exigency. *Advances: The Journal of Mind-Body Health, 14,* 207-223.

Drugan, R. C., Basile, A. S., Ha, J. H., & Ferland, R .J. (1994). The protective effects of stress control may be mediated by increased brain levels of benzodiazepine receptor agonists. *Brain Research, 661,* 127-136.

Edelstein, M. G. (1981). *Trauma, trance, and transformation: A clinical guide to hypnotherapy.* Philadelphia: Brunner/Mazel (now Brunner-Routledge).

Emery, M. (1999). *The intuitive healer: Accessing your inner physician.* New York: St. Martin's Press.

Estes, C. P. (1995). *Women who run with the wolves: Myths and stories of the wild woman archetype.* New York: Ballantine Books.

Fanning, P. (1994). *Visualization for change.* Oakland, CA: New Harbinger.

Farah, M. J. (1988). Is visual imagery really visual? Overlooked evidence from neuropsychology. *Psychological Review, 95,* 307-317.

Fawzy, F. I., Fawzy, N. W., Hyun, C. S., Elashoff, R., Guthrie, D., Fahey, J. L., & Morton, D. L. (1993). Malignant melanoma. Effects of an early structured psychiatric intervention, coping, and affective state on recurrence and survival 6 years later. *Archives of General Psychiatry, 50,* 681-689.

Ferrucci, D. (1983). *What we may be: Techniques for psychological and spiritual growth through psychosynthesis.* New York: J. P. Tarcher.

File, S. E. (1996). Recent developments in anxiety, stress and depression. *Pharmacology, Biochemistry, and Behavior, 54,* 3-12.

Fillon, M. (2000). *Tuning in to lowering stress in the ER.* [On-line]. Available: http://healthwatch.medscape.com/medscape/p/G_Library/article.asp?RecID=228642&ContentType=Library&NB=2&SP=2&Channel=nan

Finke, R. A. (1985). Theories relating mental imagery to perception. *Psychological Bulletin, 98,* 236-259.

Forisha, B. L. (1979). The outside and the inside: Compartmentalization or integration? In A. A. Sheikh & J. T. Shafer (Eds.), *The potential of fantasy and imagination.* New York: Brandon House.

Gatchel, R. J., Baum, A., & Krantz, D. S. (1989). *An introduction to health psychology* (2nd ed.). New York: Newbery Award Records.

Gendlin, E. T. (1981). *Focusing.* New York: Bantam.

Gilbert, D. G., Stunkard, M. E., Jensen, R. A., Detwiler, F. R. J., & Martinko, J. M. (1996). Effects of exam stress on mood, cortisol, and immune functioning: Influences of neuroticism and smoker–non-smoker status. *Personality and Individual Differences, 21,* 235-246.

Ginandes, C. S., & Rosenthal, D. I. (1999). Using hypnosis to accelerate the healing of bone fractures: A randomized controlled pilot study. *Alternative Therapies in Health and Medicine, 5,* 67-75.

Hannah, B. (1976). *Jung: His life and work.* New York: Putnam.

Horowitz, M. J. (1970). *Image formation and cognition.* New York: Appleton Century Crofts.

Houston, J. (1982). *The possible human: A course in enhancing your physical, mental, and creative abilities.* New York: J. P. Tarcher.

Hudetz, J. A., Hudetz, A. G., & Klayman, J. (2000). Relationship between relaxation by guided imagery and performance of working memory. *Psychological Reports, 86,* 15-20.

Irvin, J. H., Domar, A. D., Clark, C., Zuttermeister, P. C., & Friedman, R. (1996). The effects of relaxation response training on menopausal symptoms. *Journal of Psychosomatic Obstetrics and Gynecology, 17,* 202-207.

Jacobson, E. (1932). Electrophysiology of mental activity. *American Journal of Psychology, 44,* 677-694.

Jaffe, D. T. (1980). *Healing from within.* New York: Alfred A. Knopf, Inc.

Jensen, T., Genefke, I., & Hyldebrandt, N. (1982). Cerebral atrophy in young torture victims. *New England Journal of Medicine, 307,* 1341.

Jung, C. G. (1963). Mysterium coniunctunis. In *Collected works* (Vol. 14). London: Routledge & Kegan.

Kabat-Zinn, J. (1990). *Full catastrophe living.* New York: Delta.

Kiecolt-Glaser, J. K., Marucha, P. T., Marlarkey, W. B., Mercado, A. M., & Glaser, R. (1995). Slowing of wound healing by psychological stress. *Lancet, 346,* 1194-1196.

Kiecolt-Glaser, J.K., Page, G. G., Marucha, P. T., MacCallum, R. C., & Glaser, R. (1998). Psychological influences on surgery recovery: Perspectives from psychoneuroimmunology. *American Psychologist, 53,* 1209-1218.

King, D. L. (1973). An image theory of classical conditioning. *Psychological Reports, 33,* 403-411.

Kolcaba, K., & Fox, C. (1999). The effects of guided imagery on comfort of women with early stage breast cancer undergoing radiation therapy. *Oncology Nursing Forum, 26,* 67-72.

Kosslyn, S. (1987). Seeing and imagining in the cerebral hemispheres: A computational approach. *Psychological Review, 94,* 148-175.

Kosslyn, S. (1988). Aspects of cognitive neuroscience of mental imagery. *Science, 240,* 1621-1626.

Kosslyn, S. (1994). *Image and brain.* Cambridge, MA: MIT Press.

Lambert, M. J., & Bergin, A. E., (1994). The effectiveness of psychotherapy. In A. E. Bergin & S. L. Garfield (Eds.), *Handbook of psychotherapy and behavior change* (4th ed.). New York: John Wiley & Sons.

Lang, E. V., Benotsch, E. G., Fick, L. J., Lutgendorf, S., Berbaum, M. L., Berbaum, K. S., Logan, H., & Spiegel, D. (2000). Adjunctive non-pharmacological analgesia for invasive medical procedures: A randomised trial. *Lancet, 355,* 1486-1490.

Lang, P. J. (1979). A bio-informational theory of emotional imagery [1978 presidential address]. *Psychophysiology, 16,* 495-512.

Lankton, S. R., & Lankton, C. H. (1983). *The answer within: A clinical framework of Ericksonian hypnosis.* New York: Brunner-Mazel.

Lichstein, K. L., & Lipshitz, E. (1982). Physiological effects of noxious imagery: Prevalence and prediction. *Behaviour Research and Therapy, 20,* 339-345.

Locke, S., & Colligan, D. (1986). *The healer within: The new medicine of mind and body.* New York: E. P. Dutton.

Lusebrink, V. B., & McGuigan, F. J. (1989). Psychophysiological components of imagery. *Pavlovian Journal of Biological Science, 24,* 58-62.

Manuck, S. B., Kaplan, J. R., & Clarkson, T. B. (1983). Behaviorally-induced heart rate reactivity and atherosclerosis in cynomolgous monkeys. *Psychosomatic Medicine, 45,* 95-108.

Manuck, S. B., Kaplan, J. R., & Matthews, K. A. (1986). Behavioral antecedents of coronary heart disease and atherosclerosis. *Arteriosclerosis, 6,* 1-14.

Manyande, A., Berg, S., Gettins, D., Stanford, S. C., Mazhero, S., Marks, D. F:, & Salmon, P. (1995). Preoperative rehearsal of active coping imagery influences subjective and hormonal responses to abdominal surgery. *Psychosomatic Medicine, 57,* 177-182.

Marzillier, J. S., Carroll, D., & Newland, J. R. (1979). Self-report and physiological changes accompanying repeated imagining of a phobic scene. *Behaviour Research and Therapy, 17,* 71-77.

Maslow, A. (1970). *Motivation and personality* (3rd ed.). New York: Harper and Row.

May, R. (1981). *Freedom and destiny.* New York: Delta Books.

McCaffery, M., & Beebe, A. (1989). *Pain: Clinical manual for nursing practice.* Philadelphia: Mosby.

McGrady, A. V., Bush, E. G., & Grubb, B. P. (1997). Outcome of biofeedback-assisted relaxation for neurocardiogenic syncope and headache: A clinical replication series. *Applied Psychophysiology Biofeedback, 22,* 63-72.

McMahon, C. E. (1973). Images as motives and motivators: A historical perspective. *American Journal of Psychology, 86,* 465-490.

Mein, E. (1989). *Keys to health: The promise and challenge of holism.* New York: Harper & Row.

Merriam-Webster's Collegiate Dictionary (10th ed.). (1995). Springfield, MA: Merriam-Webster, Inc.

Miller, N. E. (1972). Interactions between learned and physical factors in mental illness. In D. Shapiro et al. (Eds.), *Biofeedback and self-control.* Chicago: Aldine.

Moleski, L. M., Ishii, M. M., & Sheikh, A. A. (2001). Imagery techniques in psychosynthesis. As cited in A. A. Sheikh (Ed.), *Handbook of therapeutic imagery technique.* Amityville, NY: Baywood.

Mowrer, O. H. (1977). Mental imagery: An indispensable psychological concept. *Journal of Mental Imagery, 1,* 303-325.

Naparstek, B. (1997). *Your sixth sense: Activating your psychic potential.* New York: HarperCollins.

NCCAM (National Institutes of Health, National Center for Complementary and Alternative Medicine). *Mind-body control* (Adapted from *Alternative Medicine: Expanding Medical Horizons,* a report prepared under the auspices of the Workshop on Alternative Medicine, held in Chantilly, Virginia, on September 14-16, 1992.). Retrieved March 3, 2000, from http://nccam.nih.gov/ (Overview and Imagery sections).

Nordenberg, T. (2000). The healing power of placebos. *FDA Consumer, 34,* 14-16.

Oyle, I. (1975). *The healing mind.* Berkeley, CA: Celestial Arts.

Pan, C. X., Morrison, R. S., Ness J., Fugh-Berman, A., & Leipzig, R. M. (2000), Complementary and alternative medicine in the management of pain, dyspnea, and nausea and vomiting near the end of life: A systematic review. *Journal of Pain and Symptom Management, 20*, 374-387.

Pert, C. B. (1986). The wisdom of the receptors: Neuropeptides, the emotions and bodymind. *Advances, 3*, 8-16.

Pert, C. B. (1997). *Molecules of emotion: Why you feel the way you feel.* New York: Scribner.

Pert, C. B., Dreher, H. E., & Ruff, M. R. (1998). The psychosomatic network: Foundations of mind-body medicine. *Alternative Therapies in Health and Medicine, 4*, 30-41.

Pert, C. B., Ruff, M. R., Weber, R. J., & Herkenham, M. (1985). Neuropeptides and their receptors: A psychosomatic network. *Journal of Immunology, 135*, 820s-826s.

Petrie, K. J., Booth, R. J., & Pennebaker, J. W. (1998). The immunological effects of thought suppression. *Journal of Personality and Social Psychology, 75*, 1264-1272.

Pitman, R. K., Orr, S. P., Forgue, D. F., de Jong, J. B., & Claiborn, J. M. (1987). Psycho-physiological assessment of posttraumatic stress disorder imagery in Vietnam combat veterans. *Archives of General Psychiatry, 44*, 970-975.

Posluszny, B. A. (1999). Health psychology: Mapping biobehavioral contributions to health and illness. *Annual Review of Psychology, 50*, 137-163.

Richardson, M. A., Post-White, J., Grimm, E. A., Moye, L. A., Singletary, S. E., & Justice, B. (1997). Coping, life attitudes, and immune responses to imagery and group support after breast cancer treatment. *Alternative Therapies in Health and Medicine, 3*, 62-70.

Roberts, R. J., & Weerts, T. C. (1982). Cardiovascular responding during anger and fear imagery. *Psychological Reports, 50*, 219-230.

Robertson, R. (1987). *C. G. Jung and the archetypes of the collective unconscious.* New York: Peter Lang.

Robertson, R. (1995). *Jungian archetypes: Jung, Goedel, and the history of archetypes.* York Beach, ME: Nicolas-Hays.

Rogers, C. R. (1961). *On becoming a person.* Boston: Houghton Mifflin.

Rossman, M. L. (1987). *Healing yourself: A step-by-step program for better health through imagery.* New York: Walker and Company.

Rossman, M. L. (2000). *Healing yourself: A step-by-step program for better health through imagery, with Martin L. Rossman, M.D.* Retrieved April 22, 2000 from http://www.interactiveimagery.com/index_explorer.html.

Samuels, M., & Bennett, H. (1978). *The well body book.* New York: Random House.

Sapolsky, R. M. (1986). Glucocorticoid toxicity in the hippocampus: Reversal by supple-mentation with brain fuels. *Journal of Neuroscience, 6*, 2240-2244.

Sapolsky, R. M., Krey, L. C., & McEwen, B. S. (1986). The adrenocortical axis in the aged rat: Impaired sensitivity to both fast and delayed feedback inhibition. *Neurobiology of Aging, 7*, 331-335.

Sarbin, T. R., & Coe, W. C. (1972). *Hypnosis: A social psychological analysis of influence communication.* New York: Holt.

Segal, S. J., & Fusella, V. (1970). Influence of imagined pictures and sounds on detection of visual and auditory signals. *Journal of Experimental Psychology, 83*, 458-464.

Sharpley, C. (1994). Maintenance and generalizability of laboratory-based heart rate reactivity control training. *Journal of Behavioral Medicine, 17*, 309-329.

Sheikh, A. A., & Panagiotou, N. C. (1975). Use of mental imagery in psychotherapy: A critical review. *Perceptual and Motor Skills, 41*, 555-585.

Shephard, R. N. (1978). The mental image. *American Psychologist, 33*, 125-137.

Shore, H. E. (1993). *The inner advisor technique in psychotherapy: A phenomenological analysis* (Vol. I and II). Unpublished doctoral dissertation, California School of Professional Psychology, Fresno.

Shorr, E. (1980). Discoveries about the mind's ability to organize and find meaning in imagery. In E. Shorr et al. (Eds.), *Imagery: Its many dimensions and applications.* New York: Plenum.

Shrock, D., Palmer, R. F., & Taylor, B. (1999). Effects of a psychosocial intervention on survival among patients with stage I breast and prostrate cancer: A matched case-control study. *Alternative Therapies in Health and Medicine, 5,* 49-55.

Signell, K. A. (1990). *Wisdom of the heart: Working with women's dreams.* New York: Bantam Books.

Simonton, O. C., Matthews-Simonton, S., & Creighton, J. (1978). *Getting well again.* Los Angeles: J. P. Tarcher.

Singer, J. L. (1974). *Imagery and daydream methods in psychotherapy and behavior modification.* New York: Academic Press.

Singer, J. L. (1979). Imagery and affect in psychotherapy: Elaborating private scripts and generating contexts. In A. A. Sheikh & J. T. Shaffer (Eds.), *The potential of fantasy and imagination.* New York: Random House.

Singer, J. (1994). *Boundaries of the soul: The practice of Jung's psychology.* New York: Doubleday.

Smart, G. (1997). Helping children relax during magnetic resonance imaging. *American Journal of Maternal & Child Nursing, 22,* 236-241.

Song, L. Z. Y. X., Schwartz, G. E. R., & Russek, L. G. S. (1998). Heart-focused attention and heart-brain synchronization: Energetic and physiological mechanisms. *Alternative Therapies in Health and Medicine, 4,* 44-62.

Stein, M. (1984). *Jungian analysis.* London: William Heinemann.

Susman, E. J., Dorn, L. J., Inoff-Germain, G., Nottelmann, E. D., & Chrousos, G. P. (1997). Cortisol reactivity, distress behavior, and behavioral and psychological problems in young adolescents: A longitudinal perspective. *Journal of Research on Adolescence, 7,* 81-105.

Theorell, T., Leymann, H., Jodko, M., Konarski, K., Norbeck, H. E., & Eneroth, P. (1992). "Person under train" incidents: Medical consequences for subway drivers. *Psychosomatic Medicine, 54,* 480-488.

Tiller, W. A., McCraty, R., & Atkinson, M. (1996). Cardiac coherence: A new noninvasive measure of automatic nervous system order. *Alternative Therapies in Health and Medicine, 2,* 52-65.

Tower, R. B., & Singer, J. L. (1981). The measurement of imagery: How can it be clinically useful? In P. C. Kendall & S. Hollond (Eds.), *Cognitive behavioral interventions: Assessment methods.* New York: Academic Press.

Tusek, D. L., Church, J. M., Strong, S. A., Grass, J. A., & Fazio, V. W. (1997). Guided imagery: A significant advance in the care of patients undergoing elective colorectal surgery. *Diseases of the Colon and Rectum, 40,* 172-178.

Uno, H., Tarara, R., Else, J. G., Suleman, M. A., & Sapolsky, R. M. (1989). Hippocampal damage associated with prolonged and fatal stress in primates. *Journal of Neuroscience, 9,* 1705-1711.

Watkins, M. M. (1976). *Waking dreams.* New York: Harper and Row.

Weiss, J. M. (1969). Effects of coping response on stress. *Journal of Comparative and Physiological Psychology, 65,* 251-260.

Wichowski, H. C., & Kubsch, S. M. (1999). Increasing diabetic self-care through guided imagery. *Complementary Therapy Nurse Midwifery, 5,* 159-163.

Wood, D. I., Sheps, S. G., Elveback, I. R., & Schirder, A. (1984). A cold suppressor test as a predictor of hypertension. *Hypertension, 6,* 301-306.

World Health Organization (1964). *Basic documents* (15th ed.). Geneva, Switzerland: Author.

Wynd, C. A. (1992a). Relaxation imagery used for stress reduction in the prevention of smoking relapse. *Journal of Advanced Nursing, 17,* 294-302.

Wynd, C. A. (1992b). Personal power imagery and relaxation techniques used in smoking cessation programs. *American Journal of Health Promotion, 6,* 184-190.

CHAPTER 8

Transforming the Pain Terrain: Theory and Practice in the Use of Mental Imagery for the Treatment of Pain

DAVID PINCUS, TONYA WACHSMUTH-SCHLAEFER, ANEES A. SHEIKH, AND SHIRIN EZAZ-NIKPAY

And could you keep your heart in wonder at the daily miracles of life, your pain would not seem less wondrous than your joy. (Kahlil Gibran, 1966, p. 52)

Psychotherapy is like a journey, with therapeutic change represented by movement toward some healthy destination (A. Kuchan, personal communication, April 1998). The role of the therapist is that of a trail-ready companion, prepared to move from here to there with the client. However, to get from one place to another, one needs a map, and in psychotherapy the map must be flexible enough to match the specific therapeutic terrain of pain phenomena brought in by clients, as well as the specific clients brought in by their pain. This chapter is intended to provide practitioners of imagery psychotherapy with the information to develop such therapeutic maps when treating victims of pain disorders. First, there is a brief discussion of individual causal factors, which are analogous to potentially interesting features of the clinical landscape. Next, the discussion will shift to characteristics of the clinical landscape as a whole, through the lens of systemic theories. Finally, a sample of the various techniques in imagery therapy for pain will be summarized. The use of these techniques, informed by a systemic perspective, may provide the means for empirical and practical explorations of more radical and potentially more potent pain treatments that aim beyond simple here-to-there movements, and instead aim to transform the clinical landscape itself.

PSYCHOSOCIAL FACTORS IN ISOLATION:
KEY LANDMARKS IN THE PAIN TERRAIN

Ever since Melzack's seminal *gate-control theory* of pain (Melzack & Wall, 1965, 1996) opened the theoretical gate to the impact of psychosocial factors on pain perception, a multitude of psychosocial influences on pain have been the subject of empirical investigations. Before these factors are discussed, however, it is important to point out that these psychosocial factors are only part of the picture. The identification of psychosocial causes of pain does *not* mean that physical causes are absent. Nor does the identification of physical cause mean that imagery work will not be helpful. Such oversimplified views of the separation between the mind and body have been passed down by a Cartesian philosophical legacy that no longer fits within the current scientific understanding of pain (McMahon & Sheikh, 1986).

At its worst, this mind-body split alienates and stigmatizes pain clients by leading them to believe that psychological causes imply that their pain is all in their head, that they are responsible for their pain, and/or are exaggerating to some degree. Many, if not most, pain patients, particularly those with chronic pain, will have experienced repeated failed treatments and will seek alternate treatments as a final resort. Along the way, they may pick up some of these stigmatizing beliefs, which can interact destructively with repeated treatment failures. The net effect can be a disturbance about pain treatments themselves in the form of self-blame, guilt, and hopelessness, which may then become significant causes of continuing pain themselves, as well as a hindrance to imagery treatment. Whether one takes a radical anti-Cartesian viewpoint which embraces the notion of a holistic mind-body complex, or a more moderate viewpoint of the mind and body as somewhat distinct yet highly interactive systems, it is necessary to remember that psychosocial factors have a direct impact on a person's *actual* experience of pain. Even if physical factors are ruled out, the pain is not just *in their heads*. Second, it is imperative that pain clients be assisted in modifying any outdated Cartesian pain beliefs and feelings of responsibility that they may be having at the outset of treatment.

To understand the psychosocial causes of pain one must begin simply, by examining each cause in relative isolation. Again, some of the causal factors reviewed below will be more relevant compared to others for any particular pain client. The most robust and consistent general finding in psychological pain research is that there is great variability in pain patients as a group. As such, each pain patient should be viewed as unique when one considers the vast array of causes, symptoms, and interactions between and among the two. Single causes, however, represent a starting point from which to build a more comprehensive understanding of how pain emerges, is maintained, and ultimately can be treated.

Personality Factors

One of the first and most extensive areas in the study of psychosocial factors on clinical pain has been the role of personality in pain (Gatchel & Epker, 1999; Weisenberg & Keefe, 1999). The interest in finding enduring charactero- logical patterns, as well as Axis I disorders (e.g., depression) which one can tag as a pain-prone style, is likely fed as much by the basic human bias toward dispositional attributions as by a desire to be helpful. In other words, clinicians that treat pain must be cautious not to further stigmatize pain patients through oversimplified attitudes suggesting that their personalities are *the* cause of their pain. Like most areas of pain research, the variability in specific manifestations of clinical pain has made general patterns hard to identify. Realistically speaking, there is no single pain-prone personality.

With these warnings in mind, there are some general conclusions that may be drawn from this line of research. First, both axis-I and axis-II disorders are more frequently seen in pain patients compared to matched-controls (Weisenberg & Keefe, 1999). However, causal relationships have not been established, which means that it is not clear whether the pain causes the disturbance or the disturbance causes the pain or whether both are caused by some third factor. Even within axis-II disturbances, which by definition are long-term, enduring, and present across life domains (American Psychiatric Association, 1994), there is evidence to suggest that chronic pain symptoms are frequently woven together with the axis-II diagnostic criteria (Weisenberg & Keefe, 1999). Pain personality research also suffers because of problems with the personality measures themselves, because many are biased due to questions with somatic content and because they have questionable links to DSM diagnoses (e.g., MMPI scales). A third problem is the dubious diagnostic reliabilities for DSM personality disorders as a whole.

Again, despite these limitations, there is sufficient evidence to justify that a therapist be alert to specific diagnostic categories and personality styles. Weisenberg and Keefe (1999) report a range of 31 percent to 59 percent in the prevalence of axis-I disorders in chronic pain patients. These disorders are most often mood and anxiety disorders. Again, it is not clear from the research whether axis-I disorders are a cause, effect, or both.

Axis-II disorders may be as much as three times as prevalent in pain patients as in matched controls (Reich & Thompson, 1987), a conclusion that has been broadly replicated by other researchers (Weisenberg & Keefe, 1999). Again, because of the troublesome overlap between the diagnostic criteria for different personality disorders, it is more useful to describe research results in terms of personality clusters rather than specific personality disorders (American Psychiatric Association, 1994; Widiger, Trull, Hurt, Clarkin, & Frances, 1987). Cluster C: anxious/avoidant, avoidant, dependent, and obsessive-compulsive personalities appears to be the most prevalent, followed by cluster B:

dramatic/emotional, borderline, narcissistic, and histrionic personalities. Apart from diagnostic categories, the traits that are common to both pain disorders and interpersonal dysfunction are threat avoidance, dependence, helplessness, and emotional disregulation (Weisenberg & Keefe, 1999). For the pain therapist, these four characteristics may tie a common thread between pain disorders, depression/anxiety syndromes, and the B and C personality clusters above. Therapeutic changes potentially, and perhaps necessarily, will cascade among all of these characterological processes.

Behavioral Learning Factors

Behavioral learning factors are indispensable features of a client's therapeutic map, whether one sticks to firm distinctions between operant and classical conditioning or uses a more common sense, ecological approach of asking: What function are these pain problems serving? And, how are these pain symptoms strengthened and maintained within this client's day-to-day life? Pain, although by definition uncomfortable, may be reinforced through operant conditioning if it provides some form of reward, which over-rides its negative qualities (positive reinforcement), or if it provides escape from some aversive experience which is more threatening than the pain itself (negative reinforcement). The pain becomes a relatively functional part of the client's life if its removal would lead to some greater general loss for the person. Some concrete examples of reinforcers of pain include disability wages, avoidance of work, avoidance of feared people and/or interpersonal situations, avoidance of activities such as exercise, and sympathy from others. In addition, many abstract reinforcers of pain may be particularly relevant, such as: maintaining a sense of identity (the sick-role is covered in more detail below); maintaining cognitive consistency (Festinger, 1957) around self-beliefs relating to helplessness or powerlessness; providing a means of interacting with others through pain-related topics; distraction from more threatening cognition such as lack of purpose or meaning in life; or distraction from more threatening emotional states and/or memories relating to fear, sadness, and/or anger.

Classical conditioning, with pain emerging through paired associations between pain sensations and some internal or external cue, may also be a significant factor. Classical conditioning mechanisms represent one of the most common and obvious connecting points between the mind and body. For example, seeing or imagining someone getting sick can make a person feel queasy; seeing or imagining someone eating a piece of lemon can make a person's mouth water and pucker; and talking about waterfalls and rivers can be torturous to someone who needs to urinate during a long drive. These examples of classical conditioning can be useful early in treatment for clients who have developed counter-therapeutic beliefs about psychosocial causes of pain (e.g., that their pain is not real), or that there is a firm distinction between physiological and psychological etiologies for pain. If clients have some obvious classical conditioning mechanisms involved in their pain conditions, these may be illuminated to further remoralize them at the outset of treatment, knocking out another potential cause: self-blame.

Potential classically conditioned triggers for chronic pain may include: negative emotions, various thought processes, specific behaviors, temporal-cycles (e.g., daily, monthly, etc), or even pain medications themselves. According to Salkovskis (1996), " a reduction in pain may occur in as many as 40 percent of pain patients when (prescribed and non-prescribed) medication is withdrawn" (p. 256). This effect may be particularly pronounced if pain medications have been taken in small amounts on an as-needed basis. In these situations, medications are taken when pain becomes intolerable, leading to a conditioned association between the lack of medication and increasing pain, ultimately intensifying rebound effects. In addition, medication-taking behavior is strongly negatively reinforced through operant principles, leading to increasing reliance on and need for the medication. Ideally, physicians should prescribe continual doses of pain medication at a sufficient strength to relieve pain as completely as possible (Hill et al., 1990; Portenoy, 1994) and help patients wean themselves off of medication as quickly as possible when an injury is healed (Salkovskis, 1996). In reality, though, this is frequently not the case.

The strength of a classically conditioned pain response will depend on the strength and specificity of the original pairing between the trigger and pain as well as their continued pairing over time. For example, if pain emerges during an emotionally laden experience, it may strengthen itself over time as the pain and negative emotional states are re-experienced together in subsequent episodes. Moreover, if the pain is experienced while the patient is in a wide variety of negative mood states, the conditioned link may become generalized over time. Conversely, if the associated mood is experienced without pain, counter-conditioning may occur, leading to a decrease in pain. Thus, with the simple addition of time to behavior principles, one may get a glimpse at the complex ways that pain experiences can become self-sustaining over time.

In real-life, classical and operant conditioning are inseparable and work in tandem over time, both to trigger and to maintain pain experiences. For example, imagine that a person develops leg pain due to stiffness on frequent, long drives to visit family. Originally, the pain might be due, more or less, to a physiological weakness such as bursitis. Over time, however, any long drive may come to trigger the pain through classical conditioning. At the same time, imagine that the pain becomes a serendipitous excuse, allowing the person to skip unwanted family visits, or more subtly, provides a pain-related role and emotional distance from troublesome family dynamics. Over time, this would result in greater specificity in the pairing between the pain responses and long drives. Classical and operant conditioning may, thus, reinforce one another reciprocally as reinforcements for the pain strengthen paired associations. The specific dynamics will vary with each pain patient. But already one may begin to understand how even a few simple factors, such as an avoidant personality style together with operant and classical conditioning, can interact cooperatively over time to intensify and maintain pain which would otherwise have dissipated naturally.

In a meta-analysis, Holroyd and Penzien (1986) found that behavior therapy is generally effective in the treatment of pain, with an average improvement of approximately 50 percent in the reduction in pain symptoms and a statistically significant benefit over placebo control conditions. While the analysis did not separate out imagery techniques per se, many behavioral treatments contain imaginary components (e.g., relaxation, covert desensitization, etc).

Coping Behavior

Maladaptive attempts at coping were identified briefly in the discussion of operant conditioning above, and they provide extremely salient examples of how psychosocial factors can lead to pain. Maladaptive coping occurs when a client attempts to respond to pain in a helpful manner but paradoxically makes the problem worse. The most frequent maladaptive coping behaviors are avoidant behaviors (Salkovskis, 1996), which again may exist within a broader personality style of helplessness, dependency, affective disregulation, and avoidance. An obvious example is prolonged avoidance of physical activity, which may in fact be functional in the short run, particularly if a person has pain related to some physical injury. However, prolonged inactivity can result in continued pain through direct impacts on physiological systems such as in the atrophy of muscles and/or tightening of connective tissues. Imagine a client who goes to bed every time she feels pain. As she lies there she is more and more frustrated as her attempts to get out of bed are met with increasingly severe pain experiences due to soreness and stiffness, which reinforce her continued maladaptive avoidance. Similarly, physical activity becomes harder and harder over the long-term, as her muscles lose their strength. Other maladaptive coping behaviors may include over-medicating, seeking pathological levels of support, physical overcompensation (e.g., over-reliance on a cane), quitting work, or alienating significant others.

Beliefs

Again, there has been extensive research to examine the role of cognition in pathogenic pain processes (Boothby, Thorn, Stroud, & Jensen, 1999). As with other solitary factors, a muddy picture emerges from the research, which supports general conclusions, yet contains numerous null findings and a methodological backdrop of wide client variability. Similarly, experimenters have had a difficult time manipulating mind-sets to a sufficient degree to support causal influences between beliefs and pain. Again, the issue of cause and effect is not easily settled.

General and theoretically logical patterns of results do, however, emerge and center on beliefs relating to *self-control* and *self-efficacy*. The problems of control

(Burger, 1991) are arguably at the center of the human condition and underlie every psychiatric disorder, from alcohol and other drug abuse to anxiety and mood disorders. Everyone has a limited ability to control the events in their lives, both external (e.g., obtaining food, human interactions, activities) and internal (e.g., thoughts, feelings, behavior, and bodily states). As the common motto from Alcoholics Anonymous suggests, the resulting challenge is to discern the things that can be controlled, the things that can not, and to manage most everything which falls somewhere in between (Alcoholics Anonymous World Services, 1953).

Pain is no exception. A person's sense of control over pain, or lack thereof, can contribute to the continuing problem through the mediating influence of coping behavior and/or negative emotions. For example, if a client has beliefs that support an over-developed need for control, he may set himself up for failure through misguided direct attempts to force the pain to subside. Conversely, he may believe that he has no control at all over pain and thus try nothing. In addition, people may flip-flop between styles, or eventually settle into the latter, perhaps to the point where an under-controlled style becomes somewhat characterological as described above.

A related set of beliefs is efficacy expectations (Bandura, 1977, 1986), which refers to a person's level of self-confidence. If people lack confidence in themselves and/or the ability of their treatments to help them cope with pain, the treatments generally will be less effective (Marino, Gwynn, & Spanos, 1989; Philips & Hunter, 1981; Raft, Smith, & Warren, 1986; Spanos & O'Hara, 1990). For example, Manyande et al. (1995) helped surgical patients prepare for post-operative pain through guided imagery as a means of enhancing their sense of control over the pain and their confidence in using pain management techniques. Compared to a control group, the coping-imagery patients had higher perceived coping ability, increased Noradrenaline and decreased Cortisol levels (both positive physiological signs), less post-operative pain, and less distress from the pain they did have. All of these effects were observed in the absence of group differences in self-reported anxiety and physiological arousal indexes, strengthening the conclusions that image therapy led to positive changes by way of improved coping beliefs.

Schema

In broader cognitive brush-strokes, pain schemata have been the topic of many theoretical and empirical examinations of the role of cognition and imagery in the etiology and treatment of pain. Theoretically, cognitive schemata are networks of knowledge that guide each person's construction of subjective reality (Smith, 1998), from broad reconstructive processes in memory (Bartlett, 1932), to more elemental constructive processes in perception and recognition (McClelland & Rumelhart, 1986). Furthermore, they have been shown to frame perceptual process, controlling the entry of information into consciousness. Through their ability to frame and filter experience, different schemata may either allow or disallow the experience of pain to varying degrees. Furthermore, different schemata may be invoked through some associated internal cue, such as emotional states (e.g., anger), thoughts (e.g., self-denigration), memories (e.g., episodic trauma), sensations (e.g., pain), or more generally through the paralleled activation of a number of these cognitive factors in concert within an associative network (Berkowitz, 1989, 1993; Berkowitz, Cochran, & Embree, 1981; Berkowitz & Heimer, 1989). In human terms, this means that different mindsets may either trigger and/or be triggered by pain. Experimental evidence from treatment outcome studies (e.g., Narduzzi et al., 1998; Raft et al., 1986) as well as experiments utilizing functional brain imaging (e.g., Howland, Wakai, Mjaanes, Balog, & Cleeland, 1995) support the role of schema in people's experiences of pain, as well as the potential of imagery techniques to modify those pain-related schemata.

Attentional-Perceptual Dynamics

One connecting point between people's mind-sets and pain perceptions lies in selective attention mechanisms that result in perceptual biases. Perceptual biases can lead people to experience their worlds in an excessively *top-down* (belief driven) manner, such as through the filter of a pain-related mind-set. In this way, pain may be experienced even in the absence of *bottom-up* perceptual factors like nociception (the stimulation of pain receptors). Research in the area of signal-detection theory has demonstrated clearly that perception is anything but an all-or-nothing phenomenon, but is in fact probabilistic. As a result, false perception, such as hearing something in the absence of a physical stimulus, is an everyday occurrence for most people.

Due to the constant bombardment of our sense modalities, the ability to selectively attend to some sensations while ignoring others is necessary for day-to-day functioning. Research based on signal-detection theory has demonstrated that people's attention levels will shift based on such top-down factors as expectations, beliefs, images, affective states, needs, and other motivations. For example, a child who goes to bed on Christmas Eve may hear bells or hoof-steps on her ceiling at some point during the evening. This child is not psychotic. Instead, her mind-set has created an attentional and perceptual bias, allowing her to perceive Santa-related noises in the absence of any physical sound.

These same processes are thought to underlie intractable pain or to modify the experience of nociception in some pain patients. Take a moment and scan your body for any pain that may be present. You probably will be able to locate some uncomfortable area. Follow your discovery with negative cognition relating to your ability to manage this pain, negative affect, and/or some form of maladaptive coping strategy and repeat over time. With sufficient repetitions, one has the recipe for a dysfunctional schematic mind-set for a pain disorder triggered with little or no nociceptive activity (Salkovskis, 1996). It is important to note once again that this attention-driven induction of pain happens automatically and is, thus, no more purposeful or conscious than clinical pain resulting primarily from nociception. Despite this fact, it remains relatively easy for people to grasp the idea that pain may change one's focus of attention and hard to grasp the opposite.

Researchers have not yet examined this connection between schema and attentional biases through signal-detection theory per se. However, there is ample evidence supporting the ability of simple distraction to ameliorate pain, particularly distraction from the affective/motivational dimensions of pain (e.g., Ahles, Blanchard, & Leventhal, 1983; Spanos & O'Hara, 1990: Stevens, Heise, & Pfost, 1989). Furthermore, strong support for the role of attention lies in the fact that clinical-pain patients frequently demonstrate somatic attentional biases (Barsky, Goodson, & Lane, 1988; Geisser, Gaskin, Robinson, & Greene, 1993; Okifuji & Turk, 1999). Similarly, hypochondriacal individuals tend to respond to experimental pain stimuli with more physiological arousal, stronger subjective pain reactions, and even with lower hand temperatures (from a cold water paradigm) compared to control participants (Gramling, Clawson, & McDonald, 1996). However, the specific healing mechanism(s) of distraction continues to elude pain experimenters (e.g., Farthing, Venturino, Brown, & Lazar, 1997; Johnson, Breakwell, Douglas, & Humphries, 1998), as do the specific situations, clients, and desired outcomes in which distraction will be most helpful (Boothby et al., 1999).

Affect

Negative affect serves to intensify pain not only indirectly by enacting a pain-related schema, but also directly as one of the central components in pain perception itself (Melzack & Casey, 1968). An apparent paradox lies in the outcomes of some experimental studies that have shown the efficacy of negative affect (e.g., fear and anger) in ameliorating pain. This beneficial result from induced negative affect is thought to occur due to distraction (e.g., McNeil & Brunetti, 1992) and the short-term release of endogenous Opiods and Cortisoids within a sympathetic nervous system response. However, these positive benefits for negative emotion seem limited to the rather brief arousal-response-period: approximately ten minutes. More often, when negative affect associated with pain sensations is enhanced through attention, it tends to intensify the pain experience (Ahles, Blanchard, & Leventhal, 1983), and blocking the affective dimension of pain through pleasant imagery tends to bring relief (Stevens, Heise, & Pfost, 1989; Worthington & Shumate, 1981).

Outside of the lab, it appears that any affect that serves to intensify the affective/motivational aspects of pain will intensify the experience of that pain (Robinson &

Riley, 1999). As such, longer-term feelings of sadness, anxiety, or hostility/anger will tend to make pain worse; particularly when these feelings are associated with the pain experience itself.

The Sick-Role

People learn about themselves just as they learn about others, through self-observations and the communicated observations of people around them (Baumeister, 1998). These self-referent experiences are mediated through self-schema (Markus, 1977), while experiences with others are mediated by relationship schemata (Baldwin, 1995). Again, both sets of schema are fed by the experience-filtering processes of mental-sets described above as well as by behavioral-sets, which limit a person's range of possible behaviors. Thus, a cycle emerges in which schemata limit experiences and experiences build schemata both within and across the individual and social domains. Furthermore, within this process, the self must have a sufficient degree of flexibility (Marks-Tarlow, 1999) in order to be adaptive and functional across social contexts (Turner, 1987; Turner, Oakes, Haslam, & McGarty, 1994) as well as across time-periods (Markus & Nurius, 1986).

Theoretically, one of the most insidious processes which can impinge upon a person's social and personal flexibility and upon recovery from a pain disorder is the tight coupling of the self and relationship schemata to a dysfunctional pain schemata. In other words, for some individuals pain becomes a dangerously large part of their personal and social identities, and is, thus, sustained over time by feeding off of the same social-cognition processes, which normally feed a person's sense-of-self. The pain becomes a parasite on the self, growing bigger and stronger as it devours the nutrients of a thin and weakened self-concept. These unfortunate individuals are precisely those with the Axis-II syndromes described above, exhibiting rigid cognitive and relational styles involving helplessness and dependency. In their meta-analysis of the effects of behavior therapy on clinical pain, Holroyd and Penzien (1986) found that the strongest client variable in predicting response to treatment was age, which accounted for 30 percent of the variance in treatment outcome. One reasonable explanation for this result is that pain patients adopt a stronger and stronger sick role with the passage of time, making effective treatment more and more difficult.

If this metaphor of a parasite is correct, eventually the pain schema may take over so much of these formerly healthy self and relational schema, that its removal would cause victims to lose their sense of identity, a vital organ within the psychological realm. Non-metaphorically, these clients may focus their social lives, from minute interactions all the way up to social roles, almost completely on their pain. They also might develop difficulties in imagining themselves without the pain, since it has become the focal point for movement through all of their life domains.

One life domain which is particularly influential is the financial/occupational area because vocational disability and/or financial incentives for pain represent some of the strongest barriers to the effectiveness of pain treatments (Gatchel & Epker, 1999). Again, though malingering undoubtedly occurs, it is important to point out that financial and social incentives may contribute to actual pain experiences without the conscious intent of a victim. Overall, the pain experience has a significant influence on the development of the sick-role, as well as vice versa. Therapeutically, a sufficient change in either one or both is necessary to promote health. The more difficult question is how one may promote such change(s) through imagery?

TREATMENT OUTCOME: DOES IMAGERY WORK?

The overall picture of the use of imagery techniques, both in lab-based efficacy studies on analogue pain (e.g., Fernandez & Turk, 1989) and in effectiveness studies on actual clinical pain (e.g., Achterberg, Kenner, & Lawlis, 1988; Albright & Fischer, 1990; Brown, 1984; Gauron & Bowers, 1986; Mannix, Chandurkar, Rybicki, Tusek, & Solomon, 1999; Manyande et al., 1995; Philips & Hunter, 1981; Powers, 1999; Raft et al., 1986; ter Kuile et al., 1994) is quite positive and stands in contrast to the under-utilization of imagery in combination with medical treatments (Eisenberg, Kessler, Foster, Norlock, Calkins, & Delbanco, 1993). However, answers to the process-related questions of How? How much? Which types? and For whom?, have been very illusive.

In fact, the most striking feature of experimental tests of imagery on pain are the methodological difficulties and strange results. Theoretically, these problems are the direct results of an exclusive reliance by researchers on Fisherian and nomothetic (group based) designs, which focuses on statistically significant differences between group means in an attempt to find relatively simple, reductionistic causes (Kazdin, 1992). When viewed through this Fisherian paradigmatic lens, the empirical water is extremely muddy. However, if one lends a more systemic ear, these difficulties and inconsistencies may be saying some very interesting things about pain phenomena and the potential use(s) for imagery in curing them.

The rule, in both analogue pain experiments (e.g., immersion of subjects' hands into ice water) and treatment outcome studies, is that within-subject variability in response to treatment is very pronounced. This means that within the same study (the same treatment) some people will have profound improvements in their ability to withstand pain and/or in pain reductions, while others will experience little or no effect (Mannix et al., 1999). The variability in the meta-analysis by Holroyd and Penzien (1986) ranged from 13 percent to 94 percent improvement across studies; this highlights the great differences in the pain phenomena of individuals as well as in their differential responses to specific treatments. Furthermore, some of the effective treatments have been as simplistic and palliative as relaxation training. The conclusion that people-factors are more important than treatment factors is supported even more strongly by their findings that the only significant contributions to this variability were client variables, with treatment attributes, therapeutic bond, and study attributes all unrelated to treatment outcome. Fernandez and Turk's meta-analysis (1989), as well as qualitative literature reviews (Tan, 1982; Turner & Chapman, 1982), have found the same pattern of remarkable variability in treatment response.

Within individual studies, the same variability in treatment response has been a consistent finding, with standard deviations in pain tolerance expanding between two- and four-fold following the use of various imaginal interventions (e.g., Hackett & Horan, 1980; Stevens, 1985; Stevens, Pfost, & Rapp, 1987; Worthington & Shumate, 1981). In addition, attempts to account for these variability-explosions by examining correlations between client variables and outcome or by matching particular clients to interventions have consistently generated *inconsistent* results (Beers & Karoly, 1979; Fanurik, Zelter, Roberts, & Blount, 1993; Marino, et al., 1989; Spanos & O'Hara, 1990; Stevens et al., 1987; ter Kuile et al., 1994). Again, because the nomothetic/Fisherian research paradigm relies exclusively on group averages, it is ill equipped to account for the large variability in treatment responses, if the responses are too idiosyncratic or person-specific. In fact, these designs consider these phenomena to be a major source of error and a nuisance. Again, a systemic approach may be more suitable, allowing for explanations based on causal patterns (e.g., topological patterns in the within-subject variability-explosion following treatment), rather than on isolated, individual factors and independent effects.

Another major problem with laboratory-based pain experiments (in which researchers attempt to manipulate the pain strategies of participants) is in getting people to follow instructions. In other words, people tend to use their own techniques to manage experimental pain, even when they are assigned to a no-treatment control group (Tan, 1982). In two studies employing formal manipulation checks (Stevens, 1985; Stevens et al., 1987), 68.3 percent of participants trained in, and instructed to use, specific imagery strategies generated their own strategies; 63.8 percent used multiple coping strategies across treatment groups; and only 72.5 percent of participants used their assigned strategy at all. Similarly, Hargadon, Bowers, and Woody (1995) found that only 61 percent of participants instructed to use imagery actually did so, while 14 percent of those specifically instructed *not* to use imagery did so anyway.

Hackett and Horan (1980), who made subject-bias a focus of their study, found perhaps the most comprehensive and interesting results with respect to participant recalcitrance. Overall, they found that 25 of 27 individuals across three different coping groups (relaxation training, imagery, and coping self-talk) used coping skills from all three categories at some point during the pain exposure, despite instruction and training to the contrary. They also found that people were naturally inclined to use imagery techniques aimed at regulating affect, doing so before assignment to a treatment condition in 100 percent of the cases and continuing to do so despite instructions to the contrary. Conversely, rational self-talk skills were the most frequently ignored strategy: only 55 percent of individuals in this group used their self-talk training as their primary strategy despite instructions to do so. This latter result is similar to another study in which three-fourths of participants ignored their assigned self-talk training (Worthington & Shumate, 1981). Together, these results suggest that self-talk may be a bitter pill for people to swallow.

Furthermore, these researchers found that formal manipulation checks may significantly underestimate the degree of noncompliance in pain experiments. Many more subjects admitted to non-compliance when re-questioned later on in a less formal interpersonal context. Did all of these people just hate to be told what to do? A more reasonable explanation for this subject bias is that even healthy people have idiosyncratic and automatic styles of coping with painful stimuli. Furthermore, these styles are likely a reflection of the idiosyncrasies in their underlying symbolic representations of pain as well as the ways in which they relate to these representations.

A final limitation of outcome research is such an intimate part of the research process itself that no one seems to notice it. The imaginal interventions that lend themselves most easily to empirical evaluation are also the shallowest and hypothetically the least potent. Most, if not all, experimental investigations involve two minutes or less of imagery training, which arguably does little more than distract and/or relax a person slightly. The fact that consistent positive results are found with these types of interventions at all is surprising, particularly on the backdrop of within-subject variability-explosions and messy group distinctions, both of which tie a heavy anchor onto inferential statistics that are designed to test differences in group averages. Finally, even the most flexible experiments have, at best, allowed participants only a very narrow choice of imaginal content in order to ensure the experimental control necessary to support causal inferences. The situation is similar in treatment outcome studies outside the labs, where statistical conclusion validity, internal validity, and ecological validity each rely on the provision of more or less manualized and standardized treatments (Kazdin, 1992). Taken together, these results suggest that deeper image therapies, tailored to suit actual pain victims, may hold even greater potential for healing pain. Yet to date, no rigorous study has moved beyond simple experiments to examine deeper and more comprehensive imagery work in the treatment of patients with intractable pain.

SYSTEMIC THEORIES

Beginning with the first reviews of the literature (Tan, 1982; Weisenberg, 1979), the extreme within-subject variability, imaginal idiosyncrasies, and large number of isolated psychosocial causes of pain have all contributed to the difficulty of developing a comprehensive understanding of pain etiology. As a result, researchers over the past 30 to 40 years have been developing models in which the individual factors outlined above may be conceptualized as parts of a larger pathogenic system, with the keys to therapeutic change residing within the relationships between causal factors rather than within a single factor in isolation.

Gate-Control

The gate-control theory (Melzack & Wall, 1965, 1996) was the first systemic theory linking psychosocial factors with physiological processes in pain perception. The theory had a stronger focus on the physiological side of the picture, suggesting that the dorsal horn of the Substantia Gelatinosa of the spinal cord was the connecting point, or gate, between the mind and body. Efferent (downward moving) psychological factors theoretically modified the sensitivity of the spinal cord to afferent (upward moving) nociceptive signals, thereby opening or closing the gate on the intensity of the pain experience.

On a broader scale, the theory specified three somewhat distinct yet interacting dimensions of the pain experience. The first dimension, *sensory/discriminative*, involves nerve activity at injury sites and resulting pain sensations. Imagery has been used to modify this sensory/discriminative dimension through the trans-formation of, and dissociation from, the site of pain, such as by imagining that one's arm is made of wood or rubber. The second dimension of the pain experience is *motivational/affective*, referring to the feelings and desired actions resulting from the pain experience. Imagery that produces positive affect, such as lying on a beach, has been used to decrease the intensity of the pain experience by blocking this dimension. The third dimension of pain is *cognitive/evaluative*, which refers to the meaning of the pain with respect to severity, negative implications/expectations, and other associated cognitive processes. Transforming the context of pain, such as by imagining that one is scoring the winning goal in an important football game or that one is a soldier saving a buddy in combat, has been a common treatment aimed at this dimension.

A salient example of the way these dimensions work together is in children who have not yet developed a sophisticated pain schema. Children often pause before reacting to a fall; and whether or not they cry depends upon how hard they fall (sensory/ discriminative), their moods (motivational/affective), and the reactions of the adults around them (cognitive/evaluative).

With more than 30 years of continued research into pain physiology, Melzack (1999) has proposed an updated version of the original gate-control theory: the *neuromatrix* theory. This model focused upon the body's stress-arousal systems and the functional role of pain in maintaining homeostasis within the body. He has suggested that pain and stress act together and may be adaptive in a sense, acting as a kind of emergency brake preventing dangerous fluc-tuations in body temperature or blood sugar. However, as the old saying goes, you can't get something for nothing. The body's chronic over-reliance on the pain-stress response to maintain homeostasis may lead to structural damage in skeletal, muscular, and neurological systems.

Biopsychosocial Models

The gate-control theory laid the foundations for the study of psychosocial factors by identifying an initial physiological connecting point between the mind, body, and resulting pain experience. It also implied coordination among psychosocial and physical factors in pain development within its three dimensional view of pain. However, it did not explicitly focus on these factors and the nature of their inter-relationships (Weisenberg & Keefe, 1999). Biopsychosocial models, beginning with Engel (1977), have attempted to address these higher-order systemic questions and were the first theories to describe pain phenomena as arising from the complex, non-linear (allowing for disproportional change among causes and symptoms) interactions of etiological factors (Dworkin, Von Korff, & LeResche, 1992; Turk & Flor, 1999).

Consciousness/Constructivist Theory

Chapman, Nakamura, and Flores (1999) have attempted to better account for the mind-side of the body-mind connection and pain by nesting the pain experience within the broader class of conscious experience. They wrote: "Consciousness is an *emergent* property of a *self-organizing* nervous system, and pain is an aspect of consciousness" (p. 35, italics added).

These concepts: *emergence* and *self-organization,* come from *nonlinear dynamical systems* (NDS) theory. NDS theory may be defined by looking at each term in the name separately. *Nonlinear*, again, means that causal connections are disproportional. In other words, if x is connected to y in a nonlinear manner, then a small change in x could lead to a large change in y or, conversely, a large change in x could lead to little or even no change in y. *Dynamical* refers to change over time, and thus time is always a factor in NDS models. In empirical applications, this means that change across time is more often the focus as opposed to change across groups. *System* refers to an empirical and theoretical focus on interactions between multiple causal factors, as opposed to attempts to identify simple causes and effects. In fact, systems research allows for the distinction between cause and effect to be blurred such that variables may act as both causes and effects, depending upon where and when one looks at them. In one of the most interesting systemic causal phenomena, researchers are allowed to accept the fact that variables may cause themselves over time, such as in the discussion of conditioning and pain above.

Under the theoretical umbrella of NDS, the concept of *emergence* refers to phenomena that arise from the collective behavior of underlying, smaller parts, yet as the old gestalt saying suggests, are not reducible to the behavior of those parts. *Self-organization* theory (Bak, 1996; Haken, 1984; Kauffman, 1993, 1995;

Prigogine & Stengers, 1984) describes the way in which a system develops and changes through self-determining processes and interactions with other systems over time. Common biological examples of emergent phenomena arising from self-organization include the creation of anthills, flight patterns of migrating birds, and the structural organization of the circulatory system.

Thus, a self-organized and emergent view of mind means that the mind emerges from the locally complex, yet globally coherent interaction of smaller parts (neuronal activity), with the potential to interact with these smaller parts, feeding back across the boundary of scale (Freeman, 1995; Sperry, 1993). And, of course, qualities of mind are not completely reducible to neuronal activity per se. As such, consciousness is *controlled* rather than caused, expresses a relatively narrow range of possible systemic process-structures (behavioral states), and tunes its own parameters to determine which range of processes-structures will be possible at any given time or within any situation.

According to Chapman et al., ". . . the brain deals not with reality itself but with an internal representation of reality that it constructs from moment to moment" (1999, p. 45). Thus, they view the landscape and the map as one when it comes to consciousness. Because imagery is inexorably tied to the meaning making cognitive processes described above, theoretically, if one can transform these reality-creating processes through imagery work, one will also transform the experience of pain to a greater or lesser degree. Change your clients' maps and you've changed their landscapes.

It is apparent from recent models that the trend in pain theories seems to be toward more holistic (non-reductionistic) models of pain, which include the interactions of multiple causal variables over time, and which can lead to a great variety of pain phenomena. This holistic, systemic, and ipsitive view, originally based on general systems theory (Von Bertalanffy, 1968), is explicit even in the first biopsychosocial model (Engel, 1977). If the evolution of pain theories continues in this dynamic and systemic direction, many more principles from NDS may become helpful in guiding research and practice aimed at treating pain syndromes. Because of its inherently systemic outlook, NDS theory is able to cross disciplinary boundaries from physics and meteorology through biology and into psychology. Thus, it opens the gate to searching for general principles that apply across scientific disciplines, a search that moves in the opposite direction from traditional, linear, and reductionistic research in psychology (Guastello, 1997). Furthermore, in perhaps a more practical sense, NDS methodology would not be hindered by the within-subject variability of the outcome research described above.

While Chapman et al. (1999) have relied on the NDS areas of self-organization and emergence in explaining pain phenomena, many more NDS principles may apply. Overall, the clearest hypothesis that these theoretical principles suggest is that pain is a manifestation of rigidity and inflexibility (Bak, 1996; Belaire, Glass, Ander-Heiden, & Milton, 1995; West & Deering, 1995). Just as there is tenderness, a restricted range of movement, and rigidity at the physical sites of pain, it is also likely that clients will display similar patterns of rigidity in the psychosocial process that are connected to those sites. Thus, the goal of imagery techniques may be to activate and enhance the self-correcting mechanisms within the areas of consciousness that are associated with pain. Although without more empirical backing specific to pain disorders, these ideas should be considered speculative.

ASPECTS OF IMAGERY

Imagery is generally considered to be a set of techniques rather than a theory of psychotherapy per se, and imagery work is compatible with virtually any theory of psychotherapy from cognitive-behavioral to psychodynamic theory (McMahon & Sheikh, 1986). With the systemic conceptualizations of pain in mind, the following are some theoretical ways in which imagery may ameliorate pain.

Imagery as Shadow Experience

Bandura's social-learning theory represents the most mainstream scientific view of imagery as a shadow to experience (Bandura, 1977, 1986). Bandura improved upon mechanistic radical behavioral views of human learning by stressing the role of information as opposed to learning history in guiding behavior. His theory of social learning describes four sources of information ranging in strength from largest to smallest: actual experience, vicarious experience, physiological information, and verbal persuasion. Vicarious experience means observational learning, which includes self-imagery as a relatively potent form of vicarious experience due to the obvious similarity (unity) between the subject and object.

Many of the tests of imagery on pain rely either implicitly or explicitly on images as social-learning experiences, in which a person may learn to cope better with pain through covert rehearsal of coping techniques to be used later during a pain episode (e.g., Achterberg et al., 1988), or by providing imaginal coping strategies which give a person actual coping experiences. Though these techniques have been shown to be helpful in reducing the impact of pain, they may be seen as somewhat palliative, improving self-efficacy in a person's ability to manage pain rather than transforming consciousness to a state in which pain is no longer welcome.

The Triple-Code Theory

The triple-code model (Ahsen, 1984) paves the way for deeper interventions for the treatment of pain though imagery. According to the model, images (I), somatic responses (S), and meaning (M) are inexorably linked to one another. This ISM model suggests that activation of any of the three codes will invariably lead to the emergence of the other two states to which it is linked. So if someone holds a specific image in consciousness, a specific somatic response and meaning structure will emerge; and conversely, a change to any of the coded states will lead to a change in the others. Also, any of the codes may be primary in invoking the other two. For example, meaning may invoke syntonic images, which then invoke syntonic somatic states. This theory of imagery closely parallels independent lines of empirical work in cognitive psychology known as neoassociationism (Berkowitz, 1993), which again describes the connections of emotional states, episodic memories, sensations, thought processes, and meaning structures (schemata) through the activation of theoretical nodes, which are connected, in a complicated, associationistic network. Achterberg et al., (1988) describe this theoretical process as it relates to the effectiveness of imagery treatment for reducing the intense pain associated with burn treatments:

> . . . Image, somatic response, and meaning become linked in an infinite number of complex ways and predetermine behavior, attitudes, and all manner of human functions . . . interpretation of the situation has drawn its power from the somatic-image bond . . . The current protocol [imaginal coping] apparently served to unyoke physiological and verbal expressions of fear and pain associated with burn treatment. And hence, reactions to the actual treatment were somewhat ameliorated. (p. 84)

Within the triple code model, images, sensations, and meaning enter consciousness in tandem, and may be pulled into consciousness through a change to any of the individual pieces. Thus, states of consciousness emerge like patterns of string in a game of cat's cradle (the children's game in which a string is wrapped in complicated ways around the upturned fingers of both hands). Changing the way in which a single segment of string is wrapped around even one finger invokes the emergence of a whole new pattern in the strings across both hands.

The Imagery-Sensory Lexicon of Experience

Ahsen (1984) argued against the view of imagery as an epiphenomenon or shadow experience, and assigned it a more central position in guiding meaning-making processes and somatic responses in a non-sequential and non-linear manner. Furthermore, this central position is maintained whether or not the person is currently attending to the image. From this perspective, Bandura's (1977) four sources of information may be exerting their influence by changing the dynamic flow of images, which continually underlie people's experiences. Actual experiences would then be expected to enhance efficacy expectations simply because they are the most vivid and absorbing, which gives them greater image shifting impact. Bandura's (1986) own research results may be reinterpreted to support the view that images are a central factor in guiding such aspects of consciousness as behavioral sets, affect, and somatic responses. For example, Bandura (1986) found that snake phobics' ability to handle boa constrictors was better predicted by efficacy expectations than actual past experiences. This suggests that the *current* imaginal states of individuals with respect to snake handling were the best predictors for their snake-related behaviors, whether or not they were focusing on the images per se. In other words, their state-specific snake-handler slide shows were rolling somewhere in their consciousness whether they were consciously watching them or not. Admittedly, this idea of a running slide show suggests that there is an unconscious imagery-based mind that is always active, a tricky suggestion from the scientific standpoint of falsifiability. On the other hand, it is not very different from the mainstream notion of self-talk from cognitive therapy. In fact, people's preference for imagery-based interventions over self-talk in response to painful stimulation would suggest that self-talk may in fact represent a running commentary on the content of images, as opposed to independent cognition relating to sensory input. Comparing the differential levels of attention required to attend to images versus self-talk in a controlled experiment could serve as a rather simple test of this hypothesis.

Furthermore, this running slide show interpretation may help to explain the comparable therapeutic efficacy of hypnotic analgesic suggestions with and without imagery (Hargadon et al., 1995) and some non-imaginal placebo treatments for pain. For example, Spanos et al. (1993) had an especially strong placebo effect in pain reduction, which was significantly larger than self-monitoring controls and somewhat larger than the experimental imagery/hypnosis intervention for chronic headache sufferers. Their placebo condition involved looking at four slides of random dots, flashed for one-half a second at 15-second intervals, a flashing rate that made the stimulus sufficiently ambiguous. Participants were told that the slides contained hidden messages designed to ameliorate pain by changing their unconscious autonomic processes. Finally, a specific key word was paired with the treatment to be used as a mnemonic cue during periods of stress and/or headache to trigger calmness and healing. The positive results of this rather sophisticated placebo were not related to expectations of treatment efficacy, which tended to be low at the outset of treatment. One explanation for their results is that the participants projected their own healing images on the ambiguous slides and invoked them later to modify unhealthy images associated with their headaches, all without conscious attention to the images. If this was in fact the case, the hoax may have been on the experimenters, who designed a bogus intervention and therapeutic rationale, which in fact worked just as they said it would.

The role of images as central guiding factors in current reality-making processes is also in line with research on the role of top-down processes on perception described above. The overall picture that emerges is that states of consciousness are continually constructed through the self-organized mixing of bottom-up sensory process and top-down imaginal process. Each experience emerges from the backdrop of an imagery-sensory lexicon of possible states of consciousness, and with each comes a limited range of affective, sensory, cognitive, and somatic vectors. As such, if the imagery-based factors involved in pain consciousness can be ameliorated through the direct transformation of the associative network in which they are nested, the experience of the pain disorder will no longer be possible. This explanation is in line with empirical studies that have found relationships between absorption in, but not vividness of, images and therapeutic efficacy (Kwekkeboom, Huseby-Moore, & Ward, 1998; Marino et al., 1989; Spanos & O'Hara, 1990). It is also in line with the rigidity/flexibility hypothesis suggested by NDS theory, which suggests that a pain system may dissipate if the consciousness making processes attached to it are infused with adaptive flexibility.

Imagery as a Schema Portal

Ultimately, the most efficient and effective use of imagery for pain that has a dominant psychogenic causal component is to transform the actual associative network in which pain lives, be they schema, the neuromatrix (Melzack, 1999), consciousness (Chapman et al., 1999), the ISM (Ahsen, 1984), or neoassociationistic networks (Berkowitz, 1993). For convenience, and because all of these theoretical lines are essentially describing the same process-structure(s), the term "schema" will be used to suggest that imagery may be viewed as a schema-portal, through which people may gain access to their own consciousness-making structures. Once one has entered the schema-portal, one experiences images with the same multidimensional flavor as actual experience (e.g., sights, sounds, touch, etc.). As a doorway to the abstract interconnections of consciousness, imagery therapy may provide the unique opportunity to experience one's own experience-making system and thus to modify it.

In imagery work, pain clients may be seen as astronauts who move through this schema-portal into the experiential vacuum of inner space to work on the life support systems of the self. The imagery therapist may be seen as ground control, attempting to guide the astronaut through the often-complicated procedures that must be carried out in the unique environment of imaginal space. It is clear that a variety of therapeutic imagery techniques may be helpful in facilitating the process of self-discovery and self-modification of pain within this imaginal realm. The use of systems science in describing pain processes may provide a first step for practitioners, a sort of general orientation for the selection of specific procedures for specific clients.

TREATMENT

It has been demonstrated repeatedly that, ". . . experiencing something in imagery can be considered to be in many essential ways psychologically equivalent to experiencing the thing in actuality" (Klinger, 1980, p. 5). Recall, for example, the image of sucking on a lemon described earlier. Yet, while they are somewhat equivalent to reality, images are not bound to the same rules and limitations of reality (Ahsen, 1973). Therein lies one of their greatest potential strengths in the treatment of pain disorders in conjunction with more traditional interventions.

When using imagery, it is important that clients are able to understand instructions, to concentrate on images, to achieve a fairly deep state of relaxation (Bresler, 1984), and to believe that imagery work can help to decrease their pain. Ensuring that clients are able to meet these conditions will maximize the potential benefits of imagery. In addition, imagery techniques specific to pain are generally contraindicated when there is limited motivation, time, and/or energy; when there are other, more pressing emotional issues; when clients are actively psychotic; or when they have limited concentration abilities (McCaffery & Beebe, 1989).

Potential Benefits and Limits of Pain Relief Images

As was suggested previously, the potential advantages of pain relief images are best understood by placing them within a dynamic context, where changes occur in a sequence of causal events over time (see Figure 1). McCaffery and Beebe (1989) point out one of the ways in which imagery may interrupt these pain generating cycles: "Imagery may interrupt the process here to change the image of what will happen, thereby changing the physiological response. A positive image may result in a helpful physiological response" (p. 214). Moreover, imagery may be helpful in a multitude of additional ways depending upon the specifics of a client's pain generating cycle. Indeed, with some clients the impact may be quite profound if a transformation in pain-related images is able to transform the self and/or self-pain relational schema to a substantial degree. For example, imagery may allow a person to express feelings that are attached to their pain, which may lead to corrections in erroneous ideas about the pain and ultimately to a lasting confidence in the ability to heal oneself.

Of course imagery is not always effective in pain management. For example, some clients may have substantial nociception due to tissue damage and limited abilities to use mental imagery such as those mentioned above. Other client's may have unshakable views that the use of imagery is an indication that others see their pain as merely imaginary, hindering motivation and expectations. In the worst scenarios, imagery techniques may lead to an increase in pain if intensely emotional issues are uncovered with which the person is not yet able to cope. These caveats are important for practitioners to keep in mind in order to balance creativity and optimism with caution and pragmatism.

Introducing Imagery

Again, it is imperative that the health professionals reassure patients that their pain is not merely imaginary, but is real. Syrjala and Abrams (1996) suggest doing so by simply explaining the gate-control theory to the patient and then suggesting that images may be used just as medications, to block the gates between

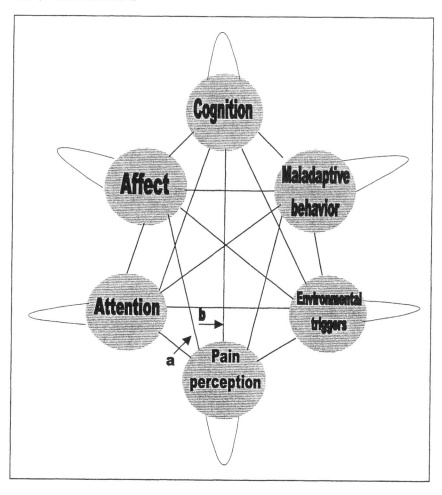

Figure 1. A conceptual illustration of the complex connections between causal factors involved in the generation and maintenance of pain disorders. The circles represent categories of causal factors: cognition (e.g., beliefs, expectations), maladaptive behavior (e.g., avoidance, inactivity), environmental triggers (e.g., conflict, loss), attention (e.g., body scanning, internal focus), and affect (e.g., helplessness, fear, anger). The thin connecting lines represent the connections between these factors over time, whereby increases in one factor at one point in time may lead to increases in any other factor through multiple pathways. The arrows, a and b, illustrate two of the ways that imagery may impact pain perception by blocking these causal connections. Arrow-a represents relaxation, which blocks the anxiety that serves to increase pain perception. Arrow-b represents positive expectations, which block negative expectations about pain. In practice, imagery techniques may have an impact at any of the causal connections within the illustration and may even impact several connections simultaneously.

the site of the pain and the brain. Furthermore, one may demonstrate the ways that attention, pain, and consciousness are connected during the natural flow of the consultation. For example, a client may be asked to rate his pain from one to ten at the start of the consultation. Later, they may be asked to rate the pain they felt during a period in the consultation process in which they were engaged in the discussion. The difference that they recognize from this simple demonstration may then be compared to the potential difference that may arise through immersion in the healing images to be discovered within treatment. Yet, no matter how elegant the examples or explanations are, it is most important that they make sense to each client. This is particularly true for clients with personality disorders, which may lead to perceptual distortions and/or concentration problems that would interfere with their ability to process such explanations. In these cases, it may even be helpful to ask clients to repeat the explanations back in their own words, or to come up with their own examples of the effect of distraction on pain.

Some Guidelines for Using Imagery for Pain Relief

The following is a list of guidelines that practitioners have found to be helpful in their work with pain patients (Korn, 1983a; McCaffery & Beebe, 1989; Syrjola & Abrams, 1996).

1. Avoid using imagery techniques if you feel uncomfortable using them.
2. Do not suggest to the client that imagery is a substitute for other appropriate pain-relieving methods.
3. Pay close attention to the client's spontaneous use of images and try to incorporate the positive ones in your approach. The negative images offered by the clients must first be transformed if they are to be helpful.
4. Even images that are anatomically or physiologically incorrect can be useful.
5. Be mindful of the potentially negative impact of certain images on the patient. For example, avoid images of strenuous exercise with a patient who requires bed rest and reduced oxygen consumption.
6. Try to determine the client's dominant sense modality and then emphasize that modality in pain relief images.
7. Encourage and help the client to use his/her own images.
8. Avoid using the word "pain" as far as possible. For example, "Your arm is becoming more comfortable and relaxed" rather than, "The pain is diminishing."
9. Do not try to force the image on the client; simply offer it using phrases such as, "If you wish, you may . . ." or "You might like to. . . ."
10. Encourage the client to have confidence in the imagery process, for changes in the beginning might be very subtle and hard to recognize.
11. Make sure the client is sufficiently relaxed before introducing specific images of pain relief.

12. To obtain full benefits from imagery procedures, one needs commitment to the process, which means regular practice.

13. Although it is very helpful if the image is vivid and lifelike, it is more important for the client to be able to control the image and be absorbed within it.

14. Using end-result imagery (image of the result the client likes to achieve) in the early stages may be more effective for some clients than process imagery (image of the process by which the desired state is achieved).

15. Just as it is in medical interventions, targeted imagery relies on knowledge of the etiology and exact location of the pain.

16. Try to measure the severity of the pain perceived by the client before and after the use of imagery, such as through the one-to-ten scaling described above.

17. Identifying previous treatments received by the patient as well as their efficacy might by very helpful. Knowledge about other treatments and illnesses the client is experiencing concurrently might also be useful.

18. How alert is the client? How well can he or she concentrate? What is his or her emotional state? How important is symptom amelioration to him or her? How strong is the client's need for control? Answers to these questions are very helpful in designing appropriate imagery treatment.

19. If family members are involved, their beliefs and attitudes can help or hinder the process of imagery.

20. For religious clients, spiritual images such as "God's healing hand" can be successfully employed.

21. It is beneficial to assess the coping style used by the client prior to choosing specific imagery techniques. People who actively cope with pain will more readily use imagery techniques in which they can participate. Others who tend to avoid or catastrophize about pain will respond to more directive imagery techniques. The client's flexibility in coping is also important in that those who are more flexible are generally easier to work with.

22. Language used by the therapist in imagery work must be action-oriented rather than passive (Watzlawick, 1978). Clients can imagine that they are doing something, while it is impossible for them to imagine themselves not-doing something.

Just as different tips from the list above will be more or less important with different clients, it is important to note that although the following imagery techniques are presented individually, a combination of them may be more effective for some clients than using one technique in isolation. Similarly, different therapists will need to attend to different guidelines, and may prefer different combinations of techniques depending upon their personal and therapeutic styles. Finally, some of the techniques presented in this section were found within the hypnosis literature. Hypnosis and imagery are generally considered to be comparable in most situations (Hilgard & Hilgard, 1994). They are both, ". . . widely agreed to be states of highly focused attention during which alterations of sensations, awareness, and perception can occur. . . . Suggestion is an integral part of hypnosis, whereas suggestion may or may not be offered in imagery." (Syrjala & Abrams, 1996, pp. 231-232). As a result, no distinctions will be made between the two in the following discussion.

Imagery and Relaxation

Generally, relaxation is considered to be a state where there is a relative absence of anxiety and skeletal muscle tension. Most relaxation procedures include a mental device to block distracting thoughts, a passive attitude, a quiet environment, a comfortable position, and behaviors previously conditioned to result in relaxation, such as deep abdominal breathing and a focus on peaceful images (Benson & Stark, 1996; Korn, 1983b; McCaffery & Beebe, 1989; Sheikh, Sheikh, & Moleski, 1985; Syrjala & Abrams, 1996).

Relaxation appears to be one of the most important prerequisites for the experience of vivid and absorbing imagery; for, it seems to allow the process of becoming aware of internal states to begin. During relaxation, the noisy, hectic world is shut out, and the inner world, the realm of imaginal experience, has a chance to become the focus of attention (Bakan, 1980; Gendlin, 1981; Sheikh, Sheikh, & Moleski, 1985).

It follows that pain-relief imagery generally is preceded by relaxation techniques. Again, relaxation is believed to increase the effectiveness of pain-relief imagery by enhancing the vividness of one's images and thereby one's absorption within them. Recall that empirical studies have demonstrated consistent effects for relaxation alone in the treatment of pain. Again, this therapeutic impact may be understood through a cyclic and systemic understanding of the pathogenesis of pain disorders (Figure 1). Numerous relaxation procedures have been developed over the years, and it is beyond the scope of the current discussion to review them. For detailed information about these methods, the reader is referred to other sources (Korn, 1983b; McCaffery & Beebe, 1989; Ost, 1987; Samuels & Samuels, 1975; Sheikh, 2001).

Following relaxation training and before introducing specific pain relief imagery, clients are often encouraged to explore pleasant, peaceful images of their special place:

> And as you enjoy this feeling of deep comfort and well-being, allow yourself to begin to create a special place of your choosing. A place where you feel safe and secure and content. It may be a place you have been before, it may be a place you would like to go now, or a place only in your imagination. All that matters is that you find a place for you right now. And begin to notice that place. Notice if it is indoors or out. Observe what is all around you. Take it in. Notice the colors, the different hues and tones of color. Perhaps there are reds

or yellows . . . the light and the dark shades, the light around you. . . . Explore the shapes in your surroundings . . . perhaps you can reach out and touch things, notice what they feel like...are they soft or hard, rough or smooth, warm or cool? Making it all real for you now, enjoying being in this pleasant, safe place, experiencing it fully. (Syrjala & Abrams, 1996, p. 252)

Exploring images of the special place serves a dual purpose: it deepens relaxation and sets the stage for the experience of more specific pain relief images (Syrjala & Abrams, 1996)

Subtle, Conversational Imagery

During routine verbal interactions with clients, healing images often emerge spontaneously. For example, clients might say that their medications *fight* their pain or a therapist might say that regular exercise *builds* pain resistance. McCaffery and Beebe (1989) offer specific guidelines for therapists in making use of these language-based images in pain treatment:

1. After choosing a particular pain relief measure one should attempt to explain how it works in a language that paints a mental picture. For example, while administering an analgesic one could say, "Now it's as if the medication is slowly floating through your body to find your pain and make it smaller and smaller, leaving feelings of comfort and healing."
2. Employ words and phrases that are likely to arouse comforting and pain-relieving imagery. Examples of these words include: floating, dissolving, quieting, releasing, loosening, soothing, healing, smaller, softer, smooth, cool or warm, and letting go.
3. If a client is offered an image of what causes his/her pain, he/she should also be provided with an image of pain relief. For example, if a client is told that the physician will make an incision to remove something, he/she should also be informed of possible comforting events, such as a soft, comfortable dressing, a soothing cold pack, medication flowing to the area to soothe it, rest and nutrients repairing and healing the wound.

Glove Anesthesia

One simple way to relieve pain is through imagery techniques suggesting that the painful body part is becoming numb (Hilgard & Hilgard, 1994). This is similar to response-transformative imagery (Fernandez, 1986), which will be discussed later. This simple technique can be expanded into a two-step imagery exercise called glove anesthesia (Bresler, 1984). First, victims learn how to develop a numbing sensation in their hand, which helps to convince them that they can have some control over the intensity of their pain. When the feeling of numbness is achieved, they learn to transfer this numbness from the hand to the pain-site by rubbing it with the anesthetized hand (Hilgard & Hilgard, 1994). This technique is demonstrated in the following example:

> And you are aware that you are unable to feel anything in your hand. It is as if your hand is numb, without sensation, and you can take your hand and move it to where you feel discomfort, gently rubbing your hand over the uncomfortable area. And as you rub this numb hand, this hand without feeling, over the uncomfortable place, you are aware that the numbness is moving, is being transferred to that place, as if you were rubbing novocaine over the affected area, making the uncomfortable sensation cease. (Meyer, 1992, pp. 229-230)

The glove anesthesia technique is especially helpful for clients who are experiencing intense pain that prevents them from using other types of guided-imagery/ hypnotic techniques (Bresler, 1984).

Displacement

Another technique that allows patients to better tolerate their pain is to displace the pain from one area of the body to another (Hilgard & Hilgard, 1994). Clients are encouraged to concentrate the pain into a smaller area, and then to move it to another body part, like their hand, where the pain is easier to tolerate. Allowing victims to choose where they want the pain to move increases this technique's effectiveness. An example of a suggestion resulting in the displacement of pain follows:

> You may have already noticed that the pain moves, ever so slightly, and you can begin to notice that the movement seems to be in an outwardly spiraling, circular direction. As you continue to attend to that movement, you may not notice until some time later that the pain has somehow moved out of your abdomen and seems to be staying in your left hand. It seems to be very much the same sensation . . . yet, for some reason, it seems less bothersome. (Barber, 1996, p. 90)

By changing the location of the pain experience, the pain becomes less disabling, and consequently, more tolerable for the patient (Barber, 1996).

Emptying the Sandbag

In this technique, clients are relaxed and then instructed to imagine their body as an empty bag that they are filling slowly with sand. Their bodies will feel heavier and heavier, until they have completely filled up the bag with sand. Next, they are instructed to focus on the area of discomfort. Once the patients have done this, they are instructed to make a small slit in the sandbag at that area and to imagine the sand slowly trickling out, until the sandbag is completely emptied and weightless. This process is repeated for each area of pain (McCaffery & Beebe, 1989).

Direct Diminution of Sensations

A very simple technique is to reduce pain intensity directly through suggestions aimed at the sensory/discriminative dimension of pain images themselves (Barber, 1996). Some possible suggestions are to *turn down the volume* or to *cool down the heat* of pain. To maximize its effectiveness, the choice of metaphor should match the pain-image of the client. The following is an example of this technique:

> You can continue to enjoy feeling increasingly well, with each breath you take . . . almost as if the discomfort is somehow gradually going away . . . as if, somehow, the feelings are getting smaller and smaller and smaller, or, perhaps, getting farther and farther and farther from your awareness. (Barber, 1996, p. 88)

In another common technique, the scaling of pain described above is used as an intervention. During imagery, a therapist can suggest that the number assigned to the pain is reduced, resulting in a decrease of pain:

> And now you can see the number seven, the number you have given to your pain. And as you see this number, you see that it is slowly, slowly changing. Now the number is six. And as you look at that number, at the number six, you are aware that your discomfort has lessened. And a six is very much like five. And as you watch, the six is changing into a five. And as you see the five, you begin to feel more comfortable. And a five is not much different from a four. And a four is very close to a three. The number is now a three. And with each change the number makes, each time the number changes into another number, your comfort becomes greater. And with only a small change, with very little effort, you can see the number three turn into a two. And as you see the two, as you experience the two, you are more and more comfortable. (Meyer, 1992, pp. 221-222)

Again, concentrating on the increase in relief, rather than focusing directly on the pain, tends to be more effective in reducing the clients' discomfort (Meyer, 1992).

Achterberg, Dossey, and Kolkmeier (1994) have suggested another diminution technique called the *ball of pain*. After some initial relaxation, the technique seeks to work with resistance rather than against it, encouraging the manifestation of pain within the client through the activation of attentional-perceptual dynamics described earlier: "Give yourself some time to relax and let go of your tension. . . . Scan your body now for any aches, pains, tightness, or discomforts, both physical and emotional" (Achterberg et al., 1994, p. 125). Next the pain is transformed, again working in the same direction as treatment resistance by making the pain brighter and larger:

> Now begin to gather up the pain into a ball, . . . a glowing, colored ball. . . . When you have the ball firmly in your mind's eye, begin to change the size of the ball, noticing how the shadings and intensity of the color change as you make the ball larger . . . and then smaller. . . . Change the size of the ball several

times, allowing it to become very large, larger than your entire body . . . and then watch and feel it shrink down to a tiny dot of color. . . . Play with the possibilities of size, intensity, and color. (Achterberg et al., 1994, p. 125).

Improvements in clients' ability to manipulate their pain in this way leads to increases in their sense of control and efficacy around the pain. At the same time, flexibility is brought to the pain system, as the pain is allowed to change in size and intensity with the ball image. This sets the stage for the complete transformation of a client's relationship with the pain, as the pain is detached from the physical body itself:

> Move the ball of pain up to the surface of your skin now, and as you do so let some or all of the ball move through your skin and feel it resting gently on the surface of your body. . . . Notice the size and color again as you image the ball beginning to float above the surface of your skin, floating up and away . . . moving across the room, and even drifting through the window or wall. (Achterberg et al., 1994, p. 105)

Incompatible Imagery

Incompatible imagery may be broken down into two types: incompatible emotive imagery and incompatible sensory imagery (Fernandez, 1986), which work by blocking the motivational/affective and sensory dimensions of pain respectively (Melzack & Wall, 1965). Incompatible emotions include happiness, confidence, and pride. The most basic examples of incompatible emotive imagery are relaxation images, such as a day at the beach or spending time in a favorite place. Deeper varieties will depend upon the specific imaginal manifestations of a victim's pain, and will involve a transformation of the motivational/affective dimension rather than simply blocking it. For example, if a victim's headaches are tied to episodic memories of being teased by other children on the playground, feelings of helplessness, fear and suppressed-anger may be transformed to confidence, and expressed-anger by changing the way she relates to her tormentors within the image.

Incompatible sensory imagery involves the use of *pure* auditory, visual, or other sensations that are incompatible with pain, but are not necessarily tied to a person's emotions (Fernandez, 1986). Pleasant imagery, such as *blue skies, gentle warmth, fluffy clouds,* and *grassy meadows,* can be used to inhibit pain (Horan, 1973). Instructing clients to use these types of images when they are experiencing pain can aid in decreasing their discomfort. One of many examples of this type of imagery given by Ferrucci (1982) involves imagining a burning flame:

> Imagine a burning flame. See it dancing, drawing ever-changing designs in the air. Look into it as it moves; seek to experience its fiery quality. As you keep visualizing this flame, think about fire and its manifestations in the psyche: personal warmth and radiance, flaming love or joy, fiery enthusiasm,

ardor. Finally, as you keep the flame in front of your inner eye, slowly imagine that you are animated by that fire, that you are becoming that flame. (p. 123)

Dissociation

Dissociation allows patients to separate themselves from their pain by directing their attention elsewhere. Dissociative techniques (Hilgard & Hilgard, 1994) allow clients to be aware of their pain without suffering from it (Barber, 1996). In one variety of dissociation, victims deny the existence of the part of the body that is feeling pain. Hilgard and Hilgard (1994) describe one example of this type of dissociative imagery:

> Think that you have no left arm. Look down and see that there is no left arm there, only an empty sleeve. An arm that does not exist does not feel anything. Your arm is gone only temporarily; you will find it amusing, not alarming, that for a while you have no left arm. (p. 66)

Kelly and Kelly (1995) present another dissociation technique called *leaving your body behind*. In this hypnotic technique, the person becomes completely dissociated from their body by removing their consciousness from their body within imagery:

> As you settle in, so peaceful, comfortable, relaxed, and at ease, you are going to allow yourself to have a curious sort of experience. You are going to allow yourself to leave your body behind. Just imagine yourself seeing your body sitting there or lying there, comfortably hypnotized, and imagine seeing a sort of translucent image of yourself stepping out from your body. (Kelly & Kelly, 1995, p. 280)

When using this technique, it is important to reassure clients that if there is information they need to know while in this state that they would find out about it immediately. This assurance allows them to more fully engage themselves in the imagery:

> You see yourself stepping away from your own body, feeling safe and secure. You are allowing your spirit, your mind, your psyche to become somewhat detached and removed from your body. You know that it's there. You know what's going on in it. It doesn't matter very much to you, however. . . . Where you are, it's comfortable and safe. It's peaceful. It's relaxed. Any sensations come to you only very slowly. . . . You get news of your body. You get information about it, but only rather slowly and sort of after the fact. (Kelly & Kelly, 1995, p. 280)

Transformative Imagery

Transformative imagery is used to change the context, stimulus, or response associated with pain (Fernandez, 1986). With contextual transformative imagery, the context or setting in which pain occurs is transformed. Fernandez

(1986) has described the use of this type of imagery during which subjects experiencing forearm pain were asked to imagine that they were spies, shot in the arm by their enemies, and were now being chased by these enemies down a treacherous mountain road.

Within stimulus-transformative imagery, the cause of the pain is changed and then transformed. For example, stomach pain could be envisioned as tight steel bands, which are then loosened in the imagination (Levendusky & Pankratz, 1975).

Finally, in response-transformative imagery, the sensations that arise from a painful stimulus can be relabeled in the imagery. This type of imagery has been used in the context of hypnosis under the label sensory substitution (Barber, 1996). Some examples of sensations that have been used for this type of imagery include numbness, insensitivity, and pressure. In order to use this technique, clients must be aware of their pain on some level, so they do not worry about failing to seek medical attention when necessary. Also, since the substitute sensation needs to be plausible to the client, it must not be too pleasant (Barber, 1996). The following case of a 42-year-old paraplegic patient experiencing burning in his legs illustrates the effectiveness of response-transformative imagery:

> The feelings that you describe (needles stabbing into his thighs) can begin to change, very slightly. Oddly enough, it may begin to seem as if the needles are becoming more and more blunt . . . broad . . . almost as if they have become tiny, massaging fingers. What an interesting sensation you can begin to have: thousands of warm, buzzing fingers, massaging your legs. Not entirely pleasant, of course, but perhaps a welcome relief. (Barber, 1996, pp. 89-90)

Mental Rehearsal

In mental rehearsal, clients envision themselves going through the steps that lead to the attainment of a specific goal (Newshan and Balamuth, 1990-91), such as when athletes wish to improve their performance. When used for pain, mental rehearsal has been applied to situations in which the goal is to reduce the pain associated with certain medical procedures, such as bone marrow aspirations (LeBaron & Zeltzer, 1996), surgeries (Meyer, 1992), burn treatment (Achterberg, Kenner, & Lawlis, 1988), or childbirth (Lindberg & Lawlis, 1988; Oster, 1994). The following is an excerpt from mental rehearsal imagery for burn treatment:

> Just let the fear go. Imagine now as the time approaches for you to get your dressings taken off and go to the bath—picture this in your imagination. Just relax, feeling deeper and deeper, breathing deeply whenever you feel uncomfortable. The nurse comes in now and starts to cut your bandages off. Imagine this happening, whenever you feel uncomfortable, breathe, relax. Imagine this happening, feeling the nurse cut the bandages off and your skin feeling the coolness. Take a deep breath and let any discomfort go, feeling relaxed and calm now . . . you begin to get out of your bed—maybe by yourself, relaxed and calm and feeling very good. . . . (Achterberg, Kenner, & Lawlis, 1988, p. 86)

Opening Around Pain

Another technique that can be used to help diminish the discomfort and pain suffered by patients is called *opening around pain* (Levine, 1982). This technique aims directly at the rigid/closed emotions, sensations, and physical reactions (e.g., muscle constriction) connected to the pain site. As the name suggests, the goal is to open these areas up, so that the client may face the pain sensations directly. If successful, self-efficacy, self-control, and flexibility are restored as the person is exposed to the pain sensations without their stereotypic coping reactions at the cognitive, emotional, and physiological levels. Ideally, this will reverse some of the fear and avoidance-based coping dynamics that paradoxically maintain and intensify pain disorders over the long-term. The following is a hypothetical example of an opening induction in guided imagery adapted from Levine (1982):

> Allow yourself to relax and become comfortable. As you relax, focus your attention on your body until you find an area of discomfort or pain. Allow your attention to completely wash over that area and feel the sensations that grow there. Notice how your body reacts to the pain. Do the muscles tighten and squeeze around the pain?. . . like a fist that squeezes tighter and tighter. . . . Allow yourself to feel the discomfort, the tightness, the squeezing of the pain, like a clenched fist closing tighter and tighter. Notice any negative emotions surrounding the pain . . . fear . . . helplessness . . . anxiety . . . guilt . . . anger . . . squeezing the pain . . . like a tight fist with white knuckles. Feel the body squeeze around the pain until it is exhausted. Why does it try to squeeze so hard? Now, allow this fist to begin to relax and to open. Moment by moment it opens around the sensations. Allow the sensations to stay, to be, to lie there calmly in the palm of the opening hand. As the hand opens the fingers move gently. Allow your fear, anxiety, anger and other negative feelings to fall away, like water flowing between its moving fingers. The final feelings melt across the open palm until the palm itself, melts back into the soft, warm, open flesh. All that is left is sensation, pure sensations floating freely in an open, soft, relaxed body.

Symbolic Representation of Pain

Symbolic representation of pain can be particularly useful in addressing the meaning of one's pain. In this technique, clients were asked to visualize the pain as a living entity in their bodies (Newshan & Balamuth, 1990-91). Further, these clients were asked to talk with the pain representation and ask it questions like, "What do you need from me?" and "What can I do to live with you?" Furthermore, the importance of listening closely to the response of the pain entity was emphasized. A case study illustrating imagery using a symbolic representation of the pain follows:

> Patient A is a woman who suffered from low back and leg pain for twenty years. She had stopped working more than a year before joining the group.

She is single, with no children, and is close to her eighty-five-year-old grandmother. At the time she entered the group, she was also investigating surgical interventions and had been through an outpatient physical therapy back program. Her initial pain creature image throughout the first two weeks of the program was of a mule facing away from her, kicking her with its hind legs. She reported suffering greatly during the first weeks. . . . In the third imagery session, she reported seeing a red devil who was laughing at her and stabbing her with a pitchfork. She was trying to beat him off with her pocketbook but was unsuccessful. During this time, she was still in a struggle about having surgery. In the fourth imagery session, the red devil returned but she was able to hide from him behind pillows. The devil searched but did not find her and she laughed at him this time. Also, in the first weeks, the mule never responded to her attempts to speak with him but the devil told her he was there to "make your life miserable." At the point when she was able to hide from the devil, she decided not to have surgery and also felt less pain. . . . In the last week, no pain creature appeared. Rather, she imagined herself looking at the beach and feeling happy—she reported that she enjoyed the beach, but had not been there in many years, and planned that as one of her upcoming goals. Her progress, although initially difficult, was steady and she reported increased socialization and activities. In the second to last week, she announced that she had taken a part-time job. (Newshan & Balamuth, 1990-1991, p. 36)

Inner Advisor

The creation of an *inner advisor* can be an extremely powerful guided-imagery technique for some victims (Bresler, 1984). Once relaxed, clients can be assisted in locating imaginary creatures in their unconscious minds that can serve as their advisors. Interestingly, these creatures may have access to all kinds of information that are unavailable to the victims. By communicating regularly with their advisors, clients can gain insight into the psychosocial causes of their pain, and discover ways to decrease or even eliminate their pain. The following case study, in which the patient, John, described his pain as a dog chewing on his spine, illustrates the potential effectiveness of the inner advisor technique:

[The] initial goal was to have the dog stop chewing on his spine. Over the next few sessions, the dog began to reveal critically important information. According to the dog (named Skippy), John never had wanted to be a physician—his own career choice was architecture—but he had been pressured into medical school by his mother. Consequently, he felt resentment not only toward his mother, but also toward his patients and colleagues. Skippy suggested that this hostility had in turn contributed to the development of his cancer and to the subsequent pain problem as well. During one session, Skippy told John, "You're a damn good doctor. It may not be the career you wanted, but it's time you recognized how good you are at what you do. When you stop being so resentful and start accepting yourself, I'll stop chewing on your spine." These insights were accompanied by an immediate alleviation of the pain, and in only a few weeks' time, John became a new person, and his pain progressively subsided. (Bresler, 1984, p. 227)

Mind-Controlled Analgesia

Mind-controlled analgesia is a technique that transforms pain experiences through the language of the unconscious (Bresler, 1984). Initially, victims were asked to draw three pictures: their pain at its worst, their pain at its best, and one symbolizing the most intense pleasure they could ever experience. The imagery exercise, which was practiced a few times per day, began with a relaxation segment, followed by an experience of the patient's pain at its worst (the first picture). Through the use of imagery, this experience was changed into the picture of pain at its best. Eventually, clients were encouraged to transform their experience even further, into the image of extreme pleasure. When successful, people were able to see that their views of the world change along with their images (Bresler, 1984).

Fantasy of In-The-Body Travel

Alexander (1971) described *fantasy of in-the-body travel* as a way that the body can communicate in a preconscious process. Once relaxed, the client focuses on the painful area. Next, the client enters this area of the body using imagery in order to explore any rigidities and tensions that resulted in pain. Furthermore, this technique may be extended to include a search for people, emotions, situations, and/or memories that are connected to the imaginary insides of the pain-site. The following is a hypothetical example:

> . . . and as you find your self more and more relaxed allow yourself to shrink down into your chest, shrinking smaller and smaller until you are small enough to enter the pain area. And now you are a tiny you, inside your chest cavity, small enough to walk around and look at the insides of your chest and find the painful spot. As you explore this new area, notice the sounds you hear, can you hear your heart beating? A relaxing thump, thump. Notice your breaths, slow and deep, can you feel them swirl around you as you look for the painful place. You can see large thick bones, like dinosaur bones, and tendons, like ropes stretching across your chest. And at last you find the site of the pain. Notice the colors and sounds that you see there. When the image becomes clear, you may describe what you see there. [Client: I see a wall of muscle . . . no, like a big woven quilt that is stretched tight. It is pulling from its edges and in the center is a bright red bulls-eye where the pain is radiating. It's like a trampoline standing on its side, but it is stretched too tight. It is right in the center of my chest.] Now, I want you to walk up to this bright, red bulls-eye and touch it with your tiny finger. When you touch this bulls-eye I want you to describe any sensation, feelings, thoughts, or memories that come to you. [It feels hot, and when I push it I feel like it will rip. It makes me feel angry and helpless.] Look around you to see what you can do to make the fabric looser,

and more flexible? [I can see a basket next to me full of fabric. I am weaving more fabric into the quilt so that it is larger and does not stretch so much.] And as you weave more and more fabric into the quilt, what happens to the bright red spot, to your feelings and your sensations? [The quilt is getting looser and looser. The wind from my lungs is blowing it around, like a sheet on a cloths-line. The red spot is cooling, and softening. I feel calmer and the pain is decreasing.]

In this idealized example, the client was able to find a remedy contained within the *basket of cloth* rather quickly. This type of healing resource may not be found as quickly in general practice. Furthermore, any number of possibilities for healing experiences may become possible once the person begins interacting with the pain site. For example, in the case above, the client may have been asked to probe for specific memories of anger and helplessness that emerged when the bulls-eye was pushed. Unleashing repressed emotions, or transforming these experiences in some other meaningful way, could result in a transformation of the imaginary landscape within the pain-site.

Eidetic Imagery

According to Ahsen (1973), an eidetic is a specific type of image that represents an episodic memory relating to a developmental situation. These images represent the unresolved traumas that lie at the heart of psychodynamic explanations for hysterical symptoms. However, rather than seeking to resolve these traumas through verbal, talk-based techniques, eidetic psychotherapy aims to identify these key experiences and transform them more directly through imagery. Again, Ahsen's triple-code model suggests that these images should ideally contain images, somatic events, and meaning. In the cases of developmental trauma, one or more of these components becomes unyoked, such as the repression of affect around the image. Thus, these images are degraded and stereotypic, like a painting without the color, or a story that goes round-and-round with no ending. Theoretically, the goal is to reconnect the dislodged elements of the image so that it may be transformed from its degraded and problematic state and re-absorbed into healthy consciousness.

The following is a summary of the basic steps, procedures, and goals of eidetic psychotherapy (for a more complete description of these procedures and their rationales, see Ahsen, 1973; Ahsen & Lazarus, 1972; and Sheikh, 1986). Eidetic psychotherapy begins with an unstructured interview that allows clients to freely discuss various aspects of their pain phenomenon such as their current life situation, symptoms, and past experiences associated with the pain. Once clients have had a chance to tell their stories, the imagery phase of treatment begins. The basic sequence in eidetic imagery is to summon the pain symptoms, to identify traumatic developmental images associated with the first emergence of the symptom (eidetics), and then to transform these images in a healing direction.

The first phase of treatment is called the *age projection test*, and is designed to find unconscious themes that are *trapped in the symptom* (Ahsen, 1973, p. 253). In the first step of this test, *composing the symptom*, the therapist gathers the information necessary to bring the symptom out in the session, like a conductor who engages various parts of an orchestra in order to conduct a symphony. The client is asked to talk about the symptom in terms of physiological sensations, psychological manifestations, and worries/concerns. It is important to direct clients to use their own language, avoiding technical jargon and diagnoses that may serve to detach them from the phenomenological aspects of their pain. The therapist keeps notes in three columns for the three areas listed above, recording the exact words to describe these aspects of the pain experience. Ahsen (1973) suggests going through a detailed checklist (e.g., How does the pain affect your head, nose, eyes, mouth, neck, shoulders, movement, talking, feelings, sleep, eating . . . ?) for less introspective clients who have difficulty describing their pain. Finally, clients are asked to list nicknames, in addition to their first and last names, that people have used for them at various phases of their life. These nicknames are used to gain access to the various parts of the self-concept, particularly those detached, forgotten selves that may have existed in the past and may have better access to possible eidetics than the current self.

Once this information is recorded, the therapist instructs clients on what they should expect from the procedure, that they will be relaxed, with their eyes open or closed, ". . . attending the therapist's words which will be spoken to him during this relaxed state of attention" (Ahsen, 1973, p. 255). Furthermore, clients are told that as the therapist repeats certain words, they will gradually see an image of themselves somewhere in the past. They are instructed to just relax and attend to the therapist, allowing this image to develop on its own with no volition of their own. Finally, the therapist *conducts* the symptom by slowly and rhythmically repeating the descriptive words from the three columns generated above together with the nicknames in sequence. The goal is to repeat these highly specific descriptions and personal nicknames in such a way as to bring the symptom, and related personal memories, to the forefront of the person's consciousness in the session. Ideally, the words are repeated until the symptoms and related discomfort is brought to a pitch. Therapists must use their intuition and sensitivity to feel the point at which this pitch is achieved, and then suddenly switch to a guided description of the *opposite* tendency as the pain. Ahsen (1973) has written, "At this stage the therapist talks about the times when the patient was healthy and happy, and he did not have these symptoms" (p. 255).

Once clients reach this step, they are guided toward self-images during their healthy year, before the onset of their pain disorders. It is often necessary to have them repeatedly see these self-images, perhaps 10 to 15 times, until they become sufficiently clear and absorbing. A useful test of vividness and immersion at this stage is to repeat the image until personal objects such as clothing become clear and vivid. Next, clients are guided through an exploration of the year following this new image to find a key eidetic experience that, ". . . discloses meaning, the origin, and the character of the symptom" (Ahsen, 1973, p. 256). If this exploration uncovers useful eidetics, the task turns to their transformation within the imaginal realm. Again, this may be done through a variety of techniques, depending upon the specifics of the eidetic, the client, and the therapist. However, these transformations usually will involve a re-experiencing of the traumatic memory with a more functional emotive, cognitive, and/or behavioral response by the client. For example, if a client uncovers a traumatic memory involving anger at an abusive parent, the client may be guided to express this anger within the safe and versatile confines of the imagination. Furthermore, clients may be guided to attend to any difference in symptoms that emerges as they shift back-and-forth between the original image and the new image. Finally, the new, healing images that are uncovered during this procedure may be rehearsed in between sessions to encourage their immersion into day-to-day consciousness.

While the above procedures may be sufficient with some clients, Ahsen (1973) described a final phase: "In the last phase of the test this image is used in association with parental images to evolve a ritualistic movement of the image. This movement finally throws light on the meaning of the symptom. This phase is useful especially in case the initial projection of the image failed to elucidate the cause of the hysterical symptom" (p. 256). In this final phase, clients face their parents, in their parental home around the time of the emergence of the symptom. First, they stand before their parents, crying in an attempt to evoke pity from them. Next, they remove an item of clothing, which again should be made vivid and bright through repetition prior to its removal. They throw this item on the floor in front of their parents and say, "Take it away! I don't want to wear it!" (Ahsen, 1973, p. 256). Following their parent, they look at where he or she has taken the item, and identify any object that stands out in its vicinity. Finally, any direct memories associated with this object are explored for ways that it may be tied to the symptoms and their possible meanings. For example, if the clothing is placed on a dresser in a client's sister's room, and her yearbook is vivid near the dresser, memories associated with the client's sister's yearbook may be explored.

While the above procedure may seem somewhat arbitrary, the rationale is rather simple. The parental images are thought to be central to a person's self-image because of their proximity to the development of the self from conception through childhood. Furthermore, these images and the home that contains them are the most stable context within the psyche because they are perceived repeatedly early in the client's development. Thus, when the parent image is used to tie the symbolic representation of the symptoms (the unwanted article of clothing) to an object within this stable schematic context, one is likely to arrive at a reliable and accurate symbolic connection for the pain disorder from the correct developmental period. Furthermore, this connection is made in a manner that is sufficiently symbolic to bypass a client's customary defenses.

Imagery Techniques for Children

When using imagery with children, the therapist first must consider children's developmental levels, along with their medical and psychological needs, in order to determine which techniques, if any, would be most beneficial (Wall, 1991). In many cases, children's pain can be effectively managed when age-appropriate imagery techniques are utilized (LeBaron & Zeltzer, 1996).

Wall (1991) has described techniques that are appropriate depending on a child's level of cognitive development (Piaget, 1972). During the *sensorimotor period* (birth to 2 years), children are unable to focus their attention on internal images and cannot develop these images into a fantasy; so any techniques that require the child to imagine an object are often too difficult for them (LeBaron & Zeltzer, 1996). Intervention strategies that direct children's attention away from the self, rather than encouraging them to have internal control of an event, seem to be the most beneficial. Distracting a child with a favorite book or toy, and comforting a child through stroking, rocking, patting, or singing are examples of techniques that are used during this developmental period (Wall, 1991).

At the *preoperational period* (2 to 7 years), techniques include: talking to the child through puppets, telling stories using toys, engaging in a favorite activity, or projecting favorable images upon a TV screen (Wall, 1991). Around the age of five years, children transition from dependence on external objects for imagination to the development of the ability to fantasize without external props (LeBaron & Zeltzer, 1996). They begin to develop the ability to form internal representation of objects, allowing imagery techniques that are closer to the adult variety to be used effectively (Wall, 1991).

Children who have reached the concrete operations phase of development (7 years to puberty) are better equipped to use techniques that employ visual imagery because their ability to hold images in their mind increases dramatically during this time (LeBaron & Zeltzer, 1996; Wall, 1991). However, abstract themes continue to be difficult for children at this age, and should be avoided in most cases. Imagery techniques that have been suggested for this age group include: pain-site rigidity (e.g. imagine your arm is a branch of an oak tree), special/favorite places, listening to music, and engaging in favorite physical activities/sports within imagery (Wall, 1991).

Individuals who reach the *formal operations* phase (puberty through adulthood) develop the capacity for abstract reasoning, allowing them to imagine and transform such abstract concepts as identity, love, and other emotions. Imagery techniques traditionally used with adults can be used with adolescents who have reached this developmental phase. It is important to note that not all individuals reach this phase completely, and that clients will differ in their levels of abstract reasoning abilities. Thus, therapists should adjust to fit their clients' level of cognitive development. Furthermore, even those with strong abstract reasoning abilities tend to have an easier time manipulating concrete, rather than abstract images. As a general rule then, therapists should attempt to help clients identify concrete metaphors that may represent both painful and healing images.

SUMMARY AND CONCLUSIONS

Good psychotherapy is artistic as well as technological because the specific *content* of pain-related images will be as unique as the person who arrives for treatment. However, one may find great similarities across patients in the *processes* of such images and the ways in which victims relate to them. At its best, systemic theories, and NDS theory in particular, may someday provide a means to unite the art and science of pain treatment by encouraging a focus on process in addition to content in both research and in treatment. Processes, such as the rigidity of pain images and people's stereotypic, predictable, and dysfunctional ways of relating to them, may be consistent across individuals no matter how much the specific content of their images varies. Once identified and brought to the magical arena of imagery (Ahsen, 1973), these rigid, closed processes may be opened and loosened in countless different ways. The acknowledgment of the role of process in research and treatment, as opposed to the search for single isolated causes, opens the door to the exploration of opportunities for transformation of pain, rather than the more limited goal of treatment.

Yet, one is still left with daunting questions about how one may best help victims to transform their pain images in the direction of healing, and to transform the ways in which they relate to these images in the direction of functional adaptation. The various approaches summarized above may provide a starting point for therapists, opening their eyes to the myriad possibilities for interventions. Furthermore, Ahsen's (1973; Ahsen & Lazarus, 1972) eidetic approach, which is based on the triple-code model, may represent the most comprehensive single approach because it provides a specific means of identifying pain-related images, yet leaves enough room for creativity in transforming those images.

Yet, with the new methodological tools and theoretical viewpoints allowed by the science of non-linear dynamical systems, even better techniques may be waiting on the horizon of scientific inquiry. Just as there are many ways to loosen up a shoulder that is stiff and sore from injury and inactivity, there theoretically are also many ways to open up a stagnant area of consciousness. Based on the theoretical analysis above, it is argued that a practitioner may make the most out of imagery techniques for pain by seeking points of rigidity and inflexibility in images that are associated with that pain. Once identified, these images may then be transformed at these points through a combination of specific techniques, a client's own healing resources, and a healthy dose of therapeutic creativity.

REFERENCES

Achterberg, J., Dossey, B. , & Kolkmeier, L. (1994). *Rituals of healing: Using imagery for health and wellness.* New York: Bantam Books.

Achterberg, J., Kenner, C., & Lawlis, G. F. (1988). Severe burn injury: A comparison of relaxation, imagery and biofeedback for pain management. *Journal of Mental Imagery, 12*(1), 71-88.

Ahles, T. A., Blanchard, E. B., & Leventhal, H. (1983). Cognitive control of pain: Attention to the sensory aspects of the cold pressor stimulus. *Cognitive Therapy and Research, 7*(2), 159-178.

Ahsen A. (1973). *Basic concepts in eidetic psychotherapy.* New York: Brandon House.

Ahsen, A. (1984). ISM: The triple code model for imagery and psychophysiology. *Journal of Mental Imagery, 8*(4), 15-42.

Ahsen, A., & Lazarus, A. A. (1972). Eidetics: An internal behavior approach. In A. A. Lazarus (Ed.), *Clinical behavior therapy* (pp. 87-99). New York: Brunzer/Mazel.

Albright, G. L., & Fischer, A. A. (1990). Effects of warming imagery aimed at trigger-point sites on tissue compliance, skin temperature, and pain sensitivity in biofeedback-trained patients with chronic pain: A preliminary study. *Perceptual and Motor Skills, 71,* 1163-1170.

Alcoholics Anonymous World Services (Pub.). (1953). *Twelve steps, twelve traditions.* New York.

Alexander, E. D. (1971). In-the-body travel: A growth experience with fantasy. *Psychotherapy: Theory, Research, and Practice, 8*(4), 319-324.

American Psychiatric Association. (1994). *Diagnostic and statistical manual of mental disorder* (4th ed.). Washington, DC: Author.

Bak, P. (1996). *How nature works: The science of self-organized criticality.* New York: Springer-Verlag.

Bakan, P. (1980). Imagery, raw and cooked: A hemispheric recipe. In J. E. Shorr, P. Sobel, P. Robin, & J. A. Connella (Eds.), *Imagery: Its many dimensions and applications.* New York: Plenum.

Baldwin, M. W. (1995). Relational schemas and cognition in close relationships. *Journal of Social and Personal Relationships, 12,* 547-552.

Bandura, A. (1977). Self-efficacy: Toward a unifying theory of behavioral change. *Psychological Review, 84,* 191-215.

Bandura, A. (1986). *Social foundations of thought and action.* New York: Prentice-Hall.

Barber, J. (1996). Hypnotic analgesia: Clinical considerations. In J. Barber (Ed.), *Hypnosis and suggestion in the treatment of pain* (pp. 85-120). New York: W. W. Norton & Company.

Barsky, A. J., Goodson, D. J., & Lane, R. S. (1998). The amplification of somatic symptoms. *Psychosomatic Medicine, 50,* 510-519.

Bartlett, F. C. (1932). *Remembering: A study in experimental and social psychology.* Cambridge, England: Cambridge University Press.

Baumeister, R. F. (1998). The self. In D. T. Gilbert, S. T. Fiske, & G. Lindzey (Eds.), *The handbook of social psychology* (Vol. I) (pp. 680-740). New York: McGraw-Hill.

Belaire, J., Glass, L., Ander-Heiden, V., & Milton, J. (Eds.). (1995). *Dynamical disease: Mathematical analysis of human illness.* Woodbury, NY: AIP Press.

Beers, T. M., & Karoly, P. (1979). Cognitive strategies, expectancy, and coping style in the control of pain. *Journal of Consulting and Clinical Psychology, 47*(1), 179-180.

Benson, H. B., & Stark, M. (1996). *Timeless healing: The power and biology of belief.* New York: Scribner.

Berkowitz, L. (1989). The frustration-aggression hypothesis: An examination and reformulation. *Psychological Bulletin, 106,* 59-73.

Berkowitz, L. (1993). Pain and aggression: Some findings and implications. *Motivation and Emotion, 17,* 277-293.

Berkowitz, L., Cochran, S. T., & Embree, M. (1981). Physical pain and the goal of aversively stimulated aggression. *Journal of Personality and Social Psychology, 40,* 687-200.

Berkowitz, L., & Heimer, K. (1989). On the construction of the anger experience: Aversive events and negative priming in the formulation of feelings. In L. Berkowitz (Ed.), *Advances in experimental social psychology* (Vol. 22, pp. 1-37). New York: Academic Press.

Boothby, J. L., Thorn, B. E., Stroud, M. W., & Jensen, M. P. (1999). Coping with pain. In R. J. Gatchel & D. C. Turk (Eds.), *Psychosocial factors in pain: Critical perspectives* (pp. 343-359). New York: Guilford.

Bresler, D. (1984). Mind-controlled analgesia: The inner way to pain control. In A. A. Sheikh (Ed.), *Imagination and healing* (pp. 211-230). Amityville, NY: Baywood.

Brown, J. M. (1984). Imagery coping strategies in the treatment of migraine. *Pain, 18,* 157-167.

Burger, J. M. (1991). Control. In V. J. Derlega, B. A. Winstead, & W. H. Jones (Eds.), *Personality: Contemporary theory and research* (pp. 287-312).

Chapman, C. R., Nakamura, Y., & Flores, L. Y. (1999). Chronic pain and consciousness: A constructivist perspective. In R. J. Gatchel & D. C. Turk (Eds.), *Psychosocial factors in pain: Critical perspectives* (pp. 35-55). New York: Guilford.

Dworkin, S. F., Von Korff, M. R., & LeResche, L. (1992). Epidemiologic studies of chronic pain: A dynamic-ecologic perspective. *Annals of Behavioral Medicine, 14*(1), 3-11.

Eisenberg, D. M., Kessler, R. C., Foster, C., Norlock, F. E., Calkins, D. R., & Delbanco, T. L. (1993). Unconventional medicine in the United States: Prevalence, costs, and patterns of use. *The New England Journal of Medicine, 328*(4), 246-252.

Engel, G. L. (1977). The need for a new medical model: A challenge for biomedicine. *Science, 196*(4286), 129-136.

Fanurik, D., Zelter, L. K., Roberts, M. C., & Blount, R. L. (1993). The relationship between children's coping styles and psychological interventions for cold pressor pain. *Pain, 53*(2), 213-222.

Farthing, G. W., Venturino, M., Brown, S. W., & Lazar, J. D. (1997). Internal and external distraction on the control of cold-pressor pain as a function of hypnotizability. *The International Journal of Clinical and Experimental Hypnosis, 45*(4), 433-446.

Fernandez, E. (1986). A classification system of cognitive coping strategies for pain. *Pain, 26,* 141-151.

Fernandez, E., & Turk, D. C. (1989). The utility of cognitive coping strategies for altering pain perception: A meta-analysis. *Pain, 38,* 123-135.

Ferrucci, P. (1982). *What we may be.* New York: Tarcher.

Festinger, L. (1957). *A theory of cognitive dissonance.* Evanston, IL: Row, Peterson.

Flor, H., Birbaumer, N., Schugens, M. M., & Lutzenberger, W. (1992). Symptom-specific psychophysiological responses in chronic pain patients. *Psychophysiology, 29*(4), 452-460.

Freeman, W. J. (1995). *Societies of brains*. New Jersey: Lawrence-Erlbaum.

Gatchel, R. J., & Epker, J. (1999). Psychosocial predictors of chronic pain and response to treatment. In R. J. Gatchel & D. C. Turk (Eds.), *Psychosocial factors in pain: Critical perspectives* (pp. 412-434). New York: Guilford.

Gauron, E. F., & Bowers, W. A. (1986). Pain control techniques in college-age athletes. *Psychological Reports, 59*(3), 1163-1169.

Geisser, M. E., Gaskin, M. E., Robinson, M. E., & Greene, A. F. (1993). The relationship of depression and somatic focus to experimental and clinical pain in chronic pain patients. *Psychology and Health, 8,* 405-415.

Gendlin, E. T. (1981). *Focussing.* New York: Bantam.

Gibran, K. (1966). *The prophet.* New York: Alfred A. Knopf.

Gramling, S. E., Clawson, E. P., & McDonald, M. K. (1996). Perceptual and cognitive abnormality model of hypochondriasis: Amplification and physiological reactivity in women. *Psychosomatic Medicine, 58,* 423-431.

Guastello, S. J. (1997). Science evolves: An introduction to nonlinear dynamics, psychology, and life sciences. *Nonlinear Dynamics, Psychology, and Life Sciences, 1*(1), 1-6.

Hackett, G., & Horan, J. J. (1980). Stress inoculation for pain: What's really going on? *Journal of Counseling Psychology, 27*(2), 107-116.

Haken, H. (1984). *The science of structure: Synergetics.* New York: Van Nostrand Reinhold.

Hargadon, R., Bowers, K. S., & Woody, E. Z. (1995). Does counterpain imagery mediate hypnotic analgesia? *Journal of Abnormal Psychology, 104*(3), 508-516.

Hilgard, E. R., & Hilgard, J. R. (1994). *Hypnosis in the relief of pain.* New York: Brunner/Mazel.

Hill, H. F., Chapman, C. R., Kornell, J. A., Sullivan, K. M., et al. (1990). Self-administration of morphine in bone marrow transplant patient reduces drug requirement. *Pain, 40,* 121-129.

Holroyd, K . A., & Penzien, D. B. (1986). Client variables and the behavioral treatment of recurrent tension headache: A meta-analytic review. *Journal of Behavioral Medicine, 9*(6), 515-536.

Horan, J. J. (1973). "In vivo" emotive imagery: A technique for reducing childbirth anxiety and discomfort. *Psychological Reports, 32,* 1328.

Howland, E. W., Wakai, R. T., Mjaanes, B. A., Balog, J. P., & Cleeland, C. S. (1995). Whole head mapping of magnetic fields following painful electric finger shock. *Cognitive Brain Research, 2,* 165-172.

Johnson, M. H., Breakwell, G., Douglas, W., & Humphries, S. (1998). The effects of imagery and sensory detection distractors and different measures of pain: How does distraction work? *British Journal of Clinical Psychology, 37,* 141-154.

Kauffman, S. A. (1993). *The origins of order: Self-organization and selection in evolution.* New York: Oxford University Press.

Kauffman, S. A. (1995). *At home in the universe.* New York: Oxford.

Kazdin, A. E. (1992). *Research and design in clinical psychology* (2nd ed.). Boston, MA: Allyn and Bacon.

Kelly, S. F., & Kelly, R .J. (1995). *Imagine yourself well: Better health through self-hypnosis.* New York: Plenum.

Klinger, E. (1980). Therapy and the flow of thought. In J. Shorr, G. Sobel, P. Robin, & J. Connella (Eds.), *Imagery: Its many dimensions* (pp. 3-20). New York: Plenum.

Korn, E. R. (1983a). The use of altered states of consciousness and imagery in physical and pain rehabilitation. *Journal of Mental Imagery, 7*(1), 25-34.

Korn, E. R. (1983b). *Visualization: Uses of imagery in the health profession.* Homewood, IL: Dow Jones-Irwin.

Kuchan, A. (1998). Personal communication.

Kwekkeboom, K., Huseby-Moore, K., & Ward, S. (1998). Imaging ability and effective use of guided imagery. *Research in Nursing & Health, 21,* 189-198.

LeBaron, S., & Zeltzer, L. K. (1996). Children in pain. In J. Barber (Ed.), *Hypnosis and suggestion in the treatment of pain: A clinical guide* (pp. 305-340). New York: W. W. Norton.

Levendusky, P., & Pankratz, L. (1975). Self-control techniques as an alternative to pain medication. *Journal of Abnormal Psychology, 84,* 165-168.

Levine, S. (1982). *Who dies? An investigation of conscious living and conscious dying.* New York: Anchor Books.

Lindberg, C., & Lawlis, G. F. (1988). The effectiveness of imagery as a childbirth preparatory technique. *Journal of Mental Imagery, 12*(1), 103-114.

Mannix, L. K., Chandurkar, R. S., Rybicki, L. A., Tusek, D. L, & Solomon, G. D. (1999). Effect of guided imagery on quality of life for patients with chronic tension-type headache. *Headache, 39,* 326-334.

Manyande, A., Berg, S., Gettins, D., Stanford, S. C., Mazhero, S., Marks, D. F., & Salmon, P. (1995). Preoperative rehearsal of active coping imagery influences subjective and hormonal responses to abdominal surgery. *Psychosomatic Medicine, 57,* 177-182.

Marino, J., Gwynn, M. I., & Spanos, N. P. (1989). Cognitive mediators in the reduction of pain: The role of expectancy, strategy use, and self-presentation. *Journal of Abnormal Psychology, 98*(3), 256-262.

Marks-Tarlow, T. (1999). The self as a dynamical system. *Nonlinear Dynamics, Psychology, and Life Sciences, 3*(4), 311-346.

Markus, H. (1977). Self-schemata and processing information about the self. *Journal of Personality and Social Psychology, 35,* 63-78.

Markus, H., & Nurius, P. S. (1986). Possible selves. *American Psychologist, 41,* 954-969.

McCaffery, M., & Beebe, A. (1989). *Pain: Clinical manual for nursing practice.* Philadelphia: Mosby.

McClelland, J. L., & Rumelhart, D. E. (Eds.), (1986). *Parallel distributed processing: Explorations in the macrostructure of cognition, Vol. 2 Psychological and biological models.* Cambridge, MA: MIT Press.

McMahon, C. E., & Sheikh, A. A. (1986). Imagination in disease and healing processes: A historical perspective. In A. A. Sheikh (Ed.), *Anthology of imagery techniques* (pp. 1-36). Milwaukee, WI: American Imagery Institute.

McNeil, D. W. & Brunetti, E. G. (1992). Pain and fear: A bioinformational perspective on responsivity to imagery. *Behavioral Research and Therapy, 30*(5), 513-520.

Melzack, R. (1999). Pain and stress: A new perspective. In R. J. Gatchel & D. C. Turk (Eds.), *Psychosocial factors in pain: Critical perspectives* (pp. 89-106). New York: Guilford.

Melzack, R., & Casey, K. L. (1968). Sensory, motivational and central control determinants of pain: A new conceptual model. In D. Kenshalo (Ed.), *The skin senses* (pp. 523-443). Springfield, IL: Thomas.

Melzack, R., & Wall, P. D. (1965). Pain mechanisms: A new theory. *Science, 150,* 971-979.

Melzack, R., & Wall, P. D. (1996). *The challenge of pain* (2nd ed.). London: Penguin Books.

Meyer, R. G. (1992). *Practical clinical hypnosis.* New York: Lexington Books: An Imprint of Macmillan, Inc.

Narduzzi, K. J., Nolan, R. P., Reesor, K., Jackson, T., Spanos, N. P., Hayward, A. A., & Scott, H. A. (1998). Preliminary investigation of associations of illness schemata and treatment-induced reduction in headaches. *Psychological Reports, 82,* 299-307.

Newshan, G., & Balamuth, R. (1990-91). Use of imagery in a chronic pain outpatient group. *Imagination, Cognition and Personality, 10*(1), 25-38.

Okifuji, A., & Turk, D. C. (1999). Fibromyalgia: Search for mechanisms and effective treatments. In R. J. Gatchel & D. C. Turk (Eds.), *Psychosocial factors in pain: Critical perspectives* (pp. 227-246). New York: Guilford.

Ost, L. G. (1987). Applied relaxation: Description of a coping technique and review of controlled studies. *Behaviour Research and Therapy, 25,* 397-410.

Oster, M. I. (1994). Psychological preparation for labor and delivery using hypnosis. *American Journal of Clinical Hypnosis, 37*(1), 12-21.

Piaget, J. (1972). *The child's conception of the world.* Totowa, NJ: Littlefield, Adams.

Philips, C., & Hunter, M. (1981). The treatment of tension headache—II EMG 'normality' and relaxation. *Behavior Research & Therapy, 19,* 499-507.

Portenoy, R. K. (1994). Opioid therapy for chronic nonmalignant pain: Current status. In H. L. Fields & J. C. Liebeskind (Eds.), *Progress in pain research and management. Pharmacological approaches to the treatment of chronic pain* (Vol. 1). Seattle: International Association for the Study of Pain.

Powers, S. W. (1999). Empirically supported treatments in pediatric psychology: Procedure-related pain. *Journal of Pediatric Psychology, 24*(2), 131-145.

Prigogine, I., & Stengers, I. (1984). *Order out of chaos: Man's new dialogue with nature.* New York: Bantam Books.

Raft, D., Smith, R. H., & Warren, N. (1986). Selection of imagery in the relief of chronic and acute clinical pain. *Journal of Psychosomatic Research, 30*(4), 481-488.

Reich, J., & Thompson, D. (1987). DSM-III personality disorder clusters in three populations. *British Journal of Psychiatry, 150,* 471-475.

Robinson, M. E., & Riley, J. L. III. (1999). The role of emotion in pain. In R. J. Gatchel & D. C. Turk (Eds.), *Psychosocial factors in pain: Critical perspectives* (pp. 74-88). New York: Guilford.

Salkovskis, P. M. (1996). Somatic problems. In K. Hawton, P. M. Salkovskis, J. Kirk, & D. M. Clark (Eds.), *Cognitive behaviour therapy for psychiatric problems: A practical guide* (pp. 235-276). New York: Oxford University Press.

Samuels, M., & Samuels, N. (1975). *Seeing with the mind's eye.* New York: Random House.

Sheikh, A. A. (1986). Eidetic psychotherapy techniques. In A. A. Sheikh (Ed.), *Anthology of imagery techniques* (pp. 179-194). Milwaukee, WI: American Imagery Institute.

Sheikh, A. (Ed.). (2001). *Handbook of therapeutic imagery techniques.* Amityville, NY: Baywood.

Sheikh, A. A., Sheikh, K. S., & Moleski, L. M. (1985). The enhancement of imaging ability. In A. A. Sheikh & K. S. Sheikh (Eds.), *Imagery in education.* Amityville, NY: Baywood.

Smith, E. R. (1998). Mental representation and memory. In D. T. Gilbert, S. T. Fiske, & G. Lindzey (Eds.), *The handbook of social psychology* (4th ed.) (pp. 391-445). New York: McGraw-Hill.

Spanos, N. P., Liddy, S. J., Scott, H., Gerrard, C., Sine, J., Tirabasso, A., & Hayward, A. (1993). Hypnotic suggestion and placebo for the treatment of chronic headache in a university volunteer sample. *Cognitive Therapy and Research, 17*(2), 191-205.

Spanos, N. P., & O'Hara, P. A. (1990). Imaginal dispositions and situation-specific expectations in strategy-induced pain reductions. *Imagination, Cognition and Personality, 9*(2), 147-156.

Sperry, R. W. (1993). The impact and promise of the cognitive revolution. *American Psychologist, 48,* 878-885.

Stevens, M. J. (1985). Modification of pain through covert positive reinforcement. *Psychological Reports, 56,* 711-717.

Stevens, M. J., Heise, R., & Pfost, K. S. (1989). Consumption of attention versus affect elicited by cognition in modifying acute pain. *Psychological Reports, 64,* 284-286.

Stevens, M. J., Pfost, K. S., & Rapp, B. J. (1987). Modifying acute pain by matching cognitive style with cognitive treatment. *Perceptual and Motor Skills, 65,* 919-924.

Syrjala, K. L., & Abrams, J. R. (1996). Hypnosis and imagery in the treatment of pain. In R. J. Gatchel & D. C. Turk (Eds.), *Psychological approaches to pain management: A practitioner's handbook.* New York: Guilford.

Tan, S. Y. (1982). Cognitive and cognitive behavioral methods for pain control: A selective review. *Pain, 12,* 201-228.

ter Kuile, M. M., Spinhoven, P., Linssen, A. C. G., Zitman, F. G., Van Dyck, R., & Rooijmans, H. G. M. (1994). Autogenic training and cognitive self-hypnosis for the treatment of recurrent headaches in three different subject groups. *Pain, 58,* 331-340.

Turk, D. C., & Flor, H. (1999). Chronic pain: A biobehavioral perspective. In R. J. Gatchel, & D. C. Turk (Eds.), *Psychosocial factors in pain: Critical perspectives* (pp. 18-34). New York: Guilford.

Turk, D., & Melzack, R. (1992). The measurement of pain and the assessment of people experiencing pain. In D. Turk & R. Melzack (Eds.), *Handbook of pain assessment.* New York: Guilford.

Turner, J. C. (with Hogg, M. A., Oakes, P. J., Reicher, S. D., & Wetherell, M. S.). (1987). *Rediscovering the social group: A self-categorization theory.* Oxford: Blackwell.

Turner, J. C., Oakes, P. J., Haslam, S. A., & McGarty, C. (1994). Self and collective: Cognition and social context. *Journal of Personality and Social Psychology, 28,* 135-147.

Turner, J. C., & Chapman, C. R. (1982). Psychological interventions for chronic pain: A critical review II, operant conditioning, hypnosis and cognitive behavioral therapy. *Pain, 12,* 23-46.

Von Bertalanffy, L. (1968). *General system theory: Foundations, development, applications.* New York: Braziller.

Wall, V. (1991). Developmental considerations in the use of hypnosis with children. In W. C. Wester II & D. J. O'Grady (Eds.), *Clinical hypnosis with children* (pp. 3-18). New York: Bruner/Mazel.

Watzlawick, P. (1978). *The language of change: Elements of therapeutic communication.* New York: Basic Books.

Weisenberg, J. N., & Keefe, F. J. (1999). Personality, individual differences, and psycho-pathology in chronic pain. In R. J. Gatchel & D. C. Turk (Eds.), *Psychosocial factors in pain: Critical perspectives* (pp. 56-73). New York: Guilford.

Weisenberg, M. (1979). Pain and pain control. *Psychological Bulletin, 84,* 1008-1044.

West, B. J., & Deering, B. (1995). *The lure of modern science: Fractal thinking.* River Edge, NJ: World Scientific.

Widiger, T. A., Trull, T. J. Hurt, S. W. Clarkin, J., & Frances, A. (1987). A multi-dimensional scaling of the DSM-III personality disorders. *Archives of General Psychiatry, 44,* 557-563.

Worthington, E. L., & Shumate, M. (1981). Imagery and verbal counseling methods in stress inoculation training for pain control. *Journal of Counseling Psychology, 28*(1), 1-6.

CHAPTER 9

Imagery in Smoking Cessation and Weight Management

COLLEEN HEINKEL, MICHELLE ROSENFELD, AND ANEES A. SHEIKH

On her son's seventeenth birthday, a mother pleadingly asked, "Promise me you'll tell me if you start smoking. Don't let me find it out from the neighbors."

"Don't worry about me, Mom," the son replied. "I quit smoking a year ago."
(Brande, 1964, p. 195)

All the things I really like to do are immoral, illegal or fattening.
Alexander Woollcott (Fanning, 1994, p. 75)

According to the Centers for Disease Control (1996), smoking and obesity result in 430,000 and 300,000 preventable deaths each year, respectively, in the United States. Not only are smoking and obesity extremely difficult to overcome, but they often are intertwined: weight gain after smoking cessation averages 6 to 9 pounds and concerns over weight gain contribute to smoking relapse, continued smoking, and the reasons why people begin smoking in the first place (Heishman, 1998; Klesges, Ward, Ray, Cutter, Jacobs, & Wagenknecht, 1998). The psychological and physiological mechanisms underlying smoking, eating behaviors, and the effects of smoking on body weight are not well understood and, as such, interventions for changing either or both behaviors have been, for the most part, either ineffective or only moderately successful.

Imagery and hypnosis have long been used as curative interventions for a host of psychological and physiological disorders and this chapter will examine their effectiveness in the treatment of smoking and weight problems. Hypnosis and imagery are commonly considered to be comparable in most cases (Hilgard & Hilgard, 1994). They are both "widely agreed to be states of highly focused attention during which alteration of sensations, awareness, and perception can occur. . . . Suggestion is an integral part of hypnosis, whereas suggestion may or may not be offered in imagery" (Syrjala & Abrams, 1996, pp. 231-232). Consequently, no special distinction is made in this chapter.

The first part of the chapter outlines the current understanding of smoking addiction and relapse, presents a brief overview of the nature of imagery from the perspective of neuroscience, summarizes some of the more rigorous scientific research on the efficacy of imagery as an intervention for smoking cessation, and presents samples of imagery-based therapeutic approaches for clinical use. The second section explores the problem of obesity and weight management by outlining current theories on the causes of obesity, reviewing the empirical findings on the role of imagery in weight loss, and presenting samples of imagery scripts for clinical use. The implications for future research will conclude the chapter.

SMOKING CESSATION

Smoking is a major health risk, causing approximately one of every five deaths annually in the United States (Henningfield, 1998). It is a major contributor to cardiovascular disease, lung cancer, stroke, and chronic obstructive pulmonary disease. In the United States, more than 430,000 people die from smoking-related illnesses annually; more die from smoking than from AIDS, vehicle accidents, alcohol, homicides, suicides, illegal drugs, and fires *combined*. Deaths from smoking are completely preventable, but, despite the awareness of its dangers and smoking prevention campaigns over the last few decades, 25.5 percent of Americans over the age of 17 smoke nonetheless (Centers for Disease Control [CDC], 1996).

It is estimated that more than 80 percent of smokers would like to quit smoking, yet only 10 percent are able to do so (Fiore et al., 1990; U.S. Department of Health Education and Welfare, 1990). Of the 10 percent of successful quitters, an estimated 90 percent did it on their own, without any prescribed smoking cessation program (Fiore et al., 1990) and those who quit "cold turkey" were more likely to remain abstinent. Studies have found that spontaneous quit rates of persons on wait-list or no-treatment controls have hovered around 10 percent, ranging between 7 to 15 percent (Bayot, Capafons, & Cardena, 1997; Green & Lynn, 2000; Valbo & Eide, 1996). The current smoking cessation programs generally only modestly improve one-year abstention rates to between 20 percent and 30 percent (Fiore et al., 1996; Lando, McGovern, & Sipfle, 1989; Powell, 1993) and sometimes they fail to show any significant effects over those found in patients in a no-treatment control group (Spanos, Mondoux, & Burgess, 1995; Valbo & Eide, 1996).

Theories of Smoking Addiction and Relapse

Determining what makes smoking so addictive may provide clues for ascertaining what might promote smoking abstinence, but, even now, the physiological effects of nicotine or the psychological effects of smoking behavior are not well understood. Nicotine is the drug found in cigarettes. Inhaled nicotine enters the lungs, mixes with blood, and travels to the brain in only seven seconds, a process twice as fast as an intravenous injection of heroin. In response to this "fix" of nicotine, the brain releases the neurotransmitters norepinephrine and dopamine. Both neurotransmitters act synergistically to selectively modulate mood: when a person is "down," nicotine will cause the neurotransmitters to stimulate and, conversely, when a person is anxious, nicotine will cause the neurotransmitters to calm them. Nicotine has also been demonstrated to enhance concentration, learning, and memory, an effect mediated through the brain's limbic system via the neurotransmitters adrenaline and dopamine.

Symptoms of nicotine withdrawal include irritability, anxiety, dysphoric mood, insomnia, difficulty concentrating, increased appetite, restlessness, and low energy levels. Perhaps the most salient symptoms of nicotine withdrawal are the intense and frequent urges and cravings to smoke. In 1991, the National Institute on Drug Abuse established that craving is a subjective state associated with drug dependence, but little is known about the determinants of craving or the best method of assessing this state (Pickens & Johanson, 1992).

Theories about addiction are varied, but most often cited are those that present either a withdrawal model, or an appetitively-based, positive-affect model, or more simply, the reward model. The withdrawal model posits that sustained drug use is associated with the avoidance and/or alleviation of the symptoms of withdrawal (Baker, Morse, & Sherman, 1987). The withdrawal-based model, favored until recently, proposes that relapse is learned through conditioned physiological responses that are opposite the effect of the drug. Cues for relapse are associated with situations previously associated with smoking, such as smoking after dinner or relaxing at home. Cravings are believed to be learned or conditioned responses to these cues—not just biological responses to the need for nicotine—and, because extinguishing learning takes time, cravings continue long after the drug has been eliminated from the body (Poulos, Hinson, & Siegel, 1981). Avoiding these situations or cues should help a smoker abstain from smoking and one of the predictors of successful abstention is the absence of another smoker at home (Frank, Umlauf, Wonderlich, & Ashkanazi, 1986).

Other models of addiction theorize that it is the rewardlike effects of the drug that promote addiction (Tiffany, 1990). These models propose that urges represent positive-affective motivational states and that the anticipation or expectancies of drug-related euphoria serve as powerful positive reinforcers of smoking behavior (Baker, Morse, & Sherman, 1987; Marlatt, 1985).

These theories correspond with the recent findings in neuroscience that stress the role of drug reward in sustaining drug use. The mesocorticolimbic dopamine pathway has been implicated as the neural pathway in drug reward (Koob, 1992; Wise, 1996). Research indicates that the reinforcing properties of nicotine are, in part, due to activation of this reward system and, in part, due to the release of dopamine in the nucleus accumbens, the brain's pleasure/reward center (Pontieri, Tanda, Orzi, & Di Chiara, 1996) In fact, Pontieri and associates (Pontieri, Tanda,

Orzi, & Di Chiara, 1996) found that the brain scans of rats given nicotine were virtually indistinguishable from the brain scans of rats given cocaine. Wise (1988) proposed that memory of dopamine-mediated positive reinforcement may be the source of drug craving.

Studies of both humans and primates using food as reward also demonstrate this theory. When humans and primates were given bananas and allowed to eat them until they were "satiated," their brain scans indicated that, although the neurons were still activated in the vision, taste, olfactory, and touch areas of the brain, satiation represented an absence of activity in the nucleus accumbens (Rolls, 1999a,b). After subjects felt satiated on bananas and could not eat any more, presenting another food stimulated this reward center, and they were able to eat again. This research indicates that our behavior and emotion are associated with what is associated with reward, and that it is the relative reward value that is important, not the stimulus itself.

Further support for the reward model can also be found in the behavioral genetics literature, where the heritability of the propensity to smoke has long been demonstrated. Shields (1962) found in one study of 42 pairs of identical twins reared apart that concordance for smoking was 79 percent, and five twin studies of over 1,000 twin pairs each found an estimated heritability of 60 percent for the propensity to smoke (Heath & Madden, 1995). However, findings from genetics research have suggested most recently that genetic variations in the dopamine receptor gene and the dopamine transporter gene may influence concentrations of and responses to synaptic dopamine, and that these responses are associated with increased smoking risk, age at smoking initiation, and the ability to quit smoking (Lerman et al., 1999; Sabol et al., 1999). These findings again implicate the role of dopamine and its role in activation of reward.

A Neuroscience Perspective of Imagery

If addiction to cigarettes is mediated also by activation of the dopamine reward pathway, as the current research indicates, then the effectiveness of imagery for smoking cessation may be enhanced by targeting this reward pathway. Yet, although imagery has been used for centuries, there is little knowledge about how it actually produces physiological and psychological changes.

Visual imagery differs from perception in that imagery is "seeing" in the *absence* of actual visual sensory inputs; whereas, perception is the act of registering the presence of *actual* stimuli. As such, imagery plays a role in abstract reasoning, skill learning and memory, information processing, and language comprehension. Interest in the cognitive neuroscience of mental imagery grew during the 1980s and 1990s principally due to the technological innovations, such as MRI (magnetic resonance imaging) or PET (positron emission tomography), that allow more than just philosophical examination of its processes (Kosslyn, Behrmann, & Jeannerod, 1995).

Researchers have begun to use neuropsychological data to explore the structure of the imagery-processing systems. Several studies have found that imagery is not confined to one area of the brain. With the help of various brain-scanning techniques, it has been determined that visual mental imagery activates the same areas of the brain used for visual perception, namely those of the occipital, temporal and parietal lobes (Kosslyn et al., 1995; Farah, 1995). Georgopoulos, Lurito, Petrides, Schwartz, and Massey (1989) found that image rotation, an aspect of visual imagery that requires the mental rotation of an image in the mind, activates areas in the motor cortex of the brain as well. Another aspect of visual imagery, the generation of images, seems to arise from an activation of information stored in short- or long-term memory. "Bits" of remembered images can be accessed as they are, or these images can be "cut and pasted" to make new images. For example, many people can visualize having lunch with their favorite movie star, even though they have never had such an encounter. The time to form images increases linearly for each additional part that needs to be visualized (a process called serial processing); thus, it seems that image generation requires the same serial processing as that found in actual perception (Kosslyn et al., 1995). Farah (1984) found that image generation was selectively disrupted by damage to the posterior left cerebral hemisphere.

Other research has found that brain activation during imagery is not found in one area or even one hemisphere of the brain, but that its tasks are shared by a number of areas and distributed over both hemispheres (Farah, 1995). In a case reported by Goldenberg, Mullbacher, and Nowak (1995), a female patient with a lesioned primary visual cortex, retained her visual mental imagery and insisted that she was not blind because these images were so vivid. The researchers theorized that the patient's visual imagery arose from her intact tactile and auditory perceptions, suggesting that connections from the nonvisual cortex play a complex role in the production of imagery. Imagery also plays a central role in abstract reasoning and there is intriguing evidence that language itself can be represented in a nonlinguistic manner (Geminiani, Bisiach, Berti, & Rusconi, 1995).

Neuroscientists now find that the mechanisms of imagery are much more complex than first thought. A review of the current research indicates that imagery is not a single, undifferentiated process, but actually involves a number of neural processes working together (Kosslyn et al., 1995). Visual imagery, like visual representation and perception more generally, cannot be conceived as a unitary concept; rather it seems to act as an organizer of neural subsystems specialized for performing particular aspects of cognitive tasks. As such, imagery activates and organizes a large number of cognitive functions, of which not all are affected concurrently (Cooper, 1995).

The research has begun to provide clearer evidence that the imaging process produces neurophysiological responses similar to those expected during an actual sensory experience. It has been found that, in addition to the physiological effects, imagining an experience evokes psychological qualities similar to an actual experience, so that mental imagery and perception seem to be *experientially equivalent* (Sheikh & Kunzendorf, 1984). This equivalence may contribute to the clinical effectiveness of imagery-based interventions in the treatment of a wide variety of problems, including blood pressure, obesity, mood disorders, chronic pain, sexual dysfunction, fibroid tumors, and cancer (Sheikh, 1983, 1984; Sheikh, Kunzendorf, & Sheikh, 1996). The use of imagery to curb tobacco use was documented as early as the 1840s and is still quite prevalent.

Research on the Use of Imagery for Smoking Cessation

Imagery studies before the 1970s focused on hypnosis interventions and were either anecdotal or reported in the form of a case study. In 1970, H. Spiegel published his brief, single-session, direct-suggestion approach that stressed that smoking was a poison, the smoker needed a body to live, and he/she owed the body respect and protection. Spiegel found that this method resulted in a cessation rate of 20 percent at 6-month follow-up.

More controlled studies began to appear, often using variants of the Spiegel method, but generally the study designs were too discrepant to allow comparisons among them. Hypnosis was often combined with other behavioral interventions, such as aversive therapies (rapid or focused smoking) or group therapy and, in most cases, the design did not isolate the effect of hypnosis alone. For example, a meta-analysis of 48 smoking cessation studies using some form of hypnotherapy revealed a quit rate of 36 percent (Viswesvaran & Schmidt, 1992). However, the hypnotherapeutic techniques were either so discrepant across studies (often combined with other behavioral interventions) or simply not reported in sufficient detail (identified only by the fact that a hypnotherapist was present) that it was difficult to clearly isolate the effect of hypnosis itself.

Green and Lynn (2000) later reviewed the literature to find if there was enough evidence to indicate that hypnosis met the standards to be classified as an empirically supported treatment for smoking cessation. The studies were reviewed to see if they randomized participants between conditions, had adequate sample sizes of over 25, used well-defined and replicable hypnotic and nonhypnotic treatments, and assessed the population to determine smoking history, previous quit attempts, social support, and hypnotizability.

The results provided evidence that a hypnosis condition was superior to a wait-list or no-treatment control group, although the results were mixed. Hypnosis was generally comparable to a variety of other nonhypnotic interventions, but it was difficult to isolate the effects of educational or behavioral interventions from those of the hypnotherapy. Most of the results were based on self-reported abstinence and, if the more stringent requirement of using a biochemical marker (e.g., plasma thiocyanate) of abstinence had been applied, most of the supportive studies would have been eliminated. Despite these factors, Green and Lynn (2000) concluded that there was sufficient evidence to classify hypnosis as a "possibly efficacious treatment" for smoking cessation; for example, if someone chose to stop smoking and wanted to choose hypnotherapy to accomplish this, hypnotherapy could be recommended. However, they recommended that more stringent studies (i.e., ones that delineated the sample population, demonstrated randomization of participants, had at least 25 or more participants per condition, and that used well-defined and replicable treatments) must be done in order to identify hypnotherapy clearly as an empirically supported intervention for the cessation of smoking.

The literature generally supports hypnotherapeutic interventions as one of many interventions that could be used in the treatment of smoking cessation. However, the quit rates continue to hover between 20 percent and 30 percent. Thirty years after Spiegel reported cessation rates of 20 percent in 1970, a study of 452 participants randomly selected from 2,810 smokers who participated in single-session, group hypnotherapy smoking cessation programs, found similar self-reported quit rates of 22 percent (Ahijevych, Yerardi, & Nedilsky, 2000).

Hypnotic versus Nonhypnotic Treatments. Smoking cessation programs involving the use of hypnosis or imagery have yielded similar cessation rates as those found in nonhypnotic interventions (Green & Lynn, 2000; Perry, Gelfand, & Marcovitch, 1979; Spanos, 1991; Spanos et al., 1995; Straatmeyer, 1984). There is some support that hypnosis combined with counseling has better outcomes than either one alone (Pederson, Scrimgeour, & Lefcoe, 1975), but pairing it with other therapies does not always enhance the abstention rates (Johnson & Karkut, 1994; Pederson, Scrimgeour, & Lefcoe, 1980).

Nonspecific Factors. In many of the hypnosis studies, the researchers often are struck by the "nonspecific" factors that may have been the agent of change in the intervention. Hyman and associates (Hyman, Stanley, Burrows, & Horne, 1986, p. 362) wrote, "The active treatment effects in smoking cessation programs are not as significant as many of the researchers have implied. Simple contact with a smoker, whether it involves treatment or not, and an expectation of success would appear to successfully modify smoking behavior."

After a review of clinical reports, Holroyd (1980) concluded that outcome was related to increased number of sessions, how individualized the hypnotic content was to the participant, and how much interpersonal contact the subject received after the intervention. Flatt (1984) also concluded that hypnosis worked best if the following four variables were present: 1) a high level of motivation; 2) at least moderate hypnotizability; 3) good client-therapist rapport and trust; and 4) the content of the hypnotic sessions carefully tailored to the individual client.

The more successful abstinence rates of 38 percent or more generally have been found in those studies that have increased the intensity of the treatment (e.g., individual rather than group sessions, live versus taped sessions, longer and/or multiple sessions, and more interpersonal contact.) Minimal treatments (e.g., brief, single session, group hypnosis treatments) generally achieve more minimal abstention rates (e.g., 20 percent) (Ahijevych et al., 2000; Bayot et al., 1997; Green & Lynn, 2000; Kottke, Battista, DeFriese, & Brekke, 1988; Lynn, Neufeld, Rhue, & Matorin, 1993), but thus far no direct correlation has been confirmed, and there are studies that do not support this (Ahijevych et al., 2000; Green & Lynn, 2000; Frank et al., 1986).

In the clinical setting, clinicians have reported that more intensive treatments are required for successful smoking cessation. Brown (1997) presented a smoking cessation program developed during 28 years of hypnosis work. He starts by determining the patients' psychodynamic reasons for smoking. He asks how they relax and then explains how hypnosis works, to raise their expectations of the treatment. "One of the most powerful, if not the most powerful factor in effective therapy is the level of belief and expectation engendered in the patient that he will be successful in his efforts to attain a cure" (Brown, 1997, p. 98). He follows this with relaxation imagery and subsequently with cognitive restructuring like that suggested by Spiegel (1970). He then requires them to do three imagery sessions daily, with the aim of replacing their old smoking habit with a new habit of autohypnosis. He tries to "reprogram" them to relax without a cigarette, to imagine ways to relax that are more healthy and enriching. A second visit is also required and includes a stress prevention and management trance with ego-strengthening. The patients call in every day for 2 months and then are asked to come back for a follow-up.

In an article invited for the "American Journal of Clinical Hypnosis Techniques of the Senior Masters," Crasilneck (1990) employs similar techniques. After 35 years of development, Crasilneck has found that hypnosis sessions 3 days in a row with a follow-up session about 3 weeks later are the most successful in helping smokers quit smoking. He reports that about 81 percent of his 4,355 patients with smoking problems have been helped and, that in three series of 100 consecutive cases, a 4-year follow-up revealed an abstention rate of 78 percent. Although the articles by Crasilneck and Brown are not empirical studies, they do provide evidence of their success over time and draw on principles of smoking cessation that have been shown empirically to be successful.

Straatmeyer's Dual Phase Model (1984) employing both hypnotic aversive and positive imagery provides an example of more intense content over multiple sessions. In the first phase, aversive imagery is applied: the stimulus of the cigarette is replaced by an aversive stimulus of a decomposing white mouse. In the second phase, age regression is employed and smokers visualize themselves for the last two years as non-smokers, looking and feeling healthy and vital, and feeling proud and pleased. This dual-stage imagery was repeated in a second session one to two weeks later. Results indicated a 35 percent abstinence rate after nine months. When dropouts were added in as recidivists, the rate dropped to 22 percent.

In a study by Wynd (1991), two forms of imagery, personal power imagery (based on a theory of client-empowerment) and relaxation imagery, were compared against a placebo control group. All three groups attended six 90-minute sessions once a week. Informational smoking cessation topics were discussed (facts about health and smoking, exploring individual reasons for smoking, behavioral techniques), and all were asked to stop smoking "cold turkey" after Session Two. The power imagery group was asked to envision themselves in a state of full awareness, with many choices, free to act and to involve themselves completely in the change from smoker to nonsmoker, to experience a time when they were confident, active, and powerful. The relaxation group imagined themselves relaxing on a beach. Both types of imagery treatments were found to be effective: 1) after the six sessions: the power imagery group had a 67 percent cessation rate, the relaxation group had a 69 percent cessation rate, and the placebo group had a 27 percent cessation rate; and, 2) at a 3-month follow-up: the power imagery group had a 52 percent abstinence rate (48 percent relapsed), the relaxation imagery group had a 55 percent abstinence rate (45 percent relapsed), and the control group had a 27 percent abstinence rate (73 percent relapsed).

Individualized hypnosis has been recommended for better results, but it is not clear from the research what it entails. Details about "tailoring" the scripts to the participants are rare and studies have not reported whether or not the imagery was meaningful to the participants. Ahsen's (1982) Triple Code Model (ISM) proposes that the images (I) draw their effectiveness and generate somatic responses (S) from that which is significant or *meaningful* (M) for the client. Current treatment outcomes may not be reaching their potential because the content of the imagery may have little meaning to the participants.

Thus far, it is not clear if participants in smoking cessation research have been asked *why* it is important to them to give up smoking, nor is it clear if the imagery was related to that content. In one study where cessation rates of those in the hypnotherapy condition were no better than those in the no-treatment condition, the subjects were placed into the smoking cessation program automatically as a part of their prenatal care, and, because they did not seek treatment themselves, may have lacked the motivation to quit (Valbo & Eide, 1996). Consequently, there may have been no meaningful answer to that question, had it been asked.

The reward model of behavior states that behavior and emotion are associated with reward and that it is the *relative* reward that is important to our actions, not the particular stimulus. Reward is that which is meaningful to us, and it is the reward that prompts us to *do* something. When smokers ask a clinician for help to quit smoking, the smokers have committed to *doing* something about their habit. It would seem reasonable that they would be assisted most by finding what is meaningful about that act, in order to complete that act. Perhaps finding the reason why they have now decided to quit smoking and creating imagery with this content may achieve more successful outcomes. A "meaning of image" rating should be obtained after the manipulation of the imagery to determine if it is the imagery/stimulus itself, or, more specifically, the meaning associated with the particular stimulus that acts as the therapeutic agent.

Green and Lynn (2000) found evidence that "what may moderate the relation between smoking-related variable and treatment outcome is expectation of perceived treatment success and motivation to quit" (p. 217). Interviews conducted by Perry, Gelfand, and Marcovitch (1979) did much to illuminate some of the possible factors at work. They found that three motivational factors—current need for cigarettes, desire to quit smoking, and the number of reasons one had for quitting—could predict outcome for 67.4 percent of the total client group and were significantly correlated with smoking levels at the 3-month follow-up. Quitters usually had less need for a cigarette (less tension, etc.), indicated a strong desire to quit on a scale of 1 to 10, and had fewer reasons for smoking as measured on a 29-item Reasons for Smoking scale.

Findings from a follow-up interview conducted after three months indicated that nearly all of those subjects who had quit reported that they had expected that they would need to make a strong personal effort to quit, had believed that hypnosis would serve as a tool in this process, had resorted to a greater number of strategies to resist urges and, when asked to visualize a relapse, did not see themselves as failures and vowed to abstain once again. Most of the nonquitters, on the other hand: 1) expected that hypnosis would work automatically and little personal effort would be required; 2) had fewer strategies from which to draw to resist urges; and 3) when asked to visualize a relapse, perceived themselves as failures.

One of the most empirically based models of change is proposed by Prochaska (1979). Lack of motivation for change, inability of the client to relate, and resistance to therapy accounted for much of the attrition and relapse found in cessation programs. Based on this finding, stages of change were developed to provide a marker for monitoring the change process and, later, five stages of change were defined specifically for those who smoked (Fava, Velicer, & Prochaska, 1995; Prochaska & DiClemente, 1983; Prochaska & Goldstein, 1991; Prochaska, Velicer, DiClemente, & Fava, 1988):

1. Precontemplation Stage—The smoker has no intention of quitting within six months and does not acknowledge having a problem.
2. Contemplation Stage—The smoker seriously considers quitting within the next six months and is aware of a problem.
3. Preparation Stage—The smoker seriously plans to quit within the next 30 days and has made at least one attempt in the past year.
4. Action Stage—The former smoker abstains from smoking for less than six months and commits time and energy to working on the problem.
5. Maintenance Stage—The former smoker has abstained from smoking for at least six months or more, indicating a stabilization of behavior change.

Empirical evidence for this model demonstrates that the pretreatment stage of change is directly associated with outcomes. Ockene, Kristeller, Goldberg, and

Ockene (1992) found that participants in the preparation or action stages stopped smoking successfully, 94 percent in one study and 66 percent in another. Regardless of treatment condition, 22 percent of those in the precontemplation stage, 43 percent of those in the contemplation stage, and 76 percent of those in both the preparation and action stages had abstained from smoking at the 6-month follow-up. Conversely, in a study in which the participants did not actively seek treatment for smoking cessation (attending treatment as a part of their prenatal care), the abstention rates were only 8 percent (Valbo & Eide, 1996). These outcomes provide evidence that it is the motivation and readiness of the smoker to quit that may play the largest part in the success of any smoking cessation program.

It has been proposed that the use of imagery may help move a smoker from one stage of readiness to another: it may move smokers who are in the contemplation stage to the preparation stage, a stage that has been shown empirically to be related to greater abstinence. Ahijevych, Yerardi, and Nedilsky (2000) found that, in 5 to 15 months after attending a treatment, 50 percent of their sample were in the preparation stage (wanted to quit smoking in the next 30 days) compared to 20 percent of smokers in general, and 14 percent were in the precontemplation stage versus 60 percent of smokers in general. Their sample represented a motivated group at follow-up, and they proposed that the effect of the hypnotherapeutic intervention used in their study "may have had an impact in moving people along the stages of change continuum and/or maintaining them in a preparation-to-quit stage" (Ahijevych et al., 2000, p. 384.) However, their study did not assess the stage of cessation prior to the intervention, and further conclusions cannot be drawn.

Urge Imagery and Its Role in Understanding Smoking Relapse. Prochaska and colleagues were drawn to develop their model because attrition and relapse in substance cessation programs were more the rule than the exception. Urges and cravings have been responsible for the high rate of smoking relapse following smoking cessation (Doherty, Kinnunen, Militello, & Garvey, 1995; Killen & Fortmann, 1997; West & Schneider, 1987) and smoking relieves the distress of these withdrawal symptoms. Killen and Fortmann (1997) found that 32 percent of those with the highest craving scores relapsed within one week, while only 15 percent of those with the lowest craving scores relapsed.

Evaluation of addiction models has been hampered by the difficulty to create self-reported urges in the laboratory; however, recent empirical studies have demonstrated that imagery can successfully generate smoking urges and cravings among subjects in a laboratory setting (Maude-Griffin & Tiffany, 1996; Tiffany & Drobes, 1990; Tiffany & Hakenewerth, 1991). Subjects reported significantly stronger urges in response to urge imagery than to neutral imagery. Urge imagery also produced physiological increases in heart rate and skin conductance, effects that are isodirectional to the agonistic properties of nicotine.

Relapse studies have found that affective states modulate urges and cravings. Negative affect states have been found to immediately precede half or more of smoking relapses (Baer & Lichtenstein, 1988), and depression has been also correlated with negative outcome in smoking cessation programs (Barbasz, Baer, Sheehan, & Barabasz, 1986). Positive affect is associated less frequently with relapse but, when it is, it is generally accompanied by smoking-related cues. Brandon, Wetter, and Baker (1996) found that affect and self-reported urges were significantly associated with one another. They also found that affect-related expectancies of reinforcement from smoking moderated the relation between affect and urge. They concluded that urge was best predicted by affect; whereas, consumption was best predicted by expectancies.

Tiffany and Drobes (1990) and later Maude-Griffin and Tiffany (1996) manipulated the affective content of urge imagery to parcel out the impact of affect on smoking abstinence. First, they found that imagery was able to produce the intended mood state, as indicated by the subjects' self-reports. They also found that affective content did have a modulating effect on urge. Negative affect with urge imagery created the highest urge ratings, followed by imagery with negative affect alone. Positive affect with urge imagery created the next highest urge ratings followed by neutral urge. Positive affect and neutral affect imagery, both used without urge imagery, produced only minimal urge for smoking.

Their findings suggest that the strength of imagery-produced urges and cravings can be influenced by both the urge and affective content of the imagery scripts. Additionally, both outcomes—the physiological response to urge and the modulating role of affect—are more congruent with the reward models that predict physiological effects isodirectional to the effects of nicotine.

Imagery Techniques for Smoking Cessation

Research continues to inform the clinician's practice and the clinician's practice continues to inform research as well. Clinicians have used a variety of scripts, each reflecting a slightly different theoretical understanding of what it takes to break the habit, to help their clients.

Wynd and Dossey (2000) try to understand individuals' bodymind responses to nicotine and their stage of change in regard to smoking cessation. Basic relaxation is used to promote inner awareness. Three types of images are used to help the bodymind prepare to see itself as smoke-free: 1) cleansing images that promote cleansing behaviors, such as deep breathing and increased liquid intake; 2) protective images designed to block negative images that have made the client smoke in the past (being aware of smoking cues, rehearsing healthy behaviors to replace urges, etc.); and 3) inner healer images.

Kelly and Kelly (1995) believe that people who have decided to quit smoking are ambivalent about their decision: a part of them wants to quit, another part does not, and both parts are struggling for control of the person's actions. A "majority" of the client must be convinced to agree to stop smoking: "The die-hard prosmoking element [in the client] need not be eradicated—just outnumbered" (p. 146). Several scripts are used to accomplish this. The first script underscores the reason why the individual has chosen to give up cigarettes and makes them aware of what to expect in the weeks ahead:

> Now that you've made the decision to stop smoking, you need to know what's going to happen, what you can expect. You're going to experience waves of desire to have a cigarette. Part of the experience of wanting a cigarette will show up in your muscles. They will tend to become tense as you physically act out ambivalence between wanting to reach for a cigarette and wanting to stop yourself. When these waves come, you have a choice of how to deal with them. What you're not going to do is to light up a cigarette because that would be to poison yourself. Instead, if the urge is very strong and you feel that you need help and support, you will have the option of putting yourself into a state of hypnosis. If you do this, it will relax your body. As your body is relaxed, you will stop fighting with yourself. (Kelly & Kelly, 1995, p. 150)

Another of their scripts is used to make a smoker more aware of others' negative responses to their cigarette smoking: "You see yourself in public lighting up and you realize that people don't want to be so near you. See people inching away from you, from the smell, people not wanting to associate with you" (Kelly & Kelly, 1995, p. 156). This imagery exercise is especially effective for those who are already aware of how they are negatively perceived while smoking.

A third script helps smokers redefine themselves as nonsmokers because it is often difficult for persons who have smoked to think of themselves as nonsmokers. Smokers are asked to imagine themselves doing things they have done before—drinking a cup of coffee or relaxing on a break at work—only without cigarettes. They are to imagine an image of the smoker stepping aside, as in the movies when "a translucent figure of a ghost leaves the body behind. . . . The smoker becomes smoke and is blown away and dispersed by a fresh spring breeze" (Kelly & Kelly, 1995, p. 158). This exercise helps them understand that they can enjoy these things equally without smoking. They are directed to go through many of the different situations in which they habitually smoked and to remove the "smoker" from each of them.

Very often when a person can no longer smoke, they remember smoking as something wonderful, something to be missed. Kelly and Kelly (1995) use imagery to remind their clients about the negatives of smoking and why they chose to quit. They ask persons to imagine themselves lighting up a cigarette and to remember the burning sensation in their throat and lungs, their nausea, their lightheadedness, etc. and then they progress to worst case scenarios, like being diagnosed with cancer or losing a lung or vocal cords. However, because they have chosen to quit smoking, the script becomes more positive at the end. They are no longer imagined as sick, but as alive and free. "You've chosen life. You've chosen well" (p. 166).

Fanning (1994) reports that imagery can help in smoking cessation by addressing the factors necessary for change. First, imagery can help the client uncover the unconscious needs that smoking fills, such as nurturance, a social lubricant, a stress reliever, weight control, or even of self-destruction. In order to uncover the particular needs, Fanning suggests beginning with a visualization that asks how the person feels in particular situations and how smoking serves them. Do they feel nurtured or relaxed? Do they gravitate toward smokers in a room? Do they receive pleasure from or avoid pain when smoking at particular times or places? They are also instructed to ask themselves if they are punishing themselves in some way by smoking.

Once the reasons for smoking are uncovered, imagery can then reinforce more healthy ways of meeting those needs. Fanning suggests short, frequent visualizations that should include: 1) an example of successfully meeting needs without smoking; 2) an image of the person as a healthy nonsmoker; and 3) an aversive image of smoking as unpleasant. This visualization should be summoned any time the client feels a strong craving. In addition to these brief visualizations, Fanning recommends longer visualizations three times a day which include two or three scenes of successfully meeting needs without smoking and elaborate the image as a nonsmoker. The instructions should be taped, and each time a client engages in visualization, he/she should listen to different segments.

A positive image of a smoker as nonsmoker is also reinforced in the nonsmoking induction created by Hadley and Staudacher (1996). The client is instructed to remember all of the positive goals they have already achieved in their life and that stopping smoking is another goal that can be achieved successfully. They are then guided through a healthy body, free of smoking:

> You have made up your mind, you have made the choice to be a nonsmoker and that feels fine, it feels fine. Your body now rejects smoking cigarettes, your lungs no longer want those poisonous fumes in them. They now want to become clean and clear and healthy once again. Your sinuses want to feel clean, fresh air. The smell of cigarettes is now disgusting, and the taste is unappealing and unappetizing. Your mouth is clear of smoke, without any trace of cigarette taste and it feels fresh. . . . There are no poisonous and unhealthy fumes in your system. You now choose to be healthy, to be strong, to breathe clean air with your lungs clean and fresh. (Hadley & Staudacher, 1996, p. 80)

At this point, clients are instructed to insert their alternative ways of dealing with their habit and to imagine that these ways are successful and allow them to go through their daily routine without smoking, enjoying the day with a smile on their face and feeling relaxed and wonderful, vital and healthy. They notice that every aspect of their life improves and that being a nonsmoker really feels fine.

Achterberg, Dossey, and Kolkmeier (1994) also use healthy images of a smoker as nonsmoker. They recommend the use of a relaxation and imagery tape for 20 minutes several times a day to help smokers form "correct biological images of being smoke-free" (p. 332). Once the clients are in a relaxed state, they are asked to "affirm to yourself at your deep level of inner strength and knowing . . . that you can stop smoking" (p. 332). Relaxation is deepened later in the visualization by repeating the words "I am calm." Clients are asked to imagine their body being cleansed of toxins and to be aware of how healthy they feel. They are also encouraged to reward themselves regularly for their efforts. Empowering phrases are used throughout the visualization, for example "you can hear your powerful inner voice repeating clear affirmations" (p. 333), and "because of the power of my unconscious mind, I am free of my addiction" (p. 333). Clients are then asked to be conscious of nutrition, excessive eating, and the need for exercise. They are reminded that they can access this inner wisdom at anytime, and that they have done their best, regardless of the outcome.

WEIGHT MANAGEMENT

Like smoking, obesity is a problem for many in today's society and, according to the CDC, over 60 percent of Americans are considered overweight or obese (Ephredra Education Council, 2001). Nearly 2 million individuals begin structured weight loss programs every year and, currently, more than $33 million dollars are spent annually on these programs (Popkess-Vawter, 2000). In addition to the financial burden associated with the treatment of obesity, there are numerous potentially dangerous health consequences, such as increased incidence of diabetes, high cholesterol, coronary disease, gall bladder disease, and immune system impairment (Kirk & Griffey, 1995-96). According to the National Institutes of Health, obesity more than doubles one's chances of developing high blood pressure and is related to nearly 70 percent of all cardiovascular disease cases (Ephredra Education Council, 2001).

Obesity is defined as "a body weight greater than 20 percent above ideal or body mass index . . ." and ranges from 30 to 38, whereas overweight is defined as "body weight 10 percent to 20 percent above ideal or body mass index" (Popkess-Vawter, 2000, p. 689). Body mass index (BMI) is a standard determined by dividing weight in pounds by height in inches squared and then multiplying by 705. A normal or healthy BMI ranges from 25 to 29 (Popkess-Vawter, 2000).

The health problems associated with obesity and its increasing prevalence in the population are especially grave in view of the difficulty in treating obesity. Only 5 percent of individuals trained in behavioral self-management weight loss programs show significant weight losses that remain over time (Kirk & Griffey, 1995-96). Goodrick and Forety (as cited in Kirk & Griffey, 1995-96, p. 146) went as far as to say that "little progress has been made in behavioral treatment [of obesity] in 24 years." Even in spite of the available knowledge about nutrition, behavior, and metabolism, the failure rate of treatment programs remains at 90 percent to 95 percent (Ritzman, 1986). Those individuals who remain in treatment may experience temporary weight loss, but the results do not appear to be long-lasting (Bolocofsky, Spinler, & Coulthard-Morris, 1985; DeBerry, 1981; Kirk & Griffey, 1995-96; Popkess-Vawter, 2000; Ritzman, 1986). In other words, for the thousands of individuals who are currently in treatment for weight management, 95 percent will drop out of treatment, remain in treatment and fail to lose the weight, or experience temporary success only and regain the weight within an average of 3 years. This difficulty in the treatment of obesity was recognized as early as 1959 when Stunkard and McLarenHume stated that, "Most obese persons will not stay in treatment for obesity. Of those who stay in treatment, most will not lose weight and of those who do lose weight, most will regain it" (as cited in Inglis, 1982, p. 35). The increase in treatment literature over the last few years attests to the continuing difficulty in addressing this problem (Cochrane, 1992).

Theories on Obesity

Problems with weight management are multifaceted and complex and no one theory provides lasting solutions or treatments. Theories of obesity currently arise from either a biological or a behavioral perspective, and many of the weight management approaches are based on and follow directly from one of these perspectives.

Biologic Theories

There are four biologic theories that attempt to explain excess weight or obesity, two from a genetic perspective and two from a metabolic/energy balance perspective (Popkess-Vawter, 2000).

Genetic Perspective. Two biologic theories propose that some individuals have a genetic predisposition to accumulate excess fat, due to either the *size* or the *quantity* of fat cells that are present in the individual's body. The adipocyte hypertrophy theory maintains that overweight or obese individuals have enlarged or hypertrophied fat cells or adipocytes (Popkess-Vawter, 2000), and the size of the fat cells regulates food consumption. In other words, when the fat cells reach their size limitation, they send a signal to stop eating. Thus, individuals who possess these larger fat cells need to eat more before the cells reach this size limitation and send the signal to stop eating. Adult onset obesity is often addressed from this perspective.

On the other hand, the adipocyte hyperplasia theory maintains that obesity arises from an overabundance of fat cells. This theory purports that obese individuals have an excess number of fat cells "resulting from fat cell proliferation, which usually happens during infancy and puberty" (Popkess-Vawter, 2000, p. 690). As a result of the higher number of fat cells, these individuals can eat more than those who have a fewer number. The degree to which the individual is overweight or obese is a function of the number of adipocytes present in childhood or adolescence. Whereas the adipocyte hypertrophy theory explains adult onset of obesity, this theory explains childhood onset. According to these theories, obesity is genetically determined and unaffected by therapeutic intervention.

Metabolic/Energy Balance Perspectives. Other biologic theories propose that obesity results from metabolic dysregulation. The set point theory introduced by Nesbitt in 1972 suggests that obese individuals have a body weight "thermostat" which is set to maintain their weight at a higher than average range (Myers, 1995). It is at this higher than normal set point that their energy expenditure is normal. In spite of temporary increases or decreases in energy expenditure, individuals will gain or lose weight to return the body to its set point (Popkess-Vawter, 2000). Certain metabolic agents are utilized to lower the set point and achieve weight loss; however, once the metabolic agent is discontinued, the set point increases to its previous level and the weight returns.

A variation of this theory, the energy balance theory, suggests that individuals gain weight when they ingest more calories than are necessary for their metabolic needs. These excessive calories, whether they are protein, carbohydrates, or fat, are transformed and stored as fat. A regular exercise program and a lower caloric intake would cause a deficit and lead to weight loss. The energy balance theory leaves more room for therapeutic interventions.

Behavioral Theories

Behavioral theories propose that individuals gain excess weight either as a response to conditioned learning to environmental stimuli or as a response to stress and arousal (Carson & Butcher, 1992; Popkess-Vawter, 2000). There are many external, environmental stimuli that have been paired with eating; for example, there are learned meal times (a stimulus) when one is expected to eat (response) regardless of hunger. People have been conditioned to eat at parties, movies, and while watching television. When individuals are anxious, angry, depressed, or stressed, they may also turn to eating as a coping mechanism. In all of these situations, the eating behavior acts as a positive reinforcer, strengthening the conditioning.

Therapeutic interventions aimed at reducing obesity by controlling the conditioned responses include stimulus-control strategies. These strategies are put in place to control eating by restricting caloric intake, locations, and timing surrounding the eating behavior. In addition, individuals are instructed to avoid stimuli that may facilitate eating outside of these restricted limitations on calories, locations, and timing. Many of the food supplements and calorie-restricted diets that individuals try independently also rely on these stimulus-control strategies. They emphasize controlling the antecedent stimuli that would affect the eating behavior, such as controlling when, where, what, and how much to eat. The goal of these diets is to eliminate, or at least to learn to avoid, hunger and when "the body's natural, physiologic, internal signals of hunger are erased, individuals are forced to focus on external cues to tell them when they need to eat" (Popkess-Vawter, 2000, p. 691). These are cues that the individual can learn and thus control. It has been argued that stimulus-control strategies address only the external causes for overeating and obesity and ignore the internal ones. Thus, permanent effects may be difficult to achieve.

Therapeutic interventions designed to address more of the internal psychological causes help individuals better control their eating in the presence of emotional stress, and also to better cope with the emotional stress. "[N]egative body image, poor self-esteem, depression, and issues of social discrimination [often] become the focus of psychotherapy, while dietary and exercise prescriptions usually receive less emphasis" (Popkess-Vawter, 2000, p. 692). Beck explained that negative and unrealistic thinking can trigger emotional responses, which can be related to overeating (Popkess-Vawter, 2000). The emotional stress may actually be present, but it may also result from negative and unrealistic thinking. Poor self-esteem and negative body image are often features of depression, and all of these have been associated with overeating, either as a cause or an effect.

Individuals need to assess and then reevaluate their negative thinking patterns. They are encouraged to "deal effectively with major, realistic problems (e.g., low self-esteem, guilt) and minor vague irritations (e.g., frustration, apathy) that seem to have no obvious external cause" (Popkess-Vawter, 2000, p. 693). These cognitive interventions to control weight emphasize an increased understanding of thinking patterns and mood changes, a broadening of the scope of coping skills to manage emotional stress, and an increased sense of personal growth (Popkess-Vawter, 2000).

Research on the Use of Imagery for Weight Management

In 1843, Robbins used aversive posthypnotic suggestions to "control a female patient's appetite for certain foods which exacerbated dyspepsia in her" (Gravitz, 1988, p. 69) and made a posthypnotic suggestion that even a small intake of tea would be followed by nausea. These suggestions were successful and remained so at 2 months following the treatment. In spite of the success noted, hypnosis did not begin to be widely cited in the literature as a treatment approach until the 1960s.

Even though hypnosis was being cited as a plausible treatment modality for weight management, Mott and Roberts (as cited in Cochrane, 1992) reviewed the existing literature and found that the research did not substantiate its effectiveness. Similar to the early research on smoking cessation, much of the research on weight management was based on uncontrolled clinical studies and anecdotal case studies. Few well-designed research studies existed to assess the long-term effectiveness (Cochrane, 1987, 1992; Davis & Dawson, 1980). Also, the hypnotic interventions utilized in the studies were not delineated clearly—imagery was often a part of the hypnotic intervention undertaken—making it difficult to determine what aspects of the interventions were useful and which were not. At times an imagery component was identified, but at other times, it was simply subsumed under the term "hypnosis."

The empirical studies to date indicate that hypnosis/imagery in the treatment of obesity and weight management holds promise, but the results are far from conclusive. The empirical rigor of the studies has improved; yet, the lack of rigorous research methodologies used in many of the studies, absence of a wait-list or attention placebo control group, and lack of long-term follow-up make it difficult to draw any viable conclusions about efficacy. Statistical analyses to determine weight management effectiveness are far less common than the simple outcome measure of percentage weight lost.

Imagery versus Control Groups. Studies that used no-treatment or attention placebo control groups provide some evidence that imagery-based interventions are more effective than no treatment. Bellack, Glanz, and Simon (1976) found, after three weeks, that imagery techniques employing self-reinforcement (positive images for resisting temptation) were as effective at promoting weight loss as those using self-punishment (aversive imagery as punishment for eating a high-calorie meal) and more effective than a minimal contact control group. Cochrane and Friesen (1986) found that both imagery-based experimental groups (with or without an audiotaped hypnosis treatment) were equally effective and had significantly greater weight loss than the control group at one- and six-month follow-ups. Kirk and Griffey (1995-96) also found a significant difference in pre- and post-weights in the imagery-based experimental group, but not in the control group.

Imagery versus Other Interventions. Those studies that compared imagery-based interventions with other treatments provide some evidence that imagery is either equally or more effective than other behavioral interventions. When combined with other interventions, imagery appears to enhance the effectiveness of other programs. A behavioral point system was found to be an equally effective intervention as imagery (Dodd, 1986) and, when an imagery component was combined with a behavioral program, the effect was enhanced: participants in the latter program had more significant weight loss at the 2-year follow-up than those using the behavioral program alone (Bolockofsky, Spinler, & Coulthard-Morris, 1985). Aversive imagery, coupled with self-management and hypnosis, was a more effective intervention at the 3-month follow-up than the self-management and hypnosis intervention or self-management alone (Barabasz & Spiegel, 1989).

Aversive Imagery. The empirical studies exploring imagery to date fall into two broad categories: 1) studies in which aversive imagery was employed, sometimes in combination with suggestions; and 2) those that employed suggestions in the absence of this aversive imagery. Clients are asked what they find aversive, and those "disgusting images" are usually paired with the problematic foods. Examples from one study include: "Imagine your infected sinuses draining down and mixing with the warm, sour, and curdled ice cream. . . . Those tape worms floating with the heavy noodles . . . hardened, smelly, rat droppings in the chocolate chip cookies . . ." (Johnson & Karkut, 1996, p. 664). It is noteworthy that, in the study that used these images, hypnosis plus aversive imagery was as effective in producing significant weight loss as hypnosis plus electric shock (Johnson & Karkut, 1996).

Hynosis with aversive imagery was found to be as effective as a behavioral point system, but the attrition rate for both groups was high (Dodd, 1986). Forty-five percent of participants did not complete the program and were excluded from the analyses. Self-management and hypnosis interventions were enhanced with aversive imagery and produced significant weight loss, while the self-management and hypnosis, or self-management intervention alone, did not (Barabasz & Spiegel, 1989).

Using a mix of success/target imagery, covert sensitization, and direct suggestions regarding food regulation and ego-enhancement, Inglis (1982) found that weight loss was directly related to the number of treatment sessions attended. However, attrition was a problem: only 5 of the 18 participants in the obese group attended all six sessions. Most of the participants only stayed through half of the sessions.

Bellack, Glanz, and Simon (1976) used both self-punishment (aversive imagery) and self-reward (positive images) and found that both were: 1) equally effective; and 2) more effective than the minimal contact control group. Other imagery studies that did not use aversive images were also found effective (Bolockofsky et al., 1985; Cochrane & Friesen, 1986; Kirk & Griffey, 1995-96) or moderately effective (Aja, 1977), and one also reported a high attrition rate of 47 percent (Bolockofsky et al., 1985).

Nonspecific Factors. Several studies were weakened by high attrition rates ranging from 45 to 75 percent of participants (Bolockofsky et al., 1985; Dodd, 1986; Inglis, 1982), a problem common with this particular population and problem. Brief treatments (e.g., three sessions or over a period of three weeks) probably accounted for depressed effects (Aja, 1977; Inglis, 1982) but, given the risk for attrition, it is difficult to say "more is better" when less stay with it.

Cochrane and Friesen (1986) found imagery and hypnosis to be effective, but they suggested that the effect actually may have been due to the clients' active participation in the weight loss treatment and not the use of the tapes per se. Compliance to interventions inside and outside therapy sessions need to be considered when assessing the effectiveness of any intervention.

Kirk and Griffey (1995-96) found similar effectiveness for the use of hypnosis/ imagery in the treatment of obesity. They also found differences in this group regarding feelings and thoughts about food. Cognitively, these participants reported a decrease in their desire to eat harmful foods and, behaviorally, they demonstrated a decreased dietary fat intake, whereas the control group experienced an increased fat intake. "Changes in feeling and thinking point to an enhanced sense of efficacy about food and the act of choosing whether or not to eat a certain thing" (Kirk & Griffey, 1995-96, p. 153). Changes in feeling and thinking often precipitate changes in behavior and the changes demonstrated in this study allow speculation that adding an imagery component into any weight loss program has promise.

Imagery Techniques for Weight Management

In general, the hypnotic interventions used in the research or in the clinical setting included relaxation exercises, exercises to put the individuals into a trance-like state, and/or suggestions to the client once in this relaxed state. At times, imagery was utilized to achieve or maintain this relaxed state.

As with any therapeutic technique, prior to its use, it is important to establish a good rapport with the client (Stanton, 1975). It is also important to emphasize the positive expectancy that hypnosis will be effective in achieving the desired goal of weight loss, because it has been established that the client's belief in a certain therapeutic technique enhances the likelihood of its success. Lazarus (as cited in Stanton, 1975, p. 95) went as far as to say that "the particular technique used is virtually irrelevant. What is important is the belief of the therapist in what he is doing and the belief of the patient that *this* therapist using *this* technique will be able to help him[/her]." It is important to discuss the clients' ideas about hypnosis and to put to rest any fears they may have.

In addition, imagery was often a component or the foundation of the suggestions that were provided. As a result of the vague distinctions made between hypnosis and imagery and the intertwining of these approaches, the techniques are usually combined. The techniques include target/success imagery, direct suggestion, and aversive imagery.

Target/Success Imagery. Target/success imagery involves prompting clients to see themselves at their desired weight (Inglis, 1982). The philosophy underlying this technique is that imaging success will help enable clients to take the actions necessary to achieve success (Cochrane, 1992). Ritzman (1986) stated that "[i]f we are going to be successful, then we must be successful in the mind, and material reality will follow. What we can conceive and truly believe, we will achieve" (p. 6). Clients are encouraged to feel gratification and a sense of accomplishment that they will be able to lose weight. As a reminder of this goal, clients are encouraged to recall the image of themselves at their desired weight after awakening (Inglis, 1982). The following is an example of a success imagery script provided by Stanton (1975):

> And now I want you to have a clear mental image, in your mind, of yourself standing on the scales and the scales registering the weight you wish to be. See this very, very, clearly for this is the weight you will be. See yourself looking the way you would like to look with the weight off those parts of the body you want the weight to be off. See this very, very vividly and summon this image into your mind many times during the day; particularly just after waking in the

morning and before going to sleep at night, also have it vividly in your mind before eating meals. And this is the way you will look, and this is the weight you will be. As you believe this, so it will happen. When you have attained this weight, you will be able to maintain it, you will find yourself eating just enough to maintain your weight at the weight you would like to be. (p. 95)

Hadley and Staudacher (1996) provide another example of a success imagery weight loss script:

Because you are now at peace and relaxed, you can be successful at reaching any goal, at losing weight. You are imagining that you have lost the amount of weight you no longer want or need and that you have maintained that weight loss. You imagine and feel and think of yourself as slimmer, slimmer, thinner, thinner, muscles tight, total body in shape. Your unconscious will now act on this image and realize and actualize this image. And you will allow yourself to lose weight, to lose the amount of weight you no longer want or need, and to maintain that weight loss. (p. 68)

This script goes on to discuss changing negative eating patterns into positive ones. It provides images of foods that are high in calories, images of rejecting those foods, and choosing healthy ones.

Kelly and Kelly (1995) provide numerous success imagery exercises that target different aspects of the weight loss process. In a visualization entitled "Learning to Eat Right," those who want to lose weight practice better eating habits imaginally; for example, they practice eating more slowly and eating smaller bites:

As you look at your plate, pick out the very best-looking bit of food. . . . Now, pick up your knife and fork and cut that small piece; put it on your fork and bring it up and place the piece in your mouth. Now, put down your knife and fork. Focus all your attention on the food in your mouth. Savor, taste, and enjoy it. That's right. Keep the food in your mouth as you chew and taste it. Continue to do so until you've extracted all the goodness, all the flavor, all the pleasure to be had from that bite. Only then do you swallow. (p. 175)

Kelly and Kelly (1995) also recommend visualizing daily food intake as a checkbook register in which clients are given a deposit of 1,100 calories that they may spend any way they wish. They could spend it all at once on something they love to eat, but they must understand that they have to choose. When they start to binge, they must realize that in the future they will have to pay back every bite that they are eating now. That realization helps to maintain control.

Direct Suggestions. Direct suggestions often address the clients' weight problem and focus on food regulation (Johnson & Karkut, 1996; Stanton, 1975). While clients are in a relaxed state, the therapist presents the suggestions and the possible benefits of following these suggestions. Clients are sometimes given an audiocassette to listen to at home for reinforcement of the suggestions made in therapy (Kirk & Griffey, 1995-96). In some cases, the suggestions are related to stimulus-control techniques. In these situations, clients are invited to attend to behaviors related to food intake and to limit these behaviors to specific reinforcers and satisfaction of hunger (Bolocofsky et al., 1985). When feelings of hunger and of eating are the target, suggestions can focus on a decreased desire to eat between meals, a feeling of satisfaction with smaller meals, a lack of desire for fattening, high-calorie foods, and an increased liking for healthy foods.

Some suggestions stress the importance of the body and the effect of overeating and are similar to those recommended by Spiegel (1970) for smoking cessation: 1) Fattening and unnecessary foods are poison for my body; 2) I need my body to live; and 3) I am going to protect and take care of my body (Aja, 1977, p. 232; Barabasz & Spiegel, 1989).

Ego-enhancing or ego-strengthening suggestions are designed to motivate clients, to encourage them to achieve the goal they set out to accomplish (Cochrane & Friesen, 1986; Inglis, 1982; Stanton, 1975), and to ask them to consider the meaning and significance of success, health, and motivation (Inglis, 1982). Positive suggestions—those that encourage relaxation, improve concentration and memory, or increase the sense of independence, energy, and confidence—also may help increase self-esteem and control eating behavior (Johnson & Karkut, 1996).

The suggestions not always are given in a relaxed or hypnotic state. One study utilized 89 suggestions printed on cards (Kirk & Griffey, 1995-96). The clients were given four preselected cards that read as follows (p. 150):

1. I go into my hypothalamus and adjust the set point to my "ideal weight."
2. Good choices are gifts to myself.
3. I imagine myself before the mirror. I can see myself looking fit, thin, and strong. I feel healthy—energetic and happy.
4. I deserve to be successful.

Clients were also invited to select five other cards that matched their situation that could be changed in the course of the study.

Fanning (1994) promotes a positive attitude about weight and good eating patterns through his visualizations about an ideal day: getting up in the morning, taking a bath or shower, getting dressed, making breakfast, leaving the house to go to work or school. Fanning encourages individuals to choose and elaborate on the images that apply to his/her life and to ignore the rest.

> Go into the kitchen and prepare some breakfast. Have some fruit, some cereal, whole grain toast, juice, or some other light, nutritious food. Take your time and enjoy. Savor your food and be sure to eat enough. Tell yourself, "I love food. Food is my friend. I eat just enough to stay healthy, active, and feeling good." (Fanning, 1994, p. 83)

Parts of this visualization also address emotional states that one might encounter throughout the day:

> Feel stressed out. Imagine that there are a million deadlines and demands on your time. Let the pressure build. Feel the intense craving to take a break for some coffee and a donut. But instead, see yourself taking a deep breath and letting it out slowly. Watch your eyes close. Feel the deep, slow breathing as it calms your body and washes away the feeling of pressure. Feel your muscles unclench as you relax. See yourself opening your eyes and calmly beginning to organize your time, all thoughts of a donut break vanished. Say the affirmation, "I am a grown-up person, intelligent and sensitive. I seldom think about food between meals." (Fanning, 1994, p. 84)

Another example of target success imagery and direct suggestions can be found in a weight loss script by Achterberg, Dossey, and Kolkmeier (1994):

> Take a few moments to image yourself at your ideal weight. You are standing in front of the mirror. Look at each part of your body. Your face looks just the way you want. And now looking at your whole body, part by part, your face, neck, arms, chest, waist, abdomen, hips, buttocks, and legs. Your body is at the ideal size for you. All parts of your body are taking on a new shape with your new eating and exercise program. Experience how this feels. Hear positive compliments about the new you from family, friends, and business associates. How does this feel? (p. 330)

Aversive Imagery and Covert Sensitization. Aversive imagery can be made very specific and individualized to the clients identified problem foods. Cautela (as cited in Inglis, 1982, p. 40) used the term "covert sensitization" and described it as "a method in which a punishing stimulus is presented in imagination in order to decrease the frequency of a sequence of behavior." While in a relaxed state, clients imagine that they are eating a certain food, and then imagine an unpleasant subjective sensation, usually nausea. As a result, the desired food is paired with an unpleasant sensation in the hopes that an aversion to this food will develop. An example follows:

> Imagine now that I am placing on your tongue in your mouth a piece of chocolate candy. You don't swallow it. The candy just sits there on your tongue. Notice the chemicals and ingredients in the candy as they begin to separate out and over your tongue. Notice the gritty and bitter taste in the chocolate. The chocolate tastes bitter, and it's growing more bitter, more and more bitter as it just sits there dissolving on your tongue. The chocolate candy is so bitter and disgusting now you can hardly keep the chemicals and taste floating around on your tongue. It tastes terrible and disgusting. Yuck! ... I am taking that bitter chocolate, chemical mess from your mouth now. Your mouth feels clean again, fresh and clean. You are glad that disgusting, bitter chocolate taste is gone, that sugary, chemical taste is gone from your mouth completely. (Johnson & Karkut, 1996, p. 663)

An aversion history can be obtained from clients to find out what they actually find aversive (Johnson & Karkut, 1996). These identified aversions can then be used to pair "disgusting images" with the problematic foods. In this same study, participants in the overt aversion treatment group were asked to bring in five of their most problematic foods. Prior to the treatment session, the foods brought in were soaked in white vinegar and mouthwash to mask the pleasurable smell and taste, thus enhancing the aversiveness. Participants were asked to put a spoonful of the food on their tongue, but not to swallow it. Then, they were instructed to close their mouth and eyes and mentally shout the following at themselves, "Make it horrible. Make it disgusting. See it turn into fat" (Johnson & Karkut, 1996, p. 664). While the participants were moving the food over their tongue, the therapist would pair the food item with the appropriate negative imagery and a shock. For example, "flour items were pasty, sticky, and gluey; rich pasta items were slimy, slippery, and wormy; ice cream items were oily, greasy, and sour; sodas were artificial, acidic and had strong, disgusting chemical tastes" (Johnson & Karkut, 1996, p. 664). Once the aversive imagery is completed and the imagined food has been removed from the mouth, rewarding sensations and feelings of well-being are suggested. In general, this method has not been found to be popular with clients (Inglis, 1982).

Whether using target success imagery, direct suggestion, or aversive imagery, losing weight takes time and patience. Kelly and Kelly (1995) address the frustrations by suggesting that clients imagine that they are traveling along a road, a mile marker marking their weight at each point, and they move along that road one mile at a time:

> So here you are, traveling down the road, slowly but steadily. You see now that this is the real way and the best way to go. It will take time to get to your destination, to the milestone that is your ideal weight, but you can get there. And you feel yourself making progress. (p. 214)

CONCLUDING REMARKS

The long-term work of clinicians (Brown, 1997; Crasilneck, 1990) supports imagery as an efficacious intervention, but the empirical research supports it only as a possibly efficacious intervention. Clinicians have found that a more intensive use of imagery is necessary for the best results: individual sessions rather than group sessions, live rather than taped sessions, increased length and number of sessions, and more interpersonal contact and follow-up after sessions. The empirical research does provide evidence that intensifying treatment does improve outcome, but the results have not been as clear.

Additionally, in an attempt to intensify treatment, clinicians begin by asking their clients why they smoke or why they overeat and why they want to change. Clinicians have long known that understanding what meaning the behavior has for the client is a necessary starting point for any successful intervention. For instance, a man began smoking just after his father, who had been a chain smoker, died. Imagery techniques uncovered that the son's desire to smoke was an attempt to continue his relationship with his father, to finish an unfinished relationship. In another case, a woman's obesity began when she was a child, shortly after her older brother died. She remembered that no one noticed her during this time of grief. Her frustrations grew as she kept trying to tell people that she was still alive, but the response to her pleas was to "grow up fast, grow big fast." So, a year after her brother died, at the age of six, she "grew big fast" and became obese (Sheikh, 2001).

The meaning of images differs from one person to another, and imagery must be tailored to the individual. Yet, empirical research is limited in its ability to measure this over groups of subjects. Its more gross design may not be able to capture the subtleties that contribute to the successful outcomes currently achieved clinically. Future imagery research in this area of smoking cessation and weight control must determine how the meaning of the behavior and the intensity of the treatment interact with outcome and, in order to examine these areas, it also must be clinical in nature.

REFERENCES

Achterberg, J., Dossey, B., & Kolkmeier, L. (1994). *Rituals of healing: Using imagery for health and wellness.* New York: Bantam.

Ahijevych, K., Yerardi, R., & Nedilsky, N. (2000). Descriptive outcomes of the American Lung Association of Ohio Hypnotherapy Smoking Cessation Program. *The International Journal of Clinical and Experimental Hypnosis, 48,* 374–387.

Ahsen, A. (1982). Imagery in perceptual learning and clinical application. *Journal of Mental Imagery, 6,* 157–186.

Aja, J. H. (1977). Brief group treatment of obesity through ancillary self-hypnosis. *The American Journal of Clinical Hypnosis, 19,* 231-235.

Baer, J. S., & Lichtenstein, E. (1988). Classification and prediction of smoking relapse episodes: An exploration of individual differences. *Journal of Consulting and Clinical Psychology, 56,* 104–110.

Baker, T. B., Morse, E., & Sherman, J. E. (1987). The motivation to use drugs: A psychobiological analysis of drug urges. In P. C. Clayton (Ed.), *Nebraska symposium on motivation: Vol 34. Alcohol and addictive behavior* (pp. 257–323). Lincoln: University of Nebraska Press.

Barabasz A. F., Baer, L., Sheehan, D., & Barabasz, M. (1986). A three-year follow-up of hypnosis and restricted environmental stimulation therapy for smoking. *International Journal of Clinical and Experimental Hypnosis, 34,* 169–181.

Barabasz, M., & Spiegel, D. (1989). Hypnotizability and weight loss in obese subjects. *International Journal of Eating Disorders, 3,* 335-341.

Bayot, A., Capafons, A., & Cardena, E. (1997). Emotional self-regulation therapy: A new and efficacious treatment for smoking. *American Journal of Clinical Hypnosis, 40,* 146–156.

Bellack, A. S., Glanz, M., & Simon, R. (1976). Self-reinforcement style and covert imagery in the treatment of obesity. *Journal of Consulting and Clinical Psychology, 44,* 490-491.

Bolockofsky, D. N., Spinler, D., & Coulthard-Morris, L. (1985). Effectiveness of hypnosis as an adjunct to behavioral weight management. *Journal of Clinical Psychology, 41*, 35-41.

Brande, J. M. (1964). *Brande's treasure of wit and humor.* Englewood Cliffs, NJ: Prentice-Hall.

Brandon, T. H., Wetter, D. W., & Baker, T. B. (1996). Affect, expectancies, urges, and smoking: Do they conform to models of drug motivation and relapse? *Experimental and Clinical Psychopharmacology, 4*, 29–36.

Brown, D. C. (1997). A hypnosis smoking cessation programme. *Australian Journal of Clinical Hypnotherapy and Hypnosis, 18*, 91–102.

Carson, R. C., & Butcher, J. N. (1992). Substance-use and other addictive disorders. In *Abnormal Psychology and Modern Life* (9th edition) (pp. 294-339). New York: HarperCollins.

Centers for Disease Control and Prevention. (1996). Cigarette Smoking among Adults—United States: 1994. *Morbidity and Mortality Weekly Report, 45*(27), 588–590.

Cochrane, G. (1987). Hypnotherapy in weight-loss treatment: Case illustrations. *American Journal of Clinical Hypnosis, 30*, 20-27.

Cochrane, G. (1992). Hypnosis and weight reduction: Which is the cart and which is the horse? *American Journal of Clinical Hypnosis, 35*, 109-118.

Cochrane, G., & Friesen, J. (1986). Hypnotherapy in weight-loss treatment. *Journal of Consulting and Clinical Psychology, 54*, 489-492.

Cooper, L. A. (1995). Varieties of visual representation: How are we to analyze the concept of mental image? *Neuropsychologia, 33*, 1575–1583.

Crasilneck, H. B. (1990). Hypnotic techniques for smoking control and psychogenic impotence. *American Journal of Clinical Hypnosis, 32*, 147–153.

Davis, S., & Dawson, J. G. (1980). Hypnotherapy for weight control. *Psychological Reports, 46*, 311-314.

DeBerry, S. (1981). An evaluation of multimodal behavior therapy, covert sensitization, and long term follow-up in the treatment of obesity. *Behavior Therapist, 4*, 17-18.

Dodd, D. K. (1986). Snacking, aversive imagery, and weight reduction. *Perceptual and Motor Skills, 62*, 313-314.

Doherty, K., Kinnunen, T., Militello, F. S., & Garvey, A. J. (1995). Urges to smoke during the first month of abstinence: Relationship to relapse and predictors. *Psychopharmacology, 119*, 171-178.

Ephredra Education Council (2001). *Obesity statistics.* [On-line] July 2001. Available: http:// www.ephredrafacts.com/obesitystats.htm.

Fanning, P. (1994). *Visualization for change.* Oakland, CA: New Harbinger.

Farah, M. J. (1984). The neurological basis of mental imagery: A componential analysis. *Cognition, 18*, 245-272.

Farah, M. J. (1995) Current issues in the neuropsychology of image generation. *Neuropsychologia, 33*, 1455-1472.

Fava, J. L, Velicer, W. F., & Prochaska, J. O. (1995). Applying the transtheoretical model to a representative sample of smokers. *Addictive Behaviors, 20*, 189-203.

Fiore, M. C., Bailey, W. C., Cohen, S. J., Dorfman, S. F., Goldstein, M. G., Gritz, E. R., Heyman, R. B., Holbrook, J., Jaen, C. R., Kottkey, T. E., Lando, H. A., Mecklenburg, R., Mullen, P. D., Nett, L. M. Robinson, L. Stitzer, M. L., Tommasell, A. C., Villejo, L.,

& Wewers, M. E. (1996). *Smoking cessation: Clinical practice guideline no. 18 (AHCPR Publication No. 96-0692).* Rockville, MD: U.S. Department of Health and Human Services, Public Health Service, Agency for Health Care Policy and Research.

Fiore, M. C., Novotny, T. E., Pierce, J. P., Giovino, G. A., Hatziandreu, E. J., & Newcomb, P. A. (1990). Methods used to quit smoking in the United States: Do cessation programs help? *Journal of the American Medical Association, 263,* 2760-2765.

Flatt, J. R. (1984) Hypnosis in the treatment of smoking: A single session success story? *Australian Journal of Clinical and Experimental Hypnosis, 12,* 58–61.

Frank, R. G., Umlauf, R. L., Wonderlich, S. A., & Ashkanazi, G. S. (1986). Hypnosis and behavior treatment in a worksite cessation program. *Addiction Behaviors, 11,* 59-62.

Geminiani, G., Bisiach, E., Berti, A., & Rusconi, M. L. (1995). Analogical representation and language structure. *Neuropsychologia, 33,* 1565- 1574.

Georgopoulos, A. P., Lurito, J. T., Petrides, M., Schwartz, A. B., & Massey, J. T. (1989). Mental rotation of the neuronal population vector. *Science, 243,* 234-236.

Goldenberg, G., Mullbacher, W., & Nowak, A. (1995). Imagery without perception— A case study of anosognosia for cortical blindness. *Neuropsychologia, 33,* 1373-1382.

Gravitz, M. A. (1988). Early uses of hypnosis in smoking cessation and dietary management: A historical note. *American Journal of Clinical Hypnosis, 31,* 68-69.

Green, J. P., & Lynn, S. J. (2000). Hypnosis and suggestion-based approaches to smoking cessation: An examination of the evidence. *International Journal of Clinical and Experimental Hypnosis, 48,* 195-224.

Hadley, J., & Staudacher, C. (1996). *Hypnosis for change.* Oakland, CA: Plenum.

Heath, A. C., & Madden, P. G. (1995). Genetic influences on smoking behavior. In J. R. Turner, L. R. Cardon, & J. K. Hewitt (Eds.), *Behavioral approaches in behavior medicine* (pp. 37-48). New York: Plenum.

Heishman, S. J. (1998). *Behavioral-Cognitive Effects of Smoking.* Conference summary from the meeting Addicted to Nicotine: A National Research Forum, National Institutes of Health, Bethesda, Maryland [On-line]. Available: http://www.nida.nih.gov/MeetSum/Nicotine/Heishman.htm.

Henningfield, J. E. (1998). *Pharmacology of Nicotine.* Conference summary from Addicted to Nicotine: A National Research Forum, National Institutes of Health, Bethesda, Maryland. [On-line]. Available: http://nida.nih.gov/MeetSum/Nicotine/Henningfield.html.

Hilgard, E. R., & Hilgard, J. R. (1994). *Hypnosis in the relief of pain.* Philadelphia, PA: Brunner/Mazel.

Holroyd, J. (1980). Hypnosis treatment for smoking: An evaluative review. *International Journal of Clinical and Experimental Hypnosis, 28,* 341–357.

Hyman, G. J., Stanley, R. O., Burrows, G. D., & Horne, D. J. (1986). Treatment effectiveness of hypnosis and behavior therapy in smoking cessation: A methodological refinement. *Addictive Behaviors, 11,* 355-365.

Inglis, S. (1982). Hypnotic treatment of obesity in a general practice. *Australian Journal of Clinical and Experimental Hypnosis, 10,* 35-42.

Johnson, D. L., & Karkut, R. T. (1994). Performance by gender in a stop-smoking program combining hypnosis and aversive imagery. *Psychological Reports, 75,* 851-857.

Johnson, D. L., & Karkut, R. T. (1996). Participation in multicomponent hypnosis treatment programs for women's weight loss with and without overt aversion. *Psychological Reports, 79,* 659-668.

Kelly, S. F., & Kelly, R. J. (1995). *Imagine yourself well: Better health through self-hypnosis.* New York: Plenum.

Killen, J. D., & Fortmann, S. P. (1997). Craving is associated with smoking relapse: Findings from three prospective studies. *Experimental and Clinical Psychopharmacology, 5,* 137-142.

Kirk, C. C., & Griffey, D. C. (1995-96). The effects of imagery and language cognitive strategies on dietary intake, weight loss, and perception of food. *Imagination, Cognition and Personality, 15,* 145-157.

Klesges, R. C., Ward, K. D., Ray, J. W, Cutter, G., Jacobs, D. R., & Wagenknecht, L. E. (1998). The prospective relationships between smoking and weight in a young, biracial cohort: The coronary artery risk development in young adults study. *Journal of Consulting and Clinical Psychology, 66,* 987–993.

Koob, G. F. (1992). Drugs of abuse: Anatomy, pharmacology, & function of reward pathways. *Tips, 13,* 177-184.

Kosslyn, S. M., Behrmann, M., & Jeannerod, M. (1995). The cognitive neuroscience of mental imagery. *Neuropsychologia, 33,* 1335-1344.

Kottke, T. E., Battista, R. N., DeFriese, G. H., & Brekke, M. L. (1988). Attributes of successful smoking cessation interventions in medical practice: A meta-analysis of 39 controlled trials. *Journal of the American Medical Association, 259,* 2882–2889.

Lando, H. A., McGovern, P. G., & Sipfle, C. L. (1989). Public service application of an effective clinic approach to smoking cessation. *Health Education Research, 4,* 103-109.

Lerman, C., Caporaso, N. E., Audrain, J., Main, D., Bowman, E. D., Lockshin, B., Boyd, N. R., & Shields, P. G. (1999). Evidence suggesting the role of specific genetic factors in cigarette smoking. *Health Psychology, 18,* 14-20.

Lynn, S. J., Neufeld, V., Rhue, J. W., & Matorin, A. (1993). Hypnosis and smoking cessation: A cognitive behavioral treatment. In J. W. Rhue, S. J. Lynn, & I. Kirsch (Eds.), *Handbook of clinical hypnosis* (pp. 555-585). Washington D.C.: American Psychological Association.

Marlatt, G. A. (1985). Cognitive factors in the relapse process. In G. A. Marlatt & J. R. Gordon (Eds.), *Relapse prevention* (pp. 128-200). New York: Guilford.

Maude-Griffin, P. M., & Tiffany, S. T. (1996). Production of smoking urges through imagery: The impact of affect and smoking abstinence. *Experimental and Clinical Psychopharmacology, 4,* 198-208.

Myers, D. G. (1995). Stress and Health. In *Psychology* (4th ed.) (pp. 573-611). New York: Worth.

Ockene, J., Kristeller, J. L., Goldberg, R., & Ockene, I. (1992). Smoking cessation and severity of disease: The coronary artery smoking intervention study. *Health Psychology, 11,* 119-126.

Pederson, L. L., Scrimgeour, W. G., & Lefcoe, N. M. (1975). Comparison of hypnosis plus counseling, counseling alone, and hypnosis alone in a community service smoking withdrawal program. *Journal of Consulting & Clinical Psychology, 43,* 920.

Pederson, L. L., Scrimgeour, W. G., & Lefcoe, N. M. (1980). Incorporation of rapid smoking in a community service smoking withdrawal program. *International Journal of the Addictions, 15,* 615–629.

Perry, C., Gelfand, R., & Marcovitch, P. (1979). The relevance of hypnotic susceptibility in the clinical content. *Journal of Abnormal Psychology, 88,* 592-603.

Pickens, R. W., & Johanson, C. E. (1992). Craving: Consensus of status and agenda for future research. *Drug and Alcohol Dependence, 30,* 127-131.

Pontieri, F. E., Tanda, G., Orzi, F., & Di Chiara, G. (1996) Effects of nicotine on the nucleus accumbens and similarity to those of addictive drugs. *Nature, 382,* 255-257.

Popkess-Vawter, S. (2000). Weight management counseling. In B. M. Dossey, L. Keegan, & C. E. Guzzetta (Eds.), *Holistic Nursing: A Handbook for Practice* (3rd ed.) (pp. 688-719). Gaithersburg, MD: Aspen.

Poulos, C. X., Hinson, R. E., & Siegel, S. (1981). The role of Pavlovian processing drug tolerance and dependence: Implications for treatment. *Addictive Behaviors, 8,* 121-127.

Powell, D. R., (1993). A guided self-help smoking cessation intervention with white-collar and blue-collar employees. *American Journal of Health Promotion, 7,* 325-326.

Prochaska, J. O. (1979). *Systems of psychotherapy: A transtheoretical analysis.* Homewood, IL: Dorsey Press.

Prochaska, J. O., & DiClemente, C. C. (1983). States and processes of self-change in smoking: Toward an integrative model of change. *Journal of Consulting and Clinical Psychology, 5,* 390-395.

Prochaska, J. O., & Goldstein, M. (1991). Processes of smoking cessation: Implications for clinicians. *Clinics in Chest Medicine, 12,* 727-735.

Prochaska, J. O., Velicer, W. F., DiClemente, C. C., & Fava, J. (1988). Measuring processes of change: Applications to the cessation of smoking. *Journal of Consulting and Clinical Psychology, 56,* 520-528.

Rolls, E. T. (1999a). *The brain and emotion.* Oxford: Oxford University Press.

Rolls, E. T. (1999b). The function of the orbiotfrontal cortex. *Neurocase, 5,* 301-312.

Ritzman, T. A. (1986). The treatment of obesity with medical hypnoanalysis. *Journal of the American Academy of Medical Hypnoanalysts, 1,* 5-32.

Sabol, S. Z., Nelson, M. L., Gunzerath, L., Brody, C. L., Hu, S., Sirota, L. A., Marcus, S. E., Greenberg, B. D., Lucas, F. R., Benjamin, J., Murphy, D. L., & Hamer, D. H. (1999). A genetic association for cigarette smoking behavior. *Health Psychology, 18,* 7-13.

Sheikh, A. A. (Ed.). (1983). *Imagery: Current theory, research and application.* New York: Wiley.

Sheikh, A. A. (Ed.). (1984). *Imagination and healing.* Amityville, NY: Baywood.

Sheikh, A. A. (2001). Personal communication.

Sheikh, A .A., & Kunzendorf, R. G. (1984). Imagery, physiology and psychosomatic illness. *International Review of Mental Imagery, 1,* 95-138.

Sheikh, A. A., Kunzendorf, R. G., & Sheikh, K. S. (1996). Healing images: From ancient wisdom to modern science. In A. A. Sheikh & K. S. Sheikh (Eds.), *Healing East and West* (pp. 470-515). New York: Wiley.

Shields, J. (1962) *Monozygotic twins brought up apart & brought up together.* London: Oxford University Press.

Spanos, N. P. (1991). Hypnosis, hypnotizability, and hypnotherapy. In C. R. Snyder & D. R. Forsyth (Eds.), *Handbook of social and clinical psychology: The health perspective* (pp. 644-663). New York: Pergamon Press.

Spanos, N. P., Mondoux, T. J., & Burgess, C. A. (1995). Comparison of multi-component hypnotic and non-hypnotic treatments for smoking. *Contemporary Hypnosis, 12,* 12-19.

Spiegel, H. (1970). A single-treatment method to stop smoking using ancillary hypnosis. *International Journal of Clinical and Experimental Hypnosis, 18,* 235-250.

Stanton, H. E. (1975). Weight loss through hypnosis. *The American Journal of Clinical Hypnosis, 18,* 94-97.

Straatmeyer, A. J. (1984). Hypnotic aversive and positive imagery in the cessation of smoking and the maintenance of nonsmoking behavior. *Journal of Mental Imagery, 8,* 57–66.

Syrjala, K. L., & Abrams, J. R. (1996). Hypnosis and imagery in the treatment of pain control. In R. J. Getchel & D. C. Turk (Eds.), *Psychological approaches to pain management: A practitioner's handbook* (pp. 231-258). New York: Guilford Press.

Tiffany, S. T. (1990). A cognitive model of drug urges and drug-use behavior: Role of automatic and nonautomatic processes. *Psychological Review, 97,* 147–168.

Tiffany, S. T., & Drobes, D. J. (1990). Imagery and smoking urges: The manipulation of affective content. *Addictive Behaviors, 15,* 531–539.

Tiffany, S. T., & Hakenewerth, D. M. (1991). The production of smoking urges through an imagery manipulation: Psychophysiological and verbal manifestations. *Addictive Behaviors, 16,* 389–400.

U.S. Department of Health, Education and Welfare. (1990). *Smoking and health: A report of the Surgeon General (DHEW Publication No. PHS79-50066).* Washington, D.C.

Valbo, A., & Eide, T. (1996). Smoking cessation in pregnancy: The effect of hypnosis in a randomized study. *Addictive Behaviors, 21,* 29–35.

Viswesvaran, C., & Schmidt, F. (1992). A meta-analytic comparison of the effectiveness of smoking cessation methods. *Journal of Applied Psychology, 77,* 554–561.

West, R., & Schneider, N. (1987). Craving for cigarettes. *British Journal of Addiction, 82,* 407–415.

Wise, R. A. (1988). The neurobiology of craving: Implications for the understanding and treatment of addictions. *Journal of Abnormal Psychology, 7,* 118-132.

Wise, R. A (1996). Addictive drugs and brain stimulation reward. *Annual Review of Neuroscience, 19,* 319-340.

Wynd, C. A. (1991). Personal power imagery and relaxation techniques used in smoking cessation programs. *American Journal of Health Promotion, 6,* 184–189.

Wynd, C. A., & Dossey, B. M. (2000). Smoking cessation: Freedom from risk. In B. M. Dossey, L. Keegan, & C. E. Guzzetta (Eds.), *Holistic nursing* (3rd ed., pp. 725–746). Gaithersburg, MD: Aspen.

CHAPTER 10

Mental Imagery in Sex Therapy

TULSI B. SARAL

> When Woody Allen was asked, if he thought sex was dirty, he replied, "Only if it is done right." (in Pope, Singer, & Rosenberg, 1984, p. 197)

We experience our environment through our senses. This sensory input is registered in our consciousness in the form of mental images. The images can be auditory, gustatory, kinetic, olfactory, and/or tactile. All imagery is, by its very nature, multi-sensory. We imagine a scene from past, present, or even a possible future, visualize it, associate it with certain sounds and voices, smells, odors and fragrances, and bitter and sweet sensations of taste and touch. We conjure up images of human intimacy and distance; movement and inactivity. We can imagine scenes that are peaceful and joyful and ones that are threatening, anxiety producing, and fearful. In other words, there are no limitations or restrictions on the nature and scope of human imagination. What makes imagery most interesting is that each individual personalizes his/her seeing, sensing, and feeling in unique images (Sheikh, 1983).

Achterberg (1985) defines imagery as the thought process that invokes and uses the senses of vision, audition, smell, taste, movement, position, and touch. It is the communication mechanism between perception, emotion, and physiological change. For example, the memory of a lover's scent can call forth not only the biochemistry of emotion but the physiology of sexual arousal as well. Klinger (1981) postulates that images carry with them emotional activity. When we imagine scenes that are happy, enraging, or sad, we feel happier, angrier, or sadder.

Mental imagery has been successfully used in psychotherapy for the past several decades. (McMahon & Sheikh, 1984; Sheikh, 1984; Shorr, 1974). It is, however, only recently that psychotherapists and sex therapists have begun to extend its use to the treatment of sexual dysfunctions (Delmonte, 1988; Miller, 1978; Saral, 1992; Shorr, 1981). This chapter will attempt to introduce systematic use of mental imagery in the treatment of the various sexual dysfunctions and propose specific imagery exercises that have been found helpful by the author in his sex therapy practice.

HISTORICAL PERSPECTIVE ON SEXUALITY

Attitudes toward sex have changed dramatically over the years, along with changes in other social and cultural mores. Our contemporaries place far greater emphasis upon sexual performance and sexual satisfaction than did our parents and grandparents. In Victorian times, sex drive was considered dangerous, and it was believed to be healthier to have little interest in sex. Sexual counseling in those days, if there was any, was carried out under the religious umbrella and was focused on reducing sexual desire, stopping masturbation, and restricting sexual expression to socially acceptable outlets, such as marital and reproductive intercourse (Singer, 1974).

Human sexual behavior has since then taken on many new dimensions. It is perfectly acceptable today not only to have sexual desires but also to actively seek ways and means to satisfy them. Unfortunately, ever since the publication of the book "Human Sexual Response" by Masters and Johnson (1966), the focus has remained solely on the physiological response patterns in sex and, subsequently, on the sexual techniques that would enhance physical pleasure. The media have popularized sex by discussing it in open forums and have, in the process, given rise to enhanced (some realistic and some unrealistic) expectations of sexual ecstasy among people, thereby fueling their performance anxiety. We have become a society in which the goal of sexual interaction is orgasm, extended orgasm, and multiple orgasms. There has been an increasing focus on immediate physical gratification rather than on development and pursuit of an enduring quality of sexual experience. This has, of course, resulted in performance anxiety and pressure to please.

The recent introduction of injection therapy, penile implants, and potency pills such as Viagra, has further changed the nature and scope of the field. Sexual dysfunctions are now viewed by many as comparable to other physical ailments that can be treated with pills, potions, or medical and surgical interventions. What is lost in the process is the fact that an experience of lovemaking between two persons involves far more than a brief union of the two body parts and the physical release of sexual tension. Drugs, injections, and implants can temporarily restore a person's physical ability to achieve sexual orgasm. However, they do nothing per se to awaken emotional intimacy, foster deeper communication, and generate genuine caring between two partners. Couples who fail to deal with the emotional and intimacy aspects of sex often end up with conflicts that could seriously strain rather than solidify their interpersonal relationships.

Sexual experience goes far beyond the physical event of two bodies connecting with each other. Relationship and intimacy issues have deep rooted emotional and interpersonal origins. A pill or a medical device cannot address the issues of interpersonal distance, distrust or conflict, and the resultant feelings of anger and frustration that are common in couples who have a history of unsatisfying sexual relationships. For any medical or therapeutic intervention to work well, the couples have to confront and change the emotional climate of their relationship (Pope, Singer, & Rosenberg, 1984; Saral, 1992).

SEX THERAPY

Sex Therapy, as we know today, is a relatively new entrant in the field of specialized therapies. It is specifically aimed at treating sexual difficulties, dysfunctions, or disorders. Its more positive contribution is in the area of enhancing and enriching sexual pleasure. Professionals differ among themselves in the definition of sexual disorders, the causes or the origins of sexually dysfunctional behaviors, the most efficient ways of treating sexual problems and restoring normal satisfying sexual behavior. Among professionals, there are as many ways to conduct sex therapy as there are clients. What renders sex therapy challenging and complex is the fact that there are no objective and value-free definitions of a normal sexual behavior, an ideal sexual behavior, an undesirable or abnormal sexual behavior, and what has come to be labeled as a sexual disorder or dysfunction. What may be considered as a sexual problem by one person or a couple may very well be seen as a perfectly normal and satisfying sexual behavior by another person or a couple.

THE NATURE AND ORIGINS OF A SEXUAL PROBLEM

Human sexual response is the result of a complex and intricate interplay between two distinct systems: the biophysical and the psychosocial. Nature has programmed into all animals certain biological processes that lead them to a subjective experience of sexual drive. Humans in their teens begin to become aware of the genital sensations that call for some sexual expression, be it masturbation, necking, petting, or intercourse with a partner. In addition, there are multitudes of psychological and sociological factors that can affect the natural expression of human sexual response. These include an individual's cultural inheritance, his/her family values and traditions, a person's moral and religious background and upbringing, and the history of his/her interpersonal interactions and sexual expectations acquired from parents, peers, and the media. All of these constitute the boundaries of sex therapy. To be successful, sex therapy must take into account the clients' background and history in both the biological and the psycho-sociological realms of sexuality (Saral, 1992).

Most sexual difficulties are the result of process (interactional) problems rather than a specific personal deficit. Modern sex therapy, however, tends to place too much emphasis on the diagnosis and treatment of sexual symptomology. Sex therapists often tend to elicit from their clients problem-oriented sexual histories, rather than gathering data on the positive nature of their interpersonal relationship and the shared joyful experiences beyond sexual encounters.

MULTI-DIMENSIONAL NATURE OF
SEXUAL EXPERIENCE

Sexual behavior is fundamentally multi-dimensional (Saral, 1992). Like any other psychological phenomenon, it is the product of an ongoing interaction among intrapersonal, interpersonal, intercultural, and transpersonal processes. Viewed from this perspective, sexual difficulties manifest when there is a communication breakdown at one or more of these four levels. For example, early childhood traumatic events or environmental circumstances (sexual abuse, unexpected or unwanted pregnancy, partner rejection) can often lead to blocking of communication at intrapersonal as well as interpersonal levels because the memories associated with such experiences are simply too painful. This may give rise to the symptoms of sexual apathy or aversion. Individuals complaining about the lack of sexual desire may very well be among those who are unable to develop and maintain healthy relationships because of their unpleasant and/or traumatic sexual experiences in their early childhood. Bringing these painful experiences into the present and open awareness can help unfreeze the blocked communication at the appropriate level and release the creative energies for more spontaneous expression.

INTRAPERSONAL SEXUALITY

Human beings have the ability to communicate with themselves while interacting with other people and/or external environment. Intrapersonal communication involves the messages that a person constantly exchanges with himself/herself while engaged in an external transaction. At a deeper level, intrapersonal communication also includes one's ever shifting internal images of oneself.

Our bodies are the expressions of what we are. Most people do not carry a very healthy opinion about their bodies and rarely look at themselves. When they do so, they tend to compare their bodies with an ideal image of an athlete or a movie star and, finding themselves deficient, stop looking at themselves.

Looking at their genitals is even more difficult for most individuals. Many people have grown up considering their sex organs as dirty, unaesthetic, and ugly. From a very early age, boys and girls learn through acculturation to keep their "private parts" covered up and keep their hands away from them. In most cultures, children are taught to wash their hands every time they urinate or inadvertently touch their penises or vaginas. Naturally, they grow up thinking that their hands, and perhaps their minds, get dirty after touching their genitals. It is ironical that the human reproductive organs remain the most unfamiliar and untouchable parts of human bodies.

INTERPERSONAL INTERACTIONS

Human sexual behavior involves a series of the interactions between two separate individuals who bring with them different definitions of sexual behavior, different beliefs and values about human sexuality, and varying expectations of a normal sexual response. A mismatch between partners' sexual expectations, symbolic meanings attached to sexuality, and the ability to give and receive affection unconditionally often result in sexual difficulties.

Humans share with the animal kingdom an inherent desire for interpersonal attachment. An individual's self-worth is, to a great extent, determined by his/her validation by the people whom he/she values and considers important. Recurrent rejection by significant people in one's life can create severe anxiety and threaten one's self-esteem. A person with low self-esteem would import this anxiety into a sexual relationship, thereby preventing spontaneous sexual enjoyment.

There is one other critical dimension of interpersonal relationships that often interferes with the spontaneity of human sexual response. An individual with diminished self-worth tends to perceive sexuality as a commodity and begins to exchange sexual favors to gain personal approval, affection, and intimacy. Such a power play between sexual partners invariably has a debilitating effect on the nature and quality of the relationship and the spontaneous flow of sexual desire and responsiveness.

INTERCULTURAL VARIATIONS

Culture is a major way in which human beings organize their experience and adapt to their environments. To accomplish this, different cultures encourage and reward different aspects of personal development and discourage others. Cultures inculcate among their people sets of beliefs, cognitions, and values that are unique to those cultures. These tenets of a culture are accepted as true and absolute by most of its people. The fact, however, remains that the most fundamental conceptions of the human body and human sexuality vary from time to time and from culture to culture. These notions give rise to the constructs of gender, modes of interpersonal interaction, and laws of morality that seem to be externally true; whereas, they actually are in a state of constant flux and are often contradictory. Nevertheless, sexual partners do bring with them their cultural assumptions and expectations, often without consciously recognizing them. These unconscious assumptions and expectations can have a major impact on the quality and nature of the sexual experience and relationship, especially if they conflict with an individual or couple's belief systems acquired as they were growing up.

TRANSPERSONAL DIMENSIONS OF
HUMAN SEXUALITY

Transpersonal communication deals with the relationship of an individual with a higher force, be it known as God, cosmic consciousness, or by any other name. How we view the cosmos is very much reflected in how we approach our bodies and our relationships with other people. Transpersonal sexuality involves the interface of sexuality and spirituality. At this level, physical orgasm is not the ultimate goal of a sexual union. Transpersonal sexuality extends much beyond that. It involves total integration of mind, body, and soul leading to an enhanced sensitivity and an enriched and unparalleled sexual communication. The sexual union at the transpersonal level resembles a trance state involving profound spiritual, emotional, and physical oneness, all at the same time.

Transpersonal sexuality involves participation with the total being: with the body, the mind, and the soul. Sex in this state is not limited to genital stimulation alone. It requires total absorption in the sexual experience and the loss of awareness of the extraneous events. The consciousness of the self and the partner is lost in such a sexual union, resulting in a mystical transformation in which the two partners momentarily merge into one another. Focus remains on the flow of energy between two partners and on experiencing the inner orgasm rather than the mere genital one.

HOW MENTAL IMAGES IMPACT SEXUAL BEHAVIOR

Humans tend to construct scripts that regulate, among other things, their sexual lives. These scripts often grow out of a variety of experiences that lead to the formation of their self-image. How persons behave in the various contexts of life greatly depends upon the images they carry about themselves. Unfortunately, they frequently carry a rather limited view of their capabilities and potential. Faced with imagined or real difficulties in a certain area of performance, they often end up developing an erroneous belief about their inability to perform. The limitations so imposed often impede their further development in the given area. This is how most people learn how to behave in their sexual relations, particularly in the area of orgasmic release (Przybyla, Byrne, & Kelley, 1983).

Almost all people entertain sexual fantasies from time to time. Some of these are aimed at converting earlier failures into imaginary triumphs. Whatever their motivation, sexual fantasies can activate the body systems that lead to sexual excitement and arousal, increased blood flow, especially in the genital areas, firmer penile erection, richer vaginal lubrication, and so on. These sexual fantasies can thus play a very significant role in managing the disorders of sexual desire. The erotic excitement generated by sexual imagery can be gently and skillfully channeled to generate and sustain greater interpersonal intimacy and produce enhanced sexual fulfillment (Pope et al., 1984).

MENTAL IMAGERY AND SEX THERAPY

As has been pointed out earlier, mental imagery is the mental creation or re-creation of an experience that resembles the actual perception of an object or the actual experience of an event, either in conjunction with, or in the absence of, direct sensory stimulation. Imagery has, therefore, been effectively used with individuals and couples suffering sexual difficulties. Sexual interaction involves all human senses, and imagery is an ideal medium to recall and revive the momentarily forgotten sensory and sexual excitement. Hogan (1975), for example, used imagery as an adjunct to implosive therapy in the treatment of frigidity. Miller (1978) explored the use of self-imagery in restoring sexual relationships and alleviating fear and tension associated with sexuality. Shorr (1981) presents empirical evidence indicating that the physiological responses elicited by sexual imagery can cause increased heartbeat, a rise in temperature, rapid breathing, vasocongestion, and even orgasm. In a controlled study carried out by Kuruvilla (1984), nine out of 13 single males suffering from psychogenic impotence were able to achieve full erections at all times, when they made use of masturbation accompanied by guided imagery, and four others reported full to partial erections on at least half of the occasions. More recent research indicates that orgasms induced by mental imagery elicit physiological and perceptual sensations identical to those produced by genitally stimulated orgasms (Whipple, Ogden, & Komisaruk, 1992). Rucker (1992) reports that positive suggestions and guided imagery can be used to enhance the experience and expression of sexuality. Purcell and McCabe (1992) discovered that the subjective sexual arousal increased significantly following imagery training. Mental imagery is thus extremely well-suited to treat sexual difficulties, disorders, and dysfunctions.

Performance Anxiety

Many sexual problems originate in performance anxiety triggered by perceived partner demands and relatively poor self-image. The very act of imagining produces a trance-like state in which external reality along with its constraints and demands can be momentarily suspended or put aside. This helps relieve the performance anxiety caused by internal expectations and perceived external demands. Mental imagery allows a person to suspend or temporarily transcend the limitations imposed by such apprehensiveness and experience the natural orgastic reflexes more spontaneously and in a nondemanding, nonrestrictive, and nonthreatening environment. It enables a person to replace the erroneously acquired beliefs about orgasmic inability with vastly expansive potential.

The relationship between a poor self-image and unsatisfactory sexual experiences has been well documented in sex therapy literature (Hartman & Fithian, 1972). Mental imagery can be of special help in enhancing one's self-image which, in turn, can lead to enhanced sexual fulfillment. Imagery is a purely subjective experience, and each person has the full freedom to create the images he/she wants without the fear of external criticism or anxiety about partner judgment or evaluation. Mental imagery can further be tailored to a person's current state of mind and, therefore, does not present a challenge to his/her self-image. Mental imagery enables a person to address the issues that are of immediate and direct relevance at a given time. It can flow at the client's own pace without the pressure of external demands and expectations.

There is an added benefit to utilizing mental imagery in sex therapy. Many of the sexual difficulties arise out of performance anxiety. The very act of imagining puts the imager in a state of deep relaxation. One cannot afford to be anxious or tense in a sexual interaction. The imagery-induced relaxation presents the client with a paradoxical dilemma. One cannot be simultaneously relaxed and tense. These are two entirely incompatible states and cannot co-occur. Skills in relaxation, acquired as a side benefit of practicing mental imagery, help the client feel comfortable and at ease in interpersonal encounters, as well as in sexual relationships (Pope at al., 1984).

In mental imagery, there is little, if any control over when, how, and what kind of images would flood into one's consciousness. A person unexpectedly may recall a series of events that may or may not have direct bearing upon the presenting problem. He/she may recapture some past events, gain a very different perspective on a present situation, and/or get a glimpse of some future possibilities. The images are usually multi-faceted and multi-dimensional and can, therefore, bring to light multiple aspects of a narrowly presented problem.

It is natural for a person to shy away from activities in which he/she has failed in the past because of the fear of repeated failure. Mental imagery provides a safe haven in which one can comfortably rehearse alternate processes and visualize attainment of the desirable outcomes in a less threatening environment.

The most notable contribution of imagery to sexual enhancement is its personalized nature. One can cultivate a repertoire of one's own unique and private images and see them flower.

Orgasmic Difficulties

Orgasm is a natural body event which is one of the most satisfying aspects of one's sexual fulfillment. The ability to be sexually responsive is inherent in each person. Sexual satisfaction depends on many factors—having a positive self-image, feeling comfortable with one's body, feeling good about one's sexuality, and having pleasurable sensations associated with fulfilling and joyous sexual experiences.

Many people mistakenly believe that an orgasm can be attained by striving and trying harder. Unfortunately, the very act of striving results in blocking of the rhythmic intensity of the orgasm, thereby interrupting its spontaneous flow. Mental Imagery can enable a person to focus more upon the flow of movement that leads to spontaneous orgastic reflexes which, in turn, can leave a person fully nourished and fulfilled. Imagery can assist an individual in building tension and energy in his/her body in a pattern that simulates the movements that precede an orgasm. With the repeated re-creation of this excitement in an imaginary experience, one can learn to generate and tolerate an extended excitement and more intense pleasure than before and to join with one's partner in producing a psycho-physiological build-up that can ultimately lead to a peak experience at both emotional and physical levels and an unconditional surrender to the abandoned flow of ultimate orgasm (Przybyla et al., 1983).

Desire Disorders

Often individuals complaining about the lack of sexual desire and dis-interest in sex have been the victims of sex abuse in their childhood, which has left them emotionally scarred and physically afraid of healthy relationships. This is carried over into their adult lives and, mostly unconsciously, they tend to play out their painful experiences in ways that are sexually dysfunctional. Active alternate imagery experiences can provide them with a safe environment in which they can break the ties that bind them to early sexual enmeshment. The carefully guided imagery can provide them with a transitory cradle in which they can resume the process of their individuation interrupted by the unwanted sexual abuse and claim the freedom to enter into interpersonally enriching, healthy, and safe sexual as well as nonsexual relationships (Saral, 1992).

Erectile Problems

Inability to achieve and maintain penile erection for a time sufficient to allow successful penetration are some of the most frequent complaints presented by men. Barring chronic medical and organic conditions, many of these erectile difficulties are caused by interpersonal conflicts, perceived partner demands, and severe performance anxiety (Saral, 2000). The very nature and process of mental imagery can go a long way in reducing, if not completely relieving interpersonal stress. An example of such imagery would be a standard relaxation procedure followed by guided instructions specifically designed around the client's personal history.

In the author's sex therapy practice, most people complaining about erectile dysfunctions have experienced, in their early years, several normal erections culminating in satisfying sexual intercourse. The challenge of a skillful imagery therapist, therefore, resides in helping them unearth some of the now-forgotten successful experiences and re-live them, in their imagery, in their entire context, richly accompanied by the associated emotions, feelings, and body sensations. With specially designed guided imagery, the clients can be encouraged to recapture their forgotten capabilities and begin to exercise them in their day-to-day life with a renewed confidence.

Premature Ejaculation

An "early" ejaculator feels that he is not able to exercise control over when to ejaculate. It is an embarrassing problem for a person who has always taken pride in remaining in control. However, the very fact that a person has labeled himself as a premature ejaculator indicates that, somewhere in his mind, he maintains certain images and expectations about exactly how long he should last before ejaculating. One way to help such a person would be to explore with him the context and circumstances in which these expectations and images first surfaced, and were subsequently ingrained into his consciousness. The person may be cherishing and holding on to some of his early ejaculatory experiences that he has come to consider "normal"; he now measures his present performance against those standards without taking into account the changes in his personal life and the nature of his relationship with his current partner. Stored away in his memory banks may be some beautiful images of his younger days when everything flowed seamlessly, and he was able to make love to his cherished partner without worrying about the "correct" or ideal duration of ejaculatory holding and releasing. An imagery therapist can help such a client explore the circumstances under which an internal or external demand variable was injected into the equation and the factors that contributed to the current perceptions of personal success, failure, and even shame.

Many of the so-called premature ejaculation problems have their origin in early adolescence. Young males often get together to masturbate in a group environment. They tend to show off to each other how quickly they can ejaculate. In another scenario, a young male may masturbate in his bedroom, garage, or the locker room under the constant fear that he may be found out by his parents, neighbors, or teachers and be punished for his biologically natural but socially unacceptable behavior. Not able to resist his natural biological urges, the young man learns to bring himself to orgasm as quickly and as unobtrusively as possible. Unfortunately, many of these young adults never manage to grow out of this unwarranted urgency. The logical role of the sex imagery therapist, under these circumstances, is to help the client to retrieve these non-functional and unproductive images and patterns of behavior and transform them into more functional, mature, and interpersonally satisfying behaviors. It should not be the task of the sex imagery therapist to tell the clients exactly how to change these images. His/her role is to help them bring those latent images into awareness and to invite them to change them into presently acceptable and desirable behaviors (Saral, 1992).

Retarded Ejaculation

Among men's sexual difficulties, one of the most difficult problems is that of retarded ejaculation. A person suffering from retarded ejaculation is able to achieve and maintain erection for a long time but in spite of his continued thrusting is unable to experience orgasmic ejaculation. The problem in most cases has its origin in restrictive upbringing and a moral code that regards sexual actions and thoughts as sinful. The sex imagery therapist, in such cases, can help the client go back in his memory bank and retrieve any images of intended or unintended ejaculations and the consequences that may have followed. It also may be helpful to have the client recall, in all its vividness, the first time the problem manifested, the circumstances around it, and the consequences that followed. It is equally important to uncover images of any successful ejaculations and explore in their minutest details the circumstances and sensory images surrounding such experiences. The therapist may need to reassure the client that he has the ability to give himself the permission to enjoy pleasurable experiences and that he has permission to let go of the old undesirable and nonfunctional injunctions from the past.

THE ROLE OF SEX IMAGERY THERAPIST

The Sex Imagery Therapist is a professional who has extensive training both in sex therapy and the therapeutic applications of mental imagery. He/she helps clients to explore and understand their own values, beliefs, and attitudes toward sexuality and to develop keen awareness of their sexual feelings, needs, and behaviors. His/her role is to take an objective look at the total sexual history of the individual/couple and assist them to examine the nature of their intrapersonal messages and the patterns of their interpersonal relationships. A critical task of the sex imagery therapist is to rule out, with appropriate medical consultation, any biological, organic, and physiological causes that may be contributing to the presenting sexual problem.

Sexuality is a very personal and sensitive subject with many people. It can elicit strong emotions both in the client and the therapist. It is, therefore, of utmost importance that the sex imagery therapist is fully aware of his/her own sexual beliefs, biases, and prejudices and exercises special care not to allow them to interfere with, or influence, the process, goals, and the outcome of therapy.

A special advantage of using mental imagery in sex therapy is that each person is unique in his/her sexual upbringing and has a unique sexual history. There are no universal causes of sexual dysfunctions, only individual and interpersonal variables that differ from person to person and from couple to couple. A seasoned imagery therapist can help the client to delve into his/her past and unearth for him/herself the actual time span when the problem first surfaced and the specific circumstances that could possibly have led to its manifestation at that particular time. The therapist may even invite the client to enter his/her personal solution house and find a course of action that is specifically suited to the present problem and helpful in regaining his/her normal and desirable sexual functioning.

MENTAL IMAGERY AS A DATA-GATHERING TOOL

Humans tend to block or forget the memories of their painful and unpleasant experiences. It is, therefore, often difficult for a client to recall all the relevant, yet critical information in a traditional face-to-face clinical interview. Mental imagery can, however, bypass this usually unconscious gate-keeping process and access information about the client's innermost beliefs, thoughts, and behaviors. Mental imagery can thus serve as an important tool to collect data about the origin, context, and nature of sexual difficulties. It can elicit critical contextual information on the client's self-image formation process and the factors that may be contributing to his/her current sexual difficulties. Mental imagery is a non-intrusive means of accessing information about the client's innermost feelings and thoughts about his/her own as well as the sexual partner's body. Further it can provide valuable information on the client's comfort level as well as performance anxiety in both sexual and non-sexual settings.

Mental imagery can help bring one's sexual expectation out in the open and trace the roots of their origin and development. It can help a person become aware of his/her latent taboos and injunctions. Also it can help clarify an individual's conscious as well as unconscious sexual role scripts.

It is important to look for the sensory configuration of emergent images. Verbal information is always incomplete. There is always an underlying undercurrent of ongoing symbolic representation. For example, focusing on a frozen body posture may open up unexpected doors to images associated with early childhood and/or more recent experiences that may be most relevant to the client's present problem.

SPONTANEOUS VS. STRUCTURED IMAGERY

Images often unfold spontaneously with little or not much help from the therapist. In some cases, however, the therapist may need to use open-ended imagery, structured imagery, or both, depending upon his/her assessment of the problem, understanding of the client, and, of course, personal philosophy of therapy. Generally, open-ended imagery is employed to collect data about the client's sexual history and the presenting problem. A great deal of information that is not shared in the clinical interview can become available through simple imagery exercises. Structured imagery exercises, on the other hand, are used mostly to help the client change his/her behavior or try out new approaches to the current behavior.

Here are some general suggestions for exploring various areas of human sexual behavior and uncovering possible antecedent factors that may underlie the current sexual difficulties, along with some possible directions for utilizing therapeutic imagery to alleviate those problems.

AUTOBIOGRAPHIC IMAGERY

Autobiographic imagery plays an important role in the enhancement of self-image and a greater appreciation of one's own body. Individuals often carry with them residual scars of their childhood traumas that prevent them from achieving their full potential. Autobiographic imagery can enable such individuals to relive these unfinished, unpleasant episodes in a safer and supportive environment, thereby bringing them to a closure and releasing the blocked energy for more productive pursuits.

In the process of their socialization, most people learn to focus more on the experiences that they have come to perceive as their failures and tend to discount, forget, minimize, or completely overlook their successful experiences. Autobiographic imagery can help an individual relive his/her forgotten positive experiences. Autobiographic imagery involves recalling the feelings associated with one's early childhood experiences. It facilitates recapturing of often forgotten memories that may have been pushed aside due to unpleasant and sometimes painful associations. Clients are encouraged to recall all of the relevant experiences, even if they may not be quite sure that certain aspects of those events actually occurred. The chronological and spatial ordering of the remembered events is not as important as the very fact of their remembrance. Clients are continually encouraged to jot down and record whatever emerges in their memory without questioning their validity or trying to make sense of their contents.

Above all, autobiographic imagery is a quick and somewhat non-threatening way to gather information about how people feel about their overall sexual expression. How do they please themselves, and how do they attempt to please their partners? What is it that they expect from their partners, and how do they convey to them these expectations? How do they sense what their partners want from them? What bio-chemical, neural, and mental images do they employ in communicating their sexual interest, desires, and preferences with potential partners?

SENSORY IMAGERY

Sex is a multi-sensory experience. Our most joyous (as well as painful) sexual encounters become associated with the auditory, gustatory, olfactory, visual, tactile, and kinetic images surrounding the experience. Clients are asked to recall their very first sexual experience and the associated sensations. They are encouraged to imagine the odors, sounds, colors, shapes, tastes, and texture of things with concrete vividness. As an example, when the vagina is healthy, most lubrication has a faint smell. This natural smell of clean healthy genitals can be a source of great stimulation for one's partner.

Clients are repeatedly, but gently, prompted to recall the various sensory experiences before, during, and after a very satisfying sexual experience. They are asked to bring alive the images, as vividly as possible, by recalling all the sensory images and sensations. Some examples would be touching and caressing the hair on one's own body, and those on the partner's body, and the sensations experienced by touching and caressing different parts of one's own body as well as those of the partner's body. How does the skin of one's own body taste when he/she touches and kisses it, and how different is it from the taste of one's partner's body? How do the person's own body and that of the partner's smell routinely, during sexual stimulation, and after a satisfying sexual experience?

What images do the various fragrances and odors evoke inside a person? What sexual images and memories do the various sights bring forth? When one hears a particular song or a melody, some of his/her sexual sensations come alive. When one smells a fragrance routinely worn by the partner, he/she may feel sexually aroused. Clients are invited to think of all of their sensory memories in an open-ended image exploration.

What are the clients' images of self-pleasure and those of partner-pleasure? How do they please themselves, and how different is it from pleasing their partners? In the area of pleasuring, what is it that they would like to receive from their partners, and what is their image of what their partners want from them?

BODY IMAGERY

Most people routinely do not look at their bodies. When they do, they view their bodies with a critical eye, often comparing them with certain idealized images unconsciously acquired from the media. When they do not measure up, they become dissatisfied and stop looking at themselves. Just the sheer act of looking at and caressing one's body can make one more comfortable with one's own and the partner's body. In the course of his extensive sex therapy practice, the author has discovered a rather creative approach to teach clients how to acknowledge and appreciate the power, potential, and the beauty of their own bodies. In this exercise, entitled Body Exchange Imagery, the client is guided through an imagery experience in which he/she assumes the body of his/her partner and makes love to the partner in this newly acquired body.

Most men find it strange, and somewhat difficult, to find themselves in a woman's body, to be on the "receiving side." It is an eye-opening experience for them to realize that somebody else is in control. In their exchanged body, it is even more difficult for them to accept the fact they someone else's penis is penetrating their vagina and gives them an entirely different perspective on the experience of love-making.

Some participants experience receptive energy that they label as female, which in their lexicon means not being in control of the situation. Different people experience the body exchange in different ways and at different levels. Men also experience not only their curiosity about being in a woman's body, but also the fact that they are, for the first time, experiencing their sexual feelings differently. They get in touch, some for the first time in their lives, with the feeling and need for interpersonal sensitivity and mutual responsiveness.

Most women, on the other hand, come out of the body-exchange experiences feeling more powerful. For the first time they sample a taste of personal power and control. For some of them, the energy begins to flow in both directions. They come to realize, some of them for the first time in their lives, that they have the ability to be aggressive and assertive as well as receptive and yielding. They begin to get in touch with their hidden strengths, as well as their vulnerabilities, their fear of oblivion, and the excitement of insurmountability. Some women even begin to empathize with men in their lives and realize, for the first time, that with the power comes the fear of failure. "Will I be able to perform when I want to or, even when my partner wants me to?" For the first time, they sample a taste of performance anxiety.

Women, when assuming male bodies, are amazed at the awkwardness of the male body, especially the penis. It has the capability of doing different things, but not necessarily under the owner's will and control. It requires interaction with another person, to provide the needed stimulation.

The body exchange experience provides both men and women with a very different understanding of, and perspective on, their partner's ways of responding to them.

PREPARING THE CLIENT FOR AN IMAGERY EXPERIENCE

Imagery is accessible all the time and in all circumstances. However, most people find it difficult to tune in to their images. It is, therefore, helpful to create a receptive environment for the clients, one in which they can tune in to their inner self without much external distraction. However, a therapist must always remember that different people respond differently to the same imagery instructions. It is, therefore, important to establish a good rapport with the client and appropriately modify the instructions to suit the needs and temperament of each client.

Following are some of the preparatory instructions that the author has found helpful in preparing clients for imagery work. They can be modified to suit the therapist's personal philosophy and style of therapy.

"Sit comfortably. Find a posture where you do not have to move or shift your muscles much. Become aware of your breathing. You will notice that as you pay attention to your breathing, it begins to slow down and your body begins to relax. A relaxed body tends to feel heavy, and you have a sensation that it is beginning to sink into the chair. Allow your body to sink deeper into the chair. As you do that, your body begins to feel more deeply relaxed. Allow that process to continue without your active effort.

"Allow your eyes to close, if they have not already done so. Become aware of the sounds and smells in the room. Continue paying attention to your breathing. You can feel your relaxation getting deeper and deeper. The relaxed body tends to feel heavy. Allow the heavy feeling, relaxed body to continue to sink into the chair."

It is helpful to have clients explore their emotional responses, as well as body sensations that surface during the imagery experience. It should be emphasized that the content of the imagery is no more important than how the clients experience it both at the emotional and the physiological level.

SOME EXAMPLES OF GUIDED IMAGERY

Following are some examples of open-ended as well as guided imagery instructions that the author has used effectively with clients experiencing sexual difficulties. It must be kept in mind that each client is unique and responds to suggestions in his/her unique way. Also, for more specific sexual complaints, the sex imagery therapist needs to have a good grounding in the basic etiology of sexual disorders, so he/she can create, modify, or re-structure the exercises targeted at specific sexual problems.

Autobiographic Imagery

Go back into your childhood. Relive some of your childhood experiences, when you had your very first sexual images or sensations. When was the first time that you touched yourself, or another person, and felt some strange body sensations? Recall your very first kiss. Recall the specific body sensations you experienced when you kissed someone or were kissed by a person of the opposite sex. What was your understanding or conception of what was happening in your body? When did you first realize that your body was sexually aroused, and how did you know that? How did you express your sexual feelings and sensations and to whom? What was the response from your peers, parents, teachers, and/or clergy to your emerging sexuality and your way of expressing it? How did you respond to their approval or disapproval of your sexual expression?

Body Imagery

Imagine that you are standing in front of a large three-way mirror. In your imagination, take off your clothes and look at your entire body from head to toe. Examine each part of your body, paying special attention to the feelings you experience in the process. Notice the changes in your feelings, as you move from one body part to the other. Now begin to gently caress each part of your body with your hands, paying special attention to the changes in your feelings, as you move from one body part to the other. As you caress your body, you may find some images beginning to unfold in your mind. Notice the sensations that are evoked by each of these images. Do any of these images involve visual, auditory, olfactory, tactile, or gustatory sensations? If so, how do these sensations change as you move from one body part to the other?

In the process of looking at and/or caressing your body, you may find that you tend to linger leisurely on certain parts of your body, while rushing or entirely skipping the others. Focus on the body parts that hold your attention longer and cherish the beauty and joy that you experience in doing so. Now, look at the body parts that you feel like avoiding or skipping. Try to pay greater attention to your feelings and sensations, as you make a special effort to stay with these parts. You may even imagine them transforming into beautiful, sensuous, and sexually appealing parts of your body—your own body.

Compare your imagined body image with your real body image. Do you notice any discrepancies? Now, repeat the same process with the body image of your partner.

Self-Pleasuring Imagery

Imagine your partner in your fantasy and have him/her interact and play with you in the ways that are pleasurable to you. Imagine that your partner is touching your body, as you would like to be touched, that he/she is caressing all of your favorite spots in exactly the way you like to be touched and caressed. Now imagine a lovemaking session that you really enjoyed. Let your mind take you back to that experience—lingering over the sexually pleasurable things that you and your partner shared. Recall the experience in as many vivid details as possible—where you were; what clothes you were wearing; what scents and sounds you were aware of; who undressed you and your partner, how the skin of your partner felt against your own skin; how your body moved in sync with your partner; and what exactly you were feeling, thinking, and sensing at that time.

Images do not have to be explicitly sexual. They can be romantic and/or sensual, such as someone stroking your hair gently, caressing your face tenderly. Recall every minute detail that left some impression on you.

Blend your sensate focus exercises with rich and sensuous imagery. As you concentrate on the feelings in different parts of your body, touch them, and imagine that your partner's hands are doing the caressing.

Joyous Sex Imagery

If you had your all the freedom and no restriction, what would the most fulfilling sexual experience be? How different would it be from your current sexual experiences? What stops you or your partner from transforming it into your ideal sexual encounter? What images of sexual stimulation come to your mind, as you think of your most joyous sexual experience?

Imagine an absolutely perfect lovemaking encounter with your partner. Start the experience from its very early stages, that is, thoughts and feelings about what is going to happen before the actual sexual encounter. Emphasize your pleasurable, emotional, and physical feelings, such as "I am very aroused as he/she is stroking my hair."

Describe the stimulation of all your five senses—touch, taste, sight, smell, and hearing. Imagine that what you experience in imagery is actually happening right now. Make it as vivid and realistic as possible. Allow yourself to experience whatever images come to your mind without censoring them. Pay special attention to how your two bodies intermingle and intertwine in a rhythmic dance, and when and how the boundaries between the two bodies begin to dissolve.

Orgasmic Imagery

Be a star in your own orgasmic imagery. Imagine your partner doing the things with you that are pleasurable to you, are exciting and stimulating, and that assist you in achieving an orgasm of your dreams. Imagine looking at yourself making love to your partner. You are the director of this play and have the freedom to provide all the required ingredients that will enable you and your partner to experience your most memorable orgasm. Re-focus your attention on what you, the central character of this play, are feeling, and how you and your partner are experiencing the orgasm. Imagine how your vagina lubricates when you feel sexually excited. Imagine having the same or similar lubrication now. Imagine feeling tension or heaviness in your genitals, legs, stomach, or arms and the sensation that your body is running away with you; that you are out of control. Imagine how this particular phase leads to the next one when the actual orgasm occurs. Imagine how this orgasmic phase brings on a series of rhythmical contractions to the muscles around your vagina and to the uterus itself. Recall the way you responded to initial stimulation and the ultimate orgasm. Recall how you allowed yourself to let go and totally immerse into the experience. Did you move your body during the orgasm, or did you choose to be absolutely still and focus on your pleasurable feelings? Did you and/or your partner make sensuous sounds or nonsensical noises? Remember the stimulation (direct or indirect) of the clitoris, sensations in the breasts, and those subtle changes occurring inside your vagina. Recall the engorgement of your breasts and the feelings associated with the experience.

You have the ability and freedom to use these sensations as your orgasm triggers. You can imagine having a full-blown orgasm—moving your hips in rhythmic and sensuous ways, saying exciting and arousing words, and even making nonsensical noises!

Spend time on yourself, create a sensual environment, enjoy your body, be patient with yourself—enjoy the process of self-stimulation without thinking about the goal of orgasm. Learn to let go; fantasize and focus in on the good feelings your body is presenting you.

Body Exchange Imagery

Imagine that you are walking in a deep forest. It is a nice fall day. The sun is bright and the air is comfortably warm. Trees are tall, thick, green, and luscious. You can hear the birds chirping and some animals growling in the distance. The grass under your feet is soft and wet; and there is sweet fragrance all around you. You are looking at trees, smelling the smell of the trees and the flowers, and breathing in the fresh air. As you are strolling, you find a log that has fallen to the ground. You sit on it, touch it, and feel its texture. You have this carefree feeling—walking, dancing, singing softly, and simply enjoying yourself, You come to a pond. The water is so clear that you can see your image in it. By impulse, you take your clothes off and begin to look at different parts of your body. Your body is alive. You begin to admire every part of your body. You feel good about yourself. All of sudden, you have an inner feeling that it would be nice if your lover, or the person you share your life with, would be there also to share your immense pleasure. The moment you get this feeling, to your great amazement, you find the person of your imagination sitting next to you. You jump with joy and want to share with him/her everything you have experienced. Now you are two people in the forest exploring the surroundings and fully enjoying yourselves. Like an excited child who has discovered a new toy, you are introducing your partner to all of the experience that you have had. You even take him/her to the clear pond and show him the image of the two of you. As you are lovingly looking at your partner, a thought emerges in your mind, "How would it be if I entered this person's wonderful body and actually felt how he/she feels residing in it." Low and behold, your partner has that same thought, at exactly the same time. Without speaking a word, you arrive at a gentle, unspoken agreement, and begin to exchange bodies with each other. Thus, if you are a woman, you are beginning to take on the male body of your partner, and if you are a male, you are changing into the female body of your partner. You are slowly beginning to experience how it feels to be the person that you have loved. You are that person. If you're a woman, you are beginning to feel the strength (and perhaps the awkwardness) of the male body, and a strange sensation of a penis between your legs. If you are a man, you begin to get a softer body, breasts on your chest and a soft, warm vagina where your penis used to be. In your newly acquired bodies, you begin to caress each other and at some point feel so aroused that you begin to make love to each other right there and then. Without rushing, taking your own time, you gently begin to return to your own original body and look at your partner with a new sense of love, understanding, and appreciation.

Erectile Imagery

Imagine your most joyful and satisfying erection experience. Recall all the sensory memories associated with that experience. Bring alive all of the sensory experiences at that moment. Recall if you were touching someone or something, if someone was touching you, and if so, where and how. Were you wearing any clothes or were you naked? How did the touch of your own body feel? Were you alone, or was there someone with you? If alone, what were you visualizing? Recall the sounds that may have been occurring at that time—music, talk, moaning, sighing, blowing of wind. Remember also the fragrances and smells that were in the air. Were you indoors or outdoors? What was your body position? Were you sitting, standing, or lying down?

Recall your most joyous and fulfilling sexual encounter. How did the erection start? How flaccid or hard was your penis? What made the erection get harder? How long did the erection last? How did the experience end? Now that you know that you have the ability to create and maintain an erection, I want you to recall a time when you had the most exciting and satisfying intercourse with a partner, maintaining your full erection.

Sexual Solution Chamber

Imagine that you are in an old spacious house. You have not been in this house for a long while, but the surroundings appear very familiar. You remember a room in this house that you used to visit frequently, when you were a young child. Whenever you felt stressed, anxious, or overwhelmed, you used to enter this room, and instantly all the worries of the world would disappear and you felt very peaceful. You also used to get in contact with your creative self in this room. Faced with a difficult or a seemingly unsolvable dilemma, you used to enter this room and spontaneously, without any effort on your part, the problem seemed to resolve itself.

Find yourself a comfortable chair in this room, and take a few minutes to settle down. Now focus on the sexual problem you are currently experiencing. Recall that situation in all its vivid details. Now allow yourself to go back in time, when you were not faced with this problem. This was the time when you experienced yourself sexually alive, capable, and fully functional. Taking your own time, slowly find yourself having all the thoughts, feelings, emotions, and body sensations that you used to experience then. If your sexual experience involved a partner, invite that person into your imagery, and relive the sexual encounter from the initial foreplay to the ultimate orgasm and the glow of a long lingering afterplay.

CONCLUSION

Sexual dysfunction is a very sensitive subject, and people experiencing problems in this area often tend to perceive it as their personal failure. Mental imagery, because of its non-threatening and non-intrusive nature, can put such persons at ease and help restore their self-confidence. It provides the therapist with opportunities to become creative in generating personalized exercises that address the needs and concerns of specific clients. One of its many strengths lies in the fact that it can be used with individuals as well as couples. By inducing deep relaxation, mental imagery can enhance sexual pleasure even in the healthy subjects.

REFERENCES

Achterberg, J. (1985). *Imagery in healing.* Boston: Shambhala.
Delmonte, M. M. (1988). The use of relaxation and hypnotically-guided imagery in therapy as an intervention with a case of vaginismus. *The Australian Journal of Hypnotherapy and Hypnosis, 9*(1), 1-7.
Hartman, W. E., & Fithian, M. A. (1972). *Treatment of sexual dysfunction: A bio-psycho-social approach.* Long Beach, CA: Center for Marital & Sexual Studies.
Hogan, R. A. (1975). Frigidity and implosive therapy. *Psychology, 12*(2), 39-45.
Klinger, E. (1981). The central place of imagery in human functioning. In E. Klinger (Ed.), *Imagery, concepts, results, and applications.* New York: Plenum.
Kuruvilla, K. (1984). Treatment of single impotent males. *Indian Journal of Psychiatry, 26*(2), 160-163.
Masters, W. H., & Johnson, V. E. (1966). *Human sexual response.* Boston: Little, Brown.
McMahon, C. E., & Sheikh, A. A. (1984). Imaging in disease and healing process: A historical perspective. In A. A. Sheikh (Ed.), *Imagination and healing.* Amityville, NY: Baywood.
Miller, E. M. (1986). *Self imagery.* Berkeley, CA: Celestial Arts.
Pope, K. S., Singer, J. L., & Rosenberg, L. C. (1984). Sex, fantasy, and imagination: Scientific research and clinical application. In A. A. Sheikh (Ed.), *Imagination and healing.* Amityville, NY: Baywood.
Purcell, C., & McCabe, M. P. (1992). The impact of imagery type and imagery training on the subjective arousal of women. *Sexual and Marital Therapy, 7*(3), 251-260.
Przybyla, D. P., Byrne, D., & Kelley, K. (1983). The role of imagery in sexual behavior. In A. A. Sheikh (Ed.), *Imagery: Current theory, research and application.* New York: Wiley.
Rucker, B. (1992). Positive suggestions and guided imagery to enhance sex therapy. *Canadian Journal of Human Sexuality, 1*(1), 29-33.
Saral, T. B. (1992). Mental imagery in sex therapy. *Journal of Communication Therapy, 5*(2), 174-185.
Saral, T. B. (2000). Impotence. In P. Roberts (Ed.), *Aging.* Pasadena, CA: Salem Press.
Sheikh, A. A. (Ed.). (1983). *Imagery: Current theory, research and application.* New York: Wiley.
Sheikh, A. A. (Ed.). (1984). *Imagination and healing.* Amityville, NY: Baywood.
Shorr, J. E. (1974). *Psychotherapy through imagery.* New York: Intercontinental Medical Book Corporation.
Shorr, J. E. (1981). The psychologist's imagination and sexual imagery. In E. Klinger (Ed.), *Imagery: Concepts, results and applications.* New York: Plenum.
Singer, J. L. (1974). *Imagery and daydream methods in psychotherapy and behavior modification.* New York: Academic Press.
Whipple, B., Ogden, G., & Komisaruk, B. R. (1992). Physiological correlates of imagery-induced orgasm in women. *Archives of Sexual Behavior, 21*(2), 121-133.

CHAPTER 11

A Guided-Imagery Treatment Approach for Eating Disorders[1]

MARY JANE ESPLEN

Diet toward life, instead of away from it. I want to take care of my body. I want to transform a heap of flesh into a conscious body. I want to listen to its wisdom. It knows how to heal itself if I give it the chance. (Woodman, 1982, p. 113)

Anorexia (AN) and bulimia nervosa (BN) are characterized by extreme attempts to control body shape and weight, a set of attitudes frequently described as a morbid fear of becoming fat, and concerns regarding weight and shape which have an undue influence in the evaluation of the self. A number of treatment approaches have demonstrated efficacy, at least in the short-term (Cox & Merkel, 1989; Garfinkel & Goldbloom, 1993; Hsu, 1990; Mitchell, 1991). However, a significant number of patients do not respond to current treatments (Fairburn, 1988; Fichter, Leibl, Rief, Brunner, Schmidt-Auberger, & Engel, 1991; Freeman, Davies, & Morris, 1990; Johnson & Connors, 1987), and treatments that have been demonstrated to be helpful often address the conceptual or cognitive and behavioral aspects of the disorders. The difficulty these people have with affect regulation, feelings of emptiness, and the experience of extreme aloneness are often less amenable to standard treatments.

The theoretical literature has suggested that at least a subgroup of individuals with eating disorders may have difficulty in modulating affects or in self-soothing (Barth, 1994; Geist, 1989; Hamburg, 1989; Swift & Letven, 1984). This conceptualization suggests the need to design treatments that specifically target the problem of affect regulation to assist these patients to comfort themselves. This chapter will review the literature on self-soothing and proposes a conceptual model of guided imagery therapy to address the difficulty of affect regulation.

---

[1] This work was partially supported by the Ontario Mental Health Foundation.

THE CAPACITY FOR SELF-SOOTHING

The ability to regulate tension or the capacity for self-soothing is believed to develop through the internalization of soothing or comforting experiences during early development. Initially, these experiences come from interactions with the mother (or other primary caregivers) and require the mother's presence. Sensations, smells, sounds, rhythms, and touch are all part of potentially soothing experiences. At first, the infant is under the illusion that mother (e.g. the breast) and infant are one and under the control of the infant. Gradually, as the mother becomes objectively perceived, a relationship develops "between what is objectively perceived and what is subjectively conceived" (Winnicott, 1965), and the child creates the illusion of the soothing experiences over and over again. According to Winnicott (1965), the infant, at the stage of recognition memory, is able to keep in awareness the soothing of the mother through the holding and feeling of a familiar object, which is reminiscent of her touch. Winnicott (1965) used the terms "transitional objects" and "transitional phenomena" to describe the repetitive objects or behaviors used for this function. For example, a transitional object, such as a blanket, can elicit soothing qualities that have become internalized and are associated with the primary caregiver: the softness of the breast, and the feeling of being stroked, held, and comforted (Adler & Buie, 1979).

The internalization of earlier soothing experiences allows the progressive separation of the child from the mother and becomes crucial in the development of the capacity to be alone (Horton, 1981; Winnicott, 1971). The child is able to leave the mother when he or she can find something of her nurturance in the external world. Therefore, the child no longer depends fully on the presence of actual people for comfort. The child is able to soothe him or herself with fantasies, images, and memories of earlier interactions with objects that resonate with the soothing maternal primary process presence.

Transitional objects in early childhood—exemplified by the blanket, stuffed animal, and favorite tune—are normally replaced by increasingly subtle and complex vehicles for growth and solace through a life-long series of progressive psychological transformations (Horton, 1981). Typical later life-stage transitional objects include music, poetry, religious figures, works of art, mentors, spouses, and friends (Horton, 1981; Winnicott, 1971).

Horton (1981) has defined the capacity "for transitional relatedness":

> Transitional relatedness is the person's unique experience of an object whether animate or inanimate, tangible or intangible in a reliable soothing manner based on the object's association or symbolic connection with an abiding mainly maternal primary process presence. In health, this relationship facilitates engagement with novel, conflictual, even frightening circumstances and mediates and catalyses psychological growth. It is a growth process and series of changes, often lifelong. It is influenced by experience through maturation and in response to influences in the environment. (p. 35)

While there is general agreement among professionals that very young children make healthy use of growth-facilitating soothers, the existence of soothing (solacing) methods at later stages of development has yet to be sufficiently researched (Horton, 1981).

The capacity for self-soothing has been directly linked to the development of the capacity to be alone (Adler, 1979; Adler & Buie, 1979; Horton, 1981; Storr, 1989; Winnicott, 1958). During alone times, the individual is left to his or her own resources for self-comforting and maintenance of a calm state. For those individuals who lack the capacity to self-soothe, being alone may lead to feelings of panic or fear or feelings of emptiness. When these painful emotions come into awareness, impulsive behaviors (e.g. bingeing or addictive behaviors) may come into play as an attempt to relieve the experienced discomfort (Adler, 1993; Ricci, 1991).

EMPIRICAL LITERATURE

Conceptualizations of early development related to self-soothing have been used to understand addictive behaviors (Horton, 1981; Khantzian, 1978; Mills, Taricone, & Bordieri, 1990), BN (Cross, 1993; Geist, 1989; Hamburg, 1989; Swift & Letven, 1984), anorexia nervosa (Bruch, 1973; Goodsitt, 1985), obesity (Glucksman, 1989), and borderline personality disorder (BPD) (Adler, 1993; Adler & Buie, 1979; Horton, 1992; Richman & Sokolove, 1992; Rosenbluth & Silver, 1992). Researchers have found that eating disorder patients have difficulties identifying, verbally expressing, and regulating all forms of physical tension (Bruch, 1973; Garner, Garfinkel, & O'Shaughnessy, 1985; Herkov, Greer, Blau, McGuire, & Eaker, 1994; Schwartz, 1988; Weisberg, Norman, & Herzog, 1987). The literature has identified a primitive inability among these patients to verbalize emotion, although they are articulate in other areas (Bruch, 1973). This difficulty leads these patients to a state which is "incommunicable" at times and experienced as an "extreme state of tension," while at other times it is characterized by feelings of emptiness which they cannot soothe (Cross, 1993; Heatherton & Baumeister, 1991). Researchers and theorists have suggested that binge eating and vomiting, as well as drug or alcohol abuse, represent an attempt to artificially modulate negative affect and in a sense serve to "numb" the pain (Bruch, 1973; Cross, 1993; Tabin & Tabin, 1988). Bruch (1973) linked the sense of loneliness, the feeling of not being listened to or understood and the pervasive sense of emptiness to eating binges and restriction. A preoccupation with food and bingeing and purging behaviors can be regarded as filling a need to relieve pain and may be relied upon for this function. The psychological pain becomes a physical one and emotional experience is concretized (Horton, Louy, & Coppolillo, 1974).

Individuals with eating disorders have been described as maintaining strong efforts directed at avoiding any arising tension; this can lead to a self-organization of extreme compliance and self-control, best exemplified by Winnicott's term "false self" (1965). The false self consists of an outer self that provides an appearance of compliance, a high level of functioning, control, and self-esteem, and serves to protect the inner self from being revealed. This way of being in the world can result in feelings of deadness, numbness, and emptiness, and a state characterized as being void of feeling and spontaneity.

Few studies have been conducted to systematically investigate these phenomena in adult clinical populations. A study by Richman and Sokolove (1992) investigated the borderline experience of extreme aloneness, suggesting an inability for self-soothing. Adler (1993) expanded upon the "empty, desperate" aloneness experienced by borderline patients, emphasizing that these patients cannot rely upon their own internal resources to hold and soothe themselves when faced with separations, and consequently, experience the panic of total aloneness and abandonment.

Generally, studies thus far have focused on borderline personality disorder (BPD) and have found that these individuals utilize more maladaptive soothing behaviors (Gunderson, Morris, & Zanarini, 1985; Sansone, Fine, & Mulderig, 1991) and that they possess fewer transitional objects, or exhibit rigid or maladaptive use of their transitional objects throughout their development (Garfinkel, Moldofsky, & Garner, 1980; Johnson et al., 1982). Studies investigating clinical populations have found an association between psychopathology and an inability for self-soothing (Johnson et al., 1982; Sohlberg et al., 1989).

In clinical populations of (BN), behaviors such as binge/purge episodes, theft, wrist slashing, substance abuse, and sexual activity are common (de Groot & Rodin, 1994; Fichter, Quadflieg, & Rief, 1994; Troop, Schmidt, & Treasure, 1995). A recent study in a clinical sample of BN has suggested a decreased capacity for soothing using a measure of soothing receptivity, as well as high levels of aloneness (Esplen, Garfinkel, & Gallop, 2000). In addition, a distinct subgroup of "multi-impulsive" bulimics have been identified, described as displaying more than one impulsive symptom and being associated with poorer prognosis and the diagnostic overlap with BPD (Schmidt, Jiwany, & Treasure, 1993). There is some empirical evidence to suggest that individuals with eating disorders have difficulty identifying, verbally expressing and regulating forms of physical tension, including hunger and emotional states (Bruch, 1973; Garfinkel et al., 1995; Schwartz, 1988). The construct of alexithymia, defined as an inability to identify and express emotions and to distinguish between emotional states and physical sensation, has been described among eating-disordered patients (Herzog et al., 1993; Winnicott, 1971). It has been suggested that this ego deficit has significant effects on the early relationship of self to body (Cross, 1993). It is not clear how this develops. Bruch identified a group of patients who believed that they had been physically or emotionally "insulted." She believed that they were particularly vulnerable to eating disorders. Recent community and clinical studies have demonstrated a significant number of women with eating disorders who have been sexually abused (Garfinkel et al., 1995; Herzog et al., 1993).

IMPLICATIONS FOR TREATMENT

Treatment approaches stemming from an object relation's framework have focused on the role of empathy and the holding environment as it relates to people with deficits in the capacity for self-comforting (Adler, 1979; Horton, 1981; Kernberg, 1975). These approaches propose that therapeutic work occurs in the transference relationship and that patients are provided with a new opportunity for the internalization of self-regulatory structures which had failed to develop in early life. The repeated working through of disruptions and events in therapy leads to a greater capacity to sustain empathic failures in relationships. Interpretations offered by the therapist assist in providing meaning and coherence for the patient and the naming of affective experiences.

While psychodynamic theorists have emphasized the value of interpretation, others have cautioned against it. Winnicott (1965) noted the danger that therapist interpretation may pose, as it may serve to repeat experiences, such as intrusiveness or lack of validation in early caregiving. He suggested that any accurate interpretation for which the patient is not ready could reach the innermost self and evoke the most primitive defenses. The most valuable interpretation has been described as one, which is "felt" and "created" by the patient (Bruch, 1973; Winnicott, 1971).

> For effective treatment, it is decisive that a patient experience himself as an active participant in the therapeutic process. If there are things to be uncovered and interpreted, it is important that the patient makes the discovery on his own and has a chance to say it first. The therapist has the privilege of agreeing or disagreeing if it appears relevant. Such a patient needs help and encouragement in becoming aware of impulses, thoughts and feelings that originate within him. (Bruch, 1973, p. 338)

Bruch believed that this approach would promote the development of untapped resources such as autonomy, initiative, and self-responsibility, and would lead to a feeling of aliveness in regard to what is going on within.

More recently, self-psychological treatment approaches have highlighted the role of validation of subjective experience, which involves assisting the patient in establishing an attitude of interest in, and a feeling of acceptance of, her/his own emotional life (de Groot & Rodin, 1994; Geist, 1989). These authors propose that such an approach strengthens affect tolerance and the growth and development of functional capacities to assist in regulating affects and impulses, resulting in a sense of mastery and enhanced self-esteem.

Adler and Buie (1979) suggest that individuals who lack sustained mental representations of others are prone to the experience of recurrent fears and panicky reactions, particularly around the notion that the therapist does not exist in the intervals between therapeutic sessions. They emphasize the importance of a sense of continuity and stability within the relationship to allow for the internalization of more stable soothing representations. For example, in the treatment of BPD, telephone contact with the patient "at the time of emergencies" between therapy sessions is a means of providing concerned attention and fulfils the patient's need to evoke soothing object representations that can offset the fear of being alone (Adler & Buie, 1979). Other techniques that may be useful for delaying interpersonal contacts include encouraging reading or other dis-tracting activities, tape-recorded therapy sessions, and encouraging increased social activities. Such activities assist patients to learn adaptive behavioral responses and lead to an increase in the tolerance for affects (Adler & Buie, 1979; Torem, 1992).

The literature on difficulty in affect regulation (self-soothing) and the inability to tolerate aloneness led to the speculation that guided imagery as a therapy may facilitate the internalization of soothing experiences and the use of a therapist for self-soothing.

Guided imagery therapy provides an ideal opportunity to address the difficulty of affect regulation in eating disorders for a number of reasons:

1. Guided imagery occurs within the context of a therapeutic relationship, thereby facilitating the role of empathy and the development of a holding environment.
2. The efficacy of guided imagery for enhancing the relaxation response and a calm affective state has been well-documented (Achterberg & Lawlis, 1978; Baider, Uziely, & Kaplan-De-Nour, 1994; Hammer, 1996; Sheikh & Jordan, 1983; Torem, 1992).
3. Guided imagery provided by the therapist can act as an "external" source of soothing and comfort, and therefore assist individuals in managing painful affective states. The use of audio-cassette tapes, written scripts, or recalled imagery exercises used in a therapeutic session provides a portable "transi-tional object" that can be used between therapeutic sessions. The imagery provided by a therapist (e.g., therapist's voice) facilitates the connection between the patient and the therapist and may promote a "therapist presence" outside of therapy.
4. The specific words and phrases of imagery are tailored within the context of the illness, and therefore can incorporate image descriptions that are relevant for soothing.
5. Imagery is the language of the inner self. It produces personal images and metaphorical themes and provides an active and "playful" approach that engages the individual in working with his/her imagination and in con-templating meaning in the experience. The subtle, non-intrusive symbolic character of imagery is less apt to trigger defenses or resistance, and frequently evokes revelations. As Hutchinson (1991) notes, "A single image can symbolize or arouse an entire constellation of meanings, which can then be explored" (p. 158).

6. The increased awareness and self-reflection during guided imagery facilitate the experience of and identification of emotions and themes that can be validated.
7. Self-experience is enhanced through various modes of expression of the imagery, including verbal and written forms and drawings.

A GUIDED IMAGERY TREATMENT APPROACH

Guided imagery has been used in a variety of clinical areas and empirical studies have supported its wide-ranging applications. Imagery has been extensively used as a therapy in oncology, particularly in symptom and stress-management (Achterberg & Lawlis, 1978; Baider et al., 1994; Mastenbroek & McGovern, 1991; Simonton, Simonton, & Creighton, 1978) and more actively as a healing imagery focusing on the cancer (Gruber et al., 1993; Gruber, Hall, Hersh, & Dubois, 1988; Simonton et al., 1978). A few well-controlled studies suggested significant improvement in performance utilizing mental rehearsal (Farrington, 1985; Gould et al., 1980; Hutchinson, 1985; Manyande et al., 1995; Ryan & Simmons, 1983; Ziegler, 1987; Skovholt et al., 1989;); in the promotion of weight loss (Farrington, 1985); for body-image disturbance (Hutchinson, 1985, 1991); and in the production of physiological changes, such as changes in cellular immune function (Zachariae et al., 1994) and alterations in skin temperature (Barber, Spanos, & Chaves, 1974; Green & Green, 1977). The use of guided imagery in the promotion of the relaxation response is well-documented (Achterberg, 1985; Butcher & Parker, 1988) and relaxation imagery remains a frequently utilized treatment either alone or with subsequent imagery exercises (Kirsch, Montgomery, & Sapirstein, 1995; Weinberger, 1991).

Imagery has been used in psychotherapy as a method for eliciting insight and feelings associated with past experiences (Blake & Bishop, 1994; Feinberg-Moss & Oatley, 1990; Reyher, 1977; Shorr, 1980). A few studies have utilized imagery as a treatment for depression (Briscoe, 1990; Burtle, 1976; Gehr, 1989; Jarvinen & Gold, 1981; Lipsky, Kassinove, & Miller, 1980; Reardon & Tosi, 1977; Schultz, 1978). These studies provide evidence that various types of directed imagery, either alone or in combination with other cognitive-behavioral approaches, can reduce both self-report and behavioral indices of depression.

There are few controlled trials of hypnotherapy in eating disorders. However, a number of case reports and anecdotal evidence suggest its usefulness as a component of a multidimensional treatment program (Hall & McGill, 1986; Holgate, 1984; Vanderlinden & Vandereycken, 1988, 1990). Bulimia patients have been found to be significantly more hypnotizable than patients with anorexia nervosa and normal age-matched populations, and a trend was found for purging subgroups of anorexics (Council, 1986; Pettinati, Home, & Staats, 1982, 1985; Vanderlinden & Vandereycken, 1988). A variety of approaches in using hypnosis/imagery have been presented. For example, its use as a relaxation or calming technique has been suggested (using nature imagery or progressive muscle relaxation) (Baker & Nash, 1987; Hall & McGill, 1986). Other suggestions in the literature include exercises geared toward increasing awareness of bodily sensations at meal times (Barabasz, 1990; Vanderlinden & Vandereycken, 1988; Yapko, 1986), age-regression techniques aimed at identifying precipitating events of the eating disorder (Gross, 1983; Torem, 1992), ego-state therapy (Torem, 1992), imagery to correct body image distortions (Baker & Nash, 1987; Gross, 1983; Hutchinson, 1991; Kearney-Cook, 1989), ego strengthening hypnotic suggestions (Gross, 1986; Torem, 1989), cognitive-restructuring (Torem, 1992), and future-oriented age-progressive hypnosis involving imagining future goals or life without an eating disorder and associated personal changes (Gross, 1986; Yapko, 1986). The therapist, therefore, has a large variety of exercises/suggestions from which to draw in tailoring a hypnotherapeutic/imagery treatment program for any given patient.

Despite the various hypnotic/imagery suggestions offered, a number of common elements are apparent, including the following: 1) the identification of the need to decrease arousal and promote comfort; 2) the recommendation to incorporate taped exercises (made by the therapist or patient) for practice outside of therapy; and 3) the identification of the use of metaphors/ symbols as being a useful way to explore personal issues (particularly for those where difficulties emerge around self-expression and impede therapeutic progress) (Hall & McGill, 1986; Torem, 1992; Vanderlinden & Vandereycken, 1988; Yapko, 1986). In addition, it has been suggested that these types of therapies enhance the development of the therapeutic alliance (Baker & Nash, 1987). Taped imagery exercises have been found to be effective and superior to self-directed practice by newly trained subjects (Hammond et al., 1988).

In summary, most of the evidence on the use of hypnotherapy, relaxation, or imagery in eating disorders is anecdotal and presents the described technique as one part of a multicomponent approach to treatment. Few details are therefore available about the specific mechanisms involved.

A MODEL OF GUIDED IMAGERY TREATMENT TO ENHANCE SELF-SOOTHING

A conceptual model of guided imagery therapy is offered which is relevant for the treatment of an impairment in self-soothing and which has been recently tested in a randomized controlled trial in BN. While the multidimensional nature of BN is recognized, the focus of the model on the role of self-soothing was utilized for two primary reasons: 1) treatments geared to affect regulation as a feature of the illness have not been extensively developed and tested in BN; and 2) the literature on imagery, hypnosis, and relaxation has demonstrated that such techniques can decrease arousal and therefore suggests their relevance in helping these individuals build skill in managing affect.

The proposed guided imagery treatment approach is conceptualized as having "layers" of active ingredients, with the view that each added layer deepens the effect (see Figure 1).

Reading the model from left to right suggests that each individual layer promotes a psychological soothing state. Reading downward indicates the additive and simultaneous nature of the layers in facilitating psychological soothing. It is not necessary to incorporate all of the layers in order to achieve a soothing experience; in fact, working with one or two levels can achieve significant results. For example, an unknown soothing voice suggesting comforting images can result in the experience of a calm state (as attested by the numerous audiocassette relaxation/imagery tapes that are commercially available). However, the addition of a familiar therapist's voice significantly enhances the effect and the imagery tape or exercise may function as a transitional object. Similarly, the further addition of soothing music (the therapeutic effects of music have been well-documented) (Hammer, 1996; Lingerman, 1983; Moleski, Ishii, & Sheikh, 1986) can complement the other components, such as voice and images, in promoting a calm state.

The specific words and phrases used in guided imagery exercises are generally designed within the context of the illness. Within a self-soothing model, one would use image descriptions that are relevant for soothing and ego strengthening. The soothing imagery provided by the therapist's voice can become internalized for self-soothing during vulnerable times, and therefore act as a transitional object outside of therapy. Individuals are encouraged to practice imagery between sessions (either with scripts or audiocassette tapes). This practice assists the individual in becoming familiar with the technique and enhances personal responsibility and self-efficacy in regulating their emotional states. The guided imagery can promote the development of internalized representations (e.g., of the therapist)

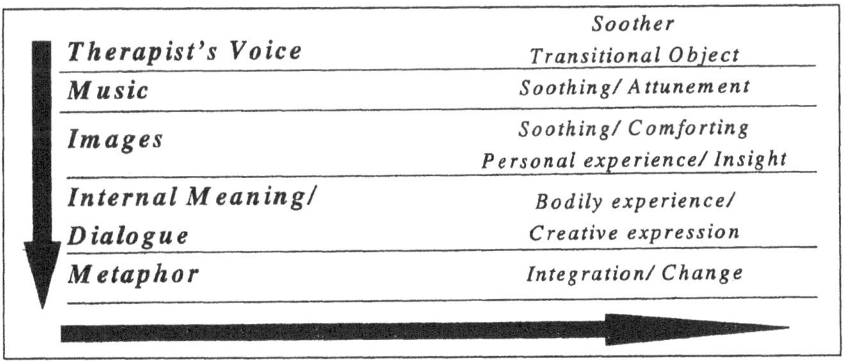

Therapist's Voice	*Soother*
	Transitional Object
Music	*Soothing/ Attunement*
Images	*Soothing/ Comforting*
	Personal experience/ Insight
Internal Meaning/	*Bodily experience/*
Dialogue	*Creative expression*
Metaphor	*Integration/ Change*

Figure 1. Guided imagery therapy.

that may provide a future and potentially permanent capacity for self-soothing. Two types of imagery can be incorporated in imagery exercises: directive, in which the image is specifically described in further detail ("imagine a meadow"), and nondirective, in which less specific description allows for the formation of more personalized and spontaneous imagery ("imagine some natural environment"; "find some special place"). Some individuals experience ambivalence or difficulty with a nondirective suggestion and prefer the more direct approach. It is important to note that directive imagery is also personal, as demonstrated by having different individuals describe the "meadow" experienced in their imaginations.

Difficulties with the technique or the imagery are explored during therapeutic sessions. Individuals who have difficulty with imagining a nondirective exercise can be encouraged to try a more directive imagery approach. Those who have experienced painful emotions through the experience are encouraged to express their feelings. They can be introduced to alternative, more soothing exercises, encouraged to build in greater safety in their imagery or, if willing, they can be encouraged to contemplate and work with the evoked images (for example, through dialogue with the imagery "Is there anything you would like to say or do with the image?").

Images used during the early stages of treatment should suggest an inner atmosphere of safety so as to establish a secure environment and raise interest in the identification of emotions and themes that will occur through the more challenging self-exploration exercises. Imagery themes that may enhance safety include soothing environments (outdoor water and meadow scenes, warmth of the sun, a golden light, and familiar places where the individual has felt safety), the construction of a protective structure, or the inclusion of a trusted individual. The imagination is embedded in bodily experience, and therefore each image is accompanied by physical and emotional sensations (Ahsen, 1984; Johnson, 1987). During the imagery therapy, personal images occur spontaneously and bring forward reactions. Feelings of fear, surprise, and recognition of earlier experiences are among the reactions that may occur. During or after the imagery exercise, the individual is encouraged to identify and comment on his/her bodily experience. The individual's attention is directed by asking questions about these reactions: "How do you feel here?" and "When you observe this image, what feelings come forward?" The therapist assists in exploring any arising themes or changes in affective states that occur.

According to this model, personal insight is promoted through soothing exercises in a relaxed state. A relaxed state is viewed as a necessary condition for self-reflection. The process of self-reflection occurs at the individual's level of readiness. It is important to allow the individual to comment on self-experience through several sessions, rather than to propose interpretations. Personal imagery will be linked to experience, and frequently individuals are able to find their own meaning in the images.

This process is congruent with Bruch's (1973) therapeutic approach, which focused on self-experience and discovery. Imagery therapy is ideal in this regard. The imagery exercises produce personal images within the individual's private imagination. These images range from the concrete, such as objects or persons, to the more abstract, such as a color or metaphor. The therapist guides the individual to concentrate and observe the experienced personal images as they are forming and this promotes a feeling of being active and creative in the therapeutic process. Such an approach results in a kind of "playful" engagement between the therapist and individual as he/she imagines and awaits the images and emotions that emerge during a given exercise. This aspect of guided imagery incorporates the elements of self-discovery and spontaneity that Bruch (1973) and Winnicott (1965) emphasized as being particularly important in the treatment of these individuals. The role of creative activities has been linked to feelings of vitality and a sense of being alive, feelings that appear to be lacking in the lives of many with eating disorders.

Personal imagery is frequently abstract, having metaphorical themes. At times, a profound sense of surprise or discovery is experienced with emerging images and themes. A particular image or metaphor may have significant meaning for an individual by being linked to an earlier memory or experience, for example, or providing insight into some behavioral pattern or emotion, or by shedding light on an important goal. The individual is encouraged to "play" with personal imagery, verbally engage with the images, rehearse behaviors or interactions, and express any corresponding feelings. Self-expression is encouraged in oral and written forms and, if the individual is willing, through more creative modes, such as drawings of the images. These multiple forms of expression promote communication and reflection of the imagery experience at cognitive and bodily levels. Encouraging drawings or written expression provides the opportunity to observe and inspect aspects of the imagery and assists in identifying emotional reactions and personal insights.

Discussing an issue or feeling through a metaphor can be experienced as less threatening because the metaphor or image is viewed in this model as providing permission and safety for the expression of feeling. At times, the individual may be unaware of what is being revealed and gradually come to identify some key insight. Further deepening of the process occurs when the identification of an important metaphor is linked to some symbol. Once a symbol is identified it can carry with it special meaning, and the therapist explores with the individual methods of integrating new discoveries into daily living. The individual is encouraged to bring this symbol into his/her life in some way. Individuals may choose to incorporate a real object that serves to remind them of an important discovery, a goal, or a new skill that is being developed, while others may choose a color or symbol in nature to represent some important theme in their imagery. This symbolic form of expression can be viewed as providing a space in the real world where meaning can be represented and stored. The symbol, in a sense, provides a type of bridge between the individual's internal world and physical reality. Once based in reality, the symbol can be utilized as a reminder of progress, personal strengths, and possibilities for the future. This symbolic representation promotes the integration of new meaning and insight into experience.

GUIDED-IMAGERY EXERCISES

Six imagery exercises that can be used for soothing and which promote a self-exploration of the individual's inner experience (recognizing that there are other possible themes that can be utilized) are presented. The first two exercises familiarize the patient with guided imagery, focus on the relaxation response, and promote increased awareness of inner feelings. As the individual becomes familiar with imagery and gains a sense of mastery with the technique, progress can be made to the more challenging self-exploration imagery exercises (exercises 3–6). It is beyond the scope of this chapter to go into detail with each exercise; a brief description of the images and goals are provided.[2]

1. *Inner Sanctuary.* This exercise has been used in the literature for having the individual create a "special" internal place for relaxation and becoming aware of feelings (Moleski et al., 1986).

2. *Exploration of a Meadow.* This exercise consists of directive imagery and has the individual explore a meadow (Leuner, 1978). Its functions include promoting the use of all senses during imagery, enhancing a relaxation response, and demonstrating to the individual her/his ability in doing imagery.

3. *Creating a Mask.* This exercise has the individual imagine discovering a box full of creative supplies and making a special mask. It assists in introducing the individual to a self-exploration exercise and at the same time involves participation in a creative act.

4. *Color of Self.* This exercise involves having the individual draw himself or herself as a color or combination of colors, called a colorform on paper. The individual is asked to imagine a painter's canvas upon which the image of the colorform is visualized. The individual is invited to experiment painting with a variety of colors of paint at the bottom of the canvas, including a special jar called the "color of aliveness." While experimenting with the colors the individual is asked to note what he/she observes (What changes are occurring? What is happening during the imagery?) Suggestions of "Kaleidoscope descriptions" may also be incorporated. This exercise is designed to be soothing and to continue with the self-exploration process in therapy in a creative and playful manner and frequently addresses body image issues in a less defensive manner than having the individual imagine their sense of their actual body size.

5. *Theater Scene.* This exercise has the individual imagine being in a theater and observing his or her "colorform" in an interaction (past, current, or future) of

---

[2] The full scripts of the exercises can be obtained from the author.

his or her choice. Its goal is to continue the self-exploration process and to bring it into the realm of interpersonal relationships.

6. *Design of a Personal Quilt.* This exercise has the individual imagine making a personal quilt through a medium of choice and to observe the pattern that is developing. The exercise is designed to be soothing, to continue with self-exploration, and to promote themes of continued growth and change. The exercise is viewed as creative and it has been found to be useful towards the end of therapy to promote an internalized feeling of continued development and growth, thereby facilitating termination of therapy.

Case 1

Helen (not her real name) is a 23-year-old woman, living with her boyfriend and attending university. She has a history of AN which developed at age 15, following a move with her parents to Denmark from Canada. At the age of 19 and after reaching her "goal weight" of 108 lbs. (she is 5'4"), which followed an intensive treatment program, she began engaging in binge eating and self-induced vomiting on a regular basis. By the age of 23, she had returned to Canada and was able to eat regular meals daily and had somewhat accepted her body weight, however had been unable to stop binge/purge episodes (reporting 3–6 episodes weekly) which prompted her to seek treatment.

Helen was introduced to imagery through individual outpatient psychotherapy in a randomized trial of guided imagery. In this trial, imagery was the focal psychotherapeutic technique with no concurrent therapy other than self-monitoring of eating symptoms. The therapist conducted the "inner sanctuary" exercise during an early session. Helen's visualized "place" where she felt comfort was a "stone house" that she imagined being located in Denmark. When asked to explore what was so special about this place, Helen eloquently described feeling "safe," "peaceful," and "protected" and in some way even "more secure." She was encouraged to practice this first scenario, daily, particularly around her bingeing and purging behaviors. Following her first week of therapy, she reported utilizing the taped exercise on several occasions and was able to discontinue three episodes of bingeing by listening to the taped version of the inner sanctuary exercise. During her sessions, she was encouraged to explore in detail her experiences in Denmark and the image of the stone house (which became a central theme during her sessions).

Her history revealed that her parents had moved from Canada to Denmark when Helen was 14, following completion of primary school. Helen recalled feeling "popular," "confident," "having numerous friends" (including a boyfriend), participating in athletics, excelling at school, and being healthy in Canada. Following her arrival to Denmark, she found herself having difficulty making friends, feeling uncomfortable in a foreign country, and began to strongly resent her parents for taking her away. She found solace only in skating and became competitive in the sport, participating in little else. It was at this time that she began to severely restrict her food intake, developing AN. She also relayed feelings of fear in relation to dating male colleagues, particularly around her feelings of sexuality, as she perceived the students in Denmark to be permissive and "more mature." She became so ill that she was hospitalized at that time, despite being successful in her competitive skating. It was several years later (after Helen returned with her family to Canada and following her treatment for Anorexia) and while she was attending university that she sought treatment for her bingeing/purging. At that time she continued to have conflictual feelings and anger toward her parents and when beginning the imagery therapy described intense negative feelings around her past experiences in Denmark.

Helen was encouraged to explore "the stone house" which presented itself consistently through many of the exercises described above (for example, during the meadow scene and when "making her mask" she was in the stone house). The therapist pointed out that the stone house appeared to be a refuge and a place of calming (according to Helen's verbalization on her imagery), and yet was in an environment that she associated with strong and intense negative feelings. Helen, too, made this observation and was encouraged over time to explore in detail what it was about the stone house that was so meaningful for her and contributed to her feeling so secure. She described the house as not being particularly familiar to her (there are many in Denmark), but reported it as being "strong," "old," "natural," and "very real," and as not being "brightly colored" or "perfect," however, having "depth," and a comforting solitude. As Helen progressed in therapy and expressed her feelings about her imagery through her drawings of images and verbally during therapeutic discussions, it became evident to her that she saw herself as "not measuring up to others," felt inadequate and wondered how her boyfriend could care for her. She would find herself alone at home, prior to his return in the evening, and experienced strong urges to binge and purge. However, over time it became clearer through her descriptions of the house that she admired the qualities of the "stone building" in contrast to personal qualities she described as being "superficial" and uncomfortable for her. Her innermost yearnings seemed to be for self-qualities that she described in terms of the house; for example, she revealed that her chief goal was to engage in academics and produce "meaningful," and "worthwhile" work that would be of enduring quality. However, she felt she could never "permit" herself to engage in courses that she desired, such as philosophy or historical literature. She believed that her family and friends did not see that she had such qualities within her. In addition, despite having participated in athletics and "the glamor of performing" she felt unfulfilled by these accomplishments and had never experienced a sense of esteem (despite many hours of preparation toward achieving goals in her skating). As the imagery therapy progressed, Helen was encouraged to visualize the "stone" building regularly in a sensory way and to explore her attachment to this image and its meaning for her. Her personal imagery became a vehicle through which she could disclose (metaphorically at first) her innermost feelings, express her pain associated with being in Denmark, and her feelings toward her parents. Over time she was able to grasp something more positive from her time there, rather than to view it as "wasted and painful years of her life." After her 6 weeks of imagery therapy, she was able to describe her experiences in Denmark as possibly contributing to the development of personal qualities such as "strength," "endurance," and "substance" that she was beginning to sense she possessed, as she explored her imagery. The therapist encouraged her to remain in touch with these qualities (e.g., "to really feel them") and to allow them to fully develop. She was encouraged to nurture the qualities that she valued and to share them with others over time, as she felt comfortable. She also came to recognize the "house" and its "special" qualities as representing "her" and her personal experience in Denmark, and interestingly, as being separate from the experience of her parents. This was an important self-discovery for her to make, given that she felt so "cheated" and "controlled" in being taken from a comforting safe environment to an unknown country, against her wishes. By the end of the 6 weeks, Helen had only occasional binge/purge episodes (one or two every few weeks) and reported a greater sense of control. She also reported an increase in her mood level and a renewed life interest. She continued to utilize the imagery for self-comforting around exams and her eating urges, and shared her personal experiences with her imagery with her boyfriend. She had also discussed her feelings more openly during a visit to her parents.

Case 1 Discussion. This case example is useful in highlighting the elements in the imagery model as well as demonstrating the patient's acceptance of the imagery therapy as a comforting device and participatory experience. Helen took an active role, the imagery was "personal," and through focusing on her specific images during the therapeutic sessions (and in her journal) *she* came to the conclusion that the stone house represented some aspect within her which was hidden from others and kept private. Perhaps because it was her own personally evoked image (rather than therapist-suggested) it became particularly meaningful and solacing for her, and she repeatedly called upon it for comforting and to inspect its meaning. The therapist acted to guide the patient to explore the imagery and, as themes emerged, asked the patient to inspect them and to describe any associated feelings or interpretations. This is similar to Bruch's (1973) "fact-finding" approach that she believes to be crucial for promoting self-discovery and autonomy. Helen, through her imagery, was able to further understand from a new perspective her development of an eating disorder and to learn about personal issues that may be contributing to her need to binge/purge, despite having normalized eating and feeling fairly comfortable with her body weight. She frequently had commented on the fact that she had gone through previous treatments and addressed other issues (e.g., weight), and yet could not understand her lack of control at times over her eating and self-induced vomiting. Helen received the guided imagery without any concurrent therapies (other than maintaining self-monitoring of her eating symptoms as part of her personal journal). However, the therapist refrained from making comments or recommendations on her eating and kept a focus on her experienced imagery, suggesting that her insights and behavioral changes appeared to have occurred as a result of the imagery therapy.

Case 2

Mary is a 28-year-old woman who had participated in numerous treatment programs and had made progress concerning her body weight and dieting behavior; however, she continued to binge and purge several times per week. She reported a history of growing up in a commune where she and her mother had lived, and she had been raised by a multitude of individuals. She reported a lack of discipline in her childhood because of the "freedom" associated with the commune. Her mother had several boyfriends. She felt that she did not have constancy in her living situation during the time of her childhood. In addition, she reported several episodes of sexual molestation as an adolescent. At the time of the study, Mary was living with her mother and felt she had achieved some progress in the relationship with her mother; however, she continued to have strong feelings concerning her sense of a "lack of mothering" during her childhood. She was in a relationship with a man that she reported as going fairly well, but she was concerned that she would experience an intense build up of emotions, at which point she would lose control and engage in bingeing and purging behavior.

During an early session in therapy, this patient was introduced to the "inner sanctuary" exercise and recorded the following experience in her journal: "I felt so relaxed going to my inner sanctuary the porch on the water. . . . I brought someone with me, though, a woman, kind of an "ideal" mother. She was comforting and loving and ethereal and encouraging. . . . I felt so good to have her with me. She is so kind and warm. . . . She gently strokes my back when I'm upset, she calms me and sometimes she holds me . . . at other times she just sits quietly." hen Mary was asked by the therapist who she believed the woman was, she stated, "She has a face like mine . . . maybe she is me." ver the course of therapy, Mary repeatedly used this exercise to manage her urge to binge and her emotional buildup. She was able to increase her sense of control over her eating symptoms and frequently utilized the imagery exercise on her own, without using the taped version, for self-comforting. By the end of the sixth week of therapy, Mary had decreased her bingeing/purging episodes to once weekly.

Case 2 Discussion.   This case suggests that the imagery operated, at least at some level, as a relaxation technique, facilitating a decrease in physical tension or discomfort. The experience of imagery as a relaxation technique is a finding consistent with previous imagery studies investigating this effect (Torem,

1992). While this is a possible explanation at the simplest level of the guided imagery model, this clinical case suggests that the treatment acted beyond the role of relaxation. For example, Mary's report of a "comforting," "loving," "ideal" mother and the role of solace and "warmth" experienced through her imagery, may highlight a deeper function of the imagery treatment, linked closely to the internal experience of being solaced or soothed. Interestingly, Mary's sense of not having had a reliable mother during her childhood may have led her to create an "ideal" type of mother. Mary repeatedly imagined this consistent image of her inner sanctuary.

Although the extent to which therapist connection was an important factor cannot be determined from the study, one might postulate this feature of the treatment as being a key component, according to the psychotherapy literature. The case example suggests that the images were called up through the patient's memories and utilized for comforting, frequently leading to an internal state of feeling serene and calm. It is possible that the repetitions, rhythmic qualities, and soothing tonal range of the voice on the taped exercise are comparable to the infant's experience of the repetitive task associated with the acquisition of soothing, internally represented transitional objects as described by Winnicott (1965).

Transitional object functions provide the patient with an external soothing device that enhances his or her ability to self-soothe and self-comfort during difficult periods or when feeling alone. These objects subsequently lead to internal representations that will be sufficient to soothe the patient. A number of supportive interventions that serve soothing functions have been identified in the literature and include the nonverbal reminder of the therapist's presence and interest (Appelbaum, 1994; Bruch, 1973; Horton, 1981). Applebaum (1994) identified the important role of the therapist in recognizing and describing an array of affects in terms close to the patient's experience and in enlisting the patient's cooperation in looking for its source and choosing a soothing device that will strengthen rather than undermine the patient's capacities for self-observation. He also identifies the therapist's need to refrain from intervening, in order to allow the patient time to discover his or her own capacity to master the anxiety.

It is interesting to note that Mary imagined a type of maternal or nurturing figure during the inner sanctuary exercise. Mary's descriptions have direct relevance to Horton's (1981) writings on the soothing experience of a maternal presence, exemplified through his clinical and literary case examples. He elaborates on specific maternal imagery as being "safely ensconced in a maternal surround," and he portrays the felt presence of a maternal object as a way forward into the future. Horton distinguishes these types of experiences from other pleasures and fantasies, describing them as "fundamentally different" because they meet criteria for transitional relatedness: "It is the special cohesion of factors that make it transitional relatedness-separation from the mother, the use of objects that in some way stand for and are connected with her, the occurrence of reliable soothing, the development of greater freedom from oppressive circumstances, internal and/or external, and the facilitation of an adaptive solution to an otherwise overwhelming conflict" (Horton, 1981, p. 78). The clinical case of Mary supports these criteria, suggesting that the personal imagery functioned as a transitional object; the imagery was specifically connected to a maternal presence (in her absence), thereby facilitating solace, and it was evoked by Mary creatively and specifically as a means to deal with stressful or challenging events.

Appelbaum (1994) has recommended teaching patients methods of self-soothing to help them restore the working state in therapy, where self-expression and observation can occur. Imagery therapy directly invites patients to find a soothing presence by linking them to previously soothing experiences, and for patients who lack such previous experience by facilitating the experience of the therapist as a soother. In addition, the creative function in the imagery treatment (for example, work with images, psychodrama, creative expression in the form of drawing the imagery) promotes self-observation, which has been identified as an important therapeutic element in addressing feelings of emptiness and numbness. Self-observation may lead to change through the alteration of the self-schema and a kind of "reconstruction" of earlier experienced events (Arntz, 1994).

Case 3

Sharon is a 26-year-old health professional who developed AN in her late teens and bulimia in her twenties. She was in a satisfactory marriage but could not gain control over her eating symptoms. When she imagined her "color of self" exercise, she visualized a wheel-like image (which she drew) that was half filled with a variety of distinct colors, while the other half remained empty. She provided a kind of "blueprint" along with her drawing of her imagery, indicating how the colors reflected different parts of her personality. For example, the color brown represented her self-esteem (a small portion of her wheel); pink, her sexuality; green, her feeling of aliveness; and so on. She described her sense of the half of the wheel that was empty as being a part of herself that she knew nothing about and wondered what it represented, suggesting that she still needed to discover it. Over the course of therapy, the color form she drew changed and began to expand in several colors within her "wheel" of self-representation. For example, the brown color expanded in size and the color yellow emerged, which she indicated as representing "hope." In addition, the colors began to take over the "uncolored" portion of the wheel. She repetitively used the exercise to view and learn more about herself and found some solace in revisiting her imagery and inspecting its changes and meaning.

When Sharon participated in the "theater scene exercise" she imagined an interaction with her father and visualized her color form on stage along with her father. What she found striking about her imagery was that she observed that her color form became very small in the presence of her father and eventually rolled off the stage. She was able to express her feelings concerning her fear of her father and to interpret her reaction as occurring as a result of his dominance and her inability to confront him about the demands he placed on her. For example, she reported that he had high career performance expectations for her. By replaying the imagery exercise involving her sense of her own color form, Sharon metaphorically experienced the possibility for change (e.g., colors changing over time, which assisted her to build confidence and to learn more about her own desires). In addition, she was able to utilize the changes observed in her imagery experience to gain the courage to begin to address the feelings of conflict she experienced with her father.

Case 3 Discussion. Therapeutic discussions on the experienced imagery occurred during each session, and the therapist encouraged Sharon to make interpretations of the imagery and to explore the experienced affect. Sharon frequently discussed the imagery in terms of metaphor or particular images that were at times interpreted by her as being symbolic of some behavior, meaning, or feeling. This therapeutic engagement between the therapist and the patient may have facilitated the patient's message and assisted in capturing what the patient was thinking and feeling. It was not unusual for patients to express feelings or insights concerning painful experiences by identifying and describing specific images, and Sharon participated in making her own interpretation concerning her imagery. These discussions in therapy may have facilitated the patient's experience of being understood, which Bruch (1973) emphasized.

SUMMARY OF THE GUIDED IMAGERY
RANDOMIZED TRIAL

The guided imagery model described above has been applied in a recent study of BN described in detail elsewhere (Esplen, Garfinkel, Olmstead, Gallop, & Kennedy, 1998; Esplen et al., 2000). A randomized controlled trial compared 6 weeks of individual guided imagery therapy (with self-monitoring of symptoms) to a control group (which controlled for therapist contact and self-monitoring of symptoms). Fifty participants who met DSM III-R criteria for bulimia nervosa completed the study. Measures of eating-disorder symptoms, psychological functioning, and self-reports associated with the experience of guided-imagery therapy were obtained. The guided-imagery treatment had substantial effects on the reduction of bingeing and purging episodes; the imagery group had a mean reduction of binges of 74 percent ($p < 0.0001$) and of vomiting of 73 percent ($p < 0.0001$). The imagery treatment also demonstrated improvement on measures of attitudes concerning eating, dieting, and body weight in comparison to the control group. In addition, the guided-imagery group demonstrated improvement on psychological measures of aloneness ($p < 0.05$) and the ability for self-comforting ($p < 0.001$). Evidence from this preliminary study suggests that guided imagery is an effective treatment for BN, at least in the short-term, and promotes psychological soothing.

SUMMARY

In summary, the eating disorders have been linked to a difficulty in the ability to modulate affects or in self-soothing. This conceptualization suggests the need to design treatments that specifically target the problem of affect regulation, which assist these individuals to comfort themselves. A model of guided imagery therapy has been proposed that can be used to describe imagery as an external source of soothing, as well as a technique that enhances self-soothing. The model suggests that imagery therapy has multiple levels of action that can assist these individuals in the regulation of affect. Case reports and evidence from a randomized trial have demonstrated its effectiveness in improving eating-disorder symptomatology and in promoting self-comforting, at least in the short-term, possibly by providing patients with a transitional object.

REFERENCES

Achterberg, J. (1985). *Imagery in healing: Shamanism and modern medicine.* Boston: New Science Library, Shambhala Publications.

Achterberg, J., Lawlis, C. F. (1978). *Imagery and cancer.* Champaign, IL: Institute for Personality and Ability Testing.

Adler, G. (1979). Psychodynamic of impulsive behavior. In H. A. Wishnie & J. Nevis-Olesen (Eds.), *Working with the impulsive person* (pp. 2-17). New York: Plenum Press.

Adler, G. (1993). The psychotherapy of core borderline psychopathology. *American Journal of Psychotherapy, 47*(2), 194-204.

Adler, G., & Buie, D. (1979). Aloneness and borderline psychopathology: The possible relevance of child development issues. *International Journal of Psychoanalysis, 60,* 83-96.

Ahsen, A. (1984). ISM: The triple code model for imagery and psychophysiology. *Journal of Mental Imagery, 8*(4), 15-42.

Arntz, A. (1994). Treatment of borderline personality disorder: A challenge for cognitive-behavioral therapy. *Behavioral Research and Therapy, 32,* 419-430.

Appelbaum, A. H. (1994). Psychotherapeutic routes to structural change. *Bulletin of the Menninger Clinic, 58,* 37-54.

Baider, L., Uziely, B., & Kaplan-De-Nour, A. (1994). Progressive muscle relaxation and guided imagery in cancer patients. *General-Hospital-Psychiatry, 16*(5), 340-347.

Baker, E. L., & Nash, M. R. (1987). Application of hypnosis in the treatment of anorexia nervosa. *American Journal of Clinical Hypnosis, 29,* 185-193.

Barabasz, M. (1990). Treatment of bulimia with hypnosis involving awareness and control in clients with high dissociative capacity. *International Journal of Psychosomatics, 37*(1-4), 53-56.

Barber, T. X., Spanos, N. P., & Chaves, J. F. (1974). *Hypnosis, imagination and human potentialities.* New York: Pergamon Press.

Barth, D. F. (1994). The use of group therapy to help women with eating disorders differentiate and articulate affect. *Group, 18*(2), 67-77.

Blake, R., & Bishop, S. (1994). The Bonny Method of guided imagery and music (GIM) in the treatment of post-traumatic stress disorder (PTSD) with adults in the psychiatric setting. *Music Therapy Perspectives, 12*(2), 125-129.

Briscoe, J. (1990). Guided imagery to affect depression and self-esteem in hospitalized adolescents. *Dissertation Abstracts International, 51*(4B), 2053-2054.

Bruch, H. (1973). *Eating disorders: Anorexia, obesity and the person within.* New York: Basic Books.

Burtle V. (1976). Learning in the appositional mind: Imagery in the treatment of depression. *Dissertation Abstracts International, 36*(11B), 5781.

Butcher, H. K., & Parker, N. I. (1988). Guided imagery within Rogers' science of unitary human beings: An experimental study. *Nursing Science Quarterly, 1*(3), 103-110.

Council, J. R. (1986). Exploring the interface of personality and health: Anorexia nervosa, bulimia and hypnotic susceptibility. *Behavioral Medicine Abstracts, 7,* 165-168.

Cox, G., & Merkel, W. T. (1989). A qualitative review of psychosocial treatments for bulimia. *Journal of Nervous and Mental Disease, 177*(2), 77-84.

Cross, L. W. (1993). Body and self in feminine development: Implications for eating disorders and delicate self-mutilation. *Bulletin of the Menninger Clinic, 57*(1), 41-68.

de Groot, J., & Rodin, G. (1994). Eating disorders, female psychology and the self. *Journal of the American Academy of Psychoanalysis, 22*(2), 299-317.

Esplen, M. J., Garfinkel, P. E., & Gallop, R. (2000). Relationship between self-soothing, aloneness and evocative memory in bulimia nervosa. *International Journal of Eating Disorders, 27,* 96-100.

Esplen, M. J., Garfinkel, P. E., Olmstead, M., Gallop, R., & Kennedy, S. (1998). A randomized controlled trial of guided imagery in bulimia nervosa. *Psychological Medicine, 28,* 1347-1357.

Fairburn, C. G. (1988). The current status of the psychological treatments for bulimia nervosa. *Journal of Psychosomatic Research, 32,* 635-645.

Farrington, G. (1985). Effects of self-hypnosis audiotapes on weight loss: Relationship with ego strength, motivation, anxiety and locus of control. *Dissertation Abstracts International, 46*(6B), 2048.

Feinberg-Moss, B., & Oatley, K. (1990). Guided imagery in brief psychodynamic therapy: Outcome and process. *British Journal of Medical Psychology, 63*(2), 117-129.

Fichter, M. M., Leibl, K., Rief, W., Brunner, E., Schmidt-Auberger, S., & Engel, R. R. (1991). Fluoxetine versus placebo: A double-blind study with bulimic inpatients undergoing intensive psychotherapy. *Pharmacopsychiatry, 24,* 1-7.

Fichter, M. M., Quadflieg, N., & Rief, W. (1994). Course of multi-impulsive bulimia. *Psychological Medicine, 24,* 591-604.

Freeman, C. P., Davies, F., & Morris, J. (1990). *A randomized controlled trial of fluoxetine for bulimia nervosa.* Fourth International Conference of Eating Disorders, New York.

Garfinkel, P. E., & Goldbloom, D. S. (1993). Bulimia nervosa: A review of therapy research. *Journal of Psychotherapy Practice and Research, 2*(1), 38-50.

Garfinkel, P. E., Lin, E., Goering, P., Spegg, C., Goldblum, D. S., Kennedy, S., Kaplan, A. S., & Woodside, D. B. (1995). Bulimia nervosa in a Canadian community sample: prevalence and comparison of subgroups. *The American Journal of Psychiatry, 152,* 1052-1058.

Garfinkel, P. E., Moldofsky, H., & Garner, D. M. (1980). The heterogeneity of anorexia nervosa: Bulimia as a distinct subgroup. *Archives of General Psychiatry, 37,* 1036-1040.

Garner, D. M., Garfinkel, P. E., & O'Shaughnessy, M. (1985). The validity of the distinction between bulimia with and without anorexia nervosa. *American Journal of Psychiatry, 142,* 581-587.

Gehr, P. (1989). Guided imagery as a treatment for depression. *Dissertation Abstracts International, 50*(2-B), 746.

Geist, R. A. (1989). Self-psychological reflections on the origins of eating disorders. *Journal of the American Academy of Psychoanalysis, 17*(1), 5-27.

Glucksman, M. L. (1989). Obesity: A psychoanalytic challenge. *Journal of American Academy of Psychoanalysis, 17*(1), 131-140.

Goodsitt, A. (1985). Self-psychology and the treatment of anorexia nervosa. In D. M. Garner & P. E. Garfinkel (Eds.), *Handbook of psychotherapy for anorexia nervosa and bulimia.* New York: Guilford.

Gould, D., Weinberg, R., & Jackson, A. (1980). Mental preparation strategies, cognitions, and strength performance. *Journal of Sport Psychology, 2,* 329-339.

Green, E., & Green, A. (1977). *Beyond biofeedback.* New York: Delacorte Press.

Gross, M. (1983). Hypnosis in the therapy of anorexia hysteria. *American Journal of Clinical Hypnosis, 26,* 175-181.

Gross, M. (1986). Use of hypnosis in eating disorders. In F. E. F. Larocca (Ed.), *Eating disorders* (pp. 109-118). San Francisco: Jossey-Bass.

Gruber, B. L., Hersh, S. P., Hall, N., Waletzky, L., Kunz, J. F., Carpenter, J. K., Kverno, K. S., & Weiss, S. M. (1993). Immunological responses of breast cancer patients to behavioral interventions. *Biofeedback and Self-Regulation, 18*(1), 1-22.

Gruber, B., Hall, N., Hersh, S. P., & Dubois, P. (1988). Immune system and psychological changes in metastatic cancer patients using relaxation and guided imagery: A pilot study. *Scandinavian Journal of Behavior Therapy, 17*(1), 25-46.

Gunderson, J. G., Morris, H., & Zanarini, M. C. (1985). Transitional objects and borderline patients. In T. McGlashan (Ed.), *The Borderline: Current Empirical Research* (pp. 45-60). Washington: American Psychiatric Press Inc.

Hall, J. R., & McGill, J. C. (1986). Hypnobehavioral treatment of self-destructive behavior: Trichatillomania and bulimia in the same patient. *American Journal of Clinical Hypnosis, 29*(1), 39-45.

Hamburg, P. (1989). Bulimia: The construction of a symptom. *Journal of the American Academy of Psychoanalysis, 17*(1), 151-171.

Hammer, S. E. (1996). The effects of guided imagery through music on state and trait anxiety. *Journal of Music Therapy, 33*(1), 47-70.

Hammond, D. C., Haskins-Bartsch, C., Grant, C. W., & McGhee, M. (1988). Comparison of self-directed and tape-assisted self-hypnosis. *American Journal of Clinical Hypnosis, 31*(2), 129-137.

Heatherton, T. F., & Baumeister, R. F. (1991). Binge eating as escape from self-awareness. *Psychological Bulletin, 110*(1), 86-108.

Herkov, M. J., Greer, R. A., Blau, B. I., McGuire, J. M., & Eaker, D. (1994). Bulimia: An empirical analysis of psychodynamic theory. *Psychological Reports, 75,*51-56.

Herzog, D. B., Staley, J. E., Carmody, S., Robbins, W. M., & van der Kolk, B. A. (1993). Childhood sexual abuse in anorexia nervosa and bulimia nervosa: A pilot study. *Journal of the American Academy of Child & Adolescent Psychiatry, 32*(5), 62-92.

Holgate, R. A. (1984). Hypnosis in the treatment of bulimia nervosa: A case study. *Australian Journal of Clinical and Experimental Hypnosis, 12,* 105-112.

Horton, P. C. (1981). *Solace: The missing dimension in psychiatry.* Chicago: University of Chicago Press.

Horton, P. C. (1992). A borderline treatment dilemma: To solace or not to solace. In D. Silver & M. Rosenbluth (Eds.), *Handbook of borderline disorders* (pp. 267-290). Madison, CT: International Universities Press.

Horton, P. C., Louy, J. W., & Coppolillo, H.P. (1974). Personality disorder and transitional relatedness. *Archives of General Psychiatry, 30,* 618-622.

Hsu, L. K. G. (1990). *Eating disorders.* New York: Guilford.

Hutchinson, M. (1985). *Transforming body image: Learning to love the body you have.* California: Freedom.

Hutchinson, M. G. (1991). Imagining ourselves whole: A feminist approach to treating body image disorders. In P. Fallon, M. Katzman, & S. Wooely (Eds.), *Feminist perspectives on eating disorders* (pp. 152-168). New York: Guilford.

Jarvinen, P. J., & Gold, S. R. (1981). Imagery as an aid in reducing depression. *Journal of Clinical Psychology 37*(3), 523-529.

Johnson, C., & Connors, M. (1987). *The etiology and treatment of bulimia nervosa: A biopsychosocial perspective.* New York: Basic Books.

Johnson, C., Lewis, L., & Stuckey, M. (1982). Bulimia: A descriptive study of 316 patients. *International Journal of Eating Disorders, 2,* 3-16.

Johnson, M. (1987). *The body in the mind.* Chicago: University of Chicago Press.

Kearney-Cooke, A. (1989). Imagining ourselves whole: A feminist approach to treating body image disorders. In P. Fallon, M. Katzman, & S. Wooley (Eds.), *Feminist perspectives on eating disorders* (pp. 152-168). New York: Guilford.

Kernberg, O. F. (1975). *Borderline conditions and pathological narcissism.* New York: Jason Aronson.

Khantzian, E. J. (1978). The ego, the self and opiate addiction: Theoretical and treatment considerations. *International Review of Psycho-Analysis, 5,* 189-198.

Kirsch, I., Montgomery, G., & Sapirstein, G (1995). Hypnosis as an adjunct to cognitive-behavioral psychotherapy: A meta-analysis. *Journal of Consulting and Clinical Psychology, 63*(2), 214-220.

Leuner, H. (1978). Basic principles and therapeutic efficacy of guided affective imagery (GAD). In J. L. Singer & K. S. Pope (Eds.), *The power of human imagination* (126-166). New York: Plenum.

Lingerman, H. A. (1983). *The healing energies of music.* London: Theosophical Publishing House.

Lipsky, M. J., Kassinove, H., & Miller, N. J. (1980). Effects of rational-emotive therapy, rational role reversal, and rational-emotive imagery on emotional adjustment of community mental health center patients. *Journal of Consulting and Clinical Psychology, 48*(3), 366-374.

Manyande, A., Berg, S., Gettins, D., Stanford, C., Mazhero, S., Marks, D. F., & Salmon, P. (1995). Preoperative rehearsal of active coping imagery influences subjective and hormonal responses to abdominal surgery. *Psychosomatic Medicine, 57*(2), 177-182.

Mastenbroek, I., & McGovern, L. (1991). The effectiveness of relaxation techniques in controlling chemotherapy induced nausea: A literature review. *Australian Occupational Therapy Journal, 38*(3), 137-142.

Mills, J. K., Taricone, P. F., & Bordieri, J. E. (1990). Oral character and alcoholism. *Psychology— A Journal of Human Behavior, 27*(3), 1-6.

Mitchell, J. E. (1991). A review of the controlled trials of psychotherapy for bulimia nervosa. *Journal of Psychosomatic Research, 35*(1), 23-31.

Moleski, L. M., Ishii, M. M., & Sheikh, A. A. (1986). Imagery techniques in psychosynthesis. In A. A. Sheikh (Ed.), *Anthology of imagery techniques* (pp. 459-478). Milwaukee: American Imagery Institute.

Norden, M. J. (1995). *Beyond Prozac.* New York: HarperCollins.

Pettinati, H. M., Home, R. J., & Staats, J. M. (1982). Hypnotizability of anorexia and bulimia patients (abstract). *International Journal of Clinical Hypnosis, 30,* 332.

Pettinati, H. M., Home, R. J., & Staats, J. M. (1985). Hypnotizability of anorexia and bulimia patients. *Archives of General Psychiatry, 42,* 1014-1016.

Reardon, J. P., & Tosi, D. J. (1977). The effects of rational stage directed imagery on self-concept and reduction of psychological stress in adolescent delinquent females. *Journal of Clinical Psychology, 33*(4), 1084-1092.

Reyher, J. (1977). Spontaneous visual imagery: Implications for psychoanalysis, psychopathology, and psychotherapy. *Journal of Mental Imagery, 2,* 253-274.

Ricci, M. S. (1991). Aloneness in tenuous self-states. *Perspectives in Psychiatric Care, 27*(2), 7-11.

Richman, N. E., & Sokolove, R. L. (1992). The experience of aloneness, object representation, and evocative memory in borderline and neurotic patients. *Psychoanalytic Psychology, 9*(1), 77-91.

Rosenbluth, M., & Silver, D. (1992). The inpatient treatment of borderline personality disorder. In D. Silver & M. Rosenbluth (Eds.), *Handbook of borderline disorders* (pp. 509-532). Madison, CT: International Universities Press.

Ryan, E. D., & Simmons, J. (1983). What is learned in mental practice of motor skills: A test of the cognitive-motor hypothesis. *Journal of Sport Psychology, 5,* 419-426.

Sansone, R. A., Fine, M. A., & Mulderig, J. K. (1991). An empirical examination of soothing tactics in borderline personality disorder. *Comprehensive Psychiatry, 32*(5), 431-439.

Schmidt, U., Jiwany, A., & Treasure, J. (1993). A controlled study of alexithymia in eating disorders. *Comprehensive Psychiatry, 34,* 54-58.

Schultz, K. D. (1978). Imagery and control of depression. In J. L. Singer & K. S. Pope (Eds.), *The power of human imagination* (pp. 281-307). New York: Plenum.

Schwartz, H. (1988). *Bulimia: Psychoanalytic treatment and theory.* Madison, WI: International Universities Press.

Sheikh, A. A., & Jordan, C. S. (1983). Clinical uses of mental imagery. In A. A. Sheikh (Ed.), *Imagery: Current theory, research and application* (pp. 391-435). Milwaukee, WI: American Imagery Institute.

Shorr, J. D. (1980). Discoveries about the mind's ability to organize and find meaning in imagery. In E. Shorr, G. E. Sobel, P. Robin, & J. A. Connella (Eds.), *Imagery: Its many dimensions and applications* (pp. 25-39). New York: Plenum.

Simonton, C., Simonton, S., & Creighton, J. L. (1978). *Getting well again.* San Francisco: J. P. Tarcher.

Skovholt, T., Morgan, J., & Negron-Cunningham, H. (1989). Mental imagery in career counseling and life planning: A review of research and intervention methods. *Journal of Counseling and Development, 67*(5), 287-292.

Sohlberg, S., Norring, C., Holmgren, S., & Rosmark, B. (1989). Impulsivity and long-term prognosis of psychiatric patients with anorexia nervosa/bulimia nervosa. *Journal of Nervous and Mental Disease, 177*(5), 249-258.

Storr, A. (1989). *Solitude.* London: Flamingo.

Swift, W. J., & Letven, R. (1984). Bulimia and the basic fault: A psychoanalytic interpretation of the bingeing-vomiting syndrome. *Journal of Child Psychiatry, 23,* 1-6.

Tabin, C. J., & Tabin, J. K. (1988). Bulimia and anorexia: Understanding their gender specificity and their complex of symptoms. In H. J. Shwartz (Ed.), *Psychoanalytic treatment and theory* (pp. 173-225). Madison, CT: International Universities Press.

Torem, M. S. (1989). Ego-state hypnotherapy for dissociative eating disorders. *Hypnosis, 16,* 52-63.

Torem, M. S. (1992). The use of hypnosis with eating disorders. *Psychiatric Medicine, 10*(4), 105-118.

Troop, N. A., Schmidt, U. H., & Treasure, J. L. (1995). Feelings and fantasy in eating disorders: A factor analysis of the Toronto Alexithymia Scale. *International Journal of Eating Disorders, 18*(2), 151-157.

Vanderlinden, J., & Vandereycken, W. (1988). The use of hypnotherapy in the treatment of eating disorders. *International Journal of Eating Disorders, 7*(5), 673-679.

Vanderlinden, J., & Vandereycken, W. (1990). The use of hypnosis in the treatment of bulimia nervosa. *International Journal of Clinical and Experimental Hypnosis, 37*(2), 101-111.

Weinburger, R. (1991). Teaching the elderly stress reduction. *Journal of Gerontological Nursing, 17*(10), 23-27.

Weisberg, U., Norman, D. K., & Herzog, D. B. (1987). Personality functioning in normal weight bulimia. *International Journal of Eating Disorders, 6*(5), 615-631.

Winnicott, D. W. (1958). The capacity to be alone. *International Journal of Psychoanalysis, 39,* 416-420.

Winnicott, D. W. (1965). *The maturational processes and the facilitating environment.* London: Hogarth Press.

Winnicott, D. W. (1971). *Playing and reality.* New York: Tavistock.

Woodman, M. (1982). *Addiction to perfection: The still unravished bride.* Toronto: City Books.

Yapko, M. D. (1986). Hypnotic and strategic interventions in the treatment of anorexia nervosa. *American Journal of Clinical Hypnosis, 28*(4), 224-232.

Zachariae, R., Hansen, J. B., Andersen, M., Jinquan, T., Petersen, K. S., Simonsen, C., Zachariae, C., & Thestrup-Pedersen, K. (1994). Changes in cellular immune function after immune specific guided imagery and relaxation in high and low hypnotizable, healthy subjects. *Psychotherapy and Psychosomatics, 61*(1-2), 74-92.

Ziegler, S. G. (1987). Comparison of imagery styles and past experience in skills performance. *Perceptual and Motor Skills, 64,* 579-586.

CHAPTER 12

Use of Imagery in the Treatment of Cardiovascular Disorders[1]

JEANNE ACHTERBERG, BARBARA DOSSEY,
LESLIE KOLKMEIER, AND ANEES A. SHEIKH

> I can see you've had a change of mind,
> but what you need is a change of heart.
>   Carole King (in Schwartz & Russek, 1999, p. 77)

It has been established that the circulatory system does not consist merely of mechanical pumps and hydraulics within our body. It is influenced by our attitudes, emotions, stress, and distress. It is affected by grief and loneliness, and feelings of love and support (Achterberg, Dossey, & Kolkmeier, 1994; Rahe & Lind, 1971). Rather than being isolated from our inner feelings, the cardiovascular system is similar to a delicate instrument on which we play the melody of our emotions (Guzetta & Dossey, 1992). Consequently, it is not surpising that our cardiovascular activities are influenced by our mental images that have been shown to have a deep connection with our world of emotions (Achterberg, 1985). The first section of this chapter first very briefly reviews research dealing with the effects of mental imagery and related procedures, such as meditation, biofeedback, and hypnosis, on several cardiovascular activities. The second section presents a number of imagery techniques that clinicians have found helpful in dealing with clients faced with cardiovascular problems (Achterberg, Dossey, & Kolkmeir, 1994; Epstein, 1989). It is hoped that both health professionals and researchers will find these techniques useful in their work.

---

[1] Several parts of this chapter are reprinted here with permission from Achterberg, Dossey, & Kolkmeier (1994).

IMAGERY AND THE CARDIOVASCULAR SYSTEM: RESEARCH FINDINGS

A substantial body of empirical research has accumulated over the last 20 years which shows quite convincingly that imagery and related procedures are capable of resulting in measurable bodily changes, and they must be treated as significant factors in disease and health (Sheikh, Kunzendorf, & Sheikh, 1996). A considerable portion of this research deals with cardiovascular activities.

Many researchers have reported that heart rate, oxygen consumption, blood pressure, cholestrol levels, angina pectoris, and premature ventricular contraction can be consciously controlled through meditative experiences (Barnes, Schneider, Alexander, & Staggers, 1997; Jevning, Wallace, & Beideback, 1992; Lichstein, 1988; Norris, 1989; Ramaswami & Sheikh, 1989; Sudsuanng, Chentanez, & Veluvan, 1991; Telles, Nagarathna, & Nagendra, 1998).

In the last thirty years, several investigations have reported heart rate increases to imagined emotional and physiological arousal (Bauer & Craighead, 1979; Bell & Schwartz, 1975; Blizard, Cowings, & Miller, 1975; Boulougouris, Rabavilas, & Stefanis, 1977; Caroll, Baker, & Preston, 1979; Caroll, Marzillier, & Merian, 1982; Craig, 1968; Gottschalk, 1974; Grossberg & Wilson, 1968; Jones & Johnson, 1978, 1980; Jordan & Lenington, 1979; Lang, Kozak, Miller, Levin, & McLean, 1980; Marks & Huson, 1973; Marzillier, Carroll, & Newland, 1979; Roberts & Weerts, 1982; Schwartz, Weinberger, & Singer, 1981; Shea, 1985; Wang & Morgan, 1992; Waters & McDonald, 1973). Heart rate decreases were noted in response to relaxing images (Arabian, 1982; Bell & Schwartz, 1975; Furedy & Klajner, 1978; McCanne & Iennarella, 1980; Shea, 1985). Also, several studies have shown a positive correlation between vividness of imagery and heart rate control (Barbaur, 1981; Carroll, Baker & Preston, 1979; Grossberg & Wilson, 1968; Kunzendorf, Francis, Ward, Cohen, Cutler, Walsh, & Berenson, 1996; Lang et al., 1980). Furthermore, a combination of imagery and biofeedback seems to successfully treat various arrythmias (Engel, 1979).

Vasoconstriction and vasodilation obviously play a significant role in cardiovascular functioning. A number of studies have demonstrated that these activities can be influenced by imagining that a certain area feels colder or hotter (Dugan & Sheridan, 1976; Kunzendorf, 1981, 1984; McGuirk, Fitzgerald, Friedman, Oakley, & Salmon, 1998; Ohkuma, 1985). There is a positive correlation between the magnitude of these changes and the degree of prevalence of visual and tactile images as measured by Kunzendorf's Prevalence of Imagery Tests (Kunzendorf, 1981).

Finally, it seems that images of anger and fear raise systolic blood pressure, whereas images of anger, but not fear, raise diastolic pressure (Roberts & Weerts, 1982; Schwartz et al., 1981). Imagined exercise elevates both systolic and diastolic blood pressure (Wang & Morgan, 1992). Also, clinical research reports indicate that relaxing images lead to lasting change in both kinds of blood pressure (Ahsen, 1978; Crowther, 1983).

Future research with large samples of cardiac patients will shed further light on the relationship between imagery and cardiac functioning. It seems that a number of such studies are currently underway (Health Journeys Website). However, findings from the clinical and experimental investigation, available thus far, strongly support that we seriously start considering the applications of imagery in this arena.

IMAGERY TECHNIQUES FOR CARDIOVASCULAR DISORDERS

This section offers a number of exercises that are considered to enhance our healing and bring various cardiovascular functions to normal levels. The following scripts are expected to help us form symbolic and correct biological images of normal cardiovascular functions. It is recommended that each exercise be preceded by training in relaxation. It is suggested that the clients record their favorite relaxation exercise followed by any of the cardiac-specific scripts that follow. Ideally, one should set aside about 20 minutes several times a day to rehearse these imagery techniques.

Imagery Script: Hypertension

As your mind becomes clearer and clearer, feel it becoming more and more alert. Somewhere deep inside of you, a brilliant light begins to glow. Sense this happening. . . . The light grows brighter and more intense. . . . This is the bodymind communication center. Breathe into it. . . . Energize it with your breath. The light is powerful and penetrating, and a beam begins to grow from it. The beam shines into your body now as you prepare to lower your blood pressure.

As your breathing slows with relaxation, feel your heartbeat also slowing and becoming more comfortable. Imagine time itself slowing down as you realize you have nothing to do in this moment but enjoy your deep relaxation.

Continue now to let the air simply flow in and out of your lungs, trusting your body to regulate your breathing. . . . Allow the wisdom of your body to breathe for you. . . .

Take some time to focus on your hands and feet getting warmer. . . . Perhaps you can imagine walking slowly along a beautiful beach, carrying a picnic basket and feeling the warmth and texture of the sand against the soles of your feet. . . . You walk to a secluded portion of the soft beach and relax in the evening sun, letting yourself sink down into the warm grass at the edge of the sand. . . . Take a few moments to listen to the breeze gently blowing the blades of grass. . . . You open the basket and take out a thermos of hot tea and pour it into a rough pottery mug. . . .

Can you feel the surface of the mug as you hold it in both hands? Can you smell the fragrance of the beverage and feel the warmth soaking deep into your hands ... ?

Perhaps you choose to wander a bit farther up the beach to a beautiful rustic cabin. ... As you open the front door of the cabin, you see a welcoming fire in the fireplace, and a big reclining chair with a handmade quilt inviting you to curl up and soak in the warm glow of the fire. ... You may even be able to smell the tang of the crackling driftwood fire and feel the soft fabric of the quilt. ...

As you succeed in warming your hands and feet, you know you are dilating your blood vessels and giving your blood a larger area in which to flow. You can almost feel the relaxation of your blood vessels as your pressure comes down to healthy, normal levels, and blood flows smoothly and freely into your fingers and toes. ...

As you return your focus to your breathing, remember the last time you took your blood pressure or had it taken by someone. ... Feel the cuff inflating around your arm and the coolness of the stethoscope at your elbow. ... As you hear the hiss of air escaping from the cuff and feel the pressure decreasing, image the numbers on the gauge coming down slowly with each breath out. ... Feel the quiet joy of knowing that you have been a part of bringing your blood pressure to healthy levels. ...

Take a few slow, energizing breaths, and as you come back to full awareness of the room, know that whatever is right for you at this point in time is unfolding just as it should, and that you have done your best, regardless of the outcome. ...

Imagery Script: Lowering Your Cholesterol

As your mind becomes clearer and clearer, feel it becoming more and more alert. Somewhere deep inside of you, a brilliant light begins to glow. Sense this happening. ... The light grows brighter and more intense. ... This is the bodymind communication center. Breathe into it. ... Energize it with your breath. The light is powerful and penetrating, and a beam begins to grow from it. The beam shines into your body now as you prepare to lower your cholesterol. ...

Begin your inner journey by following the beam of light into one of your blood vessels. ... This might be an artery that is carrying blood to your heart muscle. ... or it might be a vessel taking blood down the interior of your leg, branching into smaller and smaller divisions as it travels farther from your heart. ... As you travel into the interior of the blood vessel, notice the ruby glow of the red cells and the clearer portions of the serum in which the white cells float. ... Approach the wall of the vessel, and touch the dome-shaped accumulation of sticky cholesterol that has collected over an old injury to the blood vessel wall. ... In your mind's eye, see yourself gently peeling off the layers of fatty material and handing them over to special cells that stream by. ... Like little garbage trucks, these cells cart the cholesterol to the intestine, where it joins other unneeded materials and eventually leaves the body. ... You may continue with this process until you feel you have accomplished enough. ...

As you continue your journey, you notice the small globes of cholesterol are also free-floating in the clear liquid portion of your bloodstream. . . . On closer inspection it is apparent that there are two types of cholesterol. One is a bit darker and heavier, almost jewellike; this is your high-density lipoprotein, or HDL. The other form is lighter and opaque; it is low-density lipoprotein, or LDL. . . . As you continue to relax and learn more about your internal world, you see the HDL move toward the LDL and surround it. . . . The LDL is herded toward the garbage trucks and is taken away, some of the HDL riding along as guards. . . . After a period of time, you notice that there is far less cholesterol floating by, and what is there is predominantly the higher-density type. . . .

You may now choose to travel on the beam of light to the upper right quadrant of your abdomen, to that marvelous internal factory that is your liver. . . . The liver performs many different functions, one of which is to manufacture cholesterol. You speak with your supervisor of the cholesterol division and suggest that perhaps the workers have been under too much stress. . . . They have been turning out more cholesterol than is needed, and they deserve some time off. . . . It is agreed that they will begin to work at partial speed, and that their output will be maintained at a lower, healthier level. . . .

As you come toward the end of this journey, you feel confident that you will continue to make subtle adjustments in your lifestyle, adding pleasurable forms of exercise into your routine and eating tasty, healthy foods. . . . You can feel the warmth and peace that comes with taking time out to relax, even if it is just for a few minutes each day. . . .

Take a few slow, energizing breaths, and as you come back to full awareness of the room, know that whatever is right for you at this point in time is unfolding just as it should, and that you have done your best, regardless of the outcome. . . .

Imagery Script:
Angina, Myocardial Infarction, and Heart Surgery

As your mind becomes clearer and clearer, feel it becoming more and more alert. Somewhere deep inside of you, a brilliant light begins to glow. Sense this happening. . . . The light grows brighter and more intense. . . . This is the bodymind communication center. Breathe into it. . . . Energize it with your breath. The light is powerful and penetrating, and a beam begins to grow out of it. The beam shines into your body now as you prepare to nurture and open your heart. . . .

Travel on the beam of light to your heart, and just observe it for a while. . . . As you watch your heart, clearly see all of its structures working together in a coordinated, rhythmic dance. . . . Listen to how strong your heartbeats are, and imagine running your hand along the muscular walls, feeling the strength in them. . . . If you have had a heart attack, spend some time observing the area of scar tissue, noticing how smooth and strong the scar is . . . knowing that it is getting stronger every day. . . . .See the new collateral blood vessels beginning to form . . .

bringing blood and its healing oxygen, proteins, and other substances to the healed area. . . . Each day when you exercise you help those collateral blood vesssels grow stronger. . . .[Insert the next paragraph if you have had CABG surgery.[2]]

See how the jump grafts are healing and settling into their new job of bringing nourishing, healthy blood around the areas of blockage and to the heart muscle that is "downstream." . . . You might make a short side trip to the area from which the graft vessel was taken and note the way that area is healing as well. . . .

Allow yourself a few moments to recall your imagery for handwarming, and watch in your mind's eye as the coronary arteries begin to respond just as the blood vessels in your hands do. . . . As you feel your hands warming . . . see the muscle tissue in the coronary arteries also relaxing. . . . See how they become larger and allow more blood to flow through them. . . .

Spend a few moments now seeing how you will look when your heart healing is complete. Imagine looking at yourself in a mirror or seeing yourself on a videotape: strong, straight, and healthy. Watch yourself perhaps playing with your friends, children, or grandchilden, or throwing a ball for the family dog. . . . Hear how your voice will sound when you are completely well, and hear yourself laughing out loud. . . . Feel the strength returning to your legs and lungs. . . . Feel yourself able to walk as far as you want . . . breathing easily and feeling robust and sturdy.

As you bring your imagery to an end, sense the feeling of accomplishment that comes from being actively involved with your health. . . . Make decisions about what is right for you, taking into consideration all aspecs of the needs of your body, mind, and spirit. . . .

Take a few slow, energizing breaths, and as you come back to full awareness of the room, know that whatever is right for you at this point in time is unfolding just as it should, and that you have done your best, regardless of the outcome. . . .

Imagery Script:
Arrhythmias and Mitral Valve Prolapse

As your mind becomes clearer and clearer, feel it becoming more and more alert. Somewhere deep inside of you, a brilliant light begins to glow. Sense this happening. . . . The light grows brighter and more intense. . . . This is the bodymind communication center. Breathe into it. . . . Energize it with your breath. The light is powerful and penetrating, and a beam begins to grow from it. The beam shines into your body now as you prepare to focus on a calm, regular heartbeat. . . .

Gently place your thumbs and first fingers together and allow the air to breathe in and out of you all by itself. . . . Begin to feel the pulse of your heartbeat in your

[2] For presurgery, postsurgery, and recovery scripts, see Achterberg, Dossey, and Kolkmeier (1994).

fingertips. . . . Is it possible for you to imagine that you are resting on a beautiful, warm, sandy beach? . . . Can you feel the ocean breeze on your face, and the warmth of the morning sun on your skin? . . . As you relax on the beach, you begin to notice the waves breaking softly on the sand and a line of foam washing up the damp sand to your feet . . . and then the foam bubbles sink into the sand and the wave moves back to the edge of the water. . . . .As you continue to watch the waves, notice that they are moving up the beach as you breathe in. . . . and back down the beach as you breathe out . . . in . . . and out . . . in . . . and out. . . . Continue to focus on smooth, even body rhythms. . . .

Occasionally you may feel a variation in your heartbeat as you sense it through your fingertips, or even as you become aware of a change in rate or regularity in you chest. . . . Allow a picture to come into your mind of a healthy young animal like a horse. . . . Imagine watching that strong young horse running playfully across a field. Hear the hoof beats, and see the horse running in slow motion. . . . Once in a while, as an expression of the pure joy of living, that horse simply kicks its hind feet up into the air and keeps on running, getting stronger and more beautiful every day. . . . It is sturdy, vibrant, and full of life. . . . Visualize your heart . . . sturdy . . . vibrant . . . full of life. . . . [If you have mitral valve prolapse, continue with the rest of the script.]

In your imagination, allow yourself to become very tiny and powerful, perhaps seeing yourself as a mighty magician, wizard, or even something mechanical like a computer chip . . . tiny, but with great powers. . . . Travel on that beam of light to the interior of your heart, where you can see, hear, and touch the wonderful structures that regulate blood flow . . . valves, chambers, sparkles of electrical energy. . . . As you make your way through your heart, you can reach out and stroke the muscular walls. . . . Your can tighten up any loose cords or valve leaflets. . . . You can make any changes that you know will increase the efficiency of your heart. . . . Take all the time you need to do this. . . .

Take a few slow, energizing breaths, and as you come back to full awareness of the room, know that whatever is right for you at this point in time is unfolding just as it should, and that you have done your best, regardless of the outcome. . . .

Some Other Imagery Techniques

Naparstek (1994) offers an imagery exercise for achieving general health of the endiovascular system. After relaxing the clients, she instructs them to turn their attention inward and notice the subtle sensation of their blood moving through their body, "feeling its steady warmth . . . seeing this exquisite, intricate pattern of veins and arteries," noticing the blood's exquisite intelligence and seeing it soften the "walls of the arteries as it moves along making them into more flexible enduring stuff . . . keeping the inner lining slick and smooth and shiny . . . with no place for debris to cling to it." She further asks the clients to see the blood "strengthening and replenishing the arteries' weaker spots . . . shoring up any thin places along the walls . . . bringing everything that is needed to fortify the walls . . . gently and safely eroding whatever tiny buildup that might have accumulated in the lining. . . .safely expanding each vessel, big or small . . . dissolving any matter in the blood stream itself . . . turning any beginnings of clotting into tiny microdots . . . and dispersing them, safely and easily" (pp. 101-102).

Next, Naparstek asks the clients to visualize: "A gentle, steady river, feeding the hungry tissue along its banks . . . and just sensing how the sugar and nutrients in the blood leach out into the surrounding field of tissue . . . soaked up by the hungry cells . . . in a steady, continuous supply . . . and feeling the hungry tissue respond . . . sensing the cells plump up to full strength from this steady, generous source . . . as new life and energy return . . . organ and muscle and bone rebuilding . . . as cells replace themselves . . . and the body changes up with strengthened purpose . . . remembering its power and vitality" (p. 103).

Epstein (1989) firmly believes that the heart is the seat of love and most cardiac problems involve trouble concerning love. He offers a number of imagery exercises to help heart patients:

> *The Arrows of Hurt* Unzip your chest wall. Reach in and take out your heart. Remove all the arrows of hurt and toss them away. Clean up all the sore spots where the arrows were. Gently massage the heart. Replace it back in your chest, and rezip your chest wall. Listen to your heartbeat and sense and feel the now strengthened heart muscle becoming alive. (p. 80)

> *The Cosmic Heart* Unzip your chest wall. Reach in and take out your heart. Clean it and massage it gently. Now toss the heart straight up into the cosmos and retrieve it. See the heart now as clear crystal reflecting as a prism all the colors of the rainbow. Replace this now clean and pure heart in your chest and rezip. (p. 80)

> *Gateway to Heaven* Enter your heart. There find the gateway to heaven. See what happens. Sense and feel your heart responding. (p. 80)

Brigham (1994) offers what she calls seeds for imagery to combat various cardiovascular problems. Here are a couple of examples:

1. Imagine a river of blood going through the liver to be cleansed of cholestrol and fatty acids. The liver is an immense field of ripe dandelions with each feathery seed eager to soak up as much fat as it can. Watch with pleasure as you see the blood wind through this cleansing dandelion field and leave, clarified and purified of any harmful substance. (p. 370)
2. See a laser light flooding, not only the coronary arteries, but all the arteries of the body. This laser light totally zaps the ugly, fatty buildup on the vessels—that buildup which has to make the arteries so clogged that the nutrient blood finds it difficult to reach the muscle of the heart and other cells of the body. This intelligent, powerful laser light, however, is quite friendly to healthy tissue and actually massages the walls of the artery, heals any lesions, and leaves the tissue supple and flexible. (p. 372)

This section has covered some of the imagery techniques that deal directly with heart problems. There are numerous other imagery procedures available that may be indirectly relevant. For example, techniques that help foster emotional and spiritual growth may have a significant role to play in achieving heart health (Achterberg, Dossey, & Kolkmeier, 1994; Brigham, 1994; Naparstek, 1994; Sheikh, 2002).

CONCLUDING REMARKS

The mystique of the heart has been a major part of cultural rituals for ages. Every year we celebrate St. Valentine's Day with ritual giving of symbolic hearts to our loved ones. The heart was once thought to be the "seat of the soul" and has been incorporated into our emotional language, with phrases such as "breaking my heart." It is interesting to note that recently researchers have been suggesting that the heart is more than a mere pump. It has the capacity to learn and to remember and it plays a central role in our emotions, particularly love (Ormish, 1990; Pearsall, 1998; Schwartz & Russek, 1999).

Ormish (1990, p. 3) states "I am becoming increasingly convinced that heart disease is a metaphor as well as an anatomical illness. In poetry, art, and literature, the heart is often portrayed as the organ most affected by our emotion, and I think there is some truth in that." He suspects that emotionally opening our heart to others and experiencing mutual intimacy and love, and spiritually opening our heart to a higher consciousness may have important consequences for our heart health. If that is so, then the significance of imagery in this regard is obvious.

It goes without saying that a lot more research is needed before we can confidently and expediently apply imagery techniques in our quest for heart health. However, the clinical findings and the basic research discussed in this chapter encourage us to add relaxation, imagery, and related ways of focused attention to our health routine. It may not only empower ourselves but also add potency to medication, surgical procedures, exercise routines, and heart-healthy nutrition habits.

REFERENCES

Achterberg, J. (1985). *Imagery in healing: Shamanism and modern medicine.* Boston: Shambhala.

Achterberg, J., Dossey, B., & Kolkmeier, L. (1994) *Rituals of healing: Using imagery for health and wellness.* New York: Bantam Books.

Ahsen, A. (1978). Eidetics: Neural experiential growth potential for the treatment of accident traumas, debilitating stress conditions, and chronic emotional blocking. *Journal of Mental Imagery, 2,* 1-22.

Arabian, J. M. (1982). Imagery and Pavlovian heart rate decelerative conditioning. *Psychophysiology, 19*, 286-293.

Barbour, W. P. (1981). *Vividness of mental imagery and heart rate response to imagined anxiety evoking situations.* Unpublished honors thesis, University of Western Australia.

Barnes, V., Schneider, R., Alexander, C., & Staggers, F. (1997). Stress, stress reduction, and hypertension in African Americans: An updated review. *Journal of the National Medical Association, 89,* 464-476.

Bauer, R. M., & Craighead, W. E. (1979). Psychophysiological responses to the imagination of fearful and neutral situations: The effects of imagery instructions. *Behavior Therapy, 10,* 389-403.

Bell, I. R., & Schwartz, G. E. (1975). Voluntary control and reactivity of human heart rate. *Psychophysiology, 12,* 339-348.

Blizard, D. A., Cowings, P., & Miller, N. E. (1975). Visceral responses to opposite types of autogenic-training imagery. *Biological Psychology, 3,* 49-55.

Boulougouris, J. C., Rabavilas, D. D., & Stefanis, C. (1977). Psychophysiological responses in obsessive-compulsive patients. *Behavior Research and Therapy, 15,* 221-230.

Brigham, D. D. (1994). *Imagery for getting well.* New York: Norton.

Carroll, D., Baker, J., & Preston, M. (1979). Individual differences in visual imaging and the voluntary control of heart rate. *British Journal of Psychology, 70,* 39-49.

Carroll, D., Marzillier, J. S., & Merian, S. (1982). Psychophysiological changes accompanying different types of arousing and relaxing imagery. *Psychophysiology, 19,* 75-82.

Craig, K. D. (1968). Physiological arousal as a function of imagined, vicarious, and direct stress experience. *Journal of Abnormal Psychology, 73,* 513-520.

Crowther, J. H. (1983). Stress management training and relaxation imagery in the treatment of essential hypertension. *Journal of Behavioral Medicine, 6,* 169-187.

Dugan, M., & Sheridan, C. (1976). Effects of instructed imagery on temperature of hands. *Perceptual and Motor Skills, 42,* 14.

Engel, B. T. (1979). Behavioral applications in the treatment of patients with cardiovascular disorders. In J. V. Basmajian (Ed.), *Biofeedback: Principles and practices for clinicians.* Baltimore: Williams and Wilkins.

Epstein, G. (1989). *Healing visualization: Creating health through imagery.* New York: Bantain Book.

Furedy, J. J., & Klajner, F. (1978). Imaginational Pavlovian conditioning of large-magnitude cardiac decelerations with tilt as UCS. *Psychophysiology, 15,* 538-548.

Gottschalk, L. A. (1974). Self-induced visual imagery, affect arousal, and autonomic correlates. *Psychosomatics, 15,* 166-169.

Grossberg, J. M., & Wilson, K. M. (1968). Physiological changes accompanying the visualization of fearful and neutral situations. *Journal of Personality and Social Psychology, 10,* 124-133.

Guzzetta, C., & Dossey, B. (1992). *Cardiovascular nursing: Holistic practice.* St. Louis, MO: Mosby.

Health Journeys Website: http://www.healthjourneys.com

Jevning, R., Wallace, A. F., & Beideback (1992). The physiology of meditation: A review. *Neuroscience and Behavioral Reviews, 16,* 415-424.

Jevning, R., Wilson, A. F., & Davidson, J. M. (1978). Adrenocortical activity during meditation. *Hormones and Behavior, 10,* 54-60.

Jones, G. E., & Johnson, H. J. (1978). Physiological responding during self-generated imagery of contextually complete stimuli. *Psychophysiology, 15,* 439-446.

Jones, G. E., & Johnson, H. J. (1980). Heart rate and somatic concomitants of mental imagery. *Psychophysiology, 17,* 339-347.

Jordan, C. S., & Lenington, K. T. (1979). Physiological correlates of eidetic imagery and induced anxiety. *Journal of Mental Imagery, 3,* 31-42.

Kunzendorf, R. G. (1981). Individual differences in imagery and autonomic control. *Journal of Mental Imagery, 5,* 47-60.

Kunzendorf, R. G. (1984). Centrifugal effects of eidetic imaging on flash electroretinograms and autonomic responses. *Journal of Mental Imagery, 8,* 67-76.

Kunzendorf, R. G., Francis, L., Ward, J., Cohen, R., Cutler, J., Walsh, J., & Berenson, S. (1996). Effect of negative imaging on heart rate and blood pressure, as a function of image vividness and image "realness." *Imagination, Cognition and Personality, 16,* 139-159.

Lang, P. J., Kozak, M. J., Miller, G. A., Levin, D. N., & McLean, A. (1980). Emotional imagery: Conceptual structure and pattern of somato-visceral response. *Psychophysiology, 17,* 179-192.

Lichstein, K. L. (1988). *Clinical relaxation strategies.* New York: Wiley.

Marks, I., & Huson, J. (1973). Physiological aspects of neutral and phobic imagery: Further observations. *British Journal of Psychiatry, 122,* 567-572.

Marzillier, J. S., Carroll, D., & Newland, J. R. (1979). Self-report and physiological changes accompanying repeated imaging of a phobic scene. *Behavior Research and Therapy, 17,* 71-77.

McCanne, T. R., & Iennarella, R. S. (1980). Cognitive and somatic events associated with discriminative changes in heart rate. *Psychophysiology, 17,* 18-28.

McGuirk, J., Fitzgerald, D., Friedman, P. S., Oakley, D., & Salmon, P. (1998). The effect of guided imagery in a hypnotic context on forearm blood flow. *Contemporary Hypnosis, 15,* 101-108.

Naparstek, B. (1994). *Staying well with guided imagery.* New York: Warner Books.

Norris, P. (1986). Biofeedback, voluntary control and human potential. *Biofeedback and Self-Regulation, 11,* 1-20.

Ormish, D. (1990). *Reversing heart disease.* New York: Ballantine Books.

Ohkuma, Y. (1985). Effects of evoking imagery on the control of peripheral skin temperature. *Japanese Journal of Psychiatry, 54,* 88-94.

Pearsall, P. (1998). *The heart's code.* New York: Broadway Books.

Ramaswami, S., & Sheikh, A. A. (1989). Meditation east and west. In A. A. Sheikh & K. S. Sheikh (Eds.), *Eastern and Western approaches to healing.* New York: Wiley.

Rahe, R. H., & Lind, E. (1971). Psychosocial factors and sudden cardiac death: A pilot study. *Journal of Psychosomatic Research, 15*(19).

Ribot, T. (1906). *Essay on the creative imagination* (A. H. N. Baron, Trans.). Chicago: Open Court. (Reprinted in New York by Arno Press, 1973.)

Roberts, R. J., & Weerts, T. C. (1982). Cardiovascular responding during anger and fear imagery. *Psychological Reports, 50,* 219-230.

Schwartz, G. E. R., & Russek, L. G. S. (1999). *The living energy universe.* Charlottesville, VA: Hampton Roads.

Schwartz, G. E., Weinberger, D. A., & Singer, J. A. (1981). Cardiovascular differentiation of happiness, sadness, anger, and fear following imagery and exercise. *Psychosomatic Medicine, 43,* 343-364.

Shea, J. D. (1985). Effects of absorption and instructions on heart rate control. *Journal of Mental Imagery, 9,* 87-100.

Sheikh, A. A. (2002). *Handbook of therapeutic imagery techniques.* Amityville, NY: Baywood.

Sheikh, A. A., Kunzendorf, R. G., & Sheikh, K. S. (1996). Somatic consequences of consiousness. In M. Velmons (Ed.), *The science of consciousness.* London: Routledge.

Sudsuang, R., Chentanez, V., & Veluvan, K. (1991). Effect of Buddhist meditation of serum cortisol and total protein levels, blood pressure, pulse rate, lung volume and reaction time. *Physiology and Behaivor, 50,* 543-548.

Telles, S., Nagarathna, R., & Nagendra, H. R. (1998). Autonomic changes while mentally repeating two syllables—One meaningful and the other neutral. *Indian Journal of Physiology and Pharmacology, 42,* 57-63.

Wang, Y., & Morgan, W. P. (1992). The effect of imagery perspectives on the psycho-physiological responses to imagined exercise. *Behavioral Brain Research, 52,* 167-174.

Waters, W. F., & McDonald, D. G. (1973). Autonomic response to auditory, visual, and imagined stimuli in a systematic desensitization context. *Behaviour Research and Therapy, 11,* 577-585.

CHAPTER 13

Imagery and the Treatment of Phobic Disorders

*BEVERLY H. YAHNKE, ANEES A. SHEIKH,
AND HEIDI T. BECKMAN*

> Nothing is so much to be feared as fear.
> Henry D. Thoreau (in Peter, 1977, p. 189)

Although semanticists may be reluctant to renounce their allegiance to Whorf's hypothesis (1956), overwhelming evidence exists to dispute the notion that language is the limit of one's world. Imagistic thought integrates and processes experience. It also prompts new solutions to problems that eluded prior lexical resolution. Currently, imagistic thought is regarded to be equal in importance to man's enactive and lexical modalities (Singer & Pope, 1978). Hence, despite Watson's (1913) efforts to purge empirical inquiry of all things cognitive, imagery is enjoying an experimental, theoretical, and clinical resurrection (Sheikh, 1977; Sheikh & Panagiotou, 1975).

A diversity of psychotherapeutic techniques which use imagery prominently have become well-accepted and have served to prompt new clinical uses of imagery. Cohen (1981) observes that therapeutic ingenuity is seen perhaps with the greatest frequency in the clinical treatment of phobic disorders. Therefore, it is not surprising that the power of human imagination has been used differentially by a wide range of therapists to relieve the anxiety or fears of their phobic patients.

THE FRIGHTENING PROPERTIES OF FEAR

Fear is acknowledged universally as one of man's primary motivating drives. Although fear often serves an essential function to protect the individual and preserve the species, it has an equally powerful potential to disrupt or destroy the quality of its victims' lives.

The ultimately debilitating dimensions of fear are illustrated dramatically in Huyghe's (1982) account:

In the 1930's one celebrated doctor in India demonstrated the power of the mind and imagination in an astonishing and deadly experiment he performed on a criminal who had been condemned to death. The doctor wanted to learn whether the human imagination could kill. The convict was an assassin of distinguished rank and court permission had been obtained to bleed him to death inside the prison so that his family might be spared the disgrace of a public hanging. When the time came, the condemned man was blindfolded, led into a room, and strapped to a table. Under it a container was set up to drip water gently into a basin on the floor. The doctor pricked the skin of the man's arms and legs near his veins as if to bleed him and at the same time started the water dripping. The convict believed that the dripping he heard was his blood flowing out, and when the sound of the dripping water at length stopped, he passed out and died—without actually losing one drop of blood. (p. 20)

Hence, one deduces that fear is a formidable adversary, whether the danger is real or whether it is imaginary.

THE NATURE OF PHOBIC DISORDERS

Errera (1962) provides a historical perspective, noting that the term "phobia" is derived from the name of the Greek god, Phobos, who had the ability to terrorize the enemy. Nearly 2,000 years ago, Celsus first used the term "hydrophobia" to describe the primary symptoms of rabies. In Western Europe, until the 17th century, the treatment of phobias, regarded either as demon-phobias or theophobias, was relegated exclusively to theologians and philosophers. It was not until 1801 that the word "phobia" appeared as a generic term in the psychiatric literature. From that point forward, voluminous amounts of material documenting a wide spectrum of unreasonable fears have accumulated. Most of the early descriptions of patients' symptoms, the frequency of their occurrence, and the nature of the fears are consonant with today's clinical observations.

The Epidemiologic Catchment Area Program of the National Institute of Mental Health (Regier et al., 1984) was developed to gather uniform data on the epidemiology of specific disorders as defined by the *Diagnostic and Statistical Manual of Mental Disorders, Third Edition (DSM-III;* American Psychiatric Association, 1980). The data from this program suggested that the anxiety disorders show a lifetime prevalence rate of 14.6 percent. Within the anxiety disorders, specific phobias were most common, with a lifetime prevalence rate of 12.5 percent (Regier et al., 1988). There were significantly higher rates of anxiety disorders in female participants than in male participants. According to the most recent edition of the diagnostic manual (*DSM-IV;* American Psychiatric Association, 1994), phobic disorders fall into one of three major categories.

Agoraphobia is typified by a fear of being in places or situations where escape would be difficult or help would be unavailable. Often, this fear develops after a person has experienced an unexpected or situationally-predisposed panic attack. A typical consequence of this fear is the avoidance of being alone or the avoidance of crowded settings, such as theaters, stores, or public transportation. Agoraphobia, more frequently found among women, may progressively delimit normal activities. In the most severe occurrences of this illness, individuals may choose to remain housebound rather than to confront external, anxiety-producing situations.

Social phobias constitute the second category, the rarest of the three major phobic disorders. The prominent characteristic of this phobia is an irrational fear of being vulnerable to the scrutiny of others. Individuals will avoid those situations wherein others are likely to observe them behaving in an embarrassing fashion. Another dimension of the disorder is the fear that others will notice the anxiety. Although the individuals reason that the fear response is inappropriate, they nevertheless change their lifestyle in order to avoid the phobic situation. Some of the more frequently diagnosed social phobias include eating in public, using public lavatories, public speaking, or writing in a situation where others might observe hand tremors.

Specific phobias comprise the third category and are the most common ones. A specific phobia is evidenced by an irrational fear and avoidance of a particular stimulus object or situation (exclusive of situations defined above). The level of impairment is dependent upon the degree of proximity to the phobic stimulus and the degree to which escape from the phobic stimulus is limited. Anticipatory anxiety is a central feature of this phobic syndrome. Specific animal phobias (fear of rats, dogs, and insects), as well as fear of heights and small places, are among the most common of the specific phobias.

There are numerous discrete phobias, yet all share five basic characteristics. Phobias: 1) are persistent, pervasive, and beyond voluntary control; 2) are irrational in that the fear reaction is clearly out of proportion to any actual threat; 3) are recognized by the phobic individual to be irrational and excessive; 4) lead to an overwhelming desire for escape or avoidance; and 5) cause significant impairment or limitation in the person's life functioning (Kleinknecht, 1991).

ACQUISITION OF PHOBIAS

Early theorists claimed that phobic behavior was the result of maladaptive remnants of ancestral experience (Hall, 1897) or evidence of the nervous system's degeneration (Kraeplin, 1903; Oppenheim, 1911). Marks (1975) acknowledged that fear of certain stimuli is evident at birth, independent of experience. An infant's startle reflex occurs commonly in response to novel, unexpected, or powerful stimuli. Marks suggests that the child's experience influences the manifestation of this innate fear response; that is, learning often diminishes its impact. That innate fear mechanism, however, provides a predisposition for the formation of phobias. Empirical evidence for a genetic basis of phobias comes from: 1) twin studies; and 2) studies suggesting that infants who, during their first two years of life, show strong right frontal brain activity in response to unfamiliar stimuli are more likely to be fearful and inhibited later in their lives (Meyer & Deitsch, 1996).

The paradigm provided by learning theory affords the most precise explanation of the acquisition of specific phobias. Summarized briefly, avoidance behavior is motivated by a classically conditioned fear; the avoidance behavior helps to reduce the level of fear, and it simultaneously becomes a negative reinforcement, strengthening the avoidance behavior (Mowrer, 1960; Rachman, 1968; Wolpe, 1958). From this perspective, neurotic symptoms may be understood as maladaptive habits that have been learned (Eysenck & Rachman, 1965). Variations on the simple learning paradigm include vicarious conditioning of a phobia (observing a model's response to noxious stimuli) and informational transmission of a phobia (being warned repeatedly by significant others about the dangers of certain objects or situations) (Craske & Rowe, 1997). The learning theory paradigm *cannot* explain the more gradual acquisition of a phobia, particularly those instances when a patient is unable to recall a single traumatic event to which he or she can date the onset of the phobia (Butler, 1989). Nor has learning theory explained those cases when abreaction recalls the generative trauma to awareness and relieves the patient of phobic symptoms (Marks, 1975).

Cognitive models of phobia acquisition have become prominent in recent years, probably due to the "cognitive revolution" in psychology. Most cognitive models suggest that phobic individuals have developed characteristic patterns of thinking that reflect perceptions of harm or danger, and these interpretations then generate anxiety. For example, phobic individuals tend to overestimate the dangerousness of the feared stimulus or situation, and they engage in catastrophic thinking when confronted with it. At the same time, they underestimate their ability to cope with the feared situation. Misattribution of the common symptoms of physiological arousal, obsessional focus on distress, and catastrophic thoughts can maintain the avoidance that is prominent in phobic disorders (Butler, 1989; Craske & Rowe, 1997; Lindemann, 1994).

The psychodynamic interpretation of phobia relies upon the controversial constructs of repression and displacement to explain the origin of the fear reaction (Brehony & Geller, 1981). Psychoanalytic theory presumes that the presence of a phobia prevents the patient from understanding the true unconscious source of his or her anxiety. That is, the phobia is regarded as a set of symbols in which the genuine source of fear remains hidden from the conscious mind.

Recent research suggests that different etiological mechanisms may underlie different phobias. While some phobias may be acquired through conditioning, the development of other phobias may be linked with dispositional factors such as increased disgust sensitivity. This discovery has led to the development of treatment packages that are tailored to the unique etiological profiles of patients' phobias (Davey, 1997).

Personality Characteristics of Phobic Individuals

Most phobias appear to be much more common among women than among men. Specific Phobias of the Natural Environment Type (e.g., height phobia), the Animal Type, and the Blood-Injection-Injury type tend to begin primarily in childhood. Age at onset for Specific Phobia, Situational Type is bimodally distributed, with a peak in childhood and a second peak in the mid-20s. Social Phobia typically has an onset in the mid-teens. Agoraphobia is often related to Panic Disorder, for which the typical age of onset is between late adolescence and the mid-30s (American Psychiatric Association, 1994). There are several personality characteristics associated with phobic people:

1. Generally, they have been, since childhood, hyperreactive to a variety of stimuli, expressing their emotions in an excessive manner.
2. Already as youngsters, they have been obsessional and perfectionistic. They carry out a task either perfectly or terribly, never passably.
3. From an early age, they generally have found it difficult to cope with the unpleasant facets of life, such as suffering and death. Although they seldom are overcome by the events of the present, they suffer acutely from fears of what the future may hold.
4. Since future thinking is an essential ingredient of intelligence, it is not surprising to find that most phobic people are intelligent.
5. They are keenly sensitive to their own feelings and also to those of others, and they assume that others are equally aware. Often phobic people suffer because they feel that they have made a fool of themselves, while others did not even notice anything unusual in their behavior. Related to phobic persons' keen awareness of others is their strong need to please others and also their overwhelming concern with avoiding embarrassment (DuPont, 1982).

Seeking Treatment for Phobias

Individuals suffering from specific phobias rarely seek treatment because they suffer no serious impairment in the management of their daily lives. Yet, experimental groups frequently include volunteers with specific phobias for purposes of research. Social phobias are uncommon in clinical practice, while agoraphobia is treated with the greatest frequency (Chapman, 1997). Cohen (1981) observes that individuals seeking treatment often suffer from a variety of emotional disorders, of which phobic anxiety is only one component.

Paul and Bernstein (1979) have identified five prominent reasons why individuals suffering from phobia are motivated to seek treatment: 1) they experience frequent or extreme distress as the result of irrational fear; 2) the physiological response to anxiety prompts psychophysiological disorders, such as peptic ulcers, migraine headaches, or high blood pressure; 3) anxiety interferes with efficient cognitive and/or motor functioning; 4) the severity of the inhibitory behavior reduces nearly all external reinforcement, resulting in depressive reactions; or, 5) individuals have adopted bizarre or socially unacceptable avoidance behaviors to reduce their anxiety reactions.

A phobia, then, refers to an intricate network of affective, cognitive, behavioral, and physiological reactions that is elicited by the phobic situation or object. Given the complexity of the symptoms' configuration, it is understandable that a variety of treatment techniques have been proven to be effective. Research has been inconsistent in demonstrating the superiority of one treatment technique over others. There have been numerous studies supporting the idea of matching individual response profiles to complementary treatments (e.g., desensitization for classically conditioned fears, applied relaxation training for clients who exhibit a strong physiological fear response, cognitive treatment for fears generated by cognitive distortions, etc.), but a review article suggests that this line of research has been plagued by methodological problems (Menzies, 1996). The author argues that clinicians should not use response profile treatment matching at the expense of well-established treatment procedures.

CHARACTERISTICS OF IMAGERY PERTINENT TO TREATMENT OF PHOBIC DISORDERS

As suggested earlier, imagery is a universal human phenomenon that allows individuals to adapt to their experience in an autonomous fashion (Shorr, 1974). Imagery has progressively supplanted verbal, diagnostic, and therapeutic procedures in the treatment of phobic disorders. The superiority of imagistic thought to verbal processing has been documented in a variety of dimensions.

Imagery as Access to Right Hemispheric Functioning

Little doubt remains that the left hemisphere of the brain processes information differently than does the right hemisphere (Gazzaniga, 1970; Gazzaniga & Ledoux, 1978; Ornstein, 1972). The left hemisphere functions in a logical, linear, and semantic mode, while the right hemisphere processes information holistically, simultaneously, and spatially.

Therapeutic intervention is most commonly directed at right-hemisphere consciousness, whether the therapist is grounded in psychoanalytic, gestalt-experiential, or behavioral theory (Ley, 1979). The right hemisphere, for example, processes autonomic sensations from one's own body (Davidson & Schwartz, 1976). Furthermore, the right hemisphere is responsible for processing emotionally laden stimuli (Morrow, Vrtunski, Kim, & Boller, 1981). Perhaps of greatest importance to this discussion is the fact that the use and control of imagery is associated closely with right-hemisphere functioning (Paivio, 1971; Singer, 1974). Galin (1974) has claimed that the right hemisphere is responsible for the control of unconscious processes that affect normal behavior. Singer (1979) stresses the crucial role of right-hemisphere functioning in therapeutic settings:

> The specific events of our life, the scenes witnessed, the early childhood fantasies associated with terrors and experiences of the uncanny often have not been classified under some general category and labeled verbally. Thus, they cannot easily be retrieved on demand and may influence us without our ability to connect their occurrence with particular verbal systems. (p. 33)

Successful therapy with a phobic patient depends upon change of autonomic and affective behavior in the presence of a phobic situation or object. Inasmuch as imagery, affect, and autonomic control are right-hemisphere functions, an imagistic therapy allows for a type of processing not readily available to verbal approaches (Horowitz, 1968). Imagery, consequently, is often interpreted as the language of the unconscious (Desoille, 1965; Leuner, 1969).

Imagistic Thought Vivifies Recreation of Immediate Experience

It has been pointed out that words are not equivalent to experience; rather, words may be used to obfuscate experience or simply abstract from experience to facilitate one's communication with another (Singer, 1979). Conversely, the use of mental imagery allows the patient to plunge fully into the therapeutic experience.

If the therapist desires to create within the patient an autonomic and affective response, a mental picture of the phobic stimulus will prove to be as effective as the real phobic stimulus would be (May & Johnson, 1973; VanEgeren, Feather, & Hein, 1971). Mental pictures and physical objects are scanned and rotated in an identical fashion (Cooper & Shepard, 1978; Kosslyn, 1976; Kosslyn, Ball, & Reiser, 1978). This functional equivalence between imagery and actual stimuli is crucial to the understanding of imagery's capacity to create therapeutic change (Panagiotou & Sheikh, 1977).

Not only does imagery allow for the guided or spontaneous creation of experience, it also facilitates vivid storage and recall of significant events. When the patient has a mental image available for repeated reference, he or she speculates less, concentrates better, and is more likely to maintain an intense affective response (Singer, 1979). The visual experience is simultaneous, like the real experience, and mental images elicit a depth of emotion with greater ease than does a verbally censored recital of affect.

BEHAVIORIST AND COGNITIVE USES OF IMAGERY

Systematic Desensitization

A critical feature of desensitization therapy, as adopted first by Salter (1949) and popularized by Wolpe (1958, 1969), is the patient's reliance upon imagery rather than upon the phobic object. The technique, grounded in the classical conditioning paradigm, rests on the assumption that if a "response inhibitory of anxiety can be made to occur in the presence of anxiety-evoking stimuli it will weaken the bond between these stimuli and anxiety" (1969, p. 14). The goal of therapy is the treatment of symptomatic behavior through reciprocal inhibition.

Deep muscle relaxation training is the preliminary goal in this therapy. The need for relaxation rests upon the premise that the autonomic and muscular response of imagining a phobic stimulus is similar to the effect produced by the real phobic stimulus. Consequently, reciprocal inhibition which succeeds in imagery will transfer and influence autonomic responses in the presence of the actual phobic stimulus (Matthews, 1971).

Typically, training involves some variation of Jacobsen's progressive relaxation exercises, tensing and relaxing muscle groups in response to verbal instruction (Jacobsen, 1938). Relaxation also may be induced imagistically with Schultz and Luth's (1959) autogenic training procedure. The therapist asks the patient to visualize a particular part of his or her body, to see its shape, color, and texture vividly, as he or she simultaneously relaxes the real musculature.

Alternate means of facilitating or supplementing relaxation include administration of drugs, such as antidepressants, benzodiazepines, nonbenzodiazepine anxiolytics (e.g., Buspar), or beta-blockers (Pies, 1998). Antidepressants may work by making the individual less sensitive to aversive stimuli (Kramer, 1993). This may allow the individual to tolerate exposure to the phobic object or situation, thus permitting him or her to learn a more adaptive response. The beta-blockers are believed to block the physical symptoms of anxiety that can interfere with motor tasks or contribute to the escalation of performance anxiety (Hayward & Wardle, 1997).

Relaxation also may be induced through hypnotic suggestion. Phobics have demonstrated a relatively high hypnotic responsivity and an "unusual capacity for imagery vividness, focused attention, and flexibility in information-processing strategies" (Crawford & Barabasz, 1993, p. 311).

Another prominent means of assisting relaxation are biofeedback processes. The physiological correlates of anxiety are well known and easily measured (Van Egeren, 1971). Using feedback displays based on electrical activity of striated muscles (EMG), of the skin (GSR), or of the brain (EEG), the therapist and patient are able to assess the level of anxiety or relaxation present (Werbach, 1977). Biofeedback procedures are particularly useful in helping the patient to identify and control the internal cues that are most effective in creating a relaxation response. The technique is consonant with Wolpe's objective that systematic desensitization modify both behavioral and autonomic fear responses. In fact, Wolpe was one of the early behaviorists to use biofeedback with desensitization treatment (1958). A review of studies, however, indicates that biofeedback does not significantly enhance or retard the effectiveness of systematic desensitization (Rickles, Onoda, & Doyle, 1982).

The creation of a hierarchy is the next major component of desensitization therapy. The patient is encouraged to describe precisely the phobic stimulus. The therapist and the patient work together to identify the smallest details of the phobic stimulus as well as the variety of settings in which it may occur. The patient then translates the phobic situation into a variety of visual images, and they are labeled for convenient referencing. Those visual images then are arranged hierarchically. The image eliciting the least anxiety is presented to the patient first, and it is followed by images that elicit progressively greater anxiety. Although some therapists prefer to use carefully constructed personal hierarchies, standardized hierarchies using common images for all individuals with the same simple phobia (e.g., fear of snakes or insects) have been found equally effective and less time consuming (Emery & Krumboltz, 1967; McGlynn, 1971).

In the final step of the desensitization process, *the hierarchy is presented* to the patient. The patient is asked to relax, and then the therapist determines, either by electronic measures or by visual detection of body stillness, of breathing pattern, and of muscle tension, if the patient is prepared. Upon reaching relaxation, the patient is asked to visualize as vividly as possible the least anxiety-producing image of the hierarchy, while remaining fully relaxed. If the patient experiences any anxiety, he or she signals the therapist and is instructed to stop visualizing and to return to full relaxation. Each image in the hierarchy must be visualized without anxiety before the next image is attempted.

Wolpe's desensitization procedure is a theoretical nucleus around which divergent techniques have massed. Desensitization, which was envisioned initially as a one-to-one treatment, was first used in group therapy by Lazarus (1961). The use of self-administered procedures was reported in 1967 by Mingler and Wolpe, and soon a variety of self-teaching kits and manuals appeared on the market.

At no point in the desensitization procedure is the therapist concerned with the nature of the imagery used by the client. No effort is made to investigate the symbolism or the underlying etiology of the phobia. Wolpe is emphatic in his disregard of patients' "dynamic" ideas or attempts to interpret symbolism present in their spontaneous imagery. Wolpe remarked in regard to a client, "Even if she has got hold of some 'dynamic' ideas, since I can't see any use for them, I'm certainly not going to encourage them" (1976, p. 144).

Efficacy of desensitization treatment for many phobic disorders is claimed widely. In fact, in their review of empirically validated therapies, the American Psychological Association's Division 12 (Clinical Psychology) Task Force on Promotion and Dissemination of Psychological Procedures listed systematic desensitization as an example of a well-established, empirically-supported psychological intervention for specific phobias (Chambless et al., 1996). However, there is considerably less consensus in explaining how features of the treatment process ultimately result in anxiety reduction.

> This phenomenon of response decrement could equally well be labeled adaptation, habituation, extinction, inhibition, satiation, exhaustion, boredom, coping, or merely getting used to it. Our learned labels won't get us far until we define more precisely those conditions which decide whether exposure will lead to the response decrement usually seen in therapy, or instead to the response increment seen during acquisition and incubation. We are empirically able to treat most phobias and ritualizers by exposure methods without knowing how exposure works. (Marks, 1982, p. 74)

Despite Wolpe's preference for a learning or cognitive theoretical framework, the fundamental mechanism in his procedure is the vivid imagining of anxiety-producing scenes (Singer, 1974; Wilkins, 1971).

Most of the articles on systematic desensitization have examined whether imaginal exposure to the feared stimulus is as powerful as *in vivo* exposure. Although one evaluative review of 24 published, empirical studies found better experimental support for direct exposure than for imaginal exposure methods (Jansson & Oest, 1982), a different review highlighted some studies that do not support this conclusion (James, 1985). James suggested that "the two processes, imaginal and *in vivo* exposure, may be so inextricably confounded that they defy attempts to clearly delineate their respective influence" (1985, p. 133). Martin and Williams (1990) reasoned that because direct exposure to the feared stimulus is not a necessary prerequisite to phobia acquisition, it is not a prerequisite to anxiety reduction, either.

McLemore (1972) hypothesized that the patient's skill in manipulating imagery and treatment effectiveness were likely to be related. Wolpe (1976) acknowledged that approximately 15 percent of all subjects are unable to experience anxiety in response to an imagined stimulus and, thus, are unable to benefit from desensitization. In an investigation of imaging vividness, Dyckman and Cowan (1978) found imaging ability to be directly related to the success of desensitization. They determined that although pretherapy measures of vividness are probably of limited value in predicting therapy outcome, they are useful in identifying very low imagers who then can be marked for *in vivo* treatment. Their investigation did confirm that imaging vividness during therapy correlated highly with symptom abatement.

Emotive Imagery

Whereas some patients have difficulty in projecting images, others are likely to experience difficulty in achieving a state of relaxation, perhaps due to a feeling of increased vulnerability, a fear of losing control (where control means remaining tense and vigilant), or a fear of being trapped (e.g., feeling confined or restricted in thoughts, feelings, or actions) (Wilson, 1996). Still others, particularly children, are unable to follow sequential instructions. In such instances, the use of emotive imagery for counterconditioning anxiety is successful (Cornwall, Spence, & Schotte, 1996; King, Molloy, Heyne, Murphy, & Ollendick, 1998; Lazarus & Abramovitz, 1962).

Guidelines for the usage of emotive imagery with children have been proposed by Rosentiel and Scott (1977). They suggest that to inhibit anxiety, emotive images can be offered to the child's imagination, but these images should be tailored to fit the experience and understanding of the child. They recommend incorporating fantasy-mediated imagery, already used by Lazarus (1961). The child's most potent fantasies and cognitions, often descriptive of his or her heroes and wish fulfillment, are valuable tools. The therapist should be familiar with them, so that he or she can, for example, direct the child to call upon special heroes to help combat anxiety. Finally, Rosentiel and Scott (1977) advise that the therapist should rely on the child's nonverbal cues to supplement verbal reports.

Hence, emotive imagery often relies upon idiosyncratic and perhaps bizarre creations of the patient's imagination. The objective of evoking such imagery is to create a flood of positive feelings to counter the patient's feelings of anxiety. As in systematic desensitization, the therapist is not interested in any symbolic or diagnostic features that may be present in the patient's imagery.

King et al. (1998) considered whether enough empirical support exists for the emotive imagery treatment of childhood phobias in order to classify it as an empirically-validated intervention. They summarized the results of numerous case reports, a study that employed a multiple baseline across-subjects design, and a study that described a randomized clinical trial. All of these studies supported the effectiveness of emotive imagery. They also summarized a study that found emotive imagery to receive high acceptability ratings from students, parents, and professionals (King & Gullone, 1990). Their overall conclusion was that emotive imagery appears to be a useful treatment procedure, but more research is needed before it can be classified as "well-established." They added that a number of methodological issues need to be considered: 1) there have been no controlled trials of emotive imagery with phobias *other* than darkness phobia; 2) prior studies have not used attention-placebo controls to rule out the possibility of phobia reduction due to nonspecific factors; and 3) the long-term efficacy of emotive imagery has not been examined in controlled evaluations.

Covert Reinforcement

Some therapists prefer to work with operant shaping techniques. The framework of such procedures resembles that of systematic desensitization. The operant technique, however, provides the patient with a systematic reward for approaching the feared situation. That is, when the patient has imagined an approach behavior, he or she is then instructed to imagine a very pleasant contingent situation (Crowe, Marks, Agras, & Leitenberg, 1972).

Cautela (1970) has used covert reinforcement successfully to direct patients' approach behavior in a wide range of phobias. This technique is based upon the premise that imaginal stimuli and responses and overt stimuli and responses can be manipulated in an analogous fashion. Consequently, in covert reinforcement, Cautela instructs the patient to associate, in imagination, mental pictures of confronting the phobic situation with images of pleasurable situations. Cautela does not employ relaxation training in his technique, nor does he construct a hierarchy of progressively more threatening images. Instead, the therapist defines the logical sequence of approach responses needed to behave adaptively.

An example of Cautela's therapeutic process involves a capable doctoral student complaining of intense test anxiety and inability to concentrate while studying. After failing his qualifying exams, the student sought treatment. He was instructed to identify a reinforcing image (he chose the image of skiing with exhilaration) and to practice calling that image to mind. The therapist then began:

> Close your eyes and try to relax. I want you to imagine you are sitting down to study and you feel fine. You are confident and you are relaxed. I know you may be anxious here but try to imagine that when you are about to study you are calm and relaxed, as if you were acting a part. Start. (When the S raises his finger, the therapist delivers the word "Reinforcement," which in this case signals the image of skiing down a mountain feeling exhilarated.) Practice this twice a day and just before you study. Now let's work on the examination situation. It is the day of the examination and you feel confident. ("Reinforcement.") You are entering the building in which the exam is going to be given. ("Reinforcement.") You remember that in all these scenes you are trying to feel confident. Now you enter the building and go into the classroom. ("Reinforcement.") You sit down and kid around with another student who is taking the exam. ("Reinforcement.") The proctor comes in with the exam. You feel good; you know you are ready. ("Reinforcement.") The proctor hands out the exam. ("Reinforcement.") You read the questions and you feel you can answer all of them. ("Reinforcement.") Now let's do that again. This time you look the questions over and you are not sure about one question, but you say, "Oh well, I can still pass the exam if I flunk this one question." ("Reinforcement.") All right, this time you look over the exam, and you can see two questions about which you are in doubt, and you say, "Well, I can still pass this exam if I take my time and relax." ("Reinforcement."). (Cautela, 1970, p. 37)

The student passed his doctoral examination after ten sessions, and he reported that he had felt confident and relaxed while taking it.

The efficacy of covert reinforcement procedures for the treatment of anxiety-based problems has been established (Cautela & Kearney, 1986). Covert conditioning has been shown to be useful as an auxiliary method in behavioral treatment programs (Ascher, 1993). Also, it has been adapted for use with very young children (Cautela, 1993).

Implosive Therapy

Implosive therapy, developed by Stampfl (1961), may be regarded as material evidence for the contention that imagery is a crucial element of change in desensitization. In implosive therapy, or flooding, relaxation is not utilized (Voode & Gilner, 1971). In fact, in imagination, the patient evokes and confronts the fear-arousing stimulus without the possibility of escape, thereby extinguishing the avoidance response to that stimulus.

The mental usage of intense fear stimuli may be understood within the learning theory paradigm, which holds that neurotic behavior is comprised of learned and sustained avoidance responses which decrease anxiety (Harper, 1975). The patient is asked to imagine circumstances involving the phobic object which create the greatest degree of tension and discomfort. Typically, the anxiety produced by the stimulus image exceeds the anxiety that would be confronted in the real-life situation. For example, a client with a fear of insects may visualize an attack by a 6-foot wasp whose buzz resonates throughout the room. The therapist instructs the patient to surrender to the imagery, to focus carefully on the selected scene without seeking escape from the rush of anxious feelings by adopting a less threatening image. Ultimately, that patient experiences no primary reinforcement (real aversive consequences), and anxiety decrements are often followed by extinction.

The therapeutic effectiveness of flooding also could be explained as the reduction of fear by an unusual form of abreaction (Boulougouris, Marks, & Marset, 1971). It is not uncommon for psychiatric symptoms to remit as the patient experiences heightened affect. Therapists who adopt this understanding of Stampfl's technique are likely to introduce into the patient's imagery material that they suspect has been repressed. Sheikh and Panagiotou (1975) observe that the precise mechanism accounting for change also could be attributed to nonconscious transformations or personal defenses due to the likelihood of symbolic content in the image. Although some patients are able to acquire insight as a result of undergoing implosion, insight is not considered to be an essential objective of treatment.

An important dimension of implosion therapy is the length of time the patient remains exposed to the imagined fear stimulus. Continuous exposure during flooding has garnered more support than distributed exposure (Stern & Marks, 1973). In a literature review, Levis and Hare (1977) found that flooding for at least 100-minute intervals is characteristically found in reports of successful implosion therapy. One might reason that short and distributed exposure trials interrupt the intensity of the patient's imagery and subsequently interfere with his or her therapeutic immersion into affect (Foa & Chambless, 1978).

The relative efficacy of implosion as compared to desensitization is uncertain. Mealiea and Nawas (1971), working with snake phobia patients, concluded that implosive therapy should be used only if desensitization techniques have been unsuccessful. They found that patients treated with flooding were at greater risk of relapse than were the desensitized patients. Nevertheless, in a different study, flooding was found to be significantly superior to desensitization on GSR measures during phobic imagery, on patients' subjective assessment of anxiety, and on therapists' ratings of patients (Boulougouris et al., 1971).

Wanderer and Ingram (1990) reported that implosion therapy could be enhanced by the introduction of physiological monitoring of emotional arousal. Physiological monitoring may help ensure that patients reach a maximal level of emotional arousal during an implosion session, that their arousal level is reduced by the end of the session, and that they can receive feedback about any small improvements in their phobic symptomatology. In addition, physiological monitoring may help the clinician to pinpoint cues to clients' phobic anxiety, or it may result in beneficial placebo effects.

Covert Modeling

Bandura's theoretical and experimental work (1968, 1970, 1971, 1979; Bandura & Barab, 1973) has demonstrated convincingly that "virtually all learning phenomena that result from direct experiences can occur vicariously as a function of observing other people's behavior and its consequences for them" (1979, p. 426). In Bandura's system, phobic patients repeatedly observe models completing tasks deemed fear provoking. The models provide the phobics with repeated performance trials that are not followed by aversive consequences. The modeling may be conducted either through *in vivo* methods or *in vitro,* using pictures, slides, films, or videotapes.

Covert modeling, as discussed in Cautela's work (1970, 1972, 1976; Cautela, Flannery, & Hanley, 1974; Cautela & McCullough, 1978; Upper & Cautela, 1979), has its origin in Bandura's assumptions concerning the efficacy of vicarious conditioning. Cautela's procedure was developed to assist those patients who reported difficulty imagining themselves interacting with the phobic stimuli. Cautela discovered that these phobics were, nevertheless, able to imagine vividly a surrogate performing the fear-provoking task.

The patient is encouraged to incorporate as many sensory modalities as possible when he or she imagines the scene suggested by the therapist. Also, the therapist may suggest that the patient imagine multiple models to reduce avoidance behavior, such as coping models and mastery models (Kazdin, 1973). The use of coping models, who are depicted as anxious at the outset but fearless by the end of the scene, leads to greater avoidance reduction than the use of mastery models who perform confidently and without fear throughout the imagined scene. Kazdin has observed that the greater the degree of similarity between the patient and the imagined model, the greater the degree of patient imitation and of reduction of anxiety.

Cautela (1976) advises that in order to determine the feelings evoked during a scene, the therapist must rely upon the patient's feedback: the vividness of the scene and the rate at which the scene is presented. The therapist may need to shape the patient's imagery if it begins to reflect negative outcomes (Cautela & McCullough, 1978). Ultimately, covert modeling is as effective as overt modeling in reducing avoidance behavior (Cautela et al., 1974). There is some evidence that individuals who typically use imagery to cope with fear may benefit more from covert modeling than from more verbal treatment modalities, such as self-instructional training (Vallis & Bucher, 1986).

Mariner found that self-modeling is particularly helpful in assisting a patient who becomes fixed at some point in the desensitization hierarchy (Mariner, 1969). When this occurs, Mariner instructs the patient to visualize himself or herself as a character in a filmstrip. The patient assumes the identity of a "disembodied observer" and visualizes a caricature of himself or herself performing the next scene in the hierarchy; thus, the patient's anxiety is much attenuated. By observing this self-model engage in the scenes, the patient becomes able to imagine his or her own participation in the scene. Mariner seems to rely on a dissociation of affect from performance to resolve this impasse in therapy.

There is some evidence that covert modeling can be combined with hypnosis. Clarke and Jackson (1983) provided a brief outline of hypnotically induced covert modeling. Jackson and Francey (1985) then presented a case report of the successful application of this technique to the treatment of a woman with an escalator phobia. Covert modeling may also be supplemented with cognitive techniques. The addition of self-instructional fear reduction strategies to covert modeling procedures has been shown to enhance their effectiveness in reducing the cognitive components of fear (Tearnan, Lahey, Thompson, & Hammer, 1982).

Related Conditioning Therapies

Implosion and desensitization techniques have inspired many adaptations. Prominent among the variations is Wolpin's (1969) *guided imagining*. Unlike Wolpe, Wolpin chooses not to introduce any relaxation training exercises. Also, instead of guiding his client through a hierarchical series of incremental images, he encourages the client to visualize the fear-arousing scene in its entirety. No provisions are made for relaxation or anxiety-reduction during the imagining. Instead, the patient is advised to experience whatever rush of affect is produced by visualizing the performance of the target behavior. In contrast to the client undergoing implosion therapy, this patient is not expected to cope in imagination with levels of anxiety that exceed those produced by the actual performance.

The therapist leads the client through the imagined scene, and after each visualization of the entire scene, he or she conducts a systematic inquiry. The therapist determines what images were created by the patient during the scene. Although the therapist suggests the images for visualization, a client's idiosyncrasies may lead to meaningful variation or to absolute noncompliance. If the latter occurs, the therapist attempts to encourage the patient to shape future images in compliance with the instructions. Of equal importance during the therapist's inquiry is an examination of the feelings generated during the visualization. Wolpin (1969) reports a uniform decrement of patient anxiety after repeated visualizations.

Brown presents another related conditioning therapy (1969). He asserts that Wolpe's technique would be more effective if the therapist knew what the client actually was imagining during desensitization (1969). Brown hypothesizes that the patient's fear of an object or situation might be related to his or her conceptualization of the phobic setting. When a patient reports feeling anxious, Brown asks that patient to convert his or her feelings into a mental image, perhaps a fantasy or a cartoon. For example, when a client reported anxiety about giving a speech, he was instructed to create an image of his feelings. "He imagined an audience of straight-laced, critical women with peering eyes that extended a foot out of their heads toward him" (p. 120). Brown reports that when the patient is given an opportunity to examine such images, he or she is able to identify the idiosyncratic distortions with little or no coaching. Desensitization generally is successful after repetition of the imagery. Hence, Brown moves the client toward a clearer and more rational view of the feared setting by exposing the client's inaccurate conceptions of that setting.

Paradoxical Intention

Frankl's (1967) paradoxical technique is another short-term treatment for phobia. Frankl's phobia management consists of advising the patient to intentionally amplify the feared symptoms to levels of behavioral extravagance. In some instances, the behavior cannot be produced; for example, a person with a fear of heights would not be expected to jump from a skyscraper window and crash to the ground only to be ticketed for landing in a no-parking zone. When the symptoms cannot be produced, the client is encouraged to *wish* that the feared events would happen. The object of the paradoxical wish is to introduce the element of humor as a distancing phenomenon between the self and the external source of anxiety.

Frankl (1979) accounts for the efficacy of the technique in terms of a reduction of the client's anticipatory anxiety. When the fear of fear is eliminated, the client is able to free himself or herself from the cycle wherein "a symptom evokes a phobia and the phobia provokes the symptom. The recurrence of the symptom then reinforces the phobia" (p. 452). In addition to Frankl's rationale, other models have been proposed to explain paradoxically-induced change (reattribution, preparatory, reactance, and self-regulatory reorientation models), but the exact mechanism for therapeutic change is not yet clear (Kim, Poling, & Ascher, 1991).

Paradoxical treatment has been demonstrated to be an effective strategy for reducing somatic symptoms in social phobia (Mersch, Hildebrand, Lavy, Wessel, & Van Hout, 1992). In the treatment of social phobia, paradoxical intention may be clinically enhanced when clients are helped to change the meaning that they attribute to their symptoms and problematic behaviors (Akillas & Efran, 1995).

There is empirical support, too, for the effectiveness of paradoxical intention in the treatment of agoraphobia. This technique has been found to be more effective than no treatment and placebo treatment, and it was found to be at least as effective as other behavioral treatments (Kim et al., 1991; Michelson & Ascher, 1984; Strong, 1984). In the treatment of travel restriction in agoraphobia, paradoxical intention may be enhanced by the addition of cognitive techniques, *in vivo* exposure, and imaginal exposure. Ascher, Schotte, and Grayson (1986) described a two-part imaginal intervention that they used to supplement standard paradoxical instructions. First, participants were asked to imagine themselves employing paradoxical intention in the discomforting situations that they expected to encounter during the week after the therapy session. Then, each participant was asked to imagine:

> . . . his or her hypothesized disastrous consequence with particular emphasis on the interpersonal aspects of the final stages of the disaster. The subject was asked to produce a personal "soap opera," and was encouraged to conclude with absurd and, it was hoped, humorous consequences. In this way, each subject received imaginal exposure to his anticipated disastrous consequences with the characteristic humor of paradoxical intention. (p. 127)

Whether it is used with or without imaginal exposure, paradoxical intention does not have universal applicability simply because not all individuals are capable of self-detachment and humor appreciation. Frankl (1979) offered the following example:

> I had a man in my Department, a guard in a museum who could not stay on his job because he suffered from deadly fears that someone would steal a painting. During a round I made with my staff, I tried paradoxical intention with him: "Tell yourself they stole a Rembrandt yesterday and today they would steal a Rembrandt and a Van Gogh." He just stared at me and said, "But Herr Professor, that's against the law!" This man was too feeble-minded to understand the meaning of paradoxical intention. (p. 455)

Rational Emotive Therapy (RET)

RET, originated by Ellis, is a hybrid technique merging behavioral methods and cognitive analysis (1962). Typically, RET is an *in vivo* form of desensitization which is grounded in the theory that irrational beliefs contribute to maladaptive emotions (Ellis, 1973). Rational emotive imagery (REI) is conceptualized as a component of RET (Ellis & Harper, 1975).

The REI sessions begin with relaxation: The client takes several minutes to close his or her eyes, relax, and breathe as if he or she were trying to fall asleep. The procedure followed in REI therapy is described by Maultsby and Ellis (1974) as a process wherein the patient learns to extinguish irrational fear responses, as he or she simultaneously conditions a rational response to the phobic situation or object. The mental imagery employed in this technique is evoked initially to allow the patient an opportunity to fantasize the anxiety-producing situation. The negative imagery is to be absorbed by the client until he or she feels the maladaptive emotion. The patient is then instructed, "Change this feeling in your gut, so that instead you *only* feel keenly disappointed, regretful, annoyed, or irritated, NOT anxious" (p. 90).

Once the client has been able to transform the emotional response from debilitating anxiety to annoyance or irritation, he or she then must determine how that transformation was accomplished. That is, the therapist teaches the client to observe how he or she manipulated and controlled the affect. The negative fantasy situation is repeated in therapy and at home until the client can respond by producing the more adaptive responses automatically. Maultsby and Ellis encourage the client to fantasize how it would feel if he or she did not hold irrational fears. The patient must then vividly picture himself or herself rejecting the irrational fears and accepting rational ideas.

Maultsby (1971) proposes that three psychotherapeutic objectives are realized through the use of REI: 1) the patient deconditions himself or herself to the situation that usually elicited a fear response; 2) the patient practices and learns to make adaptive and rational responses while visualizing the phobic situation; and 3) the patient responds to the actual phobic situation automatically with a rational instead of an irrational response.

The efficacy of REI has been challenged experimentally. The REI technique was found to be not as effective in reducing test anxiety as the RET technique which relies primarily on *in vivo* verbalizations and self-talk (Hymen & Warren, 1978).

The cognitive and behavioral therapists using mental imagery to treat phobic disorders typically share a fundamental assumption: either imagined or real external stimuli can evoke neurophysiological patterns which are qualitatively and quantitatively the same (Eccles, 1957). Thus, imagery is an exposure stimulus which can be manipulated by the patient or therapist; and, unlike exposure *in vivo*, the imagery process is cost efficient and can be practiced at home.

Although the cognitive and behavioral approaches have documented success in treating a wide range of phobias, they have been the object of considerable criticism. The behaviorists have concerned themselves exclusively with symptom management. They have chosen not to muddy their theoretical waters with any exploration of the symbolic content that may be present in clients' imagery.

Disciples of the behavioral modification strategies reject the medical model and therefore disavow the notion that a symptom may emerge as the result of an underlying disease process.

SYMBOLIC ANALYSIS OF IMAGERY IN PHOBIC DISORDERS

Psychoanalytic Approach

Logical, orderly, secondary-process thought traditionally has been more highly esteemed than fantasy and imagery. Imagery has acquired the unflattering characterization as regressive and narcissistically cathected, serving id and super-ego drives (Shapiro, 1970). The presence of spontaneous imagery in psycho-analysis is interpreted, as are symptoms, to represent defenses that provide distance from an underlying impulse that receives resultant, indirect gratification.

The psychoanalytic treatment of phobia is but a narrow dimension of the analyst's broader task: major personality integration and change. In fact, although the current psychoanalytic understanding is that a phobic symptom is to be explored and "that a number of levels of meaning are likely to be found in the course of its successful unraveling" (Abend, 1992, p. 205), the customary proce-dure of disclosing the origin of the symptom has not led to uniform success.

> Freud himself saw a necessity for modification of psychoanalysis in the treatment of phobias, stressing the need for the psychoanalyst to intervene and insist that patients attempt to brave the anxiety-provoking situation...and to struggle with their anxiety while they make the attempt. (Frazer & Carr, as quoted in Chessick, 1976, p. 4021)

At the appropriate stage of transference, the patient is encouraged to undergo a desensitization experience with the help of a trusted and supportive figure. Frazer and Carr suggest that, although the process utilized casts long Wolpean shadows, its theoretical affiliation is discussed rarely.

Hence, despite Freud's early endorsement of imagery analysis as a means through which the unconscious could be excavated and accepted, the role of free association in facilitating abreaction and catharsis ultimately was accented.

Eidetic Therapy Approach

Ahsen is regarded as the first theorist to explore systematically the psychotherapeutic usefulness of eidetics (1968, 1977; Dolan, 1997). Unlike the behavioral therapist, the eidetic counterpart is not content with simple redress of symptomatic complaints; and unlike the psychoanalyst, the eidetic therapist is not compelled to explore analytically the full spectrum of the client's life experience to come to an understanding of the origin of symptoms.

Eidetic therapy relies on the elicitation and manipulation of eidetic images. Eidetic psychotherapists, in contrast to most experimental researchers in the area of eidetic imagery, view the eidetic as a semipermanent representation that has been figuratively impressed on the memory in response to the formative events in the past. Every significant event in one's developmental course is purported to implant an eidetic in the system. The visual part, the *image,* is considered to be accompanied always by a somatic pattern—a set of bodily feelings and tension, including somatic correlates of emotion—and a cognitive or experiential *meaning.* This tridimensional unity, the eidetic, displays certain lawful tendencies toward change and has specific meaningful relations to psychological processes. This description coincides to a great extent with Jung's conception of the image as an integrated unity with a life and purpose of its own (Panagiotou & Sheikh, 1977).

Eidetics are observed to be bipolarly configurated and involve ego-positive and ego-negative elements of the experience. It is believed that, among other factors, a quasi-separation of the visual part from other components, a fixation on the negative pole, or repression of a significant experience can lead to a variety of problems, including phobias. Eidetic therapists aim primarily at reviving the tridimensional unity, shifting attention to the positive pole, and uncovering appropriate healthful experiences through eidetic progression. Eidetic therapy includes a number of procedures designed to elicit the relevant eidetics.

Dolan and Sheikh (1977) report an adaptation of a specific eidetic procedure, the Age Projection Test, for use with patients suffering from phobic disorders. In this procedure, the therapist obtains all the names by which the patient has been called since childhood; these names are assumed to refer to the individual's various identities and therefore are used interchangeably throughout the procedure. The therapist instructs the patient to relax and listen carefully. Then, he or she repeats the psychological and physical features of the symptom, discovered during an initial interview, thus eliciting the symptom in its most acute form. A 5-second silence ensues.

> Suddenly the therapist starts talking about the times when the patient was healthy and happy. As the therapist talks about health in the areas in which the symptom now exists, the patient spontaneously forms a self-image and is asked to describe the following: (1) the self-image itself; (2) the clothing on the self-image; (3) the place where it appears; (4) the events occurring during the age projected in the self-image; (5) the events of the year prior to the age projected; and (6) the events of the year following the projected age. (p. 599)

The above technique generally uncovers an event that precipitated the symptom or started a series of occurrences that ultimately resulted in symptom formation. After the self-image pertaining to this event is formed, the client is asked to project it again and again until it becomes clear, and then he or she is questioned further about that critical period. On the basis of information gathered through the test, a therapeutic image is constructed and the patient is asked to project it repeatedly (Sheikh & Jordan, 1981, 1983).

It should be noted that the above procedure is used to uncover the precipitating event of a phobia of long standing. To treat a symptom that has its origin in a recent event, one which occurred less than a year previously, it is not necessary to use the Age Projection Test. The therapist begins directly with an inquiry into the experiences during the year prior to the onset of the symptom. The following case history, described by Dolan and Sheikh (1977), illustrates the use of the Age Projection Test in the treatment of phobias.

A Case History

A 35-year-old woman, Regina, had been suffering from a phobia of thunderstorms for the past ten years. She reported that her fears were severely limiting her activities, especially during the summer when electrical storms were more frequent. During a storm, she would hide in the basement, where she saw and heard less of it. Nevertheless, she experienced sweating, palpitation, mild diarrhea, and acute dread that lightning would strike her.

The Age Projection Test revealed a healthy self-image at the age of 24. Further inquiry uncovered that during the summer vacation, in the mountains, of the previous year, she had been on the front porch during a thunderstorm and had seen lightning strike nearby. At that time, she was afraid that she too would be struck by lightning and killed instantly.

Further investigation revealed that prior to this event, Regina had been in the mountains recuperating from a lobectomy to remove a benign lung cyst. The surgery had left her weak and nervous, and she had felt very vulnerable during thunderstorms.

At this point, the focus shifted from the phobia to the illness that preceded its onset. When she was told that she had a cyst that had to be surgically removed, she became very anxious. She feared that she had lung cancer and that she would not recover from the operation; therefore, she refused surgery. These feelings climaxed one evening when she became hysterical. Regina vividly saw herself sitting on her bed, with her mother and husband nearby, crying hysterically, "I'm not going to sign. I'm not going to sign." She heard her mother telling her that this hysterical behavior would only harm her and that she would benefit from the operation. The following day she signed the operative permit and underwent surgery the same day. She suffered no subsequent complications; nevertheless, she remained anxious.

Regina's phobia was interpreted in the following manner: Since she was of the hysterical type, the prospect of having surgery had filled her with acute anxiety and fear of death. This anxiety stayed with her during her convalescence and then became displaced at the time of the thunderstorm.

Regina was asked to visualize again her mother at her bedside, telling her that the hysterical behavior would only harm her and that the surgery would help. As she did so, she gradually felt her entire body relax. In fact, she almost fell asleep in her chair. Every time she focused on the positive elements of the bipolar configuration, she felt relief. Then she was encouraged to imagine herself again crying hysterically due to the prospect of surgery. She again reported a fear of death and the anxiety connected with the thunderstorm. This procedure made Regina aware of the structure of her phobia and of her ability to recreate both sides of the phobic event. This awareness was vitally important. Over the next few days, Regina repeatedly projected the positive image, and her anxiety subsided. Her fear of death, which was at the root of her fear of thunderstorms, was relieved and with it, her phobia. A follow-up indicated no recurrence of her symptoms.

Death Imagery Approach

Several researchers have proposed that the fear of death may lie at the root of many phobic disorders. For example, Eugene Shea (1978) claims that:

> It is our fear of death which accounts for the great majority of all the phobias with which humans are afflicted: acrophobia, claustrophobia, agoraphobia, etc. But these are only the symptoms of our "Dis-ease," our fear of death; dealing with them does not remove the cause of phobias. Someday we must learn to deal with the cause of ALL our phobias, our fear of death, instead of just dealing with each specific phobia. (p. 46)

Seligman (1971) notes that human phobias are largely restricted to objects that have threatened survival. Selan (1982) emphasizes the issue of death in the lives of many phobics. Seven of the 25 phobics that she treated reported confrontation with death that had occurred during their childhood or adolescence. Most of them "also revealed a great preoccupation with death, saying they dream about if often and vividly" (p. 135).

In the light of the aforementioned indications, it seems desirable to explore and to attempt to resolve the phobic patients' anxiety concerning death. A death imagery technique developed by Sheikh, Twente, and Turner (1979) may be helpful for this task. In this procedure, the client is asked to relax, confront his or her death in imagination, let go to the natural flow, and be willing to accept responsibility for whatever arises. The technique is based on the premise that purposeful life is possible only through an unflinching acceptance of death as an integral constituent of life. Confronting death draws one to the threshold of life. Several other related techniques, the aim of which is to assist the individual in coming to terms with the idea of his or her own death and the death of significant others, have appeared in the literature. The precursors of these approaches include Buddhist and Sufi meditation on death, Plato's "practicing of death," and the ideas concerning "living toward death" presented in *The Tibetan Book of the Dead* (see Sheikh, Twente, & Turner, 1979, for a review of the literature).

CONCLUDING REMARKS

Treatment of phobic disorders generally is successful with patients who report that a single phobia has caused them to become aware of increasing disease within their environment. Cohen (1981) observes that these individuals, otherwise stable, reality-centered, and functioning competently, are likely to improve with *any* kind of therapy. On the other hand, patients whose phobia is one element of a larger configuration of symptoms are less likely to respond successfully to phobia interventions. Also, certain comorbidities (alcohol dependence and personality disorders) and stressful life circumstances (marital conflict, lack of social support, job dissatisfaction) interfere with the successful treatment of phobias (Noyes, 1991).

For the past several years, an abundance of research has been carried out to determine the relative efficacy of therapeutic techniques in abating clinical phobias. Although many studies have demonstrated the superiority of certain treatments over others, many of them have produced contradictory findings or were unable to be replicated. Thus, the research has been equivocal. Still, some conservative conclusions may be offered. First, clinicians must be cautious in generalizing the results of imagery studies from one population to another. Generalization may be inappropriate because variables such as motivational state, intensity of the presenting symptom, stimulus intensity, and duration of exposure have no consistent properties among research groups (Matthews, 1979). Furthermore, the contribution of the individuals' type of phobia is becoming better understood. For example, small-animal phobics and public-speaking phobics differ significantly in the vividness and intensity of their imagery (Lang, Melamed, & Hart, 1970; Weerts & Lang, 1978).

Second, as mentioned earlier, there is still a debate whether imaginal exposure to a feared stimulus is as powerful as *in vivo* exposure. This question has become more urgent since the Task Force on Promotion and Dissemination of Psychological Procedures from the American Psychological Association listed "exposure treatment for phobias" as a well-established, empirically-validated treatment (Task Force, 1995). With the current emphasis on cost-effectiveness and accountability in health service provision, it will be important for clinicians to know whether they can achieve the same outcomes with imaginal exposure as with *in vivo* exposure. If they can, the imaginal form will be preferred, because it is more practical and easier for clients to practice on their own between therapy sessions.

Third, there has been little systematic, empirical research on the "depth-imagery" approaches to the treatment of phobias. Clinical case reports, instead of empirical analyses, are most often presented in the literature. Nevertheless, these case reports (using, for example, the eidetic approach) foreshadow empirical work which is likely to support the continued use and development of such therapeutic techniques.

There are a host of therapeutic observations which support the argument in favor of mental imagery techniques. For example, it has been shown that anxious people have enhanced imagery specifically for anxiety-related experiences. In other words, anxious individuals experience relatively more imagery for threat than for non-threat material, whereas for nonanxious individuals, non-threat material is more imageable (Martin & Williams, 1990).

Perhaps more importantly, it has been observed that patients, when introduced to the dramatic qualities of the human imagination, begin to acquire control over one of their innate abilities. The client in imagery therapy is likely not only to experience relief from symptoms, but also to experience enhanced self-esteem (Singer, 1974), and to learn to live more imaginatively, thereby increasing his or her ultimate human potential (Shorr, 1974).

REFERENCES

Abend, S. M. (1992). Phobic patients. In M. Aronson & M. Scharfman (Eds.), *Psychotherapy: The analytic approach* (pp. 203-210). Northvale, NJ: Jason Aronson, Inc.

Ahsen, A. (1968). *Basic concepts in eidetic psychotherapy*. New York: Brandon House.

Ahsen, A. (1977). *Psycheye: Self-analytic consciousness*. New York: Brandon House.

Akillas, E., & Efran, J. S. (1995). Symptom prescription and reframing: Should they be combined? *Cognitive Therapy and Research, 19,* 263-279.

American Psychiatric Association. (1980). *Diagnostic and statistical manual of mental disorders* (3rd ed.). Washington, DC: Author.

American Psychiatric Association. (1994). *Diagnostic and statistical manual of mental disorders* (4th ed.). Washington, DC: Author.

Ascher, L. M. (1993). Treating recursive anxiety with covert conditioning. In J. R. Cautela & A. J. Kearney (Eds.), *Covert conditioning casebook* (pp. 13-21). Pacific Grove, CA: Brooks/Cole.

Ascher, L. M., Schotte, D. E., & Grayson, J. B. (1986). Enhancing effectiveness of paradoxical intention in treating travel restriction in agoraphobia. *Behavior Therapy, 17,* 124-130.

Bandura, A. (1968). Modeling approaches to the modification of phobic disorders. In R. Porter (Ed.), *The role of learning in psychotherapy*. London: J. and A. Churchill.

Bandura, A. (1970). Modeling theory. In W. S. Sahakian (Ed.), *Psychology of learning: Systems, models, and theories*. Chicago: Marham.

Bandura, A. (1971). Psychotherapy based on modeling principles. In A. E. Bergin & S. L. Garfield (Eds.), *Handbook of psychotherapy and behavior change*. New York: Wiley.

Bandura, A. (1979). Factors determining vicarious extinction of avoidance behavior through symbolic modeling. *Journal of Personality and Social Psychology, 8,* 99-108.

Bandura, A., & Barab, P. (1973). Processes governing disinhibitory effects through symbolic modeling. *Journal of Abnormal Psychology, 82,* 1-9.

Boulougouris, J., Marks, I., & Marset, P. (1971). Superiority of flooding (implosion) to desensitization for reducing pathological fear. *Behavior Research and Therapy, 9,* 7-16.

Brehony, K. A., & Geller, S. (1981). Agoraphobia: Appraisal of research and a proposal for an integrative model. In M. Hersen, R. Eisler, & P. Miller (Eds.), *Progress in behavior modification* (Vol. 12). New York: Academic Press.

Brown, B. (1969). The use of induced imagery in psychotherapy. *Psychotherapy Theory, Research and Practice, 6,* 120-121.

Butler, G. (1989). Phobic disorders. In K. Hawton, P. M. Salkovskis, J. Kirk, & D. M. Clark (Eds.), *Cognitive behaviour therapy for psychiatric problems: A practical guide* (pp. 97-128). Oxford: Oxford University Press.

Cautela, J. R. (1970). Covert reinforcement. *Behavior Therapy, 1,* 35-50.

Cautela, J. R. (1972). *Covert modeling.* Paper presented to the Association for the Advancement of Behavior Therapy.

Cautela, J. R. (1976). The present status of covert modeling. *Journal of Behavior Therapy and Experimental Psychiatry, 7,* 324-326.

Cautela, J. R. (1993). The use of covert conditioning in the treatment of a severe childhood phobia. In J. R. Cautela & A. J. Kearney (Eds.), *Covert conditioning casebook* (pp. 126-134). Pacific Grove, CA: Brooks/Cole.

Cautela, J. R., Flannery, R., & Hanley, E. (1974). Covert modeling: An experimental test. *Behavior Therapy, 5,* 494-502.

Cautela, J. R., & Kearney, A. J. (1986). *The covert conditioning handbook.* New York: Springer.

Cautela, J. R., & McCullough, L. (1978). Covert conditioning: A learning theory perspective on imagery. In J. L. Singer & K. S. Pope (Eds.), *The power of human imagination.* New York: Plenum Press.

Chambless, D. L., Sanderson, W. C., Shoham, V., Johnston, S. B., Pope, K. S., Crits-Christoph, P., Baker, M., Johnson, B., Woody, S. R., Sue, S., Beutler, L., Williams, D. A., & McMurray, S. (1996). An update on empirically validated therapies. *The Clinical Psychologist, 49,* 5-18.

Chapman, T. F. (1997). The epidemiology of fears and phobias. In G. C. L. Davey (Ed.), *Phobias: A handbook of theory, research, and treatment* (pp. 415-434). Chichester: John Wiley & Sons.

Chessick, R. D. (1976). The treatment of neuroses and borderline cases. In B. Wolman (Ed.), *The therapist's handbook: Treatment methods of mental disorders.* New York: Van Nostrand Reinholt.

Clarke, J. C., & Jackson, J. A. (1983). *Hypnosis and behavior therapy.* New York: Springer.

Cohen, S. B. (1981). Editorial: Phobias. *The American Journal of Clinical Hypnosis, 23,* 227-229.

Cooper, L., & Shepard, R. (1978). Transformations on representations of objects in space. In E. C. Carterette & M. Friedman (Eds.), *Handbook of perception.* New York: Academic Press.

Cornwall, E., Spence, S. H., & Schotte, D. (1996). The effectiveness of emotive imagery in the treatment of darkness phobia in children. *Behaviour Change, 13,* 223-229.

Craske, M. G., & Rowe, M. K. (1997). A comparison of behavioral and cognitive treatments of phobias. In G. C. L. Davey (Ed.), *Phobias: A handbook of theory, research, and treatment* (pp. 247-280). Chichester: John Wiley & Sons.

Crawford, H. J., & Barabasz, A. F. (1993). Phobias and intense fears: Facilitating their treatment with hypnosis. In J. W. Rhue, S. J. Lynn, & I. Kirsch (Eds.),

Handbook of clinical hypnosis (pp. 311-337). Washington, DC: American Psychological Association.

Crowe, M. J., Marks, I., Agras, W. S., & Leitenberg, H. (1972). Time limited desensitization, implosion, and shaping for phobic patients: A crossover study. *Behavior Research and Therapy, 10,* 319-328.

Davey, G. C. L. (1997). Preface. In G. C. L. Davey (Ed.), *Phobias: A handbook of theory, research, and treatment* (pp. xiii-xvi). Chichester: John Wiley & Sons.

Davidson, R., & Schwartz, G. (1976). Patterns of cerebral lateralization during cardiac biofeedback versus the self-regulation of emotion: Sex differences. *Psychophysiology, 13,* 62-74.

Desoille, R. (1965). *The directed daydream.* New York: Psychosynthesis Research Foundation.

Dolan, A. T. (1997). *Imagery and treatment of phobias: Anxiety states and other symptom complexes in Akhter Ahsen's image psychology.* New York: Brandon House.

Dolan, A. T., & Sheikh, A. A. (1977). Short-term treatment of phobia through eidetic imagery. *American Journal of Psychotherapy, 31,* 595-604.

DuPont, R. L. (Ed.). (1982). *Phobia: A comprehensive summary of modern treatments.* New York: Brunner Mazel.

Dyckman, J. M., & Cowan, P. A. (1978). Imaging vividness and the outcome of *in vivo* and imagined scene desensitization. *Journal of Consulting and Clinical Psychology, 46,* 1155-1156.

Eccles, J. C. (1957). *The physiology of nerve cells.* Baltimore: Johns-Hopkins Press.

Ellis, A. (1962). *Reason and emotion in psychotherapy.* New York: Lyce-Stuart Press.

Ellis, A. (1973). *Humanistic psychotherapy: The rational-emotive approach.* New York: Julian Press.

Ellis, A., & Harper, R. (1975). *A new guide to rational living.* Englewood Cliffs, NJ: Prentice-Hall.

Emery, J. R., & Krumboltz, J. D. (1967). Standard vs. individualized hierarchies in desensitization to reduce test anxiety. *Journal of Counseling Psychology, 14,* 204-209.

Errera, P. (1962). Some historical aspects of the concept of phobia. *The Psychiatric Quarterly, 36,* 325-336.

Eysenck, H. J., & Rachman, S. (1965). *The causes and cures of neurosis.* London: Routledge and Paul Kegan.

Foa, E., & Chambless, D. (1978). Habituation of subjective anxiety during flooding in imagery. *Behavior Research and Therapy, 16,* 391-399.

Frankl, V. E. (1967). *Psychotherapy and existentialism: Selected papers on logotherapy.* New York: Washington Square Press.

Frankl, V. E. (1979). Logotherapy. In W. S. Sahakian (Ed.), *Psychopathology today.* Itasca, IL: F. E. Peacock Publishers.

Galin, D. (1974). Implications for psychiatry of left and right cerebral specialization. *Archives of General Psychiatry, 31,* 572-583.

Gazzaniga, M. S. (1970). *The bisected brain.* New York: Appleton-Century-Crofts.

Gazzaniga, M. S., & Ledoux, J. E. (1978). *The integrated mind.* New York: Plenum Press.

Hall, G. S. (1897). A study of fears. *American Journal of Psychology, 8,* 147-249.

Harper, R. A. (1975). *The new psychotherapies.* Englewood Cliffs, NJ: Prentice-Hall.

Hayward, P., & Wardle, J. (1997). The use of medication in the treatment of phobias. In G. C. L. Davey (Ed.), *Phobias: A handbook of theory, research, and treatment* (pp. 281-298). Chichester: John Wiley & Sons.

Horowitz, M. J. (1968). Visual thought images in psychotherapy. *American Journal of Psychotherapy, 22,* 55-57.

Huyghe, P. (1982, August). Mind. *Omni,* 20.

Hymen, S. P., & Warren, R. (1978). An evaluation of rational-emotive imagery as a component of rational-emotive therapy in the treatment of test anxiety. *Perceptual and Motor Skills, 46,* 847-853.

Jackson, H. J., & Francey, S. M. (1985). The use of hypnotically-induced covert modelling in the desensitization of an escalator phobia. *Australian Journal of Clinical and Experimental Hypnosis, 13,* 55-58.

Jacobsen, E. (1938). *Progressive relaxation.* Chicago: University of Chicago Press.

James, J. E. (1985). Desensitization treatment of agoraphobia. *British Journal of Clinical Psychology, 24,* 133-134.

Jansson, L., & Oest, L. G. (1982). Behavioral treatments for agoraphobia: An evaluative review. *Clinical Psychology Review, 2,* 311-336.

Kazdin, A. E. (1973). Covert modeling and the reduction of avoidance behavior. *Journal of Abnormal Psychology, 81,* 78-95.

Kim, R. S., Poling, J., & Ascher, L. M. (1991). An introduction to research on the clinical efficacy of paradoxical intention. In G. R. Weeks (Ed.), *Promoting change through paradoxical therapy* (Rev. ed., pp. 216-250). New York: Brunner/Mazel.

King, N. J., & Gullone, E. (1990). Acceptability of fear reduction procedures with children. *Journal of Behavior Therapy and Experimental Psychiatry, 21,* 1-8.

King, N. J., Molloy, G. N., Heyne, D., Murphy, G. C., & Ollendick, T. H. (1998). Emotive imagery treatment for childhood phobias: A credible and empirically validated intervention? *Behavioural and Cognitive Psychotherapy, 26,* 103-113.

Kleinknecht, R. A. (1991). *Mastering anxiety: The nature and treatment of anxious conditions.* New York: Plenum Press.

Kosslyn, S. (1976). Can imagery be distinguished from other forms of internal representation? Evidence from studies of information retrieval time. *Memory and Cognition, 4,* 291-297.

Kosslyn, S., Ball, T., & Reiser, B. (1978). Visual images preserve metric spatial information: Evidence from studies of imagery scanning. *Journal of Experimental Psychology: Human Perception and Performance,* 47-60.

Kraeplin, E. (1903). *Lehrbuch der Psychiatrie.* Leipzig: Barth.

Kramer, P. D. (1993). *Listening to Prozac: A psychiatrist explores antidepressant drugs and the remaking of the self.* New York: Penguin Books.

Lang, P. J., Melamed, B. G., & Hart, J. D. (1970). A psychophysiological analysis of fear modification using an automated desensitization procedure. *Journal of Abnormal Psychology, 76,* 220-234.

Lazarus, A. A. (1961). Group therapy of phobic disorders by systematic desensitization. *Journal of Abnormal Social Psychology, 63,* 504-510.

Lazarus, A. A., & Abramovitz, A. (1962). The use of 'emotive imagery' in the treatment of children's phobias. *Journal of Mental Science, 108,* 191-195.

Leuner, H. (1969). Guided affective imagery: A method of intensive psychotherapy. *American Journal of Psychotherapy, 23,* 4-22.

Levis, D. J., & Hare, N. (1977). A review of the theoretical rationale and empirical support for the extinction approach of implosive (flooding) therapy. In M. Hersen, R. M. Eisler, & P. M. Miller (Eds.), *Progress in behavior modification*. New York: Academic Press.

Ley, R. G. (1979). Cerebral asymmetries, emotional experience, and imagery: Implications for psychotherapy. In A. A. Sheikh & J. T. Shaffer (Eds.), *The potential of fantasy and imagination*. New York: Brandon House.

Lindemann, C. (1994). Phobias. In B. B. Wolman & G. Stricker (Eds.), *Anxiety and related disorders: A handbook* (pp. 161-176). New York: John Wiley & Sons.

Mariner, A. S. (1969). Resolving an impasse in systematic desensitization. *Psychotherapy: Theory, Research and Practice, 6*, 119.

Marks, I. M. (1975). *Fears and phobias*. New York: Academic Press.

Marks, I. M. (1982). Toward an empirical clinical science: Behavioral psychotherapy of the 1980s. *Behavior Therapy, 13*, 63-81.

Martin, M., & Williams, R. (1990). Imagery and emotion: Clinical and experimental approaches. In P. J. Hampson, D. F. Marks, & J. T. E. Richardson (Eds.), *Imagery: Current developments* (pp. 268-306). London: Routledge.

Matthews, A. M. (1971). Psychophysiological approaches to the investigation of desensitization and related procedures. *Psychological Bulletin, 76*, 73-91.

Matthews, A. M. (1979). Fear reduction research and clinical phobias. *Annual Review Behavior Therapy, Theory, and Practice*, 59-82.

Maultsby, M. (1971). Rational emotive imagery. *Rational Living, 6*, 24-27.

Maultsby, M., & Ellis, A. (1974). *Techniques for using rational emotive imagery*. New York: Institute for Rational Living.

May, J. R., & Johnson, H. J. (1973). Physiological activity to internally elicited arousal and inhibitory thoughts. *Journal of Abnormal Psychology, 82*, 239-245.

McGlynn, F. D. (1971). Individual versus standardized hierarchies in the systematic desensitization of snake-avoidance. *Behavior Research and Therapy, 9*, 1-5.

McLemore, C. W. (1972). Imagery in desensitization. *Behavior Research and Therapy, 10*, 51-57.

Mealiea, W. L., & Nawas, M. M. (1971). The comparative effectiveness of systematic desensitization and implosive therapy in the treatment of snake phobia. *Journal of Behavior Therapy and Experimental Psychiatry, 2*, 85-94.

Menzies, R. G. (1996). Individual response patterns and treatment matching in the phobic disorders: A review. *British Journal of Clinical Psychology, 35*, 1-10.

Mersch, P. P. A., Hildebrand, M., Lavy, E. H., Wessel, I., & Van Hout, W. J. P. J. (1992). Somatic symptoms in social phobia: A treatment method based on rational emotive therapy and paradoxical interventions. *Journal of Behavior Therapy and Experimental Psychiatry, 23*, 199-211.

Meyer, R. G., & Deitsch, S. E. (1996). *The clinician's handbook: Integrated diagnostics, assessment, and intervention in adult and adolescent psychopathology*. Boston: Allyn and Bacon.

Michelson, L., & Ascher, L. M. (1984). Paradoxical intention in the treatment of agoraphobia and other anxiety disorders. *Journal of Behavior Therapy and Experimental Psychiatry, 15*, 215-220.

Mingler, B., & Wolpe, J. (1967). Automated self-desensitization: A case report. *Behavior Research and Therapy, 5*, 133-135.

Morrow, L., Vrtunski, B., Kim, Y., & Boller, F. (1981). Arousal responses to emotional stimuli and laterality of lesion. *Neuropsychologia, 19,* 65-71.

Mowrer, O. (1960). *Learning theory and behavior.* New York: Wiley.

Noyes, R. (1991). Treatments of choice for anxiety disorders. In W. Coryell & G. Winokur (Eds.), *The clinical management of anxiety disorders* (pp. 140-153). New York: Oxford University Press.

Oppenheim, H. (1911). *Textbook of nervous diseases for physicians and students.* New York: Stechert.

Ornstein, R. E. (1972). *The psychology of consciousness.* San Francisco: Freeman.

Paivio, A. (1971). *Imagery and verbal processes.* New York: Holt.

Panagiotou, N. C., & Sheikh, A. A. (1977). The image and the unconscious. *International Journal of Social Psychiatry, 23,* 169-186.

Paul, G. L., & Berstein, D. A. (1979). Anxiety and systematic desensitization. In W. S. Sahakian (Ed.), *Psychopathology today.* Itasca, IL: F. E. Peacock Publishers.

Peter, L.J. (1977). *Peter's quotations.* New York: Bantam

Pies, R. W. (1998). *Handbook of essential psychopharmacology.* Washington, DC: American Psychiatric Press.

Rachman, S. (1968). *Phobias: Their nature and control.* Springfield, IL: Charles C. Thomas Publishing.

Regier, D. A., Boyd, J. H., Burke, J. D., Rae, D. S., Myers, J. K., Kramer, M., Robins, L. N., George, L. K., Karno, M., & Locke, B. Z. (1988). One-month prevalence of mental disorders in the United States. *Archives of General Psychiatry, 45,* 977-986.

Regier, D. A., Myers, J. K., Kramer, M., Robins, L. N., Blazer, D. G., Hough, R. L., Eaton, W. W., & Locke, B. Z. (1984). The NIMH Epidemiologic Catchment Area Program: Historical context, major objectives, and study population characteristics. *Archives of General Psychiatry, 41,* 934-941.

Rickles, W. H., Onoda, L., & Doyle, C. (1982). Task force study section report: Biofeedback as an adjunct to psychotherapy. *Behavioral Analysis and Modification, 7,* 1-34.

Rosentiel, A. K., & Scott, D. S. (1977). Four considerations in using imagery techniques with children. *Journal of Behavior Theory and Experimental Psychiatry, 8,* 287-290.

Salter, A. (1949). *Conditioned reflex therapy.* New York: Farrar, Strauss.

Schultz, J. H., & Luth, W. (1959). *Autogenic training.* New York: Grune and Stratton.

Selan, B. H. (1982). Phobias, death, and depression. In R. L. DuPont (Ed.), *Phobia: A comprehensive summary of modern treatments.* New York: Brunner Mazel.

Seligman, M. (1971). Phobias and preparedness. *Behavior Therapy, 2,* 307-320.

Shapiro, D. L. (1970). The significance of the visual image in psychotherapy. *Psychotherapy: Theory, Research and Practice, 7,* 209-212.

Shea, E. B. (1978). *The immortal "I."* Illinois: The Unprofitable Servants.

Sheikh, A. A. (1977). Mental images: Ghosts of sensations? *Journal of Mental Imagery, 1,* 1-4.

Sheikh, A. A., & Jordan, C. S. (1981). Eidetic psychotherapy. In R. J. Corsini (Ed.), *Handbook of innovative psychotherapies.* New York: Wiley.

Sheikh, A. A., & Jordan, C. S. (1983). Clinical uses of mental imagery. In A. A. Sheikh (Ed.), *Imagery: Current theory, research, and application.* New York: Wiley.

Sheikh, A. A., & Panagiotou, N. (1975). Use of mental imagery in psychotherapy: A critical review. *Perceptual and Motor Skills, 41,* 555-585.

Sheikh, A. A., Twente, G. E., & Turner, D. (1979). Death imagery: Therapeutic uses. In A. A. Sheikh & J. T. Shaffer (Eds.), *The potential of fantasy and imagination.* New York: Brandon House.

Shorr, J. E. (1974). *Psychotherapy through imagery.* New York: Intercontinental Medical Book Corporation.

Singer, J. L. (1974). *Imagery and daydreaming methods in psychotherapy and behavior modification.* New York: Academic Press.

Singer, J. L. (1979). Imagery and affect in psychotherapy. In A. A. Sheikh & J. T. Schaffer (Eds.), *The potential of fantasy and imagination.* New York: Brandon House.

Singer, J. L., & Pope, K. S. (Eds.). (1978). *The power of human imagination: New methods in psychotherapy.* New York: Plenum Press.

Stampfl, T. G. (1961). Implosive therapy: A learning theory derived psychodynamic therapeutic technique. In LeBarba and Dent (Eds.), *Critical issues in clinical psychology.* New York: Academic Press.

Stern, R., & Marks, I. M. (1973). Brief and prolonged flooding: A comparison in agoraphobic patients. *Archives of General Psychiatry, 28,* 270-276.

Strong, S. R. (1984). Experimental studies in explicitly paradoxical interventions: Results and implications. *Journal of Behavior Therapy and Experimental Psychiatry, 15,* 189-194.

Task Force on Promotion and Dissemination of Psychological Procedures, Division of Clinical Psychology, American Psychological Association. (1995, Winter). Training in and dissemination of empirically-validated psychological treatments: Report and recommendations. *The Clinical Psychologist, 48,* 3-23.

Tearnan, B. H., Lahey, B. B., Thompson, J. K., & Hammer, D. (1982). The role of coping self-instructions combined with covert modeling in specific fear reduction. *Cognitive Therapy and Research, 6,* 185-190.

Upper, D., & Cautela, J. R. (Eds.). (1979). *Covert conditioning.* New York: Pergamon Press.

Vallis, T. M., & Bucher, B. (1986). Individual difference factors in the efficacy of covert modeling and self-instructional training for fear reduction. *Canadian Journal of Behavioural Science, 18,* 146-158.

Van Egeren, L. F. (1971). Psychophysiological aspects of systematic desensitization: Some outstanding issues. *Behavior Research and Therapy, 9,* 65-77.

Van Egeren, L. F., Feather, B. W., & Hein, P. L. (1971). Desensitization of phobias: Some psychophysiological propositions. *Psychophysiology, 8,* 213-228.

Vodde, T. W., & Gilner, F. H. (1971). The effects of exposure to fear stimuli on fear reduction. *Behavior Research and Therapy, 9,* 169-175.

Wanderer, Z., & Ingram, B. L. (1990). Physiologically monitored implosion therapy of phobias. *Phobia Practice & Research Journal, 3,* 61-77.

Watson, J. B. (1913). Psychology as the behaviorist views it. *Psychological Review, 20,* 158-177.

Weerts, T. C., & Lang, P. J. (1978). Psychophysiology of fear imagery: Differences between focal phobia and social performance anxiety. *Journal of Consulting and Clinical Psychology, 46,* 1157-1159.

Werbach, M. R. (1977). Biofeedback and psychotherapy. *American Journal of Psychotherapy, 31,* 376-382.

Whorf, B. L. (1956). *Language, thought, and reality: Selected writings.* Cambridge: Cambridge Technology Press of Massachusetts Institute of Technology.

Wilkins, W. (1971). Desensitization: Social and cognitive factors underlying the effectiveness of Wolpe's procedure. *Psychological Bulletin, 76,* 311-317.

Wilson, R. R. (1996). Imaginal desensitization and relaxation training. In C. G. Lindemann (Ed.), *Handbook of the treatment of the anxiety disorders* (pp. 263-290). Northvale, NJ: Jason Aronson, Inc.

Wolpe, J. (1958). *Psychotherapy by reciprocal inhibition.* Stanford: Stanford University Press.

Wolpe, J. (1969). *The practice of behavior therapy.* New York: Pergamon Press.

Wolpe, J. (1976). *Theme and variations: A behavior therapy casebook.* New York: Pergamon Press.

Wolpin, M. (1969). Guided imagining to reduce avoidance behavior. *Psychotherapy: Theory, Research and Practice, 6,* 122-124.

CHAPTER 14

The Use of Imagery in Alleviating Depression

DAVID SCHULTZ

> Imagination is eminent in al, so most especially it rageth in melancholy persons in keeping species of objects so long, amplifying them by continuall and strong meditation, until at length it produceth reall effects, and causeth this and many other maladies.
>
> R. Burton (in *The Anatomy of Melancholy*, 1621)

In spite of William Jame's (1950) challenge to study ongoing thought in all its richness diversity, and complexity, a review of much of the literature in psychology, psychiatry, and psychotherapy since the early 1900s little serious interest in the study of our ever-changing stream of consciousness (Singer & Pope, 1978). Although Freud and other psychoanalysts drew our attention to primary process thinking, they were primarily interested in uncovering the ways in which nonverbal, irrational, wishful, childlike, fantasy-laden material intrudes into adult mental life to bring about maladaptive, self-defeating behavior and other aspects of psychopathology. Freud and many other psychoanalysts appeared to be saying that a well-analyzed adult would rely primarily on secondary process thinking and avoid primary process thinking as much as possible. Within such a framework, there was little room for the adaptive, pleasurable, creative, and therapeutic qualities of imagery-laden mentation. Instead, the value of goal-directed logical thinking was greatly underscored; and psychologists, psychiatrists, and psychotherapists developed a bias toward the use of verbal, linear thought which continues to the present.

Fortunately, since the mid-1960s this one-sidedness is gradually being counterbalanced. Aspects of the stream of consciousness have become legitimate areas of scientific research (Singer, 1966). A new appreciation for the role of imaginal processes in learning (Pavio, 1971), memory (Pavio, 1971), and perception (Segal, 1971) has developed. The clinical implications of imaginal processes have become increasingly recognized (Schwartz, 1973, Singer, 1971; Singer & Pope, 1978) and numerous imagery techniques now are being used in the treatment of various medical and psychiatric disorders (Beck, 1967; Blatt, 1974; Decker, Cline-Eisen, & Gallagher, 1992; Green, 1981; Grinder & Bandler, 1976; Schwartz, 1973; Simonton & Simonton, 1975; Singer & Pope, 1978; Van Dyck, Zitman, Corry, Linssen, & Spinhoven, 1991).

This chapter examines the major scientific models of depression and their respective treatment approaches. Then an in-depth review of systematic research regarding the psychotherapeutic use of imagery in alleviating depression is presented, and the author offers some suggestions for future research in this area. He then turns to a brief review of related research on depression and imagery and concludes with a theoretical discussion of the cognitive-affective aspects of an organismic, general systems, developmental paradigm of depressive experience.

DEPRESSION

Depression is a negative affective state which is an almost universal human phenomenon. It is characterized by feelings of despondency, despair, disinterest, and boredom and by attitudes of remorse, regret, self-blame, hopelessness, and helplessness (Beck, 1967). However, due in part to its common and frequent occurrence, a variety of definitions of depression have been proposed, and the concept has been applied to a wide range of phenomena including: 1) a temporary mood state experienced by all individuals; 2) an acute psychological disorder; and 3) a chronic character disorder. While similar in some ways, these three phenomena vary along dimensions of intensity, duration, and degree of reality distortion. Therefore, to avoid confusion, depression is herein defined as a negative affective state which can vary in intensity from relatively mild to severe and from a subtle, transitory experience to a profoundly disabling psychiatric disorder (Blatt, 1974). Furthermore, depression can represent a relatively appropriate response to an accurate appraisal of reality or it can be based on marked distortions of reality.

Theories of Depression

Widespread differences in the classification of depressive disorders may reflect the fact that psychiatric syndromes have been conceptualized historically according to "specialized frames of reference that largely depend on the training and indoctrination of the clinician or researcher" (Akiskal & McKinney, 1975, p. 275). Although the development and use of the Diagnostic and Statistical Manual IV (DSM-IV, 1994) criteria for classifying psychiatric dysfunction are positive steps toward unifying clinical and research efforts nationally and internationally, different theories of depression (and of other psychiatric disorders) are likely to prevail until clinicians and researchers utilize a holistic conceptualization of the human being to develop a more comprehensive, interdisciplinary approach to the study of well-defined psychiatric phenomena.

Currently, there are several major theories of depression: biological (physiological factors), biochemical (changes in neurotransmitters), psychoanalytic (traumatic early life experiences), cognitive (cognitive distortions of self and others), behavioral (learned helplessness), and existential (current loss of meaning). Akiskal and McKinney (1975) focused on ten different models of depression which they considered to reflect five dominant "schools of thought" as indicated in Table 1.

Akiskal and McKinney (1973, 1975) recognized the need for striving toward a more unified theory of depression and, therefore, developed an hypothesis which integrates more fully these various clinical models. Briefly, the depressive syndrome is viewed as the psychobiological common pathway of various social, psychological, and biological processes which result on a physical level in reversible dysfunction of the diencephalic mechanisms of reinforcement. The major advance introduced by their approach is the conceptualization of depression at several different levels simultaneously, which replaces the focus on a one-to-one relationship with a single event on a biological, a psychological, or a social level. Perhaps without fully recognizing it, Akiskal and McKinney took a

Table 1. Ten Models of Depression[a]

School	Model	Mechanism
Psychoanalytic	Aggression-turned-inward	Conversion of aggression instinct into depressive affect.
	Object loss	Separation: Disruption of an attachment bond.
	Loss of self-esteem	Helplessness in attaining goals of ego-ideal.
	Negative cognitive set	Hopelessness.
Behavioral	Learned helplessness	Uncontrollable aversive stimulation.
	Loss of reinforcement	Rewards of "sick role" substitute for lost sources of reinforcement.
Sociological	Sociological	Loss of role status.
Existential	Existential	Loss of meaning of existence.
Biological	Biogenic amine	Impaired monaminergic transmission.
	Neurophysiological	Hyperarousal secondary to intraneuronal sodium accumulation; Cholinergic dominance; Reversible functional derangement of diencephalic mechanism of reinforcement.

[a]Akiskal and McKinney (1975, p. 296).

346 / HEALING IMAGES

major step toward a biopsychosocial model of depression implicitly based upon general systems theory (von Bertanlanffy, 1968). It is just such a biopsychosocial model of psychiatric disorder based explicitly on general systems theory which Greenberg (1979), Gross (1981), and Schultz (1982) have found particularly useful in the diagnosis and treatment of a broad spectrum of psychiatric disorders (see Figure 1). More recently, the work of Whitehead (1969), Jordan and Streets (1973, 1978), and Bondra (1998) have contributed the development of an organismic, general systems paradigm (Schultz, 1999) useful in establishing a comprehensive understanding of the individual human being and how change, including psychopathology, occurs throughout the developmental lifespan.

Treatment of Depression

Consonant with the various theories of depression are the different approaches in the treatment of depression. Each theoretical framework has given rise to its own therapeutic modalities which unfortunately have tended to be competitive rather than complementary. Treatments range from psychoanalysis to behavior therapy and from sociopolitical activism to pharmacotherapy and electroconvulsive therapy (ECT). Since the psychotherapeutic interventions represent the major focus of this chapter, only a very brief review of these other treatment approaches will be presented here. A more detailed discussion is available elsewhere (Beck, 1967; Gallant & Simpson, 1975; Levitt & Lubin, 1975).

Biological and biochemical theories of depression have contributed to the development of various *somatic treatments,* including insulin shock therapy, ECT, and pharmacotherapy. The effectiveness of the major antidepressant medications, particularly the tricyclics, the monoamine oxidase (MAO) inhibitors, and the selective seritonin re-uptake inhibitors (SSRI), has become so well-established that insulin shock therapy is no longer used and ECT has become for many biological psychiatrists the final treatment of choice. In addition, the value of activity therapy, aerobic exercises, and running as well as light therapy and a variety of movement therapies (e.g., dance, eurythmy, etc.) in both alleviation and preventing depression is increasingly recognized. While clinical experience supports the usefulness of these approaches, a review of systematic research in this promising therapeutic area goes beyond the scope of this chapter.

Sociological and interpersonal theories of depression have contributed to *sociopolitical activism.* It aims at rectifying inequities in the social system which contribute to depression by depriving various individuals (e.g., Native Americans, African Americans, Hispanics, other ethnic minorities, women, and the elderly) of certain roles and/or freedom of choice in pursuing their interests and developing their talents. Other major *interpersonal interventions* in the treatment of depression group therapy and family group therapy clearly have an interpersonal component, they originally arose due to a shortage of clinicians and have only gradually developed their potential along with marital and family systems therapy,

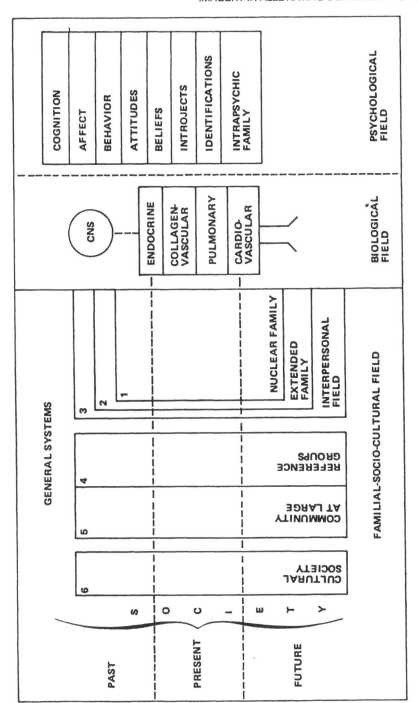

Figure 1. General systems of the biopsychosocial model. (Figure represents modifications of Greenberg's basic model [1979].)

as relationship and social system therapies. Furthermore, although considerable clinical information is available regarding the usefulness of group therapy, marital therapy, family therapy, and family group therapy in the treatment of depression and other psychiatric disorders (Gurman, 1981; Jacobson & Margolin, 1979; Wolberg & Aronson, 1980, 1981), little systematic research exists which focuses on reducing depression by resolving interpersonal conflict through either group, marital, family, or family group therapy.

Psychological theories of depression have contributed to the development of various *psychotherapeutic approaches* toward the treatment of depression. Psychotherapeutic treatment of depression ranges from minimal, once-a-month *supportive psychotherapy* to intensive, five-times-a-week *psychoanalysis.* Such treatment can range in duration from brief, time-limited psychotherapy lasting several weeks or a few months to long-term psychoanalytic psychotherapy and psychoanalysis lasting five to ten years or more. While supportive therapy aims at maintaining the individual's level of functioning and preventing further relapse, psychoanalytic treatment is geared toward major personality reorganization. The former often focuses upon crisis intervention and upon helping the individual to develop improved coping mechanisms, while the latter usually holds out the hope of a "total cure."

Dynamic, Insight-Oriented Psychotherapy. This therapy offers a more moderate alternative to both brief supportive psychotherapy and intensive psychoanalytic treatment. Like psychoanalysis, it usually involves the exploration of complex historical patterns of behavior stemming from early life experiences and it emphasizes the usefulness of insight to improvement. While there is considerable controversy regarding the efficacy of insight and the usefulness of traditional psychotherapy regardless of orientation, the fact that most traditional dynamic psychotherapies are limited to those who are more affluent, intelligent, relatively stable, and able to tolerate considerable frustration from extended periods of time lead many clinicians to explore other types of psychotherapeutic treatment for patients suffering from depression as well as other psychiatric disorders.

Behavior Therapy. This treatment of depression is based upon the theory that specific maladaptive behaviors need to be altered to restore the depressed person to a healthier level of functioning. Such interventions as assertiveness training, skills acquisition training, social skills training, parent effectiveness, sex therapy, marital therapy, role modeling, and psychodrama have been utilized in various behavioral therapy approaches to the treatment of depression with reasonably good results (Kovacs, 1979; McLean & Hakstian, 1979; Rehm, 1981).

Cognitive Psychotherapy. This psychotherapy combines the specificity of behavior therapy with the dynamic aspects of more traditional psychotherapies. Cognitive psychotherapy as a treatment of depression is based upon the theory that the depressed or depression-prone individual maintains certain unconscious idiosyncratic cognitive patterns which may become activated and/or intensified by specific stresses impinging on specific areas of vulnerability or by overwhelming, nonspecific stresses (Beck, 1967; Beck, Rush, Shaw, & Emery, 1979; Miller, Klee, & Norman, 1982; Paykel et al., 1969). Beck (1967) hypothesized the use of a cognitive psychotherapeutic approach geared toward helping the patient to gain "objectivity toward his automatic reactions and counteract them." The person's cognitive patterns (whether they are verbal or pictorial "events" in his/her stream of consciousness) are conceptualized as being based upon attitudes and assumptions (cognitive schemas) developed from pervious experiences (Beck et al., 1979). Beck regards the therapy as designed to modify these idiosyncratic cognitive patterns, thereby reducing the person's vulnerability to further depressions. Briefly, the major aspects of this approach include: 1) delineating the major maladaptive depressive patterns; 2) pinpointing the depressive cognitions; 3) examining, reality testing, and neutralizing "automatic" thoughts and images; 4) identifying idiosyncratic content; 5) distinguishing "ideas" from "facts"; and 6) weighing alternative explanation. Thus, cognitive psychotherapy of depression provides an active, directive, structured treatment approach which is time limited.

Beck (1967) reported that he has found cognitive psychotherapy to be effective during the depressed phase in mild reactive depression, but he recommended that its major application occurs during the post-depressed period, particularly for endogenous depression and reactive depression of a moderate to severe degree. He emphasized that during the post-depressed period, although the person may be feeling "blue," he/she is functioning well enough to examine objectively personal life patterns, automatic thoughts and images, and basis assumption and misconceptions. Thus, implicit in Beck's thinking is the importance of avoiding a one-sided uni-dimensional approach to the treatment of depression. The reader is, therefore, once again reminded not only of the value of the multi-dimensional organismic, general systems paradigm (Schultz, 1999; von Bertanlanffy, 1968) to the diagnosis and treatment of dysfunction but also of the importance of integrating various treatment approaches, especially complementing the more verbal aspects of various psychotherapies with nonverbal (Singer & Pope, 1978) and metaphor techniques (Witztum, Van Der Hart, & Friedman, 1988).

IMAGERY AND FANTASY TECHNIQUES IN PSYCHOTHERAPY

Historical Review

The psychotherapeutic uses of imagery can be divided according to several "schools of thought" (see review by Singer, 1974). The use of imagery techniques in *classical psychoanalysis* dates back to Freud's (Breuer & Freud, 1955) initial reliance on induced imagery in hypnotic abreaction with hysterical patients. However, after Freud abandoned induced imagery for an increased focus on verbal free associations, imagery remained important in psychoanalysis only in the re-experiencing of dream material and in the emergence of transference phenomena. More recently, however, Reyher (1963, 1978) has emphasized the usefulness of an imagery free association method in enhancing affective expression. In contrast to the implicit utilization of imagery in classical psychoanalytic work, the non-Freudian *European school of psychoanalysis* was greatly influenced by Jung (1968) and his explicit emphasis on "active imagination" in dream interpretation. After Jung, the development of mental imagery techniques in Europe was furthered by Desoille's (1938) guided daydream technique, Frétigny and Virel's (1968) "oneirodrama," and Leuner's (1969) "guided affective imagery technique." The *nonpsychoanalytic psychotherapeutic* uses of imagery in the United States include psychodrama (Moreno, 1967), transactional analysis (Berne, 1964), Gestalt therapy (Perls, 1970), the personal growth movement (Lewis & Streitfield, 1971), and psychosynthesis (Assagioli, 1965; Gerard, 1964). Finally, the psychotherapeutic use of imagery has become an integral part of various *behavior modification techniques* including systematic desensitization (Wolpe & Lazarus, 1966), positive imagery in the treatment of peptic ulcer patients (Chapell & Stevenson, 1936), noxious imagery in covert aversive therapy (Cautella & McCullough, 1978), Symbolic modeling (Bandura, 1971), Bonny's (1978a,b 1995) guided imagery and music, Lazarus' (1989) multi-modal therapy, Meichenbaum's (1975) self-regulatory techniques, and Stampfl's (Stampfl & Lewis, 1967) implosive therapy.

There currently exists, then, an ever-growing body of literature with a lengthy historical tradition indicating that induced imagery techniques play an important role in behavior change (Singer, 1974). During the 1970s a variety of publications emerged which reported the use of visual imagery in relaxation techniques for childbirth (Read, 1953), in the voluntary control of heart rate (Schwartz, et al., 1978), in improving athletic performance, in the treatment of cancer (Simonton & Simonton, 1975), in a group-oriented psychiatric treatment program (Starker, Levine, & Watstein, 1974), in the treatment of parent-child conflict (Green, 1981), and in the treatment of serious child abuse (Grinder & Bandler, 1976).

Beck (1967, 1976) and Lazarus (1968, 1977) were instrumental in identifying the use of both spontaneous and directed imagery in the treatment of various clinical disorders including depression. Although the use of cognitive therapy including imagery techniques was extended by Beck (1991) and later by Judith Beck (1995) to a broad spectrum of specific clinical, substance abuse, and personality disorders, the systematic effort to evaluate the effects of particular imagery techniques on the mood and general clinical condition of patients representative of a specific psychiatric syndrome began to emerge in the late-1970s.

Current Uses of Imagery in Alleviatin Depression

Velton (1968) and Schwartz (Schwartz, Fair, Salt, Mandel, & Klerman, 1976; Sirota & Schwartz, 1982) provided exciting evidence indicating that different affective states can be induced systematically and altered through various imagery procedures. Schultz (1976, 1978) narrowed the field of investigation to a specific affective disorder (i.e., depression) and reviewed the use of imagery in its treatment. He suggested that directed imagery might either distract the depressed person from his/her depressed affective state and/or help him/her to contact and discharge suppressed affect, which would lead to a reduction in underlying conflict and a corresponding decrease in level of depression. In view of the fact that the study of imaginal processes previously had focused primarily on non-patient populations and that the use of imagery in the treatment of depression had not yet been systematically evaluated, Schultz (1976, 1978) conducted a study designed to investigate the immediate changes in the affective state of depressed psychiatric patients in response to specific imagery content. The short-term and longer-term changes in level of depression as a result of imagery therapy were subsequently investigated and will be reviewed later.

Immediate Changes. Schultz (1976, 1978) studied the immediate changes in level of depression of 60 depressed male psychiatric patients who experienced a brief induction procedure of either aggressive, socially gratifying, positive, or free imagery. Each patient was seen individually within the first week after the beginning of psychiatric treatment and was encouraged to regard the use of imagery as a skill which can be learned. After being instructed to get as comfortable as possible, he was asked to close his eyes or to focus his gaze at a point. The patient was then instructed to follow one of the four imagery procedures by visualizing the entire experience in his "mind's eye" in as much detail as possible. The *aggressive imagery* procedure directed the patient to recall someone saying/doing something which angered him. In the *socially gratifying imagery* procedure the patient was instructed to recall someone saying/doing something which made him feel very pleased. The *positive imagery* procedure requested the patient to recall a place in nature he used to visit in order to relax. In the *free imagery* procedure the patient was instructed to report all images, thought, fantasies, and ideas which occurred to him without consciously trying to direct his stream of consciousness. After participating in the imagery induction procedure which last about 10 minutes, each patient was instructed to complete a series of cognitive, affective, and perceptual measures which have been shown to be related to one's level of depression.

Findings indicated that : 1) directed imagery (*aggressive, socially gratifying, and positive*) produced significantly lower levels of depression than *free imagery*;

and 2) more socially oriented imagery (*aggressive* highest, *socially gratifying* second, *positive* third, and *free* lowest[1]) produced significantly lower levels of depression than less socially oriented imagery. Furthermore, particular types of depressives responded differently to the various imagery contents: 1) those patients whose depression was characterized by themes of dependency achieved lower levels of depression after aggressive and socially gratifying imagery; 2) those patients whose depression centered around self-criticism attained lower levels of depression after socially gratifying and positive imagery; and 3) those depressives who experienced considerable guilty dysphoric themes in their daydreaming showed more signs of depression after positive imagery. Clearly, not only did directed and socially oriented imagery serve to reduce the level of depression but also different types of depressed patients improve more after some directed imagery contents than after others.

In a somewhat related study, Burtle (1976) investigated the immediate changes in level of depression of eight depressed patients (with psychomotor retardation) who experienced either *positive imagery training* or *relaxation training*. Those depressives in the positive imagery training experienced a three-stage procedure which included perceptual training using Thematic Apperception Test (TAT) cards, relaxation training with practice in imaging TAT cards, and a period of making self-generated positive changes in the TAT images. Those depressives who experienced positive imagery training showed lower levels of depression than those who experienced relaxation training only and a considerable increase in imagery production.

The findings from these two studies indicated that different types of directed imagery can help seriously depressed people to reduce their level of depression for a brief period of time and that different types of depressives are likely to improve more after experiencing some directed imagery contents than after others. However, the question whether directed imagery could produce positive changes in level of depression which would persist for a more extended period of time required further investigation.

Immediate, Intermediate, and Longer-Term Changes. Extending the work of Schultz (1976, 1978), Jarvinen and Gold (1981) studied the immediate and longer-term changes in level of depression of 53 mildly to moderately depressed female undergraduate students who practiced either neutral, positive, or self-generated positive imagery or who were assigned to a no-treatment control condition. Those students in the *neutral* or *positive imagery* group were given five neutral scenes and five positive scenes, respectively, which they were asked to visualize throughout the day and picture at least twice daily. Each student in the *self-generated positive imagery* condition generated five positive scenes (which

---

[1] This ordering along a continuum of social involvement was determined on the basis of the patients' behavior during the various imagery sessions (Schultz, 1976, 1978).

matched the scenes in the positive imagery condition) and these students where asked to visualize these five scenes throughout the day and to picture them at least twice daily. The students in the *no-treatment control* condition were given no scenes to practice. All students were asked to make daily mood ratings for a two-week period.

After two weeks, the students in the three imagery conditions reported lower levels of depression, as measured by the Beck (1967) Depressive Inventory, than the students in the no-treatment condition. Gold, Jarvinen, and Teague (1982) subsequently found that more vivid imagery produced greater therapeutic benefit. Jarvinen and Gold (1981) further reported lower levels of depression on the Zung (1965) Self-Rating Depression Scale and higher mood ratings, but these findings did not reach significance. Six months later, the 31 students who responded to a follow-up questionnaire reported no significant differences in level of depression. Nevertheless, of the 21 students in the three *imagery* conditions, 57 percent reported noticing a change in mood as a result of the study; whereas, of the eight students in the no-treatment condition, only 13 percent reported noticing such a change. Sixty-two percent of the students in the *imagery* conditions also reported that they were applying what they had learned through the study, but only 38 percent of those in the *no-treatment* condition reported so doing. Thus, while the initial changes in level of depression as a result of practicing directed imagery for a two-week period are quite promising, the degree of benefit appeared to diminish gradually over time. Such a finding in a 6-month follow-up study is not surprising. What is indeed impressive and encouraging, however, is that mildly depressed students are likely to report noticing a change in mood even six months after experiencing a two week directed imagery practice period.

Subsequent research explored the capacity for older adults to utilize imagery. Hamm and King (1984) found that geriatric patients who utilized visual imagery as a pain control technique reported a decrease in self-perceived pain. Casler (1985) demonstrated that nursing home residents who were given positive verbal instructions about health and longevity lived four times longer than matched control subjects. Giray, Roodin, Altkin, Flagg, and Yoon (1985) determined that adults between the ages of 60 and 94 were able to produce *eidetic imagery* at a significantly higher frequency than younger adults and were equally as capable as 5- to 7-year-old children. Leja (1989) utilized *guided imagery* to combat post-surgical depression in older adults and found that when compared to controls those utilizing *guided imagery* reported a significant decrease in depression immediately following the intervention. The findings, however, were limited by the fact that the number of subjects in each condition was small ($N = 10$) and the effect did not persist after discharge from the hospital.

DeBerry, Davis, and Reinhard (1989) provided either *relaxation-meditation imagery, cognitive-behavioral therapy,* or *pseudo-treatment* to 65- to 75-year-olds who indicated complaints of anxiety and depression but who did not evidence any major affective disorder or major medical illnesses and did not receive psychotropic medication. All treatment was provided in groups which met for 45 minutes twice a week for 12 weeks. Although those practicing meditation-relaxation imagery reported a significant reduction from pre- to post-treatment state anxiety, positive clinical trends indicated that significant reductions in depression and anxiety may have occurred if group treatment had continued for a total of 24 weeks.

The potential benefit of *cognitive-behavioral, focused visual imagery,* and *education discussion* group therapy on cognition, depression, hopelessness, and dissatisfaction with life among depressed nursing home residents was evaluated by Abraham, Neundorfer, and Currie (1992). Self-report measures were completed serially on four occasions: 4 weeks prior to treatment, 8 weeks after the beginning of treatment, 20 weeks after treatment initiation, and 4 weeks after termination of treatment. Findings indicated no significant changes in level of depression, hopelessness, or life satisfaction for any of the treatment conditions. Nevertheless, the cognitive performance of those receiving either cognitive-behavioral or visual-imagery group therapy improved after 8 weeks of treatment and persisted through 20 weeks of treatment and 4 weeks following the end of treatment, with those in the visual imagery group demonstrating greater improvement. Although cognitive-behavior and visual imagery group therapy may not be effective in reducing levels of depression among multiply-impaired, institutionalized older adults, the improvement in cognition underscores the importance of focused cognitive and visual imagery stimulation for institutionalized elderly who are generally intact to mildly impaired cognitively.

An earlier study by Watts, McLeod, and Morris (1988) evaluated the short-term effects of a *focused imagery formation* technique versus *relaxation training* versus *simple concentration instructions* on post-intervention measures of memory, number of lapses in concentration, and ratings of a series of concentration problems. Findings indicated that the focused visual imagery formation technique subsequently improved objective memory for a passage of prose especially for non-endogenously depressed non-elderly adults. Although no comparable effects, however, were noted on subjective measures, adults with lower state anxiety evidenced the fewest lapses of concentration after the imagery procedure. Thus, the findings of Abraham et al. (1992) and Watts et al. (1988) remain encouraging and are consistent with earlier findings of some benefit in using *imagery strategies* to improve the memory performance of anxious subjects (Edmundson & Nelson, 1976), neurological patients (Powell, 1981), and the elderly (Kausler, 1982).

Although not designed to study imagery approaches in the treatment of clinical depression, several studies have explored the efficacy of imagery-related interventions in the treatment of a variety of medical and/or psychological disorders and related emotional sequelae. Neidhardt, Krakow, Kellner, and Pathak (1992) provided adults who suffered from chronic nightmares with either a month period of *nightmare recording only* or *nightmare recording followed by a brief imagery rehearsal technique training session* to treat their nightmares. The 4-step imagery technique focused on consciously changing the nightmare followed by rehearsal of the changed version at least once daily for three days and repeating the process as necessary. Nightmare frequency and symptom distress scales were completed prior to the month-long treatment intervention process and three months after the completion of the intervention period. Although nightmare frequency decreased in both treatment groups, the imagery rehearsal procedure resulted in not only a more significant decrease in nightmare frequency but also significant decreases in anxiety, depression, hostility, somatization, and overall distress.

In a related study VanDyck, Zitman, Linssen, and Spinhoven (1991) investigated the effect of a 4-session 7-week treatment period of *autogenic training* or *future-oriented, reduced-pain hypnotic imagery* on the treatment of tension headache sufferers. Pre- and post-treatment measures indicated a reduction in headache intensity, pain medication, state anxiety, and depression in both treatment conditions. Further analyses indicated that depth of relaxation, degree of imagery skills, and hypnotizability were associated with lower headache ratings at post-treatment regardless of treatment condition.

Although a previous report (Auerbach, Oleson, & Solomon, 1992) indicated that a variety of cognitive-behavioral interventions were ineffective in reducing depression among individuals diagnosed with AIDS or ARC, Eller (1995) investigated the effect of a 6-week treatment period of daily practiced *guided imagery* or daily practiced *progressive muscle relaxation (PMR)* versus *standard medical treatment only* for HIV seropositive individuals blocked by illness stage. Pre- and post-treatment measures of fatigue, depression, and cellular immunity indicated that guided imagery produced a significant decrease in depression and fatigue whereas PMR resulted in a reduction in depression and an increase in CD4+ T-lymphocyte count.

Propst (1980a,b) studied the immediate and intermediate changes in level of depression of 33 female and 11 male mildly depressed undergraduate students who scored moderately high on a religiosity scale. Interested in systematically investigating the use of religious imagery reported in the Bible (1953) and by various Christian counselors (McNutt, 1974; Peale, 1982; Scanlon, 1974), Propst assigned each depressed religious student to one of the four following treatment conditions: *nonreligious imagery, religious imagery, self-monitoring plus nondirective discussion*, and *self-monitoring only*. Each student showed a mildly depressed mood for a baseline period of two weeks and then experienced two one-hour group therapy sessions per week for a four-week period (for a total of eight group therapy sessions).[2] Those students in the *nonreligious imagery* group

---

[2] Therapists were one first- and one second-year graduate students. Neither was religious and both reported feeling less comfortable though not antagonist to the religious treatment.

were asked to relive their depressive episodes, to describe their accompanying images, and to develop an awareness of their depression-engendering images. They also were instructed to record their moods and accompanying mental images five times daily between sessions as added self-awareness practice. Usually in Session 3, students were given a list of coping statements and images directed toward modifying the three components of Beck's (1976) cognitive triad of depression (negative self, environment, and future), and they were instructed to select statements and images from this list to reduce their depression. The students then relived their depressive images and attempted to modify them using their selected coping imagery and statements. Students in the *religious imagery* group followed an identical procedure except that a list of religious images and coping statements were used in modifying their depressive images (e.g., "I can visualize Christ going with me into that difficult situation in the future as I try to cope"). Students in the *self-monitoring plus nondirective discussion* group were permitted to discuss whatever they wanted with little therapist intervention, were asked to keep track of their daily mood, and were given homework which consisted of recording items for group discussion on their mood cards. Students in the *self-monitoring only* condition were informed that they were in a control condition, a very important part of the project, and were asked to fill out daily mood cards.

Findings indicated that: 1) students who experienced either religious imagery or self-monitoring plus nondirective discussion reduced their level of depression as compared to those who experienced self-monitoring only; 2) only 14 percent of the students who had experienced religious imagery still scored in the depressed range as compared with 60 percent of the nonreligious imagery and 69 percent of the self-monitoring only condition[3]; and 3) students who experienced religious imagery also showed a greater increase in group interaction than the students in the other conditions. Furthermore, a 6-week follow-up study indicated that students who experienced religious imagery continued to show a trend ($p < .10$) toward decreased global psychopathology and decreased depression as compared to students in the other conditions. Unfortunately, there was no longer any significant difference among the four conditions in the proportion of students who still scored in the depressed range or in the degree of group interaction.

Thus, similar to the finding reported by Jarvinen and Gold (1981), mildly depressed students are able to reduce their level of depression through participating in an 8-session directed imagery therapy group for a 4-week duration, but the degree of benefit appears to diminish gradually over a 6-week period following the end of treatment. Of particular interest in the Propst (1980a,b) study are two additional factors. First, the reduction in level of depression as a result of directed

---

[3] Twenty-seven percent of those students in the self-monitoring plus nondirective discussion group still scored in the depressed range.

imagery therapy was indicated by behavioral as well as self-report indices of depression, thus minimizing the likelihood that demand characteristics produced the decrease in depression. Second, and even more important, is the fact that Propst demonstrated the increased therapeutic efficacy of imagery which is geared specifically to the individual's value system.

A somewhat related but more recent study (Richards, Owen, & Stein, 1993) evaluated a group counseling intervention emphasizing *religious-spiritual psycho-education and religious imagery* for the treatment of self-defeating perfectionism among devout Mormon college students. A total of 15 students completed an 8-week counseling group which provided three major treatment components: 1) discussion of the relationship between religious beliefs and perfectionism using an adaptation of concepts from Propst's Cognitive Therapy Mediation Manual (1980c); 2) assigned reading followed by group discussion of several religious bibliotherapy articles which emphasized acceptance in spite of imperfections, forgiveness, grace, Christ's atonement, and the lifelong process of spiritual growth; and 3) the use of religious imagery (Propst, 1980a,b) in relaxation exercises conducted in the last portion of two group counseling sessions. Pre- and post-treatment measures of perfectionism, depression, self-esteem, existential well-being, and spiritual well-being, and very significant increase in self-esteem with a trend ($p = .063$) toward an increase in religious well-being. Although these findings are quite positive and encouraging, the lack of an intervention control group and the attrition of six clients who did not complete the intervention and post-treatment measures leave unclarified which aspects of the group counseling intervention were most effective and whether clients who dropped out prematurely were not benefiting from the intervention, were spontaneously feeling better, or left for some other reason.

Interested in the differential effectiveness of various aspects of Ellis' (1973) Rational Emotive Therapy (RET), Lipsky, Kassinove, and Miller (1980) investigated the immediate post-treatment changes in level of anxiety, depression, hostility, and neuroticism among 37 female and 13 male mental health clinic patients. All patients were diagnosed as neurotic or suffering from adjustment reaction of adulthood, and they were assigned to one of five treatment conditions which were then divided into high and low IQ groups. Patients in the *Rational Emotive Therapy (RET)* condition were taught the basic principles of RET and how to use these principles to cope with emotional upsets which brought about the need for treatment. These patients also were given a minimum of 12 ABC statements to analyze, were taught the 11 irrational ideas postulated by Ellis (1973), and were given bibliotherapy and behavioral homework assignments when appropriate. Patients in the *RET plus Rational Role Reversal (RRR)* condition were treated similarly to those in the RET condition but they also were given one RRR exercise consisted of the therapist and patient reversing roles for 15 minutes. At the end of the 12-week treatment period, each patient had participated in 10 RRRs. Patients in the *RET plus Rational-Emotive Imagery (REI)* condition were treated similarly to those in the RET condition, but they also were given one REI scene per therapy session. Each REI scene lasted approximately 15 minutes; during period the patient imagined a disturbing event to which he/she usually responded with an irrational thought and excessive emotion. H/she then imagined responding with rational thoughts which led to the experience of a new feeling which was less negative, excessive, and counterproductive. At the end of the 12-week treatment period, each patient had participated in 10 REI scenes. Patients in the *alternate treatment (AT)* control condition received a combination of supportive therapy and deep muscle relaxation training. Relaxation training exercises began with the third treatment session an lasted for approximately 20 minutes each session. At the end of the 12-week treatment period each patient had received 2 sessions of supportive therapy and 10 sessions of combined supportive therapy and relaxation training. Patients in the *no contact (NC)* control condition were informed that they had been placed on a treatment waiting list. Patients in the three RET conditions and the AT condition met individually with one of two experienced therapists[4] for a 45-minute therapy session once per week for total of 12 weeks. Patients in all five conditions were administered the dependent measures immediately before and after the 12-week period. Both therapists were blind to the patients' pre-treatment scores and remained so throughout the entire study.

Findings indicated that: 1) patients who participated in any of the three RET treatment conditions reported more RET content acquisition, less depression, and less neuroticism than those in the AT and NC conditions; and 2) patients in the RET plus RRR and RET plus REI conditions reported lower state anxiety than those in the AT and NC conditions and lower trait anxiety than those is the RET, AT, and NC conditions. Also of particular interest is the finding that although high and low IQ patients acquired the principles and concepts of RET equally well, they responded differently to some of the treatment conditions: 1) low IQ patients reported lower depression than high IQ patients regardless of treatment modality; 2) high IQ patients in the RET plus REI conditions reported less trait anxiety than low IQ patients in the same condition; and 3) low IQ patients in the AT condition reported less trait anxiety than high IQ patients in the same condition. Thus, once again, the use of directed imagery in therapy is demonstrated not only to be very effective in reducing depression but also to be particularly helpful in enhancing the therapeutic benefit of more purely verbal psychotherapeutic approaches. Also, of particular interest is the fact that although IQ does not seem to be a major factor affecting therapeutic benefit in this study, there is sufficient evidence to indicate the importance of balancing IQ across different treatment conditions.

---

[4] Each therapist had more than two years of training and supervised clinical experience in RET and behavior therapy. Both reported being equally committed to behavior therapy and RET.

A related study by Reardon and Tossi (1977) investigated the immediate post-treatment effects and intermediate follow-up changes in self-concept and level of depression of 32 adolescent delinquent females who had experienced on the following five conditions: 1) *Rational State Directed Imagery (RSDI)*[5]; 2) a *cognitive behavioral treatment* approach which utilized vivid emotive imagery and intensive muscle relaxation; 3) a *cognitive treatment* utilizing rational re-structuring; 4) a *placebo treatment*; or 5) *no treatment*. All patients in the four treatment conditions met one hour per week in their respective groups for six consecutive weeks during which time homework assignments also were utilized. At the end of six weeks, self report measures of self-concept and level of depression were obtained for patients in all five conditions.

Findings indicated that: 1) patients who had participated in the RSDI group reported a higher self-concept and a lower level of depression than patients in the remaining four conditions; and 2) patients who had participated in the cognitive rational restructuring group reported somewhat similar improvement. A 2-month follow-up study, however, indicated that only those patients in the RSDI group still reported higher self-concept and lower depression. Thus, directed-imagery therapy can be useful not only in reducing level of depression but also in improving deficiencies in more global aspects of personality, such as self-concept and self-esteem, which are often characteristic of more chronic depressive disorders. Furthermore, it is encouraging that such gains can be maintained for at least two months after the cessation of a relatively brief six-week treatment period.

Taken together, the studies by Lipsky et al. (1980) and Reardon and Tossi (1977) offer encouraging evidence for the usefulness of imagery therapy in the treatment of patients whose difficulties include but are not limited to symptoms of depression. Of particular interest is the finding that therapeutic modalities which integrate nonverbal imagery techniques with verbal approaches appear to produce more extensive and long-lasting improvements, including lowered depression, less neuroticism, and improved self-concept. A related intervention study which has been recognized as helping people identify and explore less accessible emotional experience utilizes music-guided imagery. A specific music psychotherapy approach developed by Bonny (1978a,b), Guided Imagery and Music (GIM), combines specific classical music (as a catalyst to unfold imagery and related inner experience to access significant emotional concerns) with an ongoing dialogue between therapist and client to provide grounding, focus, conscious working through, and eventual resolutions (Goldberg, 1995).

[5] RSDI is a synthesis of sensory imagery, deep relaxation or hypnosis, and rational or cognitive restructuring which also includes the use of directed imagery to bring the patient through various developmental states (e.g., increased awareness of self and environment, re-experiencing through imagery of real life situations, etc.). It, therefore, has much in common with the previous RET plus REI condition (Lipsky et al., 1980).

Several proponents have reported that this dynamic process has helped people integrated previously disconnected aspects of self (Clark, 1991; Weiss, 1994), develop insight and cognitive-emotional reorganization (Blake, 1994), and contribute to a renewal of meaning and purpose (Wrangsjo & Korlin, 1995). A variety of case studies reported the use of GIM in the treatment of individuals with such diverse diagnoses as multiple personality disorder (Picket, 1991a; Picket & Sonnen, 1993), PTSD (Blake, 1994; Blake & Bishop, 1995), the co-occurrence of depression and substance abuse (Picket, 1991b), and individuals recovering from physical, emotional, and/or sexual abuse (Borling, 1992; Rinker, 1991; Tasney, 1993; Ventre, 1995). Others have reported the use of GIM for a variety of medical conditions including pregnancy (Short, 1993), AIDS (Bruscia, 1991), uterine fibroid tumors (Picket, 1987), and individuals recovering from mastectomy (Hale, 1992).

Encouraged by these promising case reports, several researchers have more recently developed more controlled studies of the treatment effects of GIM. For example, Wrangsjo and Korlin (1995) found that 14 individuals who sought GIM therapy reported a significant pre- versus post-session decrease in both depression and total distress whereas Jacobi (1994) reported that a series of 10 individual GIM significantly reduced depression and arthritis symptoms for 27 rheumatoid arthritis patients. McKinney, Antoni, Kumar, and Kumar (1995) also noted that generally healthy individuals experienced a significant decrease in depressed mood after a series of six individual GIM sessions. Music with imagery suggestions was reported by Rider, Floyd, and Kirkpatrick (1985) to have a significant positive effect on urinary corticosteroids in nurses working the night or alternate day and evening shifts. A series of six weekly GIM sessions was found by McDonald (1990) to be effective in decreasing both systolic and diastolic blood pressure of unmedicated hypertension patients whereas the blood pressure of those participating in the 6-session verbal psychotherapy and no-treatment control conditions was unchanged. McKinney, Tims, Kumar, and Kumar (1997) also found individuals who participated in a single group music imagery session demonstrated decreased plasma beta-endorphin levels, whereas those who listened to music without imagery suggestion, those who imaged in silence, and those in the no-treatment condition evidenced unchanged beta-endorphin levels. A second study by McKinney, Antoni, Kumar, Tims, and McCabe (1997) investigated the effects of GIM on mood and cortisol in generally healthy adults. A series of six individual GIM sessions every two weeks significantly lowered pre- versus post-treatment measures of depressed mood, fatigue, and total mood disturbance which continued to be significantly lower at least seven weeks following the final GIM session as indicated by pre- versus follow-up comparisons. The GIM intervention also lowered pre- versus post-treatment resting serum cortisol levels so that pre- versus follow-up levels were significantly decreased seven weeks after the final session. Furthermore, the pre- versus follow-up mood was strongly associated with changes in cortisol levels and was found to predict cortisol change above and beyond pre-treatment cortisol levels and independent of group assignment.

Although no further systematic studies of the use of imagery in alleviating depression were identified, a clinical case report by Brunell (1990) underscored the benefit of a multi-modal cognitive-behavioral intervention including resolution of ideal-real self discrepancy imagery and the use of note-taking to focus on positive experiences and rehearsal of positive cognitions and imagery with considerable improvement within two to three months. Another paper by Witztum, Van Der Hart, and Friedman (1988) provided a general overview of the use of metaphoric imagery in psychotherapy, reviewed both strategic and tactical applications of metaphors in guided metaphoric imagery work, story-telling and metaphoric tasks, and detailed the efficacy of metaphoric imagery in the treatment of individuals with highly anxiety-provoking, traumatic, and/or depressive concerns and especially at times of significant therapeutic impasse. Clearly a variety of both systematic research and detailed case studies indicate that therapeutic modalities which utilize both non-verbal metaphor and imagery techniques with verbal approaches appear to produce more significant and long-lasting improvements including lowered depressed mood, anxiety, and fatigue as well as positive changes in a variety of physiological measures.

Summary. Although there is clearly a wealth of research indicating the usefulness of imagery techniques in alleviating depression in individuals with a variety of medical and emotional concerns, only six of the studies reviewed above (Burtle, 1976; Gold, Jarvinen, & Teague, 1982; Jarvinen & Gold, 1981; Lipsky et al., 1980; Propst, 1980a; Reardon & Tossi, 1977; Schultz, 1976, 1978) provide evidence directly relevant to the systematic use of imagery in alleviating depression. The fact that few studies of this nature have been conducted is not surprising, since such studies ideally require the collaborative efforts of several researchers and clinicians committed and well-trained in the use of imagery procedures in verbal psychotherapy who provide coordinated care to individuals meeting specific DSM-IV criteria for major depression over an extended period of time with pre-, post-, and follow-up indices. Most of these studies were originally conducted as dissertation research projects prior to the advent of managed health care and behavioral health services which have contributed to brief treatment interventions with narrowly defined short-term objectives and specified goals.

Of the six studies only four (Burtle, 1976; Lipsky et al., 1980; Reardon & Tossi, 1977; Schultz, 1976, 1978) utilized patient populations; and only two (Burtle, 1976; Schultz, 1976, 1978) of these four studies utilized moderately to severely depressed psychiatric patients. Nevertheless, the findings from these six studies offer clear evidence that various types of directed imagery procedures, either alone or in combination with other cognitive and behavioral approaches, can reduce both self-report and behavioral indices of depression for mild to moderately depressed college students (Gold, Jarvinen, & Teague, 1982; Jarvinen & Gold, 1981; Propst, 1980a,b), mental health center patients whose symptoms included depression (Lipsky et al., 1980), adolescent delinquent females whose symptoms included depression (Reardon & Tossi, 1977), and moderately to severely depressed psychiatric patients (Burtle, 1976; Schultz, 1976, 1978). Furthermore, three studies (Gold et al., 1982; Jarvinen & Gold, 1981; Propst, 1980a,b; Reardon & Tossi, 1977) provided evidence that, although the initial improvement in level of depression gradually diminishes over time, there are still some indications of continued improvement in level of depression six weeks (Propst, 1980a,b), two months (Reardon & Tossi, 1977), and even six months (Gold et al., 1982; Jarvinen & Gold, 1981) after the cessation of relatively brief therapeutic interventions. Finally, it remains important in evaluating the efficacy of various imagery procedures in alleviation depression to consider the level of skill and experience of the clinicians providing the treatment. While further research may determine the stability of the therapeutic benefit over time and clarify the extent of benefit for more seriously depressed individuals, there is now considerable evidence indicating immediate, intermediate, and longer-term improvement in level of depression after relatively minimal directed-imagery therapy interventions lasting for as little as 2 to 6 weeks and as long as 24 weeks. In addition, of particular interest is the finding in a variety of studies during the past 25 years that *therapeutic interventions which integrate nonverbal imagery techniques with verbal approaches appear to produce more extensive and long-lasting improvements.*

Implications for Future Research. The current review offers considerable encouragement for further systematic study as well as the clinical practice of the use of imagery in alleviating depression. Of particular clinical relevance is the development of comprehensive interdisciplinary research teams focusing on different ways in which directed imagery techniques may be integrated with more verbal psychotherapy approaches. It may also be possible to study the integration of these approaches with a variety of interpersonal, artistic, creative, psychopharmacological, holistic, and other lifestyle interventions. Such an endeavor represents a complex interaction of potentially relevant approaches and is, therefore, not likely to come about through the efforts of a single research team. In any case, collaborative investigator teams and independent researchers may continue to provide some answers through considering the following suggestions in designing and conducting further research.

Population. It is particularly important that future research in this area utilize depressed psychiatric patients. With the continued use of the DSM-IV (1994), greater uniformity in diagnostic criteria is readily available nationally and internationally. Depressed psychiatric patients[6] who meet the DSM-IV diagnostic criteria for major unipolar depressive disorder and those who meet the criteria for dysthymic disorder could be studied by researchers nationally and internationally, thereby not only facilitating the possibility of establishing a comprehensive research network but also fostering the comparison of studies among different researchers. Furthermore, depressed psychiatric patients who meet various DSM-IV criteria in the future should be subdivided according to current level of depression as measured by the Beck Depressive Inventory (1967) or the Zung Self-Rating Depression Scale (1965). One could thereby determine whether depressed psychiatric patients differ in their response to the various imagery procedures according to their current level of depression (Beck, 1967).

In addition, various researchers already have indicated a number of other population variables which may affect therapeutic outcome and which, therefore, are worthy of further investigation. Such population variables include IQ (Lipsky et al., 1980), sex (Schwartz, Brown, & Ahern, 1980), types of depression (Schultz, 1976, 1978), daydreaming patterns (Schultz 1976, 1978), and attitudes toward various imagery procedures (Propst, 1980a,b).

Therapists. Another crucial variable which requires greater attention in future research concerns the level of experience and training of the therapists who provide treatment. The minimal criteria for therapist inclusion would be at least two to four years of experience in the particular cognitive, behavioral, or imagery modality, and in lieu of a clearly demonstrable level of competence. The inclusion of yet more experienced therapists would be even better.

The attitude of therapists toward a particular treatment modality is also a crucial variable. Propst (1980a,b) was interested in controlling for therapist expectancies and therefore chose therapists who were not committed to the use of religious imagery. However, generally it is advisable to utilize therapists who are not only experienced in a particular modality but also convinced of its therapeutic efficacy. It is the author's contention that in actual practice, therapists cannot hope to be truly neutral or objective in providing treatment nor would one prefer a therapist to have no conviction about the efficacy of a particular treatment for a particular concern. Clearly, more naturalistic research is essential and should be conducted. Such research should take into consideration the fact that therapists generally become committed to a limited number of therapeutic modalities and develop their skills in these modalities to the exclusion of others; and that, where choice is available, patients often seek out a particular therapist who is known to be committed to a particular point of view.

---

[6] It is particularly important to be certain that there are no undiagnosed and/or untreated medical illnesses which could contribute to depression, and, therefore, could diminish the likelihood of clinical improvement regardless of the therapeutic intervention(s) employed.

Finally, therapeutic differences which may arise secondary to the gender of the therapist also should be given greater attention in future research.

Cognitive, Behavioral, and Imagery Modalities. A major factor in future research concerns the types of therapeutic modalities which will be compared and contrasted with each other. Currently, there is sufficient evidence to indicate that most types of therapeutic interventions, including cognitive, behavioral, and directed imagery modalities, have been useful in alleviating depression in some instances. But the question that requires further investigation is whether a particular cognitive, behavioral, or imagery approach is better, either singly or in combination, than another for a particular type of depressed individual (depending upon, for instance, gender, age, IQ, severity of depression, type of depression, attitude about treatment, etc.). Another question that needs to be addressed is: What should be the minimal length of a therapeutic intervention to bring about meaningful and enduring improvement? Furthermore, will a particular cognitive, behavioral, or directed imagery approach be more or less effective if antidepressant medications also are prescribed or if exercise, activity, artistic, or creative therapies are also a focus of treatment? Will differences arise if antidepressant medications or exercise, activity, or creative therapies are prescribed before or after the beginning of a particular cognitive, behavioral, or imagery intervention?

It is also important to determine whether certain cognitive, behavioral, and directed imagery approaches produce better results through individual therapy, group therapy, or a combination of the two.

Furthermore, there is some evidence to suggest that the therapeutic efficacy of various directed imagery approaches may be improved if relaxation training and/or hypnotic procedures are utilized to enhance the imagery experience. Therefore, future research may include a consideration of the importance of comparing the use of various directed imagery approaches with and without the use of relaxation training and with and without the use of hypnotic procedures.

Finally, while directed imagery clearly seems to be consistently more effective in alleviating depression than non-directed imagery approaches, there is considerable work to be done in determining the particular imagery content (e.g., aggressive, socially gratifying, positive, socially-oriented, religious, neutral, etc.) which is more suitable for alleviating depression in particular sub-types of depressed people.

Control Groups. Future research not only should include more comparable treatment groups as outlined above, but also should include at least two treatment control conditions. Although one control condition often has been a no-treatment waiting list condition, ethical considerations underscore that the provision of no treatment should be avoided unless there truly is a lack of providers. Additional control conditions should consist of patients who are seen individually or as a group in consonance with the main treatment conditions but not exposed to a particular cognitive, behavioral, or directed imagery intervention.

Indices of Depression. Considerable evidence indicates that future therapy outcome depression research should utilize behavioral indices of depression as well as self-report measures. Of particular interest is the work of Schwartz (1973) and his colleagues (Schwartz et al., 1976, 1980; Sirota & Schwartz, 1982) who have utilized changes in facial electromyography (EMG) activity as a measure of current affective state. Research in the future may be conducted utilizing such behavioral such as: facial EMG activity, localization of gaze, time productions, verbal productions (e.g., creating a dream), mirth response (Schultz, 1976, 1978), and/or level of interpersonal interaction (Propst, 1980a,b). In addition, future research may benefit from the use of weekly observational checklists for the presence or absence of various neurovegetative signs of depression as another behavioral index of degree of clinical improvement.

Although there are numerous self-report measure of affective state and trait, the most promising and widely used measures of level of depression include the Beck Depressive Inventory (Beck, 1967), the Zung (1965) Self-Rating Depression Scale (ZSDS), the MMPI-D Scale (Overall, Butcher, & Hunter, 1975), the Multiple Affect Adjective Checklist (MAACL) (Zuckerman, Lubin, & Robins, 1965), and the Differential Emotions Scales (DES) (Izard, 1971). The ZSDS offers the rater flexibility in stating on a 4-point scale the degree to which 20 particular statements are presently true for him/her. Although 20 years ago the ZSDS appeared to offer some advantages over other self-rating depression scales, the Beck Depression Inventory appears to have become more widely used and accepted among a variety of researchers and clinicians. The DES also offers the rater flexibility in stating on a 5-point scale the degree to which 30 emotions are presently true for him/her. As such the DES has particular advantages over the MAACL, which contains 132 adjectives which the rater must check or not depending on whether the adjective currently applies to him/her.

Other Issues Relevant to Research Design. It is particularly important to establish a similar level of expectancy and mental set among subjects across all treatment conditions. All subjects initially should be informed that one of the major purposes of the research project is to determine which individuals are more likely to show greater improvement in level of depression in the various treatment categories. As long as facilities establish a treatment waiting list whenever appropriate services temporarily can no longer be provided, clients who are placed on a waiting list can be given the same initial expectancy and then later provided with a particular treatment approach as openings arise.

Furthermore, it is crucial that all subjects who participate in any research project be informed that they will be expected to complete various questionnaires and participate in various tasks to assess systematically the degree and rate of improvement attained; and that they will be asked to do so at 3-, 6-, and 12-month follow-up intervals as well. Of course, any client who later decides not to do so should complete the therapy without interruption. However, in all research of this nature, the attempt should be made to minimize subject attrition as much as possible. Therefore, paying clients to be subjects by completing the questionnaires and participating in tasks (or reducing their therapy charges, in some instances) may help to reduce attrition during the treatment phase as well as during the follow-up phase.

This leads to another crucial issue in clinical treatment and research design. The importance of follow-up contact in clinical care has now become increasingly recognized as a standard of practice. Therefore, the need for follow-up studies in clinical research parallels the clinical needs of many populations served. Perhaps follow-up research studies could divide subjects into two groups: 1) those who complete follow-up measures without additional review of previous therapeutic interventions; and 2) those who complete follow-up measures but with additional review and rehearsal of the previous therapeutic interventions (e.g., the particular cognitive, behavioral, or imagery approach previously employed).

Summary. Clearly, although the suggested future imagery therapy research would provide necessary information, many of the suggestions are difficult to bring into practice unless comprehensive, multidisciplinary clinical research teams are developed to design and conduct integrated studies with practitioners committed to each particular intervention being investigated. From an organismic, general systems paradigm perspective[7], it is just such a research project which would provide the most fruitful information (Schultz, 1982, 1999). It is more likely that several research teams will continue to contribute to the study of imagery techniques and that both individual and collaborative teach researchers may contribute to comparability across various research studies by endeavoring to follow any of the present suggestions which prove to be relevant as well as establishing additional common guidelines in the future.

Depressive Affect and Imaginal Processes

Although the following areas of research do not specifically investigate the systematic use of imagery to alleviate depression, a limited review of the relevant findings is warranted to provide a basis for theoretical considerations regarding the relationship between depressive affect and imaginal processes.

Daydreaming Patterns. Much of the work on daydreaming patterns and imaginal processes accomplished thus far has been concerned with establishing normative data on nonpatient samples (Singer, 1966; Singer & Antrobus, 1970;

---

[7] For example, the organismic, general systems paradigm of dysfunction postulates that all areas of an individual's life must be considered when attempting to resolve dysfunction and to maximize personal growth (see Figure 1).

Starker, 1973). Work relating specific daydreaming patterns to aspects of psychopathology is limited (Cazeralon & Epstein, 1966; Streissguth, Wagner, & Weschler, 1969). Starker and Singer (1975a) found the daydreaming of psychiatric patients to be less positive and less vivid with greater emphasis on fear of failure than the daydreams of college students. Streissguth et al. (1969) also reported more dysphoric daydreaming among psychiatric patients than among nonpsychiatric medical patients and normals. Another study by Starker and Singer (1975b) found that psychiatric patients whose presenting symptoms included signs of depression reported fewer positive daydreams and fewer guilt daydreams as compared with psychiatric patients having few or no signs of depression. Level of depression has, therefore, been found to relate positively to dysphoric daydreaming patterns and negatively to positive daydreaming patterns in college students (Traynor, 1974), male prisoners (Traynor, 1974), and depressed psychiatric patients (Schultz, 1976). Taken together, these findings are clearly consistent with clinical evidence of the presence anhedonia and ruminative doubt in depression. Of particular interest is the fact that moderate to severe levels of depression appear to result in an inability to experience positive daydreams and memories spontaneously. This inability may underscore the important of induced directed imagery training in disrupting negative introspection and thereby reducing painful inner experience.

Neuropsychological Functioning and Imagery Capacity. Research conducted by Schwartz and colleagues (Schwartz et al., 1976, 1980; Sirota & Schwartz, 1982) focused on the study of involuntary facial muscle patterning response to various types of affective imagery. One study (Schwartz et al., 1976) compared the changes in electromiography (EMG) activity from selected regions of the face of 12 nondepressed nonpatient females, six depressed nonpatient females and six depressed female patients when asked to imagine happy, sad, and angry situations which strongly evoked these emotions in the past. Each person was asked to imagine each emotional situation for three minutes with the instruction to attempt to re-experience the feelings associated with imagery. Also included as a nonspecific emotional control condition was the instruction to think for three minutes about the activities in a typical day with no requirement to experience any particular emotion. As might be expected, findings indicated that: 1) each discrete emotional imagery period produced a different facial EMG activity pattern; and 2) depressed subjects showed an attenuated EMG pattern for happiness as compared to normals. In addition, whereas nondepressed subjects more reliably generated a happy EMG pattern, depressed subjects more reliably generated the sad EMG pattern. Of particular interest is the finding that the typical day EMG pattern for nondepressed subjects is similar to the happy EMG pattern, while the typical day EMG pattern for depressed subjects is similar to the sad EMG pattern. Finally, subjective reports of experienced emotion generally mirror the differences found in facial EMG activity; nondepressed subjects report more happiness during happy imagery and typical day mentation than do depressed subjects. These findings were also replicated by Schwartz, Mandel, Fair, Salt, Mieske, and Klerman (1978) who also found that depressed patients who showed decreases in resting corrugator muscle tension (an EMG indicator of decreased level of depression) after 2 weeks of antidepressant treatment, showed corresponding improvements in clinical symptoms. Taken together, these findings not only underscore the importance of facial EMG activity as an indicator of current affective state but also stress the importance of utilizing directed imagery and other structured cognitive techniques to disrupt typical daily patterns of negative introspection among depressives.

Additional studies by these researchers have indicated that: 1) females show greater affective response to imagery and elicit greater facial EMG activity changes (Schwartz et al., 1979); 2) females show greater laterality in zygomatic facial activity for positive versus negative emotions (Schwartz et al., 1979); and 3) right-handed females show greater zygomatic activity on the right side of their faces for positive emotions (Schwartz et al., 1976, 1979, 1980). One of the major implications of such findings is the hypothesis that the left cerebral hemisphere in right-handed subjects may play a special role in positive emotions.

Similarly, several studies by Tucker, Stenslie, Roth, and Shearer (1981) indicated that: 1) college students who reported greater levels of depression also had less vivid visual imagery; 2) right-handed college students who experienced hypnotic induction of depressed mood as compared to hypnotic induction of euphoric mood reported a right-ear attentional bias and poor visual imagery but no difference in arithmetical calculation ability; and 3) right-handed college students who experienced an induced depressed mood as compared to an induced euphoric mood showed less EEG activation of the right frontal hemisphere. Taken together, these studies indicate that depression may coincide with a decrement in the information processing capacity of the right hemisphere. Such findings parallel the evidence of right hemisphere dysfunction in depressed psychiatric patients in visuospatial task performance (Flor-Henry, 1976; Goldstein, Filskov, Weaver, & Ives, 1977; Kronfol, Hamsher, Digire, & Waziri, 1978) and dichotic listening (Yozawitz & Bruder, 1978). These studies also suggest that "there may be a functional and transient relationship between depressive affect and decreased information processing capacity of the right hemisphere" (Tucker et al., 1981, p. 173). This possibility is consistent with another study which found that patients who showed alleviation of depressed mood after ECT also showed improvement in right task performance (Kronfol et al., 1978).

Thus, mounting evidence indicates that the left cerebral hemisphere may play a special role in positive emotions (Schwartz et al., 1976, 1979, 1980); whereas, the right frontal cerebral hemisphere may play a special role in negative emotions (Flor-Henry, 1976; Goldstein et al., 1977; Kronfol et al., 1978; Tucker et al., 1981;

Yozawitz & Bruder, 1978). Of particular interest as well is the finding in several different kinds of studies (Starker & Singer, 1975a; Tucker et al., 1981) that depressives have a decreased imagery capacity, suggesting that the effectiveness of imagery approaches in alleviating severe levels of depression may be enhanced with specific imagery training procedures. Furthermore, the finding that improvement in right hemispheric functioning corresponded with alleviation of depressed mood suggests that imagery approaches may be more effective in reducing depression when utilized in consonance with other treatment interventions (Beck, 1967).

Depressive Affect, Memory, and Attributions of Life Events. Several studies have reported that memories which are inconsistent with induced mood are retrieved more slowly than memories which are consistent with induced mood (Frost, Graf, & Becker, 1979; Teasdale, Taylor, & Fogarty, 1980). In addition, Clark and Teasdale (1982) found that depressed patients were more likely to recall memories of unhappy experiences on occasions when they were more depressed than on less depressed occasions. Furthermore, they noted that depressed patients rated the current pleasantness of a recalled experience more negatively than the original level of pleasantness depending upon the current level of depression. Another study (Raps, Peterson, Reinhard, Abramson, & Seligman, 1982) reported that when unipolar depressed patients were asked to imagine vividly six good and six bad events, they were more likely to attribute bad events to internal, stable, and global causes than were nondepressed medical patients. A related study found that depressed patients showed greater depressive attributions in response to their most stressful life events than did nondepressed psychiatric patients, but there was no difference in their attributions in response to either hypothetical or experimental tasks (Miller, Klee, & Norman, 1982). These findings are consistent with clinical evidence that depressed patients are characterized by a negative attributional style in which bad outcomes are attribute to self-deficiencies which are chronic and pervasive, whereas good outcomes are more likely to be related to external circumstances which are unstable and likely to be limited to a specific situation. Furthermore, Sirota and Schwartz (1982) have reported the interesting finding that for nondepressed normal females, EMG zygomatic activity increases immediately during elation and decreases over time, whereas facial EMG corrugator activity grows over time in response to depressive statements. Thus, it may well be that the subjective and physiological experience of happiness as an emotion peaks and diminishes over time while depression as an emotion gradually builds over time. In the case of depressed patients, however, their experience of the depressive emotion persists and perhaps grows so pervasively over time that their feeling state stands in marked contrast to that of others around them who are experiencing normal fluctuations in their emotional life. Thus, depressed patients may be unable to find any suitable explanation for this contrast other than causes which reflect chronic, pervasive, self-deficiencies.

THE COGNITIVE-AFFECTIVE ASPECTS OF AN
ORGANISMIC GENERAL SYSTEMS PARADIGM
OF DEPRESSION

The reader will recall an earlier discussion in this chapter of some of the major theories and models of depression. While a comprehensive consideration of the many models of depression is beyond the scope of this chapter, a brief discussion of some of the implications of imagery research for current theories and models of depression will be pursued. The reader is already somewhat acquainted with the author's present commitment (Schultz, 1982, 1999) to the organismic general systems paradigm which provides the context within which one may develop an understanding of the factors which contribute to the development and maintenance of dysfunction (see Figure 1). Since a more thorough discussion of the organismic general systems paradigm is available elsewhere (Schultz, 1982, 1999) and in forthcoming papers, the following remarks will primarily be confined to a specific aspect of the paradigm—that is, the interaction between what happens intrapsychically on a cognitive and affective level in the depressed individual and what takes place externally.

Considerable research has underscored a cognitive-affective circular feedback model of depression (Beck, 1967; Schultz, 1976), and some evidence suggests that individuals may rehearse certain attitudes, beliefs, and themes (e.g., life scripts) in their fantasy life and thereby make them integrated aspects of their reality. Some researchers have emphasized the role of undesirable recent life events in the onset of depression (Paykel et al., 1969) while other theorists have emphasized the role of previous losses and past traumatic life events in the development of depressive disorders. Incorporating many of the findings from cognitive, behavioral, and imagery approaches to the treatment of depression, Schultz (1978) suggested that undesirable recent life events may serve as cues to memories of more traumatic life events in the individual's past. Such memories (whether verbal or visual-pictorial in nature) may then further exacerbate negative affect and further confirm the enduring aspects of the negative self-image, leading eventually to increased belief in the "reality" of the negative cognitive. Figure 2 illustrates this process pictorially.

While the etiology of depression may remain controversial, there is considerable evidence that the conceptualization represented in Figure 2 is a useful and accurate model of the maintenance of depressive affect in seriously depressed individuals. Furthermore, this model is also supported by related research regarding the chronic, pervasive self-deprecatory attributional style of depressives (Clark & Teasdale, 1982; Miller et al., 1982; Raps et al., 1982), their increased retrieval of negative experiences with increased depression (Clark & Teasdale, 1982), and the rating of recalled experiences as more negative at times of increased depression (Clark & Teasdale, 1982). Additional research relevant to the neuropsychology of emotions suggests that the left cerebral hemisphere may play a

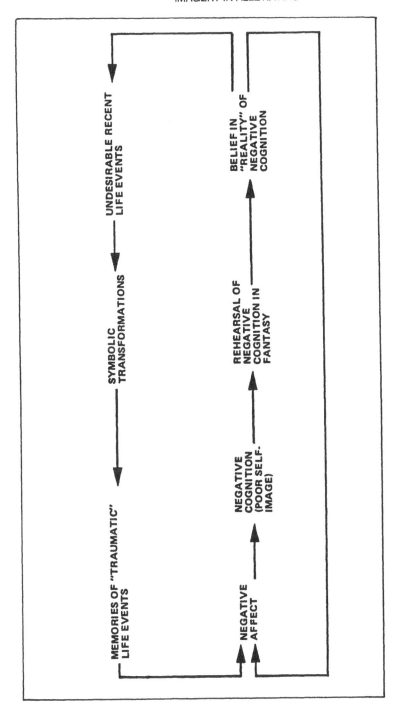

Figure 2. The cognitive-affective aspects of a biopsychosocial model of depression.

special role in positive emotions (Sirota & Schwartz, 1982), whereas the right frontal hemisphere may play a special role in negative emotions (Flor-Henry, 1976; Goldstein et al., 1977; Kronfol et al., 1978; Tucker et al., 1981). Further evidence suggest a possible transient functional relationship between depressive affect and decreased information-processing capacity of the right hemisphere (Kronfol et al., 1978; Tucker et al., 1981;). Thus, one implication of various treatment interventions, such as anti-depressant medication, ECT, exercise, artistic, creative, and activity therapy, and cognitive, behavioral, and imagery approaches, is that they all may serve eventually to disrupt the final common pathway (Akiskal & McKinney, 1973, 1975) of the individual's cognitive-affective feedback cycle, perhaps even at a metabolic or biochemical level in various cortical and/or subcortical areas of the brain. Whether various psychological treatment strategies may be useful only for less severe levels of depression (Beck, 1967) and more biological-biochemical interventions may be necessary initially in the treatment of more severe levels of depression remains to be established by further research.

If one were to utilize the organismic general systems paradigm in trying to understand an individual's function and dysfunction, the various biological, psychological, social, and spiritual interventions would not need to be seen as competitive but as complimentary, with each factor serving a useful purpose as it is identified as relevant to a particular individual at a particular point in time. It may become well-established that severe levels of depression initially require a more biological-biochemical intervention. Nevertheless, current clinical experience as well as various research findings clearly indicate that various psychological (especially cognitive, behavioral, and imagery approaches) and social interventions are absolutely necessary in reducing other factors which contribute to depression and also are important in helping those who have resolved the acute phase of their depressive disorder to maintain their present level of functioning and lessen the likelihood of a relapse. Also, if further research regarding the use of imagery in alleviating depression can establish which types of depressed individual respond better to which types of imagery contents and procedures as well as to other cognitive and behavior approaches (either singly or in combination), clinicians will be able to assign more individuals to the best-suited psychological intervention, just as biological psychiatrists are now somewhat better able to determine which individuals will respond better to different types of antidepressant medications. Clearly, this is an exciting field of research with both pure scientific and applied practical implications for improvement of the quality of life of many people throughout the world.

CONCLUSION

Considerable attention already has been focused upon the use of various imagery approaches in alleviating depression and upon the different theories and models of the etiology of depression and the maintenance of depressive affect. Such concerns are the major focus of this chapter but it would be deficient if it did not include some remarks relevant to the potential role of imagery approaches in health care regardless of one's particular theoretical orientation.

Those who seek psychotherapy are likely to vary not only in their current awareness of the effects of verbal and imagery experience on affective state but also in their current ability to utilize imagery as a cognitive coping device. Thus, the practitioner's initial step in using imagery in therapy is drawing attention to inner experience and verbal-imaginal processes and emphasizing the possibility of utilizing imagery as a resource in treatment. Also, the emphasis on imagery and stream of consciousness encourages the individual to become more aware of the many thoughts, fantasies, expectations, and judgments about people and situations which represent distorted and poorly integrated childhood experiences that no longer correspond appropriately to current life circumstances. Furthermore, imagery approaches in psychotherapy can serve to augment rather than replace more traditional verbal approaches. Of particular importance to the person seeking help, however, is not only the discovery of a new capacity to use imagery in generating positive affect and/or in shifting away from certain negative affective patterns, but also the realization that such a capacity is a skill which can be learned, developed, and utilized as a resource.

REFERENCES

Abraham, I. L., Neundorfer, M. M., & Currie, L. J. (1992). Effects of group interventions on cognition and depression in nursing home residents. *Nursing Research, 41*(4), 196-202.

Abraham, I. L., Neundorfer, M. M., & Terris, E. A. (1993). Effects of focused visual imagery on cognition and depression among nursing home residents. *Journal of Mental Imagery, 17*(3 & 4), 61-76.

Akiskal, H. S., & McKinney, W. I. (1973). Depressive disorders. *Science, 182,* 20-29.

Akiskal, H. S., & McKinney, W. I. (1975). Overview of recent research in depression: Integration of ten conceptual models into a comprehensive clinical frame. *Archives of General Psychiatry, 32,* 285-305.

American Psychiatric Association. (1994). *Diagnostic and statistical manual of mental disorders* (4th ed.). Washington, DC: Author.

Assagioli, R. (1965). *Psychosynthesis: A manual of principles and techniques.* New York: Hobbs, Dorman.

Auerbach, J. E., Oleson, T. D., & Solomon, G. F. (1992). Biofeedback, guided imagery, and hypnosis as an adjunctive treatment for AIDS and AIDS-related complex. *Proceedings of the Third National Conference on the Psychology of Health, Immunity, and Disease* in Storrs, CT: The National Institute for the Clinical Application of Behavioral Medicine, 50.

Bandura, A. (1971). *Psychological modeling.* New York: Atherton.

Beck, A. T. (1967). *Depression: Causes and treatment.* Philadelphia: University of Pennsylvania Press.

Beck, A. T. (1976). *Cognitive therapy and emotional disorders.* New York: International Universities Press.

Beck, A. T. (1991). Cognitive therapy: A 30 year perspective. *American Psychologist, 46,* 368-375.

Beck, A. T., Rush, A. J., Shaw, B. F., & Emery, G. (1979). *Cognitive therapy of depression.* New York: Guilford Press.

Beck, J. S. (1995). *Cognitive therapy: Basics and beyond.* New York: Guilford.

Berne, E. (1964). *Games people play.* New York: Grove.

Blake, R. L. (1994). Vietnam veterans with post-traumatic stress disorder: Findings from a music and imagery project. *Journal of the Association for Music and Imagery, 3,* 5-17.

Blake, R. L., & Bishop, S. R. (1995). The Bonny method of guided imagery and music (GIM) in the treatment of post-traumatic stress disorder (PTSD) with adults in a psychiatric setting. *Music Therapy Perspectives, 12,* 125-129.

Blatt, S. J. (1974). Levels of object representation in anaclitic and introjective depression. *Psychoanalytic Study of the Child, 29,* 107-157.

Bondra, G. (1998). *Toward a science of persons: New instrumentation for understanding the individual.* Unpublished manuscript. Institute for Self-Managed Success, Torrington, Connecticut..

Bonny, H. (1978a). *Facilitating guided imagery and music sessions.* Bonny Foundation, 2020 Simmons, Salina, KS 67401.

Bonny, H. (1978b). *The role of taped music programs in the GIM process.* Bonny Foundation, 2020 Simmons, Salina, KS 67401.

Bonny, H. L. (1995). Twenty-one years later: A GIM update. *Music Therapy Perspectives, 12,* 70-74.

Borling, J. E. (1992). Perspectives on growth with a victim of abuse: A guided imagery and music (GIM) case study. *Journal of the Association for Music and Imagery, 1,* 85-98.

Breuer, I., & Freud, S. (1955). Studies in hysteria. In J. Strachey (Ed.), *The standard edition* (Vol. 2). London: Hogarth.

Brunell, L. F. (1990). Multimodal treatment of depression: A strategy to break through the "strenuous lethargy" of depression. *Psychotherapy in Private Practice, 8*(3), 13-22.

Bruscia, K. E. (1991). Embracing life with AIDS: Psychotherapy through guided imagery and music. In K. E. Bruscia (Ed.), *Case studies in music therapy* (pp. 581-602). Phoenixville, PA: Barcelona.

Burtle, V. (1976). Learning in the appositional mind: Imagery in the treatment of depression. *Dissertation Abstracts International, 36*(II-B), 5781.

Burton, R. (1621). *The anatomy of melancholy.* Oxford: John Lichfield and James Short.

Casler, L. (1985). A simple verbal procedure for reducing the rates of psychosomatic enfeeblement and death in an aged population. *Death Studies, 9,* 295-307.

Cautela, J. R., & McCullough, L. (1978). Covert conditioning: A learning theory perspective on imagery. In J. L. Singer & K. S. Pope (Eds.), *The power of human imagination* (pp. 227-254). New York: Plenum Press.

Cazeralon, J., & Epstein, S. (1966). Daydreams of female paranoid schizophrenics. *Journal of Clinical Psychology, 22*(1), 27-32.

Chappell, M. N., & Stevenson, T. I. (1936). Group psychological training in some organic conditions. *Mental Hygiene of New York, 20,* 588-597.

Clark, M. F. (1991). Emergence of the adult self in guided imagery and music (GIM) therapy. In K. E. Bruscia (Ed.), *Case studies in music therapy* (pp. 321-332). Phoenix-ville, PA: Barcelona.

Clark, D. M., & Teasdale, J. D. (1982). Diurnal variation in clinical depression and accessibility of memories of positive and negative experiences. *Journal of Abnormal Psychology, 91*(2), 87-95.

DeBerry, S., Davis, S., & Reinhard, K. E. (1989). A comparison of meditation-relaxation meditation and cognitive-behavioral techniques for reducing anxiety and depression in a geriatric population. *Journal of Geriatric Psychiatry, 22,* 231-247.

Decker, T. W., Cline-Eisen, J., & Gallagher, M. (1992). Relaxation therapy as an adjunct in radiation oncology. *Journal of Clinical Psychology, 48*(3), 388-393.

Desoille, R. (1938). *Exploration de l'affectivité subconsciente par la méthode du rêve é veillé.* Paris: D' Autry.

Edmunson, E. D., & Nelson, D. L. (1976). Anxiety, imagery and sensory interference. *Bulletin of the Psychonomic Society, 8,* 319-322.

Eller, L. S. (1995). Effects of two cognitive-behavioral interventions on immunity and symptoms in persons with HIV. *Annals of Behavioral Medicine, 17*(4), 339-348.

Ellis, A. (1973). *Humanistic psychotherapy: The rational emotive approach.* New York: Julian Press.

Flor-Henry, P. (1976). Lateralized temporal-limbic dysfunction and psychopathology. *Annual of the New York Academy of Science, 280,* 777-797.

Fretigny, R., & Virel, A. (1968). *L'imagerie mentale.* Geneva: Mont-Blanc.

Frost, R. O., Graf, M., & Becker, J. (1979). Self-devaluation and depressed mood. *Journal of Consulting and Clinical Psychology, 47*(5), 958-962.

Gallant, D. M., & Simpson, G. M. (1975). *Depression: Behavioral, biochemical, diag-nostic, and treatment concepts.* New York: Spectrum Publications.

Gerard, R. (1964). Psychosynthesis: A manual for the whole man. *Psychosyntheseis Research Foundation, 14.*

Giray, E. F., Roodin, P., Altkin, W., Flagg, P., & Yoon, G. (1985). A life span approach to the study of eidetic imagery. *Journal of Mental Imagery, 9,* 21-32.

Gold, S. R., Jarvinen, P. J., & Teague, R. G. (1982). Imagery elaboration and clarity in modifying college students' depression. *Journal of Clinical Psychology, 38,* 312-314.

Goldberg, F. S. (1995). The Bonny method of guided imagery and music. In T. Wigram, G. Saperston, & R. West (Eds.), *The art and science of music therapy: A handbook* (pp. 112-124). Chur, Switzerland: Harwood Academic.

Goldstein, S. G., Filskov, S. B., Weaver, L. A., & Ives, J. O. (1977). Neuropsychological effects of electroconvulsive therapy. *Journal of Clinical Psychology, 33,* 789-806.

Green, R. J. (1981). Visual imagery and behavior prescription in the treatment of parent-child conflict. In A. S. Gurman (Ed.), *Questions and answers in the practice of family therapy* (pp. 426-430). New York: Brunner/Mazel.

Greenberg, I. M. (1979). *General systems: Social and biological interactions.* Unpublished manuscript.

Grinder, J., & Bandler, R. (1976). *The structure of magic II.* Palo Alto, CA: Science and Behavior Books, Inc.

Gross, D. A. (1981). Medical origins of psychiatric emergencies: The systems approach. *International Journal of Psychiatry in Medicine, 11*(1), 1-24.

Gurman, A. S. (Ed.). (1981). *Questions and answers in the practice of family therapy*. New York: Brunner/Mazel.

Hale, S. E. (1992). Wounded woman: The use of guided imagery and music in recovering from a mastectomy. *Journal of the Association for Music and Imagery, I,* 99-106.

Hamm, B. H., & King, V. (1984). A holistic approach to pain control with geriatric clients. *Journal of Holistic Nursing, 2,* 32-36.

The Holy Bible. (1953). New York: Thomas Nelson and Sons.

Izard, C. E. (1971). *The face of emotions*. New York: Appleton-Century-Crofts.

Jacobi, E. M. (1994). *The efficacy of the Bonny method of guided imagery and music as experiential therapy in the primary care of persons with rheumatoid arthritis.* Unpublished doctoral dissertation, Union Institute, Cincinnati, Ohio.

Jacobson, N. S., & Margolin, G. (1979). *Marital therapy*. New York: Brunner/Mazel.

James, W. (1950). *The principles of psychology* (Vols. I and II). New York: Dover.

Jarvinen, P. J., & Gold, R. S. (1981). Imagery as an aid in reducing depression. *Journal of Clinical Psychology, 37*(3), 523-529.

Jordan, D. C., & Streets, D. T. (1973). The anisa model: A new basis for educational planning. *Young Children, 28,* 289-307.

Jordan, D. C., & Streets, D. T. (1978). *Releasing the potentialities of the child: A new conceptual basis for comprehensive educational planning.* Amherst, MA: University of Massachusetts.

Jung, C. G. (1968). *Analytical psychology: Its theory and practice*. New York: Vintage Books.

Kausler, D. H. (1982). *Experimental psychology of human aging*. New York: Wiley.

Kronfol, Z., Hamsher, K., Digre, K., & Waziri, R. (1978). Depression and hemispheric functions: Changes associated with unilateral ECT. *British Journal of Psychiatry, 132,* 560-567.

Kovacs, M. (1979). Treating depressive disorders: Efficacy of behavior and cognitive therapies. *Behavior Modification, 3*(4), 496-517.

Lazarus, A. A. (1968). Learning theory and the treatment of depression. *Behavior Research and Therapy, 6,* 83-89.

Lazarus, A. A. (1977). *In the mind's eye*. New York: Rawson.

Lazarus, A. A. (1989). *The practice of multimodal therapy*. Baltimore: Johns Hopkins University Press.

Leja, A. M. (1989). Using guided imagery to combat postsurgical depression. *Journal of Gerontological Nursing, 15*(4), 6-11.

Leuner, H. (1969). Guided affective imagery (GAI): A method of intensive psychotherapy. *American Journal of Psychotherapy, 23,* 4-22.

Levitt, E. E., & Lubin, B. (1975). *Depression: Concepts, controversies, and some new facts*. New York: Springer.

Lewis, H. R., & Streitfield, S. (1971). *Growth games*. New York: Harcourt.

Lipsky, M. J., Kassinove, H., & Miller, N. J. (1980). Effects of rational-emotive therapy, rational role reversal, and rational-emotive imagery on the emotional adjustment of community mental health center patients. *Journal of Consulting and Clinical Psychology, 48*(3), 366-374.

McDonald, R. G. (1990). *The efficacy of guided imagery and music as a strategy of self-concept and blood pressure change among adults with essential hypertension.* Unpublished doctoral dissertation, Walden University, Minneapolis, Minnesota.

McKinney, C. H., Antoni, M. H., Kumar, A., & Kumar, M. (1995). The effects of guided imagery and music (GIM) on depression and beta-endorphin in healthy adults: A pilot study. *Journal of the Association for Music and Imagery, 4,* 67-78.

McKinney, C. H., Antoni, M. H., Kumar, M., Tims, F. C., & McCabe, P. M. (1997). Effects of guided imagery and music (GIM therapy on mood and cortisol in healthy adults. *Health Psychology, 16*(4), 390-400.

McKinney, C. H., Tims, F. C., Kumar, A., & Kumar, M. (1997). The effect of selected classical music and spontaneous imagery on plasma beta-endorphin. *Journal of Behavioral Medicine, 20,* 85-99.

McLean, P. D., & Hakstian, A. R. (1979). Clinical depression: Comparative efficacy of outpatient treatments. *Journal of Consulting and Clinical Psychology, 47*(5), 813-836.

McNutt, F. (1974). *Healing.* Notre Dame: Ave Maria.

Meichenbaum, D. (1975). Toward a cognitive theory of self-control. In G. Schwartz & D. Shapiro (Eds.), *Consciousness and self-regulation: Advances in research.* New York: Plenum Press.

Miller, I. W., Klee, S. H., & Norman, W. H. (1982). Depressed and nondepressed inpatients' cognitions of hypothetical events, experimental tasks, and stressful life events. *Journal of Abnormal Psychology, 91*(1), 78-81.

Moreno, J. L. (1967). Reflections on my method of group psychotherapy and psychodrama. In H. Grunwald (Ed.), *Active psychotherapy.* New York: Atherton.

Neidhardt, E. J., Krakow, B., Kellner, R., & Pathak, D. (1992). The behavioral effects of one treatment session and recording of nightmares on chronic nightmare sufferers. *Sleep, 15*(5), 470-473.

Overall, J., Butcher, J., & Hunter, S. (1975). Validity of the MMPI-168 for psychiatric screening. *Educational and Psychological Measurement, 35,* 393-400.

Pavio, A. (1971). *Imagery and verbal processes.* New York: Hold, Rinehart, and Winston.

Paykel, E. S., Myers, J. K., Dienelt, M. N., Klerman, G. L., Lindenthal, J. J., & Pepper, M. P. (1969). Life events and depression: A controlled study. *Archives of General Psychiatry, 21,* 753-760.

Peale, N. V. (1982). *Dynamic imaging.* Old Japan, NJ: Fleming Revell.

Perls, F. (1970). *Gestalt therapy verbatim.* New York: Bantam.

Pickett, E. (1987). Fibroid tumors and response to guided imagery and music: Two case studies. *Imagination, Cognition and Personality, 7,* 165-176.

Pickett, E. (1991a). *Guided imagery and music (GIM) in the treatment of multiple personality disorder.* Paper presented at the annual conference of the Association for Music and Imagery, Sonoma, California.

Pickett, E. (1991b). Guided imagery and music (GIM) with a dually diagnosed woman having multiple addictions. In K. E. Bruscia (Ed.), *Case studies in music therapy* (pp. 497-512). Phoenixwille, PA: Barcelona.

Pickett, E., & Sonnen, C. (1993). Guided imagery and music: A music therapy approach to multiple personality disorder. *Journal of the Association for Music and Imagery, 2,* 49-72.

Powell, G. E. (1981). *Brain function therapy.* Aldershot, England: Gower.

Propst, L. R. (1980a). A comparison of the cognitive restructuring psychotherapy paradigm and several spiritual approaches to mental health. *Journal of Psychology and Theology, 8*(2), 107-114.

Propst, L. R. (1980b). The comparative efficacy of religious and nonreligious imagery for the treatment of mild depression in religious individuals. *Cognitive Therapy and Research, 4*(2), 167-178.

Propst, L. R. (1980c). *Cognitive therapy mediation manual.* Unpublished manuscript, Department of Counseling Psychology, Lewis and Clark College, Portland, Oregon.

Raps, C. S., Peterson, C., Reinhard, K. E., Abramson, L. Y., & Seligman, M. E. P. (1982). Attributional style among depressed patients. *Journal of Abnormal Psychology, 91*(2), 102-108.

Read, G. D. (1953). *Childbirth without fear.* New York: Harper.

Reardon, J. P., & Tossi, D. J. (1977). The effects of rational stage directed imagery on self-concept and reduction of psychological stress in adolescent delinquent females. *Journal of Clinical Psychology, 33,* 1084-1092.

Rehm, L. P. (Ed.). (1981). *Behavior therapy for depression: Present status and future directions.* New York: Academic Press.

Reyher, J. (1963). Free imagery: An uncovering procedure. *Journal of Clinical Psychology, 19,* 454-459.

Reyher, J. (1978). Emergent uncovering psychotherapy: The use of imagoic and linguistic vehicles in objectifying psychodynamic processes. In J. L. Singer & K. S. Pope (Eds.), *The power of human imagination* (pp. 51-93). New York: Plenum Press.

Riccio, C. M., Nelson, D. L., & Bush, M. A. (1990). Adding purpose to the repetitive exercise of elderly women through imagery. *American Journal of Occupational Therapy, 44,* 714-719.

Richards, P. S., Owen, L., & Stein, S. (1993). A religiously oriented group counseling intervention for self-defeating perfectionism: A pilot study. *Counseling and Values, 37,* 96-104.

Rider, M. S., Floyd, J. W., & Kirkpatrick, J. (1985). The effect of music, imagery and relaxation on adrenal corticosteroids and the re-entrainment of circadian rhythms. *Journal of Music Therapy, 22,* 46-58.

Rinker, R. L. (1991). Guided imagery and music (GIM): Healing the wounded healer. In K. E. Bruscia (Ed.), *Case studies in music therapy* (pp. 309-320). Phoenixville, PA: Barcelona.

Scanlon, M. (1974). *Inner healing.* New York: Paulist.

Schultz, K. D. (1976). *Fantasy stimulation in depression: Direct intervention and correlational studies.* Unpublished doctoral dissertation,. Yale University, New Haven, Connecticut.

Schultz, K. D. (1978). Imagery and the control of depression. In J. L. Singer & K. S. Pope (Eds.), *The power of human imagination* (pp. 281-307). New York: Plenum Press.

Schultz, K. D. (1982). Humanistic psychology and general systems theory: Toward a humanistic general systems model of mental health care. *Division of Humanistic Psychology, APA-Division 12 Newsletter, 10*(2).

Schultz, K. D. (1999). *The organismic general systems paradigm and the individual's actualization of potentiality.* Unpublished manuscript, Woodbury, Connecticut.

Schwartz, G. E. (1973). Biofeedback as therapy: Some theoretical and practical issues. *American Psychologist, 28,* 666-673.

Schwartz, G. E., Ahern, G. L., & Brown, S. L. (1979). Lateralized facial muscle response to positive versus negative emotional stimuli. *Psychophysiology, 16,* 561-571.

Schwartz, G. E., Brown, S. L., & Ahern, L. (1980). Facial muscle patterning and subjective experience during affective imagery: Sex differences. *Psychophysiology, 17,* 75-82.

Schwartz, G. E., Fair, P. L., Salt, P., Mandel, M. R., & Klerman, G. L. (1976). Facial muscle patterning to affective imagery in depressed and nondepressed subjects. *Science, 192,* 489-491.

Schwartz, G. E., Mandel, M. R., Fair, P. L., Salt, P. Mieske, M., & Klerman, G. L. (1978). Facial electromiography in the assessment of improvement in depression. *Psychosomatic Medicine, 40,* 355-360.

Segal, S. J. (Ed.). (1971). *Imagery: Current cognitive approaches.* New York: Academic Press.

Short, A. E. (1993). GIM during pregnancy: Anticipation and resolution. *Journal of the Association for Music and Imagery, 2,* 73-86.

Simonton, O. C., & Simonton, S. S. (1975). Belief systems and management of the emotional aspects of malignancy. *Journal of Transpersonal Psychology, 7,* 28-47.

Singer, J. L. (1966). *Daydreaming.* New York: Random House.

Singer, J. L. (1971). Imagery and daydream techniques employed in psychotherapy: Some practical and theoretical implications. In C. Spielberger (Ed.), *Current topics in clinical and community psychology.* New York: Academic Press.

Singer, J. L. (1974). *Imagery and daydream methods in psychotherapy and behavior modification.* New York: Academic Press.

Singer, J. L., & Antrobus, J. S. (1970). *Imaginal processes inventory: Revised.* New York: Authors.

Singer, J. L., & Pope, K. S. (1978). The use of imagery and fantasy techniques in psychotherapy. In J. L. Singer & K. S. Pope (Eds.), *The power of human imagination: New methods in psychotherapy* (pp. 3-34). New York: Plenum Press.

Sirota, A. D., & Schwartz, G. E. (1982). Facial muscle patterning and lateralization during elation and depression imagery. *Journal of Abnormal Psychology, 91*(1), 25-34.

Stampfl, T. G., & Levis, D. J. (1967). Essentials of implosive therapy: A learning theory based psychodynamic behavior therapy. *Journal of Abnormal Psychology, 72,* 496-503.

Starker, S. (1973). Aspects of inner experience: Autokinesis, daydreaming, dream recall, and cognitive. *Perceptual and Motor Skills, 36,* 663-673.

Starker, S., Levine, I. R., & Watstein, G. J. (1974). *The subjective focus in a group oriented treatment program: A preliminary report.* Unpublished manuscript.

Starker, S., & Singer, J. L. (1975a). Daydreaming and symptom patterns of psychiatric patients: A factor analytic study. *Journal of Abnormal Psychology, 84,* 567-570.

Starker, S., & Singer, J. L. (1975b). Daydreaming patterns of self-awareness in psychiatric patients. *Journal of Nervous and Mental Disease, 163,* 313-317.

Streissguth, A. P., Wagner, N., & Weschler, J. (1969). Effects of sex, illness, and hospitalization on daydreaming. *Journal of Consulting and Clinical Psychology, 33*(2), 218-225.

Tasney, K. (1993). Beginning the healing of incest through guided imagery and music: A Jungian perspective. *Journal of the Association for Music and Imagery, 2,* 35-48.

Teasdale, J. D., Taylor, R., & Fogarty, S. T. (1980). Effects of induced elation-depression on the accessibility of memories of happy and unhappy experiences. *Behavior Research and Therapy, 18,* 339-346.

Traynor, J. D. (1974). *Patterns of daydreaming and their relationship to depressive affect.* Unpublished masters thesis,. Miami University, Oxford, Ohio.

Tucker, D. M., Stenslie, C. E., Roth, R. S., & Shearer, S. L. (1981). Right frontal lobe activation and right hemisphere performance decrement during depressed mood. *Archives of General Psychiatry, 38,* 169-174.

Van Dyck, R., Zitman, F., Corry, A., Linssen, G., & Spinhoven, P. (1991). Autogenic training and future oriented hypnotic imagery in the treatment of tension headache: Outcome and process. *The International Journal of Clinical and Experimental Hypnosis, 29*(1), 6-23.

Velton, E. (1968). A laboratory task for induction of mood states. *Behavior Research and Therapy, 6,* 473-482.

Ventre, M. E. (1995). Healing the wounds of childhood abuse: A guided imagery and music case study. *Music Therapy Perspectives, 12,* 98-103.

Von Bertanlanffy, L. (1968). *General systems theory. Foundations, development, applications.* New York: Braziller.

Watts, F. N., MacLeod, A. K., & Morris, L. (1988). A remedial strategy for memory and concentration problems in depressed patients. *Cognitive Therapy and Research, 12*(2), 185-193.

Weiss, J. E. (1994). Accessing the inner family through guided imagery and music. *Journal of the Association for Music and Imagery, 3,* 49-58.

Whitehead, A. N. (1969). *Process and reality.* New York: Free Press.

Witztum, E., Van Der Hart, O., & Friedman, B. (1988). The use of metaphors in psychotherapy. *Journal of Contemporary Psychotherapy, 18*(4), 270-290.

Wolberg, L. R., & Aronson, M. L. (Eds.). (1980). *Group and family therapy 1980.* New York: Brunner/Mazel.

Wolberg, L. R., & Aronson, M. L. (Eds.). (1981). *Group and family therapy 1981.* New York: Brunner/Mazel.

Wolpe, J., & Lazarus, A. A. (1966). *Behavior therapy techniques: A guide to the treatment of neuroses.* New York: Pergamon Press.

Wrangsjo, B., & Korlin, D. (1995). Guided imagery and music as a psychotherapeutic method in psychiatry. *Journal of the Association for Music and Imagery, 4,* 79-92.

Yozawitz, A., & Bruder, G. E. (1978). *Dichotic listening assymmetries and lateralization deficits in affective psychosis.* Presented at the American Psychological Association Annual Convention, Toronto, August 29, 1978.

Zuckerman, M., Lubin, B., & Robins, S. (1965). Validation of the multiple affect adjective check list in clinical situations. *Journal of Consulting Psychology, 29,* 594.

Zung, W. W. K. (1965). A self-rating depression scale. *Archives of General Psychiatry, 12,* 63-70.

CHAPTER 15

Imagery: Its History and Use in the Treatment of Posttraumatic Stress Disorder

JO M. WEIS, MERVIN R. SMUCKER,
AND JANE G. DRESSER

> Traumatic memory consists of images, sensations, affective and behavioral
> states that are invariable and do not change over time.
> Pierre Janet (in van der Kolk & Fisler, 1995, p. 520)

Imagery experiences in posttraumatic stress disorder (PTSD) have been
explored for more than a century, initially through the psychoanalytic context of
dreams, and later, driven by an awareness of intrusive images during wakeful
states, through the work of Horowitz and Kaltreider (1979). PTSD related images
are generally multi-sensorial in nature that include visual as well as auditory,
kinesthetic, olfactory, tactile, and gustatory experiences. Traumatic images tend to
be emotionally charged memories that feel so overwhelming to the PTSD sufferer
that they are difficult to integrate into already existing schemata (Janoff-Bulman,
1992). These unassimilated and unaccomodated (Piaget, 1952) memories continue
to intrude, unbidden and unwanted, through recurring images, flashbacks, and
dreams—with concomitant heightened emotion and physiological arousal—and
continue to "assault" the psyche until the information is adequately processed and
integrated (Horowitz, 1986).

HISTORICAL OVERVIEW

Since the late 1800s the study of trauma has alternated between periods of
open investigation and almost total abandonment. As natural disasters and human
perpetrated atrocities come increasingly into public view, society's awareness of
psychological trauma and sensitivity to human vulnerability also increases. At
times, however, when human barbarity and suffering become part of a hidden and

secret "underground" (Hermann, 1992), violations of social contracts may also affect society at large and become too horrifying to speak about. As such, the powers that be in a society (e.g., the media, government institutions) may manifest the very symptoms of denial and dissociation that plague many traumatized individuals. As a result, the study of trauma has been shrouded in controversy, as it forces society to address the dissonance that ensues when individuals are confronted by the divergence between the actuality of society as it is and the ideal of how people believe it should be. In the same manner that the traumatized individual must reclaim, understand, and integrate the past, so too must the rich and abundant history of trauma and treatment be redis-covered and integrated by social scientists, mental health professionals, and society at large.

Documents of traumatized patients from over 100 years ago are strikingly similar to symptoms and treatments that appear in journals today. Both diagnosis and treatment of trauma appear to have come full circle to support the sus-pected neurobiological underpinnings for psychological phenomena and subse-quent treatment interventions. In the late 1800s, Pierre Janet wrote in his dis-sertation *Psychological Automatism* that traumatic experiences leave indelible memories to which the individual continually returns. These memory traces of the hysteric unfold as terrifying perceptions, obsessional preoccupations, and somatic sensations. Janet referred to these mental images as "idees fixes" because of "their stereotypic nature, separation from normal mental processes and relative imperviousness to change" (Janet, 1898). These "idees fixes" lead eventually to depersonalization, depression, apathy, and social withdrawal. Janet characterized a posttraumatic syndrome as the incapacity to integrate memory and experience (van der Hart, Brown, & van der Kolk, 1989) and postulated that integration is further prevented by dissociation, which may occur when the individual perceives the presence of overwhelming threats.

French neurologist and contemporary of Pierre Janet, Jean-Martin Charcot initially treated and defined hysteria in terms of neurological functioning such as amnesia, convulsions, and paralyses, while paying little attention to the sub-jective experiences of his patients. However, he eventually came to recognize that hysteria was psychological in origin because symptoms could so easily be triggered, and then relieved, through the use of hypnotic images and suggestions (Hermann, 1992).

Sigmund Freud was among Charcot's followers in Vienna who continued the clinical observation of hysterics. He found that classification of symptoms alone was not enough and began intense interviewing of patients. Freud and Josef Breuer, in their *Studies on Hysteria,* reported that hysterics "suffer mainly from reminiscences." They hypothesized that traumatic events were split off from conscious awareness and later reappeared in the form of disguised representations or images. Explorations of patients' pasts often revealed appalling accounts of incest, abuse, and sexual assault. Social consciousness rose against this hypothesis and Freud eventually recanted (Freud, 1896/1962; Hermann, 1992).

Freud collaborated with Carl Jung on issues of analysis and theory development until their final split over Jung's insistence that dissociation was the result of the psyche coping with trauma and did not represent id impulses. Jung described consciousness as consisting of three elements: cognitive awareness, sensations, and affect (Jung, 1955; Kalsched, 1996). He further believed that dissociation, the splitting of these parts of consciousness, was a normal part of the psyche's defense against the overwhelming impact of trauma. While this response is normal and protective, the split (dissociated) parts move into unconsciousness and create unmitigating pain in the form of distressing dreams, intrusive images, and "annoying resentments" (Jung, 1955, p. 495) in the conscious life of the traumatized individual. Jung described the process of healing as irrational, for it required the individual to face in the present those very traumatic images he has been working to avoid. Jung wrote

> The "solvent" can only be of an irrational nature. In nature the resolution of opposites is always an energic process: she acts *symbolically* in the truest sense of the word, doing something that expresses both sides, just as the waterfall visibly mediates between above and below. . . . In an open and unresolved conflict dreams and fantasies occur which, like the waterfall, illustrate the tension and nature of the opposites, and thus prepare the synthesis. (Jung, 1955, p. 495)

There was a hiatus from the focus on traumatic experiences until the emergence of combat neuroses or "shell shock" among World War I and World War II combatants (Griffin, Nishith, Resick, & Yahuda, 1997). The extensive numbers of people affected by these wars again brought trauma and posttraumatic symptomology to the forefront of public awareness. The work of Abram Kardiner (1941) and his collaborative work with Herbert Spiegel delineated the core diagnostic criteria for PTSD, which remains essentially unchanged today (van der Kolk, McFarlane, & Weisaeth, 1996). Yet, despite these advances in diagnostic clarification, scientific interest in the study of trauma appeared to fall off significantly following the end of World War II.

During the next 25 years, relatively little emerged in the trauma literature. Interest in trauma was resurrected during the Vietnam conflict and the resurgence of the women's movement in the 1970s (Foy, Resnick, Sipprelle, & Carroll, 1987; Hermann, 1992). Trauma as the primary etiologic force for the hysterical symptomology of intrusive images, avoidance, and heightened arousal that had been documented in the late 1800s by Charcot, recapitulated by Freud and Janet, was again being acknowledged and studied by scientists and clinicians nearly a century later.

TRAUMATIC IMAGERY AND MEMORY ENCODING

There are three systems for processing and encoding memory experiences: somatic, imagery, and linguistic which involves the labeling of abstract symbolizations (Ahsen, 1982; Bruner, as cited in van der Kolk, 1994; Zilberg, Weiss, & Horowitz, 1982). The earliest organization of information occurs through the interplay of the somatic and imagery systems creating the initial self structure (Suler, 1996). Memories are encoded and revived through the interaction of images and somatic patterns of experience. As language develops, all incoming sensorial information is classified and organized linguistically. From adolescence on, people tend to synthesize normal non-traumatic sensory experiences linguistically into symbolic form that develop into the personal narratives of their lives (van der Kolk, 1994; van der Kolk & Fisler, 1995).

Van der Kolk proposed that during high sympathetic nervous system arousal associated with traumatic stressors, memories are stored iconically (somatic and imagery systems) because linguistic encoding of traumatic events fails to occur (Hermann, 1992; van der Kolk, 1994; van der Kolk & Fisler, 1995). Many scientific observers, beginning with Janet, have noted that emotional experiences are often relived through the non-linguistic symptoms of intrusive images, avoidance, and hyperarousal long after the original traumatic event (Foa & Hearst-Ikeda, 1996). The non-linguistic nature of these symptoms appears central to maintaining these reliving experiences.

Horowitz and Kaltreider (1979) proposed that stressful events require massive processing of internal and external stimuli. Accordingly, when information overload results in images, thoughts, and emotions that cannot be integrated into the self, they remain unprocessed and defense mechanisms such as dissociation, numbing, and denial are employed (Horowitz & Kaltreider, 1979). The innate need to maintain a balance between retention of old schemas and acceptance of new ones demands that the unprocessed information become integrated (Alexander, 1999). Thus, periods of intrusive recurring flashbacks and repetitive nightmares may reflect an attempt, albeit at a subconscious level, to complete this process.

The observations of Pierre Janet in the late 1800s have been demonstrated over and over again. Janet stated that, "traumatic memory consists of images, sensations, affective and behavioral states that are invariable and do not change over time" (van der Kolk & Fisler, 1995, p. 520). He further suggested that memories cannot be summoned at will and that they are state dependent. By contrast, narrative memory is semantic and symbolic and can be assimilated or accommodated into existing schemata according to social and personal demands. As such, successful integration of these traumatic images may need to be the primary focus of treatment.

TREATMENT MODALITIES USING IMAGERY

Psychodynamic Applications of Imagery

Psychodynamic theorists have attempted to account for posttraumatic symptomology using terms such as abreaction, catharsis, and denial. Janet was the first clinician to formulate a treatment of trauma based on clinical examinations. The stages of treatment in Janet's model are as follows (van der Hart et al., 1989):

1. the stabilization and reduction of symptoms, oriented toward preparation for the liquidation of the traumatic memories.
2. the identification, exploration and modification of traumatic memories.
3. reintegration of the personality and rehabilitation.

This "talking cure" was perhaps the most parsimonious explanation for the treatment of recurring images experienced by hysterical patients in early PTSD theoretical evolution. This treatment approach was the earliest documentation of "imagery substitution." Freud reconceptualized the process as "remembering, repeating, and working through" (Spiegel, 1988, p. 26). Jung recommended the use of "active imagination" (Jung, 1955, p. 526) to confront the images and ideas that, through the therapeutic process, take on " a dramatic character" (Jung, 1955, p. 496). This confrontation moved the interaction with the intrusive images from one of passivity to action and mastery. Jung also insisted that a running commentary of this process of action and mastery be kept so that the individual had tangible evidence of this knowledge and could no longer maintain avoidance and self-deception. This conceptualization of the need for and process of reintegrating cognitive awareness, affect, and imagery in consciousness (Kalsched, 1996) served as the primordial fuel for contemporary imaginal and reprocessing therapies (Jung, 1955).

Contemporary hypnotherapists contend that by creating a trance-like state and inducing emotional arousal, intrusive images and avoidant behaviors evoked by traumatic events can be reexperienced and reduced in a controlled situation (Brom, Kleber, & Defares, 1989; Spiegel, 1988). Appel (1999) contends that, through directed attention, hypnotherapy aids in the accommodation and assimilation, not only of the affect but also the traumatic images associated with the event. The therapeutic goal may be further extended to include the integration of a new worldview and an accompanying change in cognitive schema. While hypnosis allows for a level of relaxation that is likely to minimize avoidance and facilitate desensitization to the traumatic images, it also leaves the patient vulnerable to suggestion. Indeed, individuals' reports of their victimization are sometimes thought to be iaetrogenically induced through the use of suggestion in treatment, which in turn has fed and fueled the false memory controversy.

Behavioral Applications of Imagery

From a behavioral perspective, it is the severe anxiety accompanying the reexperiencing of traumatic events that hallmarks PTSD symptomology. Often individuals are unable to recall many of the details surrounding the traumatic event. Indeed, it appears that "traumatic memories are so aversive and anxiety-provoking that the motivation to enhance the consolidation of the memory is compromised by the extreme aversion associated with the memory" (Saigh, Yule, & Inamdar, 1996). Yet, because traumatic memories are stored in a state of high physiological arousal, recollection will likely be hampered unless they are recalled in a similar emotional state (Keane, Zimering, & Caddell, 1985). Thus, behaviorists contend that PTSD serves to block the needed exposure that promotes extinction by preventing the individual from accessing the original state of the traumatic arousal.

Traditionally, behaviorists have conceptualized anxiety as the attempt to avoid fear-evoking stimuli. As such, behavioral treatments have focused on exposure principles to facilitate extinction of the fear response. Imagery techniques used by behaviorists for the deconditioning of anxiety responses fall upon a continuum ranging from flooding or implosive therapy at one end to systematic desensitization on the other (Lyons & Keane, 1989; Saigh et al., 1996).

Systematic desensitization is based on the conditioning of incompatible responses (Wolpe, 1973). The patient is first taught a form of progressive deep muscle relaxation while simultaneously developing pleasant imagery (Bernstein & Borkovec, 1973), which is designed to later increase the patient's ability to engage in imaginal exposure of the traumatic event. Visual scenes of the traumatic event are arranged hierarchically from the least anxiety-arousing to the most distressing and are presented to the patient one scene at a time, interspersed with relaxation imagery, until habituation occurs. This back-and-forth from distressing imagery to relaxation imagery is continued until habituation and desensitization (i.e., an absence of anxiety) to all scenes of the hierarchy have been achieved (Foa, Rothbaum, & Molnar, 1995; Frueh, Turner, & Beidel, 1995; Lyons & Keane, 1989; Peterson, Prout, & Schwarz, 1991).

At the other end of the behavioral spectrum, flooding (imaginal or in vivo exposure) has also been successful in the treatment of anxiety in PTSD patients. Flooding involves prolonged exposure to distressing, trauma-related cues until the patient habituates and anxiety associated with these cues is extinguished. Keane, Fairbank, Caddell, and Zimering (1989) contend that the more visual cues generated during imaginal exposure, the greater the improvement in memory and subsequent greater deconditioning and anxiety reduction. Their treatment consists of relaxation training, practice in pleasant imagery and imaginal exposure (flooding) to the traumatic memories (Keane et al., 1989; Saigh, 1989). Boudewyns and Hyer (1990) have also reported success using a visual flooding exposure with Vietnam veterans. Similarly, Lyons and Keane (1989) outlined an implosive (flooding) therapy treatment for combat-related PTSD, identifying shifts that take place from direct re-experiencing to more symbolic representations of the traumatic event. These cognitive shifts appeared to add a dimension for which behavioral conditioning theories did not account.

Cognitive Behavioral Applications of Imagery

Foa and Kozak (1986), in their seminal article, noted limitations to the behavioral conceptualization of stimulus-response associations. They postulated that "fear is represented in memory structures that serve as blueprints for fear behavior, and therapy is the process by which these structures are modified" (Foa & Kozak, 1986, p. 21). Lang's (1979) bio-informational theory describes a fear network that includes emotional information about the "stimulus," "response," and "meanings" (Saigh et al., 1996). Thus, a fear structure is identified not only by physiological changes (responses) to a representational stimulus, but by the *meaning* given to that stimulus. This model includes both cognitive and affective components of the fear network (Foa, Steketee & Rothbaum, 1989; Kreitler & Kreitler, 1988).

Foa and Kozak (1986) further expanded Lang's theory by suggesting that imaginal exposure to traumatic stimuli corrects (by deconditioning) PTSD-related maladaptive evaluations. According to Foa and Meadows (1997), corrective emotional processing "requires the activation of the fear structure via introduction of feared stimuli, and the presentation of corrective information that is incompatible with the pathological elements of the fear structure" (p. 462). Therefore, because of the intensity of their responses, the prevalence of the stimulus generalization, and the low threshold required to activate the fear structure, trauma victims are thought to be significantly more vulnerable to anxiety and PTSD. Indicators of corrective emotional processing include: (a) a decrease in physiological reporting of fear activation during imaginal exposure, (b) a decrease in physiological reactions (habituation) within imaginal exposure sessions, and (c) a decrease in reaction to feared stimulus across imaginal exposure sessions (Foa & Kozak, 1986).

Many studies demonstrate that prolonged, repeated imaginal exposure to traumatic events, including combat, rape, and sexual assaults, ameliorates PTSD symptomology (Brett & Ostroff, 1985; Bryant & Harvey, 1996; Bryant, Harvey, Dang, Sackville, & Basten, 1998; Foa et al., 1995; Foa, Riggs, Massie, & Yarczowier, 1995; Foa & Rothbaum, 1990; Foa, Rothbaum, & Steketee, 1993; Friedman, 1997; Grigsby, 1987; Jaycox, Foa, & Morral, 1998; Pitman, 1997; Pitman et al., 1996; Riggs, Rothbaum, & Foa, 1995). Brief relaxation training is generally a precursor to the use of imaginal exposure during which patients are asked to imagine in great visual and sensory detail the complete sequence of their traumatic memories using the first person and the present tense. Patients rate their discomfort using a 0 percent to 100 percent Subjective Units of Distress (SUDs) (Wolpe & Lazarus, 1966) rating scale throughout the imaginal exposure process. The exposure is audio taped and used for practice at home between sessions. The length of each exposure session varies, usually between 60 and 90 minutes. However, it must be long enough to allow for reduction in physiological arousal and habituation both within and across sessions (Foa & Kozak, 1986; Orr, 1997; Shalev, Orr, & Pitman, 1992). In work with rape victims, Foa and colleagues (1995) suggest that as prolonged imaginal exposure decreases anxiety associated with traumatic experiences, a reevaluation of the meanings surrounding the events can occur. Reliving the traumatic event imaginally over and over facilitates the organizing of memories so they can fit into existing schemas (Resick, Jordan, Girelli, Hutter, & Morhoefer-Dvorak, 1988; Resick & Schnicke, 1990; Rothbaum, Foa, Riggs, Murdock, & Walsh, 1992).

Stress inoculation training (SIT) has a more direct effect on the traumatized individual's schema (Meichenbaum, 1994). Treatment focuses on teaching strategies to help problem solve, control anger, and relax so the victim can come to view himself/herself as a "coper" and survivor (Rothbaum et al., 1992). In addition to the intrusive ideations, many people diagnosed with PTSD experience a variety of related clinical problems including depression, panic attacks, anger reactions, interpersonal anxiety, and other generalized stress responses. With the use of SIT, clients have the opportunity to practice coping behaviors for addressing both the intrusions and related anxiety features in the form of imagery rehearsal. SIT affords the opportunity for more graduated exposure than more direct exposure therapies. This is done through helping the client to identify and isolate more specific stressors from the global experience of stress. Integration can then occur through gradual imaginal and in vivo rehearsals (Meichenbaum, 1994). Early identification of anxiety provoking cues and use of appropriate coping skills can greatly reduce anxiety (Sherman, 1998). Thought stopping, guided self-dialogue, biofeedback, social-skills training, and distraction are further examples of techniques used in anxiety management programs for PTSD (Foa & Meadows, 1997).

Another exposure-based strategy is eye movement desensitization reprocessing (EMDR). Francine Shapiro (1989) describes this approach as an integrated treatment that directs the client's attention to an external stimulus (e.g., eye movements, alternating hand taps, auditory tones) while focusing on the traumatic images or thoughts. Many characteristics of flooding and desensitization are shared with EMDR techniques (Cahill & Frueh, 1997; Shapiro, 1996). Recent studies have questioned the efficacy of this treatment approach, however (Feske & Goldstein, 1997; Foa & Meadows, 1997; Muris, Merckelbach, Holdrinet, & Sijsenaar, 1998; Sherman, 1998; Vaughn, Wiese, & Tarrier, 1994). Macklin et al. (2000) published a 5-year follow-up study of EMDR efficacy with Vietnam veterans. Their findings indicated no long-term gains from this treatment modality and in some cases there were increases in PTSD symptomology.

Recently, imagery rescripting and reprocessing therapy (IRRT) has been developed as an empirically based treatment intervention for adult survivors of childhood sexual abuse suffering from PTSD (Smucker, 1997; Smucker & Dancu, 1999; Smucker, Dancu, Foa, & Niederee; 1995; Smucker & Niederee, 1995) and expanded to traumatic injury victims (Grunert, Weis, & Rusch, 2000; Smucker, Weis, & Grunert, 2001). The goal of IRRT is to replace victimization imagery with mastery and self-nurturing imagery. IRRT includes three phases: imaginal exposure, mastery imagery, and self-nurturing/self-calming imagery as part of the treatment protocol. Individuals are trained in relaxation and SUDs ratings are used throughout the process to help the clinician identify, not only the point of most distress, but also the resolution of the distress. The role of the clinician remains non-directive and facilitative at all times. This is insured by the use of Socratic questioning. Socratic questioning during imaginal reenactment allows the participant's active imaginal engagement of the traumatic event in the present and facilitates the generation of new mastery images that confront and counter the traumatized individual's experiences of victimization and helplessness. These self-generated responses challenge and transform the images of victimization and powerlessness into images of mastery and competence. These transformed images provide an entrée for the development of not only mastery images, but also the cognitive and emotive experiences of mastery. These are then followed by the development of self-nurturing competence across this cognitive and emotive spectrum. A further goal of IRRT is for these mastery and self-nurturing/self-calming images to generalize to, and be activated in, other stressful situations while becoming a permanent part of the individual's cognitive coping repertoire.

CONCLUSION

The historical use of imagery in the treatment of posttraumatic stress disorder has been brief, sporadic, and fraught with what contemporary researchers would call methodological flaws. PTSD is a relatively new diagnosis, first appearing in the Diagnostic and Statistical Manual of Mental Disorders in 1980 (American Psychiatric Association, 1980). It would be difficult to imagine that trauma and the symptoms of PTSD have not plagued human existence since our inception in prerecorded time. To be sure, the absence of a diagnosis does not mean the absence of the experience.

Human history shows that people have used images throughout time to make meaning and record life experiences. Inherent in human nature is the need to order, label, and understand experiences in a way that leads to mastery in a safe and predictable world. Undoubtedly, overcoming trauma has been part of the evolutionary process of individual emotional and social competence since the "birth" of the human species. The newness herein thus lies not in the existence or non-existence of trauma, but rather in the understanding of this common human experience.

By contrast, the study of the psyche—as well as the active use of imagery in the treatment of trauma—is so new as to be all but invisible in the brief span of recorded history. Trauma is an aversive event for both the individual and the greater society. No doubt, it is this aversion that has contributed to the waxing and waning of efforts to understand trauma over the past century, as well as to the relative paucity of scientific data on the subject prior to 1980. This paucity speaks loudly to the urgent and dramatic expansion of research that has occurred in the last two decades.

Contemporary research can clearly be traced from the work of Janet, Jung, Kardiner, and Horowitz and is now being expanded by a plethora of committed scientist practitioners. To date, exposure-based techniques in a behavioral or cognitive setting comprise the majority of PTSD studies. Sherman (1998), citing other studies (Boudewyns, Hyer, Woods, Harrison, & McCranie, 1990; Foa & Rothbaum, 1990; Freuh et al., 1995; Gerrity & Solomon, 1996; Hyer, McCranie, Boudewyns, & Sperr, 1996), concluded that imaginal exposure-based therapies appear to be the most effective treatments currently available for PTSD.

These empirically supported cognitive behavioral interventions also appear to corroborate the treatment model proposed by Janet in the late 19th century; that is, in order for individuals diagnosed with PTSD to improve they must be able to stabilize, identify, explore, modify, and reintegrate the trauma experience (van der Hart et al., 1989). The use of imagery has been the critical factor in each effective treatment modality. As the study of the human psyche and PTSD continues, and our awareness of the precedence and power of images in the human experience increases, it is difficult to imagine that the role of imagery in the treatment of PTSD will not expand exponentially.

REFERENCES

American Psychiatric Association (1980). *Diagnostic and statistical manual of mental disorders* (3rd ed.). Washington, DC: Author.

Ahsen, A. (1982). Imagery in perceptual learning and clinical application. *Journal of Mental Imagery, 6,* 157-186.

Alexander, D. A. (1999). The presentation of adult symptoms. In E. D. Hickling & E. B. Blanchard (Eds.), *Road traffic accidents & psychological trauma: Current understanding treatment and law.* Oxford: Pergamon.

Appel, P. (1999). A hypnotically mediated guided imagery intervention for intrusive imagery: Creating ground for figure. *American Journal of Clinical Hypnosis, 41*(4), 327-335.

Bernstein, A. D., & Borkovec, T. D. (1973). *Progressive relaxation training: A manual for the helping professions.* Champaign, IL: Research Press.

Boudewyns, P. A., & Hyer, L. (1990). Physiological response to combat memories and preliminary treatment outcome in Vietnam veteran PTSD patients treated with direct therapeutic exposure. *Behavior Therapy, 21,* 63-87.

Boudewyns, P. A., Hyer, L., Woods, M. G., Harrison, W. R., & McCranie, E. (1990). PTSD among Vietnam Veterans: An early look at treatment outcome using direct therapeutic exposure. *Journal of Traumatic Stress, 3*(3), 359-367.

Brett, E. A., & Ostroff, R. (1985). Imagery and posttraumatic stress disorder: An overview. *The American Journal of Psychiatry, 142*(4), 417-424.

Breuer, J., & Freud, S. (1895/1955). Studies on hysteria. In J. Strachey (Ed. and Trans.), *The standard edition of the complete psychological works of Sigmund Freud* (Vol. 2). London: Hogarth Press. (Original work published 1895.)

Brom, D., Kleber, R. J., & Defares, P. B. (1989). Brief psychotherapy for posttraumatic stress disorders. *Journal of Consulting and Clinical Psychology, 57*(5), 607-612.

Bryant, R. A., & Harvey, A. G. (1996). Visual imagery in posttraumatic stress disorder. *Journal of Traumatic Stress 9*(3), 613-619.

Bryant, R. A., Harvey, A. G., Dang, S. Y., Sackville, T., & Basten, C. (1998). Treatment of acute stress disorder: A comparison of cognitive-behavioral therapy and supportive counseling. *Journal of Consulting and Clinical Psychology, 66*(5), 862-866.

Cahill, S. P., & Frueh, B. C. (1997). Flooding versus eye movement desensitization and reprocessing therapy: Relative efficacy has yet to be investigated—Comment on Pitman et al. (1996). *Comprehensive Psychiatry, 38*(5), 300-303.

Feske, U., & Goldstein, A. J. (1997). Eye movement desensitization and reprocessing treatment for panic disorder: A controlled outcome and partial dismantling study. *Journal of Consulting and Clinical Psychology, 65*(6), 1026-1035.

Foa, E. B., & Hearst-Ikeda, D. (1996). Emotional dissociation in response to trauma: An information-processing approach. In L. K. Michelson & W. J. Ray (Eds.), *Handbook of dissociation: Theoretical, empirical, and clinical perspectives* (pp. 207-224). New York: Plenum Press.

Foa, E. B., & Kozak, M. J. (1986). Emotional processing of fear: Exposure to corrective information. *Psychological Bulletin, 99*(1), 20-35.

Foa, E. B., & Meadows, E. A. (1997). Psychosocial treatments for posttraumatic stress disorder: A critical review. *Annual Review of Psychology, 48,* 449-480.

Foa, E. B., Riggs, D. S., Massie, E. D., & Yarczowier, M. (1995). The impact of fear activation and anger on the efficacy of exposure treatment for posttraumatic stress disorder. *Behavior Therapy, 26,* 487-499.

Foa, E. B., & Rothbaum, B. O. (1990). Rape: Can victims be helped by cognitive behavior therapy? In K. Hawton & P. Cowen (Eds.), *Dilemmas and difficulties in the management of psychiatric patients* (pp. 197-204). Oxford: Oxford University Press.

Foa, E. B., Rothbaum, B. O., & Molnar, C. (1995). Cognitive-behavioral therapy of posttraumatic stress disorder. In M. J. Friedman, D. S., Charney, & A. Y. Deutch (Eds.), *Neurobiological and clinical consequences of stress: From normal adaption to PTSD* (pp. 483-494). Philadelphia: Lippincott-Raven.

Foa, E. B., Rothbaum, B. O., & Steketee, G. S. (1993). Treatment of rape victims. *Journal of Interpersonal Violence, 8*(2), 256-276.

Foa, E. B., Steketee, G., & Rothbaum, B. O. (1989). Behavioral-cognitive conceptualizations of posttraumatic stress disorder. *Behavior Therapy, 20,* 155-176.

Foy, D. W., Resnick, H. S., Sipprelle, R. C., & Carroll, E. M. (1987). Premilitary, military, and postmilitary factors in the development of combat-related posttraumatic stress disorder. *The Behavior Therapist, 10*(1), 3-9.

Freud, S. (1896/1962). *The aetiology of hysteria* (in Standard Edition, Vol. 3, trans. J. Strachey). London: Hogarth Press.

Friedman, M. J. (1997). Posttraumatic stress disorder. *Journal of Clinical Psychiatry, 58*(9), 33-36.

Frueh,·B. C., Turner, S. M., & Beidel, D. C. (1995). Exposure therapy for combat-related PTSD: A critical review. *Clinical Psychology Review, 15*(8), 799-817.

Gerrity, E. & Solomon, S. (1996). The treatment of PTSD and related stress disorders: Current research and clinical knowledge. In A. Marsella & M. Friedman (Eds.), *Ethnocultural aspects of posttraumatic stress disorder: Issues, research, and clinical applications*. Washington, DC: American Psychological Association.

Griffin, M. G., Nishith, P., Resick, P. A., & Yehuda, R. (1997). Integrating objective indicators of treatment outcome in posttraumatic stress disorder. In R. Yehuda & A. C. McFarlane (Eds.), *Psychobiology of posttraumatic stress disorder—Annals New York Academy of Sciences, 821* (pp. 388-409). New York: New York Academy of Sciences.

Grigsby, J. P. (1987). Single case study: The use of imagery in the treatment of posttraumatic stress disorder. *The Journal of Nervous and Mental Disease, 175*(1), 55-59.

Grunert, B. K., Weis, J. M., & Rusch, M. D. (2000). *Imagery rescripting after failed imaginal exposure for PTSD following industrial injury*. Paper presented at the Third World Conference for the International Society for Traumatic Stress Studies, Melbourne, Australia.

Hermann, J. L. (1992). *Trauma and recovery*. New York: Basic Books.

Horowitz, M. J. (1986). *Stress response syndromes* (2nd Ed). Northvale, NJ: Jason Aronson.

Horowitz, M. J., & Kaltreider, N. B. (1979). Brief therapy of the stress response syndrome. *Psychiatric Clinics of North America, 2*(2), 365-377.

Hyer, L., McCranie, E., Boudewyns, P., & Sperr, E. (1996) Modes of long-term coping with trauma memories: Relative use and associations with personality among Vietnam veterans with chronic PTSD. *Journal of Traumatic Stress, 9*(2), 299-316.

Janet, P. (1898). *Nervoses et idees fixes*. Paris: Alcan.

Janoff-Bulman, R. (1992). *Shattered assumptions: Towards a new psychology of trauma*. New York: The Free Press.

Jaycox, L. H., Foa, E. B., & Morral, A. R. (1998). Influence of emotional engagement and habituation of exposure therapy for PTSD. *Journal of Consulting and Clinical Psychology, 66*(1), 185-192.

Jung, C. G. (1955). *The collected works* (Bollingen Series XX), R. F. C. Hull (trans.), H. Read, M. Fordham, & G. Adler (Eds.), Princeton, N.J.: Princeton University Press.

Kalsched, D. (1996). *The inner world of trauma: Archetypal defenses of the personal spirit*. New York: Routledge.

Kardiner, A. (1941). *The traumatic neurosis of war*. New York: Hoeber.

Keane, T. M., Fairbank, J. A., Caddell, J. M., & Zimering, R. T. (1989). Implosive (flooding) therapy reduces symptoms of PTSD in Vietnam combat veterans. *Behavior Therapy, 20*(2), 245-260.

Keane, T. M., Zimering, R. T., & Caddell J. M. (1985). A behavioral formulation of posttraumatic stress disorder in Vietnam veterans. *The Behavior Therapist, 8*(1), 9-12.

Kreitler, S., & Kreitler, H. (1988). Trauma and anxiety: The cognitive approach. *Journal of Traumatic Stress*, *1*(1), 35-57.

Lang, P. G. (1979). A bio-informational theory of emotional imagery. *Psychophysiology*, *16*, 495-512.

Lyons, J. A., & Keane, T. M. (1989). Implosive therapy for the treatment of combat-related PTSD. *Journal of Traumatic Stress*, *2*(2), 137-152.

Macklin, M. L., Metzger, L. J., Lasko, N. B., Berry, N. J., Orr, S.P., & Pitman, R. K. (2000). Five-year follow-up study of eye movement desensitization and reprocessing therapy for combat-related posttraumatic stress disorder. *Comprehensive Psychiatry*, *41*(1), 24-27.

Meichenbaum, D. (1994). *A clinical handbook / practical therapist manual: For assessing and treating adults with post-traumatic stress disorder (PTSD)*. Ontario, Canada: Institute Press

Muris, P., Merckelbach, H., Holdrinet, I., & Sijsenaar, M. (1998). Treating phobic children: Effects of EMDR versus exposure. *Journal of Consulting and Clinical Psychology*, *66*(1), 193-198.

Orr, S. P. (1997). Psychophysiologic reactivity to trauma-related imagery in PTSD. In R. Yehuda & A. C. McFarlane (Eds.), *Psychobiology of posttraumatic stress disorder—Annals New York Academy of Sciences, 821* (pp. 114-124). New York: New York Academy of Sciences.

Peterson, K. C., Prout, M. F., & Schwarz, R. A. (1991). *Post-traumatic stress disorder: A clinician's guide*. New York: Plenum Press.

Piaget, J. (1952). *The origins of intelligence in children*. New York: International Universities Press.

Pitman, R. K. (1997). Overview of biological themes in PTSD. In R. Yehuda & A. C. McFarlane (Eds.), *Psychobiology of posttraumatic stress disorder—Annals New York Academy of Sciences, 821* (pp. 1-9). New York: New York Academy of Sciences.

Pitman, R. K., Orr, S. P., Altman, B., Longpre, R. E., Poire, R. E., Macklin, M. L., Michaels, M. J., & Steketee, G. S. (1996). Emotional processing and outcome of imaginal flooding therapy in Vietnam veterans with chronic posttraumatic stress disorder. *Comprehensive Psychiatry*, *37*(6), 409-418.

Resick, P. A., Jordan, C. G., Girelli, S. A., Hutter, C. K., & Morhoefer-Dvorak, S. (1988). A comparative outcome study of behavioral group therapy for sexual assault victims. *Behavior Therapy*, *19*(32), 385-401.

Resick, P. A., & Schnicke, M. K. (1990). Treating symptoms in adult victims of sexual assault. *Journal of Interpersonal Violence*, *5*(4), 488-505.

Riggs, D. S., Rothbaum, B. O., & Foa, E. B. (1995). A prospective examination of symptoms of posttraumatic stress disorder in victims of nonsexual assault. *Journal of Interpersonal Violence*, *10*(2), 201-214.

Rothbaum, B. O., Foa, E., Riggs, D. S., Murdock, T., & Walsh, W. (1992). A prospective examination of post-traumatic stress disorder in rape victims. *Journal of Traumatic Stress*, *5*, 455-475.

Saigh, P. A. (1989). The use of an in vitro flooding package in the treatment of traumatized adolescents. *Journal of Developmental and Behavioral Pediatrics*, *10*(1), 17-21.

Saigh, P. A., Yule, W., & Inamdar, S. C. (1996). Imaginal flooding of traumatized children and adolescents. *Journal of School Psychology*, *34*(2), 163-183.

Shalev, A. Y., Orr, S. P., & Pitman, R. K. (1992). Psychophysiologic response during script-driven imagery as an outcome measure in posttraumatic stress disorder. *Journal of Clinical Psychiatry, 53*(9), 324-326.

Shapiro, F. (1989). Eye movement desensitization: A new treatment for post-traumatic stress disorder. *Journal of Behavior Therapy & Experimental Psychiatry, 20*(3), 211-217.

Shapiro, F. (1996). Eye movement desensitization and reprocessing (EMDR): Evaluation of controlled PTSD research. *Journal of Behavior Therapy & Experimental Psychiatry, 27*(3), 209-218.

Sherman, J. J. (1998). Effects of psychotherapeutic treatments of PTSD: A meta-analysis of controlled clinical trials. *Journal of Traumatic Stress, 11*(3), 413-433.

Smucker, M. R. (1997). Posttraumatic stress disorder. In R. L. Leahy (Ed.), *Practicing cognitive therapy* (pp. 193-200). Northvale, NJ: Jason Aronson.

Smucker, M. R., & Dancu, C. V. (1999). *Cognitive behavioral treatment for adult survivors of childhood trauma: Rescripting and reprocessing.* Northvale, N.J.: Jason Aronson.

Smucker, M. R., Dancu, C., Foa, E. B., & Niederee, J. L. (1995). Imagery rescripting: A new treatment for survivors of childhood sexual abuse suffering from posttraumatic stress. *Journal of Cognitive Psychotherapy: An International Quarterly, 9*(1), 3-17.

Smucker, M. R., & Niederee, J. (1995). Treating incest-related PTSD and pathogenic schemas through imaginal exposure and rescripting. *Cognitive and Behavioral Practice, 2,* 63-93.

Smucker, M. R., Weis, J. M., & Grunert, B. K. (2001). Imagery rescripting therapy for trauma survivors with PTSD. In A. A. Sheikh (Ed.), *Handbook of therapeutic imagery techniques.* Amityville, NY: Baywood.

Spiegel, D. (1988). Dissociation and hypnosis in post-traumatic stress disorders. *Journal of Traumatic Stress, 1*(1), 17-33.

Suler, J. (1996). Mental imagery in the organization and transformation of the self. *Psychoanalytic Review, 83*(5), 657-672.

Van der Hart, O., Brown, P., & van der Kolk, B. A. (1989). The psychological treatment of posttraumatic stress of Pierre Janet. *Annales Meico-Psychologiques, 147*(9), 976-982.

van der Kolk, B. A. (1994). The body keeps the score: Memory and the evolving psychobiology of posttraumatic stress. *Harvard Review of Psychiatry, 1*(5), 253-265.

van der Kolk, B. A., & Fisler, R. (1995). Dissociation and the fragmentary nature of traumatic memories: Overview and exploratory study. *Journal of Traumatic Stress, 8*(4), 505-525.

van der Kolk, B. A., McFarlane, A. C., & Weisaeth, L. (1996). *Traumatic stress: The effects of overwhelming experience on mind, body, and society.* New York: The Guilford Press.

Vaughan, K., Wiese, M., & Tarrier, N. (1994). Eye-movement desensitization: Symptom change in post-traumatic stress disorder. *British Journal of Psychiatry, 164,* 533-541.

Wolpe, J. (1973). *The practice of behavioral therapy.* New York: Pergamon Press.

Wolpe, J., & Lazarus, A. A. (1966). *Behavior therapy techniques.* New York: Pergamon Press.

Zilberg, N. J., Weiss, D. S., & Horowitz, M. J. (1982). Impact of event scale: A cross-validation study and some empirical evidence supporting a conceptual model of stress response syndromes. *Journal of Consulting and Clinical Psychology, 50*(3), 407-414.

CHAPTER 16

Imagery in the Treament of Trauma

JAN TAAL AND JOHN KROP

> It appears your complaint stems from all these things that you told me that
> happened, all these memories that you have of these things that you say
> happened; and so would you be different today, would your situation be
> different today, if your memories were different?
>
> David Grove (in Grove & Panzer, 1984, p. 99)

A trauma is a psychological wound, which time did not heal. That
wounding has not been integrated adequately in the person's organism and continues to influence the person's life in a negative way. The negative experience
continues to hurt and is reactivated periodically. Most of the time the person
has dissociated from the memories or feelings of the occurrence or series of
occurrences. This is particularly true if the pain is unbearable. The dissociation
is a psychological rescue attempt to escape the painful feelings. The person is
"somewhere else" so that he/she can continue to live his/her life (van der Hart,
Steele, Boon, & Bliss, 1986).

That "going away" or splitting from the pain has two major consequences:
The person will try to avoid everything that is associated with the trauma
(generalization) and, paradoxically and unintentionally, will thereby maintain
the presence of the trauma. It helps the client to feel the pain less acutely, but
it also will result in the wound remaining infected and continuing to exert
negative psychological and often physical influence. These feelings and memories
often occur in the form of images. Images are building stones of the human
psychological experience, and negative images often play a dramatic and central
role in Posttraumatic Stress Disorder (PTSD). It is therefore understandable and
logical that imagery is widely used in the treatment of trauma. Exposure to
traumatic memories through the use of imagery is frequently and effectively used
as a procedure in many therapeutic approaches. However, therapeutic approaches

using imagery also can have serious dangers. These methods can destabilize a client and therefore should be handled by the therapist with great care and in continuous consideration of the needs and possibilities of the client. Confrontation with traumatic images is not a medicine by itself and should not be a goal in itself. When it is used, it always should be embedded in the overall goal, which is better adaptation and functioning in the client's present life situation (Taal, 1994).

WHY IMAGERY?

Imagery is a particularly useful and effective method in the treatment of trauma because of several reasons:

1. Spontaneous images related to the traumatic events often are an important part of the person's complaints, psychological and social suffering, and therefore constitute an important psychological field to work in. An example may illustrate this: Every time Fred drove his car near the particular town where his best friend died in a motorcycle accident, he "saw" images of the accident and of his friend dead on the ground, although in reality Fred had not been present when it had happened. Each time great sadness would rise up in him, he would start to tremble and would have to stop his car.

2. Words only partly express and represent a person's inner experience. Images provide a more comprehensive picture of what matters.

3. Extremely distressful and frightening situations can be expressed and worked on in a metaphorical and symbolic form, without the necessity to mention all the details. What a client verbally does not dare to say or is unable to do, often can be expressed in images or in a metaphor of some sort. Another example: Carol talks about this dark shadow she so often feels on herself, immobilizing her. Without telling exactly what the dark shadow represented, she was able to gradually deal with the shadow. In the beginning she did not fully know what or whom the shadow represented. During the imagery work (like drawing the shadow, talking to the shadow, taking the place of the shadow), her understanding of it became clearer.

Eventually she came to see how the shadow played a role in her history. Even though she was not able to verbally express the related historical events until much later, she was able to stand her ground vis-a-vis the shadow, even push the shadow away and become less immobilized by it.

Some clients will never get to the "exact facts" related to the trauma from which they are suffering; yet, they become much better in dealing with it through imagery. These images may not truly represent what actually happened; however, the historical truth is not as important as what the client thinks happened. The client will not react to the historical truth but rather to what he/she imagines it to be. When that becomes apparent to the therapist, it is usually not productive to confront the discrepancy. Historical truth and inner experience belong to two different realms. It is wiser to stay with the image the client presents, historically accurate or not. For a client it may be essential to be "believed" by the therapist. When the client asks the therapist, whether he/she believes that it really happened this way, the latter may say: "I believe that what you tell me, is what you believe has happened. Whether this is historically true does not matter to me." Ours is not a legal profession.

4. Certain symbolic images may exert a beneficial influence on the client and help the client to fortify his/her identity. The image of the sun often helped Carol in difficult times. Concentrating on the internal image of a sun and on a drawing she made of a sun helped her in two ways. It helped her counter the negative emotional influence of "the shadow," and it promoted feelings of warmth and trust in herself.

THE IMPORTANCE OF I-STRENGTH
AND STRUCTURE IN DAILY LIFE

The procedure most mentioned in literature on treatment of trauma is "imaginary exposure." However, as an isolated procedure, it is usually not effective and even can be harmful. This can be the case when the I-strength of the person (ego-strength) is not sufficient. The "I" is the faculty within a person that takes care of the integration of experiences and emotional balance. In order to help the person to cope better with the traumatic images, the person needs to be trained to integrate the emotional and psychological influences the images exert. He/she needs capability and strength to handle these contents. A client wrote this reflection: "As long as I was not conscious of the traumas that had occurred in my life, I was in a frozen state, stagnant. In the course of my life only more ice accumulated. Now, as I am thawing, I start to see and feel what happened. That hurts a lot and scares me. Maybe in a while, new things will develop or latent qualities come to life, but now I need 'grip.' I need a goal for the future or else I become overcome by depression and intense pain."

Treatment of trauma should initially focus on better coping with day-to-day life, thus creating the right conditions to approach traumatic psychological material directly. In cases where there is not enough I-strengh and an exploration of traumatic content could lead to decomposition of the personality, any direct approach to traumatic content is to be avoided.

Therapy should then restrict itself to coping with concrete day-to-day life issues. It is necessary for the client to develop a structured basis on which to fall back and from which to derive strength.

Dealing with traumatic material and using revealing imagery comes later. An example again: John, a shy, unkemp 40-year-old man, was having difficulty with relations and finding a proper place in society; he had no job, for instance. In the first interview John mentioned that he had lost his father at the age of 7. The death of his father, the person he had been very fond of, changed his life dramatically. His mother was unable to run her family of John and his four brothers and sisters.

John, who was also handicapped by a vision problem, was put in a residential home. When he came out of the residential home, at age 15, he was emotionally withdrawn and felt unwanted and inadequate.

It seemed evident that the loss of his father was one of the major sources of his problems today. But talking with the therapist about that event and remembering what happened then, caused him great distress. When he came home after the session, he did not eat for days, did not wash, and did not show his face to anyone. Only when he did not show up for his appointment the next week, did the therapist realize the gravity of John's condition. Talking about the death of his father brought up such an overwelming flood of images and feelings of loneliness that he was literally unable to move or take care of ordinary daily actions.

During the following 2 years, the focus of the therapy was on helping John to structure his life, to learn to take care of himself, to learn the importance of taking the time and trouble to wash his body and his clothes regularly, to cook a proper meal at least five times a week, and to clean up his house. Eventually John, stimulated by the therapist, found some voluntary work in a home for the aged. During all that time, the death of his father was never brought up.

What was needed first was to establish more structure in his day-to-day life. Although the historical source of his distress was not treated directly, his strength and position in life had improved to the point that John could develop some friendships and even found a job that satisfied him.

I-STRENGTHENING STRATEGIES

For this phase of the therapy, the following strategies may be of use:

1. Promote and repair the adaptive capacities in daily life. Pay attention to meals, personal hygiene, keeping a clean house, safety, etc.
2. Enhance self-esteem.
3. Develop positive perspective; improve areas of complaint. Foster new hope.
4. Stabilize symptoms and complaints, check medication if indicated, possibly in tandem with the client's physician.
5. The therapist should practice active listening ("I hear you").
6. Focus on positive aspects of the present and the future.
7. Practice healing imagery. For example, after some relaxation: "Imagine yourself in a comfortable place, maybe in nature, maybe somewhere else. Go where you really feel safe and at ease . . . . Notice how this place looks . . . . Feel the beneficial atmosphere . . . . Let it enter your body . . . your cells . . . relax in the safety of this place . . . smell the smells . . . hear the sounds . . . . Make this a place you always can come back to, for comfort and to deeply relax."

8. Give homework (writing and other assignments). Be sure to come back to it at the next session. Honor the work done.
9. Redefine the client from "victim" to "survivor."
10. Make use of transpersonal energies. In the literature various names are given to these—for instance, center core, internal self-helper, higher self, spiritual helper, guide. It is amazing how many severely traumatized people mention the presence of transpersonal energies. Example: A client who had been misused by her father during a substantial portion of her childhood, reported that there always had been "an angel singing psalms to her." She felt it had helped her survive. Another client reported seeing a light: it would appear when she needed it most. Others find solace in going to a place where there is no pain and no suffering. A good way to access these energies in a client is to ask: "What helped you survive, what sustained you?"

Transpersonal energies can nourish and support clients and can help them to develop meaning and identity. Sometimes, however, transpersonal energies can cause an unbalance. They can facilitate dissociation. In those cases the client can be helped to develop other capacities as a counter force. For instance, by learning to be more assertive, a client who generally seeks refuge in "heavenly visions" will have the option to stand his/her ground rather than to flee.

DEALING WITH THE TRAUMA ITSELF

Imagination can be an eminent technique in the healing of traumas. The work-through consists of contacting the original events, feelings, and/or traumatic images and then correcting what seemed to be dysfunctional in the response of the client at that time. The following steps can be discerned in the process:

1. Recognizing and Acknowledging the Importance of the Trauma. Is there still a negative influence in the present life of the client? Often the client is unclear about the extent of the damage, denies or diminishes the influence the trauma still has. This often springs out of powerlessness and fear. Only when the person is sufficiently convinced of the seriousness of the trauma, can he/she develop the necessary motivation to venture the work-through.

2. Context and Diagnosis.
a. Evaluate the client's context, background, daily life.
b. What trauma does it concern? How much insight and awareness is there? What are any situational triggers? What are the physical sensations or complaints?
c. Is the client motivated to work through?
d. What is the desired state? What can be achieved? How feasible is a work-through?

3. Anchoring. Before commencing the actual viewing of the traumatic events, the client needs to be taught to "anchor" in his/her body and in the here and now. This will make it possible for the client to come back when being overwhelmed. He/she knows how to return to his/her body and this "safe spot." A procedure to do this follows: The client, sitting in a chair, is helped to become aware how the feet rest on the ground, how the body is supported by the chair, how the breath flows in and out. Once the client has reached a satisfactory degree of relaxation, he/she can be asked to touch a part of the body (the pulse, the elbow) and symbolically anchor this feeling of relaxation. Whenever he/she becomes too tense or overwhelmed in the work-through, he/she can now touch this spot and return to relaxation. It is also possible for the therapist to provide anchoring by touching the client, when it seems necessary.

4. Admitting the Feelings Related to the Traumatic Events. Is the person prepared to face the feelings that possibly could emerge? Ask for instance: "What is the worst you could discover?" "And do you think you can handle that?" Explore little step by little step the association with the feelings that are related to the traumatic events and the gradual letting go of dissociation.

5. Reliving or Reviewing the Traumatic Events. Various forms and gradations are possible. Initially it may be necessary to keep a distance from the traumatic experience. The client can regress and slip back into the "overwhelmed victim" position. That is usually not desirable. Keeping distance may be achieved by instructing the client to let the images appear on a film screen. Or the therapist can emphasize that "the current 45-year-old Sandy from her safe position in the chair with her current resources looks at what the 6-year-old Sandy goes through and experiences." Or the therapist can ask the client to imagine that he/she has push-buttons to control the film, when he/she wishes.

Some therapists ask the client to go back and reexperience what happened. That requires much I-strength from the client. The therapist in that case may end up becoming a good parent who helps the client recover from the painful experience.

It is important to pay close attention to the decisions the client makes under the influence of the trauma. The therapist should distinguish between a "bad experience" and a trauma. In a "bad experience," the belief system of the client stays intact and the client can integrate the experience without major changes in his/her belief system. In a trauma, the client can no longer maintain his/her belief system. It shatters, and for his/her own protection the client now makes a life decision that may be life-denying and seriously narrows the choices that are available. Again an example: Jannie, 30, was not able to establish a meaningful relationship with a man. Every time the encounter with a man, even a desirable man, came to the point that sex became a possibility, she froze and had to interrupt the experience, even walk out of the room. She consciously wanted to have sex but could not handle it. In the therapy, she made a connection between her fear of sex and being molested when she was 8 and 9 years old by an uncle who lived with her family.

She was asked to review one of these episodes and she reluctantly agreed. She was afraid to "go back to the scene of the crime." She was sure that she would fall apart.

The therapist, noticing this fear, decided not to go ahead, even though she had agreed. He explained that it was not necessary to feel the way she felt at the time of the molestation. In fact that would be undesirable. She would not relive the experience. She would review what had happened to the 8- and 9-year-old Jannie, while the 30-year-old Jannie remained in the safety of her chair and in possession of her current resources. At any time that the experience became too much, she or the therapist could stop the experience and relax again.

She now indeed was able to review a whole episode without too much trouble. Two or three times the therapist had to say, "as the 30-year-old Jannie in her chair in this room now sees what 8-year-old Jannie goes through . . . ," to prevent her from regressing. When the uncle had left the room and 8-year-old Jannie was left bewildered, the therapist now asked 30-year-old Jannie to see what was going on for the 8-year-old Jannie. What did she think, feel, and what decisions did she make? Adult Jannie thought that 8-year-old Jannie felt she was dirty, that her genital area was dirty, and that she never wanted to touch "that" again. Also she never wanted to be in a room alone with a man.

It was not difficult for the therapist to see the connection between those decisions and her inability to engage in anything that came close to sex. But this was not the time to try to make that connection overt. Instead, the therapist now asked Jannie what she thought the 8-year-old needed to hear. Jannie needed to hear that she was not dirty, that it was O.K. to touch her genitals, and that later, when she was grown up, she could have sex any time she wanted and enjoy that.

Now the therapist asked Jannie to say that directly to young Jannie, which she did. The therapist then asked Jannie, if she thought young Jannie understood. "Yes, except for that about enjoying sex; she is too young to grasp that." "What do you want to say now to young Jannie?" Jannie was not quite sure how to respond to Jannie. The therapist offered: "Would it be O.K. to say to Jannie that it is O.K. that she does not understand that now, but to just remember that for later?" Jannie nodded and said to young Jannie, "Your uncle was wrong in what he did. This is your body and no one should touch it the way your uncle did. But when you grow up, I hope that you can remember what I tell you now. You can enjoy this with the right person. Remember that for later." "Does young Jannie get that now?" "No, but that is all she can now understand about it." "Anything else you want to tell her?" "Yea, I love you, you are O.K."

This dialogue between little Jannie and adult Jannie is in essence a repro-gramming of the belief system that was scrambled at the time of the molestations. For the therapist, it is essential to see to it that adult Jannie does not regress and start feeling like 8-year-old Jannie. The therapist can facilitate that by always addressing the adult Jannie. For instance, the therapist should not ask, "How do you feel?" but rather "What do you think 8-year-old Jannie feels now?" The whole process is conducted via adult Jannie. Also the therapist should try to make the dialogue between the adult and the 8-year-old Jannie as direct as possible; for example, "Tell her that . . ." (Krop, 1981, 1997).

6. Recovery and Reintegration. It is evident that one experience like this, impactful as it is, is not enough to establish a new belief system that is life affirming. It may be necessary for the client to repeat the process a number of times and maybe even to go through scenes, later in her life, where she experienced the same feelings. It also may be possible now for the client to imagine future scenes, where she is able to have a positive intimate encounter with a man. It is not possible to forget the traumatic experiences or to pretend that they did not happen. But where there was a wound, there is now a scar, and people can live quite well with a scar.

7. Implementation. It is necessary now to try out if the changes indeed show up in the daily life of the client. Therapist and client now can explore possible scenarios where the client exposes himself/herself to a clearly delineated experience. For instance, in the case of Jannie, to allow receiving or giving a massage that can include as much or as little of her body as she wants can be helpful.

Of course these steps do not always follow in this sequence. Another example, in which the elements mentioned above can be recognized, though not necessarily in sequence, follows. Anita is 43 years old. At the age of 6, she was lured to the attic by her neighbor and sexually abused. Only recently did she remember that this took place. It was repressed for years.

Thinking back to this event is accompanied by great anxiety; she hardly dares tell me what happened. It is the first time that she shares this with someone. Repeatedly her throat tightens; as if she is being strangled. Later Anita tells me that her neighbor indeed throttled her throat to prevent her from screaming. It is not essential for the therapist to hear every detail of what happened. Anita can make contact with what occured in her own way.

As Anita talks about what happened, she occasionally disconnects from what she tells. She "floats away to a far land where she is alone and feels nothing." The exploration of this experience through the images and accompanying feeling occupies a number of sessions. Anita notices that "not being there" in a way provides safety but also causes her to "not always live fully." She realizes that this also occurs in her sexual life. She detaches, feels nothing, and floats around in that far land.

At the time of this occurrence, Anita's mother was seriously ill and not available to Anita, and she did not feel that she could tell her father what had happened. The inability to talk to anyone about this added significantly to the pain and anxiety of the sexual abuse. That she now can talk about this is of great importance in itself. Later in imaging what happened, the therapist goes with her to the attic and protects her against this neighbor, and thus takes the position of the available, protective adult—a kind of "ideal parent." Holding her hand, in a combination of imagery and psychodrama, the therapist goes with her up the stairs to the attic and she describes the terrible things the neighbor does.

In the beginning she slips readily back into the pain and fear, becomes the child of then. She cannot feel the therapist's helping presence and "floats away" again. Gradually she comes to see the therapist as the adult who interferes and protects her, and she can allow herself to stay and see what happens between the girl and the neighbor. She begins to develop some perspective on what happened.

In the next phase, the therapist asks Anita to take the position of the "ideal parent." Gradually Anita learns to become an "ideal mother" for the traumatized child. This brings her to a crucial phase where her I-strength allows her now to do the confrontation herself. For the first time she manages to open her throat, express her anger, and scream. In her fantasy, she kills the neighbor and cuts him to pieces. (In reality the man had died years ago.) Now that she is operating out of her own adult position toward the trauma, the therapist can step out of the role of "ideal parent."

More and more she experiences herself as an adult and can take care of the 6-year-old who had suffered so much and had felt so alone. She also made a number of real changes in her life. A year later she moved into a new flat, and for the first time in her life she felt that this flat was really hers; she also went back to school. She reported that she was beginning to have faith in herself and to believe in a future. Her circle of friends also changed drastically. In a follow-up 2 years later, Anita said that she had started a relationship with a man and that, contrary to her old relationships, she felt that in this relationship she maintained her identity and self-worth.

THE ROLE OF THE THERAPIST

Dealing with a trauma is a complex and delicate matter with many traps, and requires a great deal of sensitivity on the part of the therapist and a careful step-by-step approach. When confronting the trauma, the therapist provides emotional support as an empathetic presence, without in any way forcing the client. A balance has to be achieved between too much and too little stimulation in confronting the traumatic events (Taal, 1994).

A metaphoric picture of the client/therapist relationship could be that of the therapist walking with the client, one step behind, hand on the shoulder of the client. The client leads. When the client stops, the therapist stops and may inquire what is going on. When the client wants to back off, the therapist backs off with the client. When the client does anything peculiar, like holding his/her breath, raising an arm, turning away, the therapist asks, "What is going on now?" Thus the client is not led or pushed by the therapist, the therapist is behind the client and helps him/her find out what is going on. The therapist is not in front of the client pulling him/her along.

At times, when the client needs protection, the therapist can leave the position behind the client and take an active role, for example, going up the stairs to the attic with Anita. In traumas that occurred at an early age, in particular incest, there is often a serious developmental disturbance. The "I" in relation to the trauma still functions on the traumatized-child level, still feels the same powerlessness in relation to what happened and often has split off from it (dissociation).

It is necessary in the first phase of the therapy to develop a bond with the client. This bond facilitates filling the gaps in the development of the child so that the adult becomes equipped to deal with what needs to be processed. The therapist assumes temporarily the role of a protecting, nurturing supportive parent, who was needed, but was sorely lacking, when the traumatic experience(s) took place.

This has far reaching consequences for the client/therapist relationship. It requires an emotional engagement of the therapist, much patience, and ability to handle aggression or distrust. A great deal of the therapeutic work takes place in the transference with the therapist. Fortunately the countertransference issues that play a role here are more and more recognized. When there is little "I" strength in the client, the therapist can "lend ego" to help the client find the way in all the turmoil inside. Again an example: Gerard was haunted by images of his father pursuing him with an axe. When the client was a child, his father had been aggressive and violent. After the divorce of his parents, which occurred when Gerard was 6, he was raised by his mother. The images of his father with the axe were still so strong, that Gerard locked himself up in his room a great deal of the day. During the night, Gerard at times had violent outbursts during which he broke things and sometimes injured himself. When he was in the last year of his studies, he had quit.

The confrontations with the pictures of his father wielding the axe were intense. In the beginning, Gerard screamed and trembled. It was as if his father were present in the therapy room. At those times, the therapist became a protective, supportive parent to him and, on occasions, would scream loudly at that imaginary father to leave Gerard alone.

His anxiety level decreased bit by bit. The threat of his father, however, remained until Gerard, in an imaginary confrontation with his father, frantically tried to wrest the axe from his father's hands. Initially he did not succeed; yet the efforts, guided by the therapist's support and coaching, gave him more self-confidence. For instance, Gerard now began to ask advice about resuming his studies.

It is possible, and often very valuable, to use a combination of mental imagery and artistic expression (Taal, 1998; Wertheim-Cahen, 1998). Instead of describing the images to the therapist, the client can express his/her emotions and inner experience, and discharge tension. Creative expression provides room for feelings or experiences that—consciously or unconsciously—are unacceptable to the client. It is often necessary to emphasize that artistic or aestethic performance is not the aim of the expression. Sometimes clients feel hampered in expressing themselves creatively because of memories of negative experiences, when their work was judged negatively, for instance in school.

To counteract these negative expectations, it is useful to emphasize that the creative work is not supposed to be beautiful. It may also be helpful to do some liberating excercises, such as making "ugly paintings" on purpose.

The choice of materials is important. Each expressive medium has its own possibilities. A client who has a tendency to lose himself/herself in images, can be offered clay, which will help in grounding himself/herself more. Paint gives the client a great variety of shapes and colors. The choice of the size of paper is relevant. The client may be too timid to use a large sheet and may start using a small sheet or the corner of a large sheet; later the client can become more venturesome and draw bolder. Creative expression is an act and asks concrete action of a client.

Thus the ability to participate and take a stand is mobilized. Concretely dealing with the materials, actively choosing an art form and materials increase the client's participation in the healing process and enhance problem-solving capacities. Combining mental imagery and expressive means can make mental images more visible; and vice versa: a drawing, painting, or a created object can in turn lead to further mental images. It often happens that a client's artistic expression already shows what the client is not yet aware of. Six months later the client may say, "Oh, that's what that meant."

There is no question that the expression itself has healing value. There are diverging opinions in the field how much interpretation of the expressive product or the process is useful. It seems safe to ask the client's opinion or even to ask the client to take the place of the objects or drawings and speak for them. It is unwise for the therapist to presume to know what an image means and to insist that the client consider or even buy the explanation.

An example of combined use of mental images and creative expression follows: Vera grew up with much loneliness and anxiety. She sees herself as "a rose that is broken and has fallen on the ground." She is not able to see herself in any other way. The suggestion of the therapist to visualize a stronger, more ideal image is of no avail. The image of the broken rose comes back all the time.

Only when she starts working with paint, a change starts to occur. The therapist asks her to mix colors that for her represent power. Then he asks her to smear these colors on a sheet, then on another sheet which is bigger. She happens to like working with paint and chooses one painting to take home with her to hang on her wall.

In the following sessions she continues doing art work. She works with crayons, paint, cut-outs, and collages around the themes "power" and "rose." The rose remains unrooted, however. On a suggestion of the therapist, she changes the rose into a rosebush. But the rosebush is continually being pruned back, even leveled to the ground. In a further exploration of how this takes place, "a man with shears who comes to do that in the night" appears. When these images appear she becomes nauseated. After excercises in anchoring (I-strength), she at last feels strong enough to paint this man and, subsequently, with thick stripes to put him behind bars.

Almost always the work with traumatized clients proceeds slowly. In small steps, one thing leads to another. In Vera's case, after the session in which she "crossed out the man," she reported that she had effected a change in her work situation. When that was successful, it reinforced her feeling of power and that manifested itself again in a change in the image of the rosebush. It was no longer pruned back, and new branches and buds began to appear.

SUMMARY

Imagery is particularly useful in the treatment of trauma. Extreme, distressful, and frightening situations can be expressed and worked through in a metaphorical and symbolic form, without the necessity to mention all the details. The treatment entails discovering what is needed to heal the trauma and diminish the pain and the continual regression and dissociation.

In order to effectuate a succesful recovery it is usually necessary to introduce new helpful elements into the images. Special attention needs to be given to the "I"-strength of the subject. One can proceed only if the subject is present enough in the here-and-now and is able to assimilate the emerging material. When the trauma originates from a young age (e.g., incest) there is often a serious disturbance in the development of the personality, which needs to be addressed first.

REFERENCES

Bliss, E. 1986. *Multiple personality, allied disorders and hypnosis*. Cambridge: Cambridge University Press.

Grove, D., & Panzer, B. I. (1984). *Resolving traumatic memories*. New York: Irvington.

Krop. J. (1981). *Actiemethoden*. Baarn: Nelissen.

Krop. J. (1997). *Using metaphors in therapy*. 3 videotapes. Available through ENVISION, tel. 831-4797667.

Taal, J. (1994). Imaginatie therapie. *Tijdschrift voor Psychotherapie, 4*, 227-246.

Taal, J. (1997, January). Innerlijke beelden die helen. Imaginatie bij ziekte. *Prana*, 33-39.

van der Hart, O., Steele, K., Boon, S., & Brown, P. (1993). The treatment of traumatic memories: Synthesis, realization and integration. *Dissociation, 6*(2/3), 162-180.

Taal, J. (1998). *Coping with cancer through artistic expression and imagery*. www.kankerinbeeld.nl.

Wertheim-Cahen, T. (1998). Art therapy with asylum seekers. In D. Dokter (Ed.), *Art therapists, refugees and migrants* (pp. 80-93). London: Jessica Kingsley.

CHAPTER 17

Imagery and Cancer

HOWARD HALL

[Cancer] is a word—not a sentence
R. F. Jevene (in Jevene & Levitan, 1989, p. 51)

Imagery techniques were one of the earliest means of treating physical diseases. There is evidence that such procedures were employed in ancient Babylonia and Summaria (Samuels & Samuels, 1975). Around the 1960s, however, imagery techniques began to receive serious scientific scrutiny (Holt, 1964), and there were efforts to incorporate imagery techniques into the practice of cognitive behavior therapy (Craighead, Kazdin, & Mahoney, 1981; Lazarus, 1978).

Another development was the use of imagery in facilitating physiological change with such techniques as autogenic training (Schultz & Luthe, 1969), hypnosis, biofeedback, relaxation procedures, and meditation (Pelletier, 1979). These techniques were employed for what might be termed stress-related illnesses (Selye, 1974). Imagery and relaxation techniques have also been utilized within primary medical care settings in the treatment of medical conditions that are associated with stress, such as chronic pain, headaches, hypertension, and the emotional aspects of cancer (Chiaramonte, 1997). Imagery and hypnotic approaches have also been helpful non-pharmacological means of addressing the distress associated with multiple invasive cancer treatment procedures (Chen, Joseph, & Zeltzer, 2000).

A controversial area is the suggested relationship between the development and course of cancer with psychological factors such as stress (Bammer & Newberry, 1981; Holden, 1978; Tache, Selye, & Day, 1979). Although retrospective studies do not allow for inferences of causal relationships, Achterberg and Lawlis (1978) reviewed about 50 studies in this area and summarized them by stating that:

> There are two general conclusions that are evident from this research. First, regardless of instrumentation, there are enough replications to formalize the notion that a relationship does exist between the course of the disease and the

psychological dimensions. Second, several premorbid psychological factors consistently appear. For example, the memory of an early home life inadequate to needs of support and security, a pre-disease event of an emotional loss and feelings described as helplessness or hopelessness all emerged in several independent investigations. (Achterberg & Lawlis, 1978, p. 17)

THE SIMONTONS' EARLY IMAGERY WORK

On the basis of the relationship between psychological factors and cancer, Carl Simonton, a radiation oncologist, and Stephanie Matthew-Simonton, a psychotherapist, developed a comprehensive treatment approach to cancer. Included in this package was one of the first reported uses of imagery and relaxation in the treatment of cancer. In addition to imagery exercises and the patient's regular cancer medication, the Simontons also conducted intensive psychotherapy to explore emotional issues surrounding the onset and course of the disease.

The Simontons first employed imagery and relaxation in 1971 with a 61-year-old man whose diagnosis was cancer of the throat (Simonton, Matthews-Simonton, & Creighton, 1978). The man's physical condition was very poor and his weight had dropped from 130 to 98 pounds. He also had difficulty breathing and swallowing his saliva. When the Simontons saw this patient, his prognosis was less than a 5 percent chance of surviving five years.

A program of imagery and relaxation was developed for this patient to practice three times a day. He was instructed to first concentrate on relaxing his muscles from his head down to his feet. Next he was to visualize being in a calm, pleasant place, such as the woods. Then he was to vividly picture the cancer in his body and to visualize his radiation treatment as "millions of tiny bullets of energy" striking all cells in his body, both the normal and the cancerous cells. The cancer cells were seen as being "weaker and more confused" than the normal cells, and thus would die from radiation, whereas the healthy cells would be capable of repairing the damage. Then the patient was asked to imagine his white blood cells carrying away the dead cancer cells through his kidneys and liver. Finally, he was able to picture his body as healthy and normal with the cancer tumors decreasing in size.

The results of this first case were remarkable. Halfway through the treatment, the cancer began to disappear and the patient started to eat and gain weight. Additionally, there were few negative side effects from the radiation treatment. After two months of continued improvement, there were no signs of cancer. It is interesting to note that this man successfully employed imagery on his own to decrease his arthritis symptoms and to restore full sexual activity after a 20-year problem of an erectile dysfunction.

After this case, the Simontons clinically tested this imagery/relaxation procedure with 159 highly selected patients diagnosed to have medically incurable cancer and given one year to live. Of the original 159, 63 patients were alive two years after their diagnosis—that is, one year beyond their original prognosis. Furthermore, of those 63 patients who had practiced the imagery/relaxation technique and had survived beyond their prognosis, 22 percent demonstrated no evidence of cancer, 19 percent showed tumor regression, while 27 percent had stabilized. There was some new tumor growth for 38 percent of this group. This study had no untreated control groups, thus definitive conclusions could not be reached.

The Simontons argued that their approach to cancer treatment provided a means of actively involving patients in their own treatment. They also suggested that the imagery/relaxation component of their program led to an enhancement of the patients' immune system. This intriguing hypothesis, however, was never directly tested as no blood measures of immune functioning were taken during the course of this initial study.

After extensive work with imagery in the treatment of cancer, the Simontons identified eight features that they felt were important in altering the course of cancer. They noted that patients who did not do well often lacked one or more of these features.

1. The cancer cells are imagined as weak, confused, soft, and easily broken down. It is encouraging when the cancer cells are imagined to resemble hamburger meat or fish egg, for example. On the other hand, ants or crabs, for example, are regarded as poor images, since they are quite tenacious.
2. The treatment is viewed as "strong and powerful" and able to interact with and destroy the cancer.
3. In the imagery, the healthy cells easily repair any treatment-related damage. The cancer cells, on the other hand, being "weak and confused," are not able to recover and consequently are destroyed.
4. The body's immune system or army of white blood cells are imagined to greatly outnumber and overwhelm the cancer cells.
5. Along the same lines, the white blood cells are viewed as aggressive and eager to destroy the cancer cells, and their victory seems inevitable.
6. It is important to visualize the dead cancer cells being flushed out of the body in a biologically natural way.
7. Patients should see themselves as healthy and disease free.
8. Finally, patients are to imagine themselves fulfilling their life's goals.

The Simontons recognized the importance of monitoring the content of their patients' imagery. After one individual's medical condition continued to deteriorate even though he was practicing imagery three times a day, it turned out that many of the above eight features were absent from his visualizations. The patient described his cancer as a "big black rat." Clearly this rat was neither weak nor confused. His treatment, however, was viewed as "small yellow pills." The patient reported that occasionally the rat would eat one of these pills and become sick for a while but then recover and bite him even harder. In other words, the cancer was visualized as stronger than the medical treatment. In addition, the white blood cells were described as eggs in an incubator waiting to be hatched. The Simontons pointed out that this patient had, in essence, visualized total suppression of his immune system. Thus, if a patient practiced imagery regularly yet medically regressed, the content of the imagery might provide a key to understanding the lack of improvement.

Although the Simontons helped to launch the broad use of imagery with the aim of altering the course of cancer, this approach has subsequently been severely criticized on several grounds. Specifically, their cancer patients may not have been representative of the cancer population, but may have reflected a highly select sample of patients. Also, their claim that the use of imagery extended survival time in cancer patients has not been statistically substantiated. In addition, their intensive 5-day psychotherapy treatment program was quite costly. It has also been argued that the program made patients feel guilty that they had brought on their own disease. Susan Sontag (1978) criticized psychological approaches to cancer, such as the use of imagery, on the grounds that they place blame on the patient for the development of his/her illness. Finally, the immune surveillance of cancer cells, on which their imagery was based, has been seriously questioned (Friedlander, 1985).

THE IMAGE-CA TECHNIQUE AND CANCER PREDICTIONS

Building on the suggestion that specific features of the patient's imagery may be associated with cancer outcome, Achterberg and Lawlis extended the Simontons' work on the content analysis of imagery with the development of the Image-CA technique (Achterberg & Lawlis, 1978). This psychological instrument was employed to evaluate the effectiveness of the patient's imagery and also to predict the future development of the disease.

The Image-CA has 14 dimensions that include: 1) vividness; 2) activity; and 3) strength of the cancer cells. The less vivid, less active, and weaker these cells were imagined to be, the higher the person's score. Dimensions (4) through (8) measured the imagery for the white blood cells (i.e., the immune system). Specifically, they assessed the vividness, activity, proportions of white blood cells to cancer cells, the size, and the strength of the white blood cells. The white blood cells should be seen vividly, they should appear active, large, and stronger than the cancer cells, and they should outnumber the enemy. Dimensions (9) and (10) evaluated the imagery of the medical treatment in terms of its vividness and effectiveness. Again, the more vividly the treatment was imagined and the more effective it was seen to be, the higher the score.

Imagery also was assessed along the dimension of (11) concrete or symbolic. The more symbolic the imagery was, the higher the score. For example, visualizing the white blood cells as white knights would be considered highly symbolic.

Dimension (12) evaluated the overall strength of the imagery on a scale ranging from weak to very strong. Dimension (13) dealt with the patient's regularity in practicing imagery or thinking about his/her disease. This scale ranged from not imaging to imaging extremely frequently.

Finally, the last dimension (14) was the examiner's prognosis on a scale ranging from a continued active disease state to rapid remission. This last dimension required a certain degree of clinical judgment, and it was omitted for inexperienced examiners. With all 14 dimensions, a total score ranged from 247 or greater to 109 or less. With only the 13 dimensions, the range was from 165 or greater to 86 or less.

The administration of the Image-CA initially involved tape-recorded relaxation exercises, followed by instructions to visualize the white blood cells, cancer cells, and medical treatment. Unlike the Simontons' approach, however, the Image-CA evaluation did not provide any suggestions concerning the form the images should take.

Achterberg and Lawlis had their patients draw images of their tumors, white blood cells, and medical treatment (Achterberg & Lawlis, 1978). Subsequently, a structured interview was given so that the 14 dimensions could be scored on the 5-point scale with 1 representing "weak or ineffective" visualization and 5 indicating "strong or most desirable" imagery (Achterberg & Lawlis, 1978).

The reliability and validity of the Image-CA was examined within two normalization studies (Achterberg & Lawlis, 1978) employing samples from two different populations of cancer patients. The first study employed a group of 58 patients having metastasized cancer with roughly 0.05 chance of surviving five years. This group was composed of mostly white, middle class, highly educated individuals. The second study involved a group of 21 racially mixed cancer patients from a low socioeconomic level.

When the Image-CA was administered to these two different populations, good intercorrelational and interrater reliability for both groups was obtained. Of greater interest, however, was the validity data from these two studies. In the first study, an attempt was made to predict the patient's health status with the Image-CA at a two-month follow-up. When a multiple regression analysis was performed on all 14 dimensions of the Image-CA scale, it made correct predictions for 93 percent of the patients who showed a favorable prognosis at a two-month follow-up. The individuals in this category scored 198 or above on the Image-CA. This instrument also predicted correctly for 100 percent of the patients who showed an unfavorable prognosis at the follow-up period. In this group, all subjects who scored 150 or below on the Image-CA demonstrated new cancer growth or died. The middle range of the Image-CA (i.e., 198-150) was not reliably predictive.

When the clinical opinion dimension was omitted from the total score, the predictive validity of the tool was still good for the uppermost and lowermost range of the Image-CA scale, but it was more powerful when the full assessment was used (Achterberg & Lawlis, 1980).

In the second study, concurrent validation was attempted by correlating the Image-CA with social workers ratings of the patient's general activity, working ability, and social adjustment. A Patient Status Form was employed to obtain these ratings. The results of the second study revealed significant concurrent validity between the Image-CA and these ratings.

The observation that the Image-CA predicted future disease conditions was supported by findings from an early study (Achterberg, Lawlis, Simonton, & Matthews-Simonton, 1977) that demonstrated that psychological instruments, including the Image-CA, accurately predicted the follow-up disease status, whereas the blood chemistry data only provided information about the current disease state and was not predictive of later disease conditions. The other psychological tests employed within this battery were the Minnesota Multiphasic Personality Inventory, Locus of Control Scales, Fundamental Interpersonal Relations Orientation Test, Bem's Sex Role Inventory, and the Profile of Mood States. The blood chemistry data included measurements of complete blood count: free fatty acids, cortisol, cholesterol, acid phosphatase, lactic dehydrosenase, and alkaline phosphate.

Achterberg and Lawlis (1978) employed imagery not only for assessment purposes, but also for the treatment of cancer and other diseases (Achterberg & Lawlis, 1980). They, like the Simontons, felt that imagery provided patients the opportunity to participate in their rehabilitation process (Simonton, Matthews-Simonton, & Creighton, 1978). Also, they stated that counterproductive imagery could be altered, although sometimes with difficulty (Achterberg & Lawlis, 1978).

Attention to the specific nature of imagery employed would continue with the work of Belleruth Naparstek on prescriptive imagery for specific conditions (Naparstek, 1994). She pointed out that imagery had come a long way after the Simontons:

> But since those early days, we've all learned a lot more about imagery. We know now that it needs to be a multisensory experience, accessed in the altered state, and probably most effective when felt as sensation in the body. In the sixties and seventies, imagery was something essentially visual and two-dimensional. Imagery meant flat, disembodied pictures produced in the head. One problem with this view was that people who weren't particularly "visual" didn't do well with it; those with auditory and kinesthetic imaginations, for example, were at a disadvantage. Secondly, for physical and emotional well-being, imagery needs to be experienced in the body for maximum impact. This was the lesson that Elmer and Alyce Green, two tireless biofeedback pioneers from the Menninger Foundation, and their gifted psychologist daughter, Patricia Norris, taught us. (Naparstek, 1994, p. 41)

Naparstek outlined a range of different levels of imagery: feeling state imagery, end-state imagery, energetic imagery, cellular/immune imagery, physiological imagery (e.g., cardiovascular imagery, metaphoric imagery, psychological imagery, and spiritual imagery). Imagery exercises were also outlined for emotional conditions such as depression as well as common complaints such as headaches, allergies, pain, sleeplessness, fatigue, and a sluggish metabolism.

In the years following the early work of the Simontons and Achterberg, President Nixon declared a war on cancer waged on the molecular front. At the same time, but below the radar screen of modern medicine, an alternative paradigm was emerging. Relaxation and imagery techniques were being employed by the people as some of the most frequently used alternative/unconventional medical approaches for treating chronic non-life threatening medical conditions (Eisenberg et al., 1993). The use of imagery techniques for treating cancer were becoming more popular within the emerging field of mind-body medicine. The American Institute of Stress, established in 1978, worked to promote an understanding of this relationship between stress and its effects on health and illness. Some of the individuals involved with this early movement included: Peter Rosch, president of the institute; pioneering stress researcher, Hans Selye; as well as Flanders Dunbar who introduced the term "psychosomatic" into American medicine. Trustees of the institute included such prominent individuals as: Norman Cousins and Kenneth Pelletier, who wrote in the area of imagery and healing; as well as mind-body researcher Marvin Stein. In 1982, the field of mind-body medicine was advanced by a symposium sponsored by the institute to promote thinking in this controversial field. This symposium focused on why and how we get sick or stay well as well as what the relationship was between stress, emotions, behavior, and the immune system with special reference to cancer. The meeting brought together some of the most prominent researchers and clinicians who would later shape the landscape of the mind/body field over the next decade. This distinguished group of researchers and clinicians included: Jeanne Achterberg and G. Frank Lawlis; Robert Ader, the father of psychoneuroimmunology; Herbert Benson, who did extensive research on the relaxation response; Lawrence LeShan, who pioneered the notion that illness often follows some loss or disruption in one's life; Patricia A. Norris, who made major contributions to the field of biofeedback at the Menninger Foundation; and Caroline B. Thomas, who presented her classic study on prediction of cancer and other disorders by personality traits. I also spoke on the effects of hypnosis on the immune system. Following this pivotal meeting, we witnessed the emergence of the field of psychoneuroimmunology and attention to how psychological factors could influence immune activity and the development and/or course of a disease such as cancer.

PSYCHONEUROIMMUNOLOGY

Robert Ader (1981) helped to pioneer the field of "psychoneuroimmunology" which provided evidence of clinically significant interactions between the central nervous system (CNS) with various immune processes.

A decade later revealed abundant data regarding the neuroanatomical, neuro-chemical, and neuroendocrine pathways with the immune system (Ader, Felton, & Cohen, 1991). This CNS influence on immune activity provided a mechanism to account for how, in part, psychological and cognitive factors such as imagery techniques might facilitate healing processes (Hall, 1983).

My colleagues and I (Hall, Mumma, Longo, & Dixon, 1992) conducted a study to examine the effects of imagery and hypnosis on immune responses as assessed by traditional measures of lymphocyte function. Hypnosis, instead of relax-ation, was employed for several reasons. For one, it is very similar to the relax-ation technique used by the Simontons and Creighton (Bowers & Kelly, 1979; Simonton, Matthews-Simonton, & Creighton, 1978). Secondly, I was experienced in the use of hypnosis for pain reduction with cancer patients. Also, there was both clinical and experimental evidence in the literature that suggested that hypnosis could result in an enhancement of immune reactions (Hall, 1983). In addition, Bowers and Kelly argued that the patients who improved in the Simontons' study might have been highly hypnotizable individuals (Bowers & Kelly, 1979). Thus, the Simontons may have inadvertently selected for such subjects (Bowers & Kelly, 1979). However, they did not assess for hypnotizability to determine the importance of this factor. Given the above factors, an experiment was designed to examine the effects of hypnosis and imagery on T and B cell immune functions.

EXPERIMENTAL STUDIES ON IMAGERY AND BLOOD MEASURES OF IMMUNE RESPONSES

Hall, Mumma, Longo, and Dixon (1992) investigated the use of hypnosis to increase immunity function in 19 healthy individuals ages 22 to 85. This broad age range was employed because research has shown that increas-ing age appears to be associated with decreased immune functioning. Also, as one grows older there is an increase in the production of cancer cells possibly due to an immune deficiency (Weksler & Hutteroth, 1974).

The first step involved taking a 25cc sample of blood from each subject to provide pre-hypnosis baseline data of immune activity. Subsequently, subjects were hypnotized with relaxation induction. During hypnosis, they were asked to imagine their white blood cells as "strong," "powerful" sharks with teeth that attacked and destroyed "weak," "confused" germ cells that caused colds and flu. Following hypnosis, subjects were given written and verbal instructions in self-hypnosis and asked to practice twice a day until the second scheduled session one week later. One hour after the end of hypnosis, another 25cc post-hypnosis blood sample was drawn. The purpose of this second session was to determine the effects of practice on hypnosis and immune activity. After completing both hypnosis sessions, each subject was individually assessed on hypnotizability with the Stanford Hypnotic Susceptibility Scale, Form C (Weitzenhoffer & Hilgard, 1962).

In this study, it was demonstrated that 14 of 19 healthy adults increased lymphocyte responses to stimulation with Pokeweed mitogen after practicing relaxation with suggestions for increasing immune activity (Hall, Mumma, Longo, & Dixon, 1992). An interaction of age and hypnotizability with changes in white cell counts from pre- to post-intervention was noted. It should be pointed out that these changes were quite modest and only detectable with the above interaction.

In accord with the hypothesized role of imagery impacting the immune system in her early work, Stephanie Simonton went on to examine the effects of relaxation and imagery training to enhance the immune recovery for 17 cancer patients with advanced head, neck, breast, and lung cancer who were immunosuppresive following radiation treatment. It should be noted that this study was not designed to extend survival time of advanced cancer patients, but to examine the impact of imagery on immune activity. The intervention involved randomly assigned subjects to either a treatment group or a delayed treatment condition. Treatment involved a 3-week baseline period for blood immune measures of lymphocyte stimulation by Varicella Zoster (VZ) viral antigen. This baseline period was followed by a 3-week intervention phase. During this part of the study, patients received group sessions twice weekly of relaxation and imagery of their cancer, their immune system, and their treatment. Simonton observed an increase on in vitro lymphocyte stimulation measure from baseline to the end of treatment for the immediate treatment group (4.8 to 7.2 units), but for the delayed control group there was little change during this period prior to their intervention with VZ antigen levels during these two periods at (3.5 to 4.8). Following treatment, the VZ measure increased to six units for the delayed treatment group (Simonton-Atchley, 1993). Frequency of imagery practice was correlated with immune VZ changes, but level of hypnotic susceptibility was not related (Simonton-Atchley, 1993). Simonton-Atchley followed six of these subjects a year later and found that all had discontinued imagery practice and that their immune levels had returned to pretreatment baseline values (Simonton-Atchley, 1993). Our research group continued to explore the relationship between imagery and immune changes within healthy individuals.

Voluntary Immunomodulation in Adolescents Using a Cyberphysiologic Strategy

A subsequent study by our research group examined the effects of prior training in relaxation/imagery before subjects attempted to alter immune activity (Hall, Minnes, Olness, & Tosi, 1992). In this study, high school students and undergraduate college students were randomly assigned to one of three groups.

Group A (the control group) had blood sampling before and after a rest condition for two sessions spaced one week apart. Peripheral temperature and pulse recordings were also taken before and after the rest intervention to explore psychophysiologic responses associated with voluntary immunomodulation. Group B (the untrained experimental group) had blood, peripheral temperature, and pulse recordings taken before and after a self-regulation (relaxation/imagery) exercise with imagery focused on increasing neutrophil adherence. Group C was an experimental group that received four training sessions prior to their attempts to increase neutrophil adherence. The results of this study revealed that neither the control group (Group A) nor the untrained experimental group (group B) demonstrated increased neutrophil adherence in either session. In fact, the post-adherence measures actually decreased during session one for group B. The experimental group that received training (Group C) had an increase in their adherence for the second session. Consistent with the hypnosis and physiology literature, the psychophysiologic measures in the study revealed that only the resting control Group (A) demonstrated a psychophysiologic profile suggestive of relaxation with decreased pulse rates for both sessions and an increase in peripheral temperature during the first session after resting. The trained experimental group increased neutrophil adherence on the second session and demonstrated no changes on the psychophysiologic measures during either session (Hall, Minnes, & Olness, 1993).

Directional Changes in Neutrophil Adherence Following Relaxation/Imagery (Self-Regulation) Training

This study examined the effects of self-regulation training on directional changes in neutrophil adherence (Hall, Papas, Tosi, & Olness, 1996). This study also employed undergraduate college students who were randomly assigned to one of three groups. Group 1 (a new control group that had prior resting experience) ($N = 9$), received four training sessions where they were asked to rest without any formal instructions, two sessions each week for two weeks. This was followed by two experimental sessions one week apart where blood samples were taken before and after a rest period. Pulse rate and peripheral temperature recordings were also made before and after a rest period. It should be pointed out that this control group differed from the one in the prior study in that the subjects in the control group (Group A) had no prior instructions to rest before the experimental session. Group 2 (decrease experimental group, $N = 4$) and Group 3 (increase experimental group, $N = 3$) received four self-regulation training sessions followed by two experimental sessions where blood samples, pulse rate, and peripheral temperature recordings were made before and after a self-regulation exercise with a focus on decreasing or increasing neutrophil adherence. It should be noted that the subjects were strongly encouraged to focus on imagery that was associated with directional changes in neutrophil adherence.

The results from this pilot study revealed that the two experimental groups (Groups 2 and 3) demonstrated pre- to post-intervention decreases in neutrophil adherence. The trained control group (Group 1) demonstrated a sizable increase in neutrophil adherence during both sessions. This finding was contrary to initial expectation. Directional changes were observed in neutrophil adherence, but not in the expected experimental groups. The results from the psychophysiologic measures helped to clarify this finding. The two groups that demonstrated the greatest opposite changes in neutrophil adherence (Groups 1 and 3) also demonstrated opposite psychophysiologic alterations. For example, in both sessions Group 1 demonstrated pre- to post-resting increases in neutrophil adherence along with psychophysiologic changes suggestive of relaxation, with decreases in pulse rates and increases in peripheral temperature during both sessions. Group 3, which demonstrated decreases in adherence, however, had psychophysiologic measures suggestive of cognitive activity with increases in pulse rates and decreases in peripheral temperature. Group 2 showed little variation in pulse or peripheral finger temperature during either session. The results from this pilot study suggest that it may be possible to behaviorally engineer directional changes in neutrophil adherence. It does appear, however, that the psychological factor associated with the increase in adherence for both studies was the deep relaxation and not the imaging. Active imaging appears to be associated with decreases in adherence. Given the emphasis in this study for directional changes, imaging was highly emphasized for the two experimental groups. During the prior study, subjects in the trained experimental group (Group C) had more relaxation training than either the untrained experimental group (Group B) or the untrained control group (Group A). Group C also demonstrated initially a decrease in adherence during session one, which was probably associated with imaging. Thus, it appears that deep relaxation is associated with increases in neutrophil adherence and active imaging is associated with decreases on this measure.

This research on attempting to produce bi-directional changes on neutrophil adherence with particular images cautions against too much focus on producing an image designed to produce a specific image directional physiologic change. As noted earlier when the subjects actively imaged their neutrophils increasing in adherence, they actually did the opposite and decreased. There was the suggestion that such intense imaging may result in a physiologic stress response, with its corresponding down regulation on some components of immune activity. While on the other hand, just resting without imaging was associated with increases in adherence. This was probably mediated via a physiologic state of parasympathetic relaxation versus the direct ability of imagery to alter specific physiologic changes. Clearly this is a complicated issue where continued research is needed.

HYPNOTIZABILTY

High hypnotic susceptibility has been proposed to account for the ability of individuals to alter their physiology (Bowers & Kelly, 1979). In my initial study, age, hypnotizability, and their interaction, was associated with changes in immune measures (Hall, Mumma, Longo, & Dixon, 1992). In a subsequent study with neutrophil adherence, no evidence for an association between hypnotizability and immune changes was found (Hall, Minnes, Olness, & Tosi, 1992). It should be recalled that there was also no association between hypnotizability and increases on immune measure in the Simonton-Atchley's study (1993). Experimental evidence for hypnotizability being associated with immune alterations, has met with mixed results, with both positive support (Ruzyla-Smith, Barabasz, Barabasz, & Warner, 1995) and negative findings (Locke et al., 1994). Thus, the role of hypnotizability and changes in immune activity does not appear to be very robust. It has also been suggested that high hypnotic ability, with its association with altered perceptions, may actually interfere with an individual's ability to alter his/her physiology (Hall, 1986).

PSYCHOSOCIAL INTERVENTIONS AND CANCER

Beyond imagery, it is now clear that psychosocial interventions can have a major impact on the course of cancer. Researcher David Spiegel approached the idea of imagery and cancer with a great deal of skepticism. Spiegel (1991) noted:

> Throughout the United States, patients were joining programs in which they were taught to visualize their white cells killing their cancer cells and were being asked questions such as, "Why did you want your cancer to spread?" This so irritated me that I conceived what I thought would be the perfect negative experiment: I had a group of patients with cancer who had been helped psychologically. If I could show that there was no difference in survival time between this group and groups that had not received such psychotherapy, the "mind-over-matter" issue could be put to rest once and for all. (p. 62)

In this study, 86 patients with metastatic breast cancer were randomly assigned to either a one-year intervention condition where subjects would receive weekly supportive group therapy and self-hypnosis for pain management or a control condition where subjects received routine oncological care (Spiegel, Bloom, Kraemer, & Gottheil, 1989). Much to Spiegel's surprise, 48 months into the study, a third of the patients who had received the intervention were still alive, whereas all of the control patients had died. At the 10-year follow-up there were only three patients alive, but the mean survival time for the intervention group was 36.6 months, whereas the mean survival for the control group was only 18.9 months. The Spiegel study had a major impact in the field of psychosocial intervention and increased survival time for metastatic cancer patients. It should be noted that this study did not prove that imagery extended the survival time of cancer patients, but more broadly, psychosocial interventions had a major impact on not only the psychological adjustment to cancer, but also to how long patients lived.

Psychosocial support has been associated with lower levels of depression, fatigue, and confusion and increases in vigor, active coping strategies, as well as enhanced immune activity in terms of large granular lymphocytes and natural killer cells activity compared to a non-intervention control group (Fawzy et al., 1990a,b). Thus, psychosocial interventions may result in a number of wide ranging psychological and physiological benefits that suggest the need for inclusion of other components to a cancer treatment program beyond just imagery.

INTEGRATED CANCER PROGRAMS

Deirdre Brigham (Brigham & Davis, 1994) has incorporated prescriptive imagery approaches within a comprehensive 28-day program incorporating stress management, expressive therapies, group and individual therapy, play and laughter, exercise and nutrition, along with high-level awareness and other approaches. Brigham (Brigham & Davis, 1994) outlines her imagery approach to cancer below as she notes:

> Cancer is actually many conditions. Imagery will need to take into account the type of cancer being dealt with. For example, imagery for leukemia might be very different from imagery for a lung tumor. Cancer is a disease with a complex web of causality. One very significant factor in cancer is stress, with its destructive effect on the immune system. In the case of most cancers, high doses of stress chemicals destroy or inactivate immune cells, allowing cancer cells to develop into potentially life-threatening tumors. (p. 337)

Clearly, this type of comprehensive program taps into the therapeutic benefit of interventions beyond imagery and relaxation. The psychosocial support aspects are clearly evident from the literature.

Several decades ago, imagery was employed with the hope of directly altering the course of cancer given some initial uncontrolled case histories by the Simontons. It is now known that such a dramatic impact of imagery is not routine. Additionally, imagery approaches to cancer have generated a great deal of controversy. A 1980 *Psychology Today* article entitled: "Images that Heal: A doubtful idea whose time has come" attacked the underlying assumptions of the Simontons' approach, particularly the relationship of stress, the immune system, and human cancers (Scarf, 1980).

On the other hand, psychosocial interventions such as comprehensive programs that include imagery and social support are associated with improved psychological functioning as well as increased survival time. Can the prescriptive use of imagery result in specific physiologic changes? It is not clear, however, that such intentional use of particular images can have specific effects. It is clear that specific physiologic changes can be produced via different behavioral operations that result in either activation of the sympathetic nervous system with its accompanying physiologic effects or via relaxation with its associated parasympathetically mediated outcomes. Thus, if one desires to either up regulate or down regulate certain immune responses that are mediated via the sympathetic or parasympathetic nervous system, then one could design behavioral interventions that would activate the appropriate autonomic nervous system response. This might involve simple relaxation without imagery or active imaging to elicit a more sympathetically based system. Whether intentional imagery of specific physiologic changes produces specific outcomes independent of the sympathetic and parasympathetic nervous system is not clear. Hopefully, more research will clarify this issue in the future. It should be pointed out that there are reports in the literature of cancer regression due to procedures that do not employ imagery, such as intensive nonfocused meditation (Meares, 1978, 1979, 1983) and an imageless type of deep hypnotic inductions (Newton, 1983). These types of relaxation procedures are apparently very different from those employed in the imagery/relaxation techniques reviewed in this chapter. They are also quite different from the progressive relaxation variety employed in behavior therapy programs (Bernstein & Borkovec, 1973). The question of how these non-imagery procedures work or how they are similar to imagery techniques cannot be answered at this time.

In the 1980s, Achterberg and Lawlis (1980) addressed critics who questioned the use of these imagery procedures as an adjunct to cancer treatment. They stated that:

> Our bias is that treatment must be as well grounded in a database as possible but that to withhold psychological intervention until "all the facts are in" is unethical. The facts may never be "all in." However, there are sufficient data currently available to warrant pursuing a psychological approach, together with medical treatment, in the best interests of patients with malignancy. (p. 129)

It is clear today that the literature supports the inclusion of an imagery approach as a viable adjunct within an integrative medical program for cancer treatment. Thus, imagery as psychosocial component to an integrative cancer treatment is no longer "a doubtful idea" but an important component whose time has come. Beyond imagery, the field continues to offer new directions for healing.

NEW DIRECTIONS: THE META-PSYCHOLOGY OF HEALING

Vitalism or Healing Energies

The progression of thinking about physical diseases has moved from a lack of attention to psychological factors in disease and healing process, including the germ theory of infectious diseases, to the field of mind-body medicine for stress-related conditions. The emergence of Acquired Immune Deficiency syndrome (AIDS) along with advanced forms of cancer, however, have revealed some limitations of both the current biomedical and mind-body models. Such challenges have encouraged the evolution of new thinking regarding healing and disease processes. Concepts of "vitalism" or healing energies appears to be influencing and gently transforming the mind-body field within complementary and alternative medicine (Kaptchuk, 1996). As noted by Kaptchuk (1996), "Practitioners of most alternative healing believe that one source of their intervention is a kind of "vital energy" their system uses still not appreciated by conventional biomedical science. Subtle health-promoting influences pervade the alternative healing world" (p. 35). Modern alternative and complementary healing approaches that posit energy healing practices are Non-Contact Therapeutic Touch (Krieger, 1975) within the United States, as well as practices borrowed from other cultures which are thousands of years old, such as Indian (Ayurveda) medicine and Chinese traditional medicine. These cross-cultural traditional healing practices are recognized and practiced throughout the world as well as within the United States.

For example, in Zigaching, China "The Center," one of the largest hospitals in China, offers an ancient 5,000-year-old healing tradition known as Qigong or Chi Kung, a type of energy healing (Chan, 1996). Since it was established in 1988, the center has reported treating tens of thousands of individuals that presented with over 180 types of diseases. They report an overall success rate of more than 95 percent, although this has not been evaluated by western scientific standards.

In the United States, a modern approach to the ancient practice of energy healing is Non-Contact Therapeutic Touch (TT) (Krieger, 1975). This therapy has its historical roots in the ancient practice of laying on of hands. Therapeutic Touch is widely used primarily by nurses throughout the United States and is available in some hospitals. Research conducted on Therapeutic Touch demonstrates its impact on immunologic parameters, such as diminution of the percentage of suppressor T cells following TT intervention (Quinn & Strelkauskas, 1993). A double-blind study observed an increased rate of full thickness dermal healing from experimentally induced wounds following TT as compared to sham treatment interventions (Wirth, 1990). In vitro measures have also demonstrated the impact of Therapeutic Touch. For example, the growth and motility of bacteria in culture was altered following TT (Rauscher 1990) as was alterations in infrared spectra in water (Schwartz, DeMattei, Brame, & Spottiswoode,1990). TT has also been observed to provide benefits for symptom reduction of pain and anxiety for persons with AIDS (Newshan, 1989).

Since the late 1980s, researchers at Paramann Programme Laboratories (PPL) in Amman, Jordan have done extensive investigations of the unusual healing abilities of followers of a Sufi school known as Tariqa, Casnazaniyyah (Al-Dargazelli, 1993-94; Hussein, Fatoohi, Al-Dargazelli, & Almuchtar, 1994a, 1994b, 1994c). Practitioners have been reported to respond to induced wounds with either no or minimal bleeding and wound healing within 4–10 seconds with no pain or infection. PPL researchers report that these unusual healing phenomena are reproducible under controlled laboratory conditions. Also, these researchers report that this healing ability is accessible to anyone and is not restricted to a few talented individuals who have spent years in training. These phenomena do not appear to be related to hypnosis, meditation, relaxation, altered states of consciousness, or trance states, but are described in terms of healing energies (Hall, 2000; Hussein, Almukhtar, Fatoohi, and Al-Dargazelli, 1996; Hussein, Fatoohi, Hall, and Al-Dargazelli, 1997).

Similar healing phenomena have been observed by Brazilian trance surgeons who often cut into a patient's body for therapeutic purposes (Don & Maura, 2000). Despite the lack of anesthesia or sterile procedures, there is apparently no post-operative infection, the absence of pain, minimal bleeding, and the patient often claims that they were healed (Don & Moura, 2000). This type of treatment has also been described in terms of "energy healing." Although such phenomena have received scant attention from the Western scientific community, they have profound implications for healing serious diseases such as cancer and AIDS and may add to our understanding of the meta-psychology of healing. Perhaps the future will witness a transition from imagery and relaxation procedures to the incorporation of subtle energy in healing.

REFERENCES

Achterberg, J., & Lawlis, G. F. (1978). *Imagery and disease.* Champaign, IL: Institute for Personality and Ability Testing.

Achterberg, J., & Lawlis, G. F. (1980). *Bridges of the bodymind: Behavioral approaches to health care.* Champaign, IL: Institute for Personality and Ability Testing.

Achterberg, J., & Lawlis, G. F., Simonton, O. C., & Matthews-Simonton, S. (1977). Psychological factors and blood chemistries as disease outcome predictors for cancer patients. *Multivariate Experimental Clinical Research , 3*(3), 107-122.

Ader, R. (Ed.). (1981). *Psychoneuroimmunology.* New York: Academic Press.

Ader, R., Felton, D., & Cohen, N. (Eds.). (1991). *Psychoneuroimmunology.* New York: Academic Press.

Al-Dargazelli, S. (1993-94). New findings in healing research. *The Doctor-Healer Network Newsletter, 7,* 12-17.

Bammer, K., & Newberry, B. H. (Eds.). (1981). *Stress and cancer.* Toronto: C. J. Hogrefe, Inc.

Bernstein, D. A., & Borkovec, T. D. (1973). *Progressive relaxation: A manual for therapists.* Champaign, IL: Research Press.

Bowers, K. S., & Kelly, P. (1979). Stress, disease, psychotherapy and hypnosis. *Journal of Abnormal Psychology, 85,* 490-505.

Brigham, D. D., & Davis, A. (1994). *Imagery for getting well: Clinical applications of behavioral medicine.* New York: Derry Cameron-Samper.

Chan, L. (1996). A visit to a unique Qigong hospital. *Tai Chi, 19*(5), 34-35.

Chen, E., Joseph, M. H., & Zeltzer, L. K. (2000). Acute pain in children: Behavioral and cognitive interventions in the treatment of pain in children. *Pediatric Clinics of North America, 47*(3), 513-525.

Chiaramonte, D. (1997). Complementary and alternative therapies in primary care: Mind-body therapies for primary care physicians. *Primary Care; Clinics in Office Practice, 24*(4), 787-807.

Craighead, W. E., Kazdin, A. E., & Mahoney, M. J. (1981). *Behavior modification: Principles, issues, and applications.* Boston: Houghton Mifflin.

Don, N. S., & Moura, G. (2000). Trance surgery in Brazil. *Alternative Therapies in Health and Medicine, 6*(4), 39-48.

Eisenberg, D. M., Kessler, R. C.,Foster, C., Norlock, F. E., Calkins, D. R., & Delbanco, T. L. (1993). Unconventional medicine in the United States. *The New England Journal of Medicine, 328*(4), 246-252.

Fawzy, I. F., Cousins, N., Fawzy, N. W., Kemeny, M. E., Elashoff, R., & Morton, D. (1990a). A structured psychiatric intervention for cancer patients. I. Changes over time in methods of coping and affective disturbance. *Archives of General Psychiatry, 47*(8), 720-725.

Fawzy, I. F., Kemeny, M. E., Fawzy, N. W., Elashoff, R., Morton, D., Cousins, N., & Fahey, J. L. (1990b). A structured psychiatric intervention for cancer patients. II. Changes over time in immunological measures. *Archives of General Psychiatry, 47*(8), 729-735.

Friedlander, E.R. (1985). Dream your cancer away: The Simontons. *Examining Holistic Medicine.* New York: Prometheus Books.

Hall, H. R. (1983). Hypnosis and the immune system: A review with implications for cancer and the psychology of healing. *American Journal of Clinical Hypnosis, 25,* 92-103.

Hall, H. R. (1986). Hypnosis, suggestion, and the psychology of healing: A historical perspective. *Advances, 3*(3), 29-37.

Hall, H. (2000). Deliberately caused bodily damage: Metahypnotic phenomena? *Journal of the Society for Psychical Research, 64*(861), 211-223.

Hall, H., Minnes, L., & Olness, K. (1993). The psychophysiology of voluntary immuno-modulation. *International Journal of Neuroscience, 69,* 221-234.

Hall, H., Minnes, L., Olness, K., & Tosi, M. (1992). Voluntary modulation of neutrophil adhesiveness using a cyberphysiologic strategy. *International Journal of Neuroscience, 63*(3-4), 287-297.

Hall, H., Papas, A., Tosi, M., & Olness, K. (1996). Directional changes in neutrophil adherence following passive relaxation versus active imaging. *International Journal of Neuroscience, 85,* 185-194.

Hall, H. R., Mumma, G. H., Longo, S., & Dixon, R. (1992). Voluntary Immunomodulation: A preliminary study. *International Journal of Neuroscience, 63*(3-4), 275-285.

Holden, C. (1978). Cancer and the mind: How are they connected? *Science, 200*(23) 1363-1369.

Holt, R. R. (1964). Imagery: The return of the ostracized. *American Psychologist, 19,* 254-264.

Hussein, J. N., Almukhtar, N., Fatoohi, L. J., & Al-Dargazelli, S. (1996). The role of ambiguous terminology of consciousness in misunderstanding healing phenomena. *Frontier Perspectives, 6*(1), 27-32.

Hussein, J. N., Fatoohi, L .J., Al-Dargazelli, S., & Almuchtar, N. (1994a). The deliberately caused bodily damage phenomena: Mind, body, energy or what? (Part I). *International Journal of Alternative and Complementary Medicine, 12*(9), 9-11.

Hussein, J. N., Fatoohi, L. J., Al-Dargazelli, S., & Almuchtar, N. (1994b). The deliberately caused bodily damage phenomena: Mind, body, energy or what? (Part II). *International Journal of Alternative and Complementary Medicine, 12*(10), 21-23.

Hussein, J. N., Fatoohi, L. J., Al-Dargazelli, S., & Almuchtar, N. (1994c). The deliberately caused bodily damage phenomena: Mind, body, energy or what? (Part III). *International Journal of Alternative and Complementary Medicine, 12*(11), 25-28.

Hussein, J. N., Fatoohi, L. J., Hall, H., & Al-Dargazelli, S. (1997). Deliberately caused bodily caused bodily damage phenomena. *Journal of the Society for Psychical Research, 62*(849), 97-113.

Jevne, R. F., & Levitan, A. (1989). *No time for nonsense: Self-help for the seriously ill.* San Diego, CA: Luramedia.

Kaptchuk, T. J. (1996). Historical context of the concept of vitalism in complementary and alternative medicine. In M. S. Micozzi (Ed.), *Fundamentals of Complementary and Alternative Medicine* (pp. 35-48). New York: Churchill Livingston.

Krieger, D. (1975). Therapeutic touch: The imprimatur of nursing. *American Journal of Nursing, 75*(5), 784-787.

Lazarus, A. (1978). *In the mind's eye: The power of imagery for personal enrichment.* New York: Random House.

Locke, S. E., Ransil, B. J., Zachariae, R., Molay, F., Tollins, K., Covino, N. A., & Danforth, D. (1994). Effect of hypnotic suggestion on the delayed-type hypersensitivity response. *Journal of American Medical Association, 272*(1), 47-52.

Meares, A. (1978). Regression of osteogenic sarcoma metastasis associated with intensive meditation. *The Medical Journal of Australia, 2,* 433.

Meares, A. (1979). Regression of cancer of the rectum after intensive meditation. *The Medical Journal of Australia, 2,* 539-540.

Meares, A. (1983). A form of intensive meditation associated with the regression of cancer. *American Journal of Clinical Hypnosis, 25,* 114-121.

Naparstek, B. (1994). *Staying well with guided imagery: How to harness the power of your imagination for health and healing.* New York: Warner Books, Inc.

Newshan, G. (1989). Therapeutic touch for symptom control in persons with AIDS. *Holistic Nursing Practice, 3*(4), 45-51.

Newton, B. W. (1983). The use of hypnosis in the treatment of cancer patients. *American Journal of Clinical Hypnosis, 25,* 104-113.

Pelletier, K. R. (1979). *Mind as healer mind as slayer: A holistic approach to preventing stress disorders.* New York: Delta.

Quinn, J. F., & Strelkauskas, A. J. (1993). Psychoimmunologic effects of therapeutic touch on practitioners and recently bereaved recipients: A pilot study. *Advances in Nursing Science, 15*(4), 13-26.

Rauscher, E. A. (1990). Human volitional effects on a model bacterial system. *Subtle Energies, 1*(1), 21-41.

Ruzyla-Smith, P., Barabasz, A., Barabasz, M., & Warner, D. (1995). Effects of hypnosis on the immune response: B-cells, t-cells, helper and suppressor cells. *American Journal of Clinical Hypnosis, 38*(2), 71-79.

Samuels, M., & Samuels, N. (1975). *Seeing with the mind's eye: The history, techniques and uses of visualiza*tion (p. 28). New York: Random House.

Selye, H. (1974). *Stress without distress* (p. 6). New York: Signet.

Scarf, M. (1980, September). Images that heal: A doubtful idea whose time has come. *Psychology Today,* 32-46.

Schultz, J. H., & Luthe, W. (1969). *Autogenic therapy volume 1, Autogenic methods.* New York: Grune and Stratton.

Scwhartz, S. A., DeMattei, R. J., Brame, E. G., & Spottiswoode, J. P. (1990). Infrared spectra alteration in water proximate to the palms of therapeutic practitioners. *Subtle Energies, 1*(1), 43-72.

Simonton, O. C., Matthews-Simonton, & Creighton, J. L. (1978). *Getting well again: A step-by-step, self-help guide to overcoming cancer for patients and their families* (p. 114). New York: Bantam Books.

Simonton-Atchleye, S. (1993). The influence of psychological therapy on the immune system in patients with advanced cancer. (Doctoral dissertation, The Fielding Institute.) *UMI Dissertation Services,* Order Number 9419254.

Sontag, S. (1978). *Illness as metaphor.* New York: Vintage Books.

Spiegel, D. (1991). Mind matters: Effects of group support on cancer patients. *The Journal of NIH Research, 3,* 61-63.

Spiegel, D., Bloom, J. R., Kraemer, H. C., & Gottheil, E. (1989). Effect of psychosocial treatment on survival of patients with metastatic breast cancer. *The Lancet,* October 14, 888-891.

Tache, J., Selye, H., & Day, S. B. (Eds.). (1979). *Cancer, stress, and death.* New York: Plenum.

Weitzenhoffer, A. M., & Hilgard, E. R. (1962). *Stanford hypnotic susceptibility scale, Form C.* Palo Alto, CA: Consulting Psychologists Press.

Weksler, M. E., & Hutteroth, T. H. (1974). Impaired lymphocyte function in aged humans. *Journal of Clinical Investigations, 53,* 99-104.

Wirth, D. P. (1990). The effect on non-contact therapeutic touch on the healing rate of full thickness dermal wounds. *Subtle Energies, 1*(1), 1-20.

CHAPTER 18

How to Use Mental Imagery for Any Clinical Condition

GERALD EPSTEIN[1]

> Imagination is more important than knowledge. Knowledge is limited. Imagination encircles the world.
>
> Albert Einstein (in Viereck, 1929, p. 17)

Over the years, numerous imagery exercises have been developed by clinicians to deal with a variety of diseases (Achterberg, Dossey, & Kolkmeier, 1994; Sheikh, 2002). This chapter offers suggestions to create imagery procedures regardless of the name of the disease, for names of diseases are merely descriptors of the physical or emotional situation that is diagnosed. They do not inherently convey information beyond that, unlike other medical systems where patterns are discerned by taking pulses (Chinese), looking at the face (Hebraic), or smelling bodily excretions (Tibetan). However, these descriptors are useful in guiding us. Once the area for action has been defined, we can then devise an imagery exercise.

BASIC IMAGERY EXERCISE: CLEANING THE AIRWAYS

Close your eyes and breathe out three times slowly. Take a light with you, and enter your body through your mouth and see your way to your bronchial tree. See the mucus that has accumulated there and its color. Now see a big glass syringe with a golden bulb at the end, suck up and out all the mucus deposits, and put the waste in a container that you have with you. After finishing, imagine a golden air gun and spray a jet of warm air throughout the bronchial tree, making the whole

---

[1]For information about teaching and training in imagery and allied techniques, Dr. Epstein can be reached at: 16 East 96th Street, New York, New York 10128, or by fax (212-369-5648), phone (212-369-4080), email (jerry@drjerryepstein.org), or Web (www.drjerryepstein.org).

area dry. Use your light to see everything that you are doing. Then, breathe in pure oxygen in the form of white light. See and sense your chest wall and rib cage expanding, the lungs expanding like a bellows in all directions—up and down, front to back, left to right—allowing your lungs to fully expand and fill with this white light. Sense your diaphragm descending to receive the full lungs. Then, see your lungs contracting, as the bellows contracts, forcing out all the carbon dioxide that comes out as a black stream. At the end of exhalation, squeeze your lungs with transparent fingers to get rid of the last bit of trapped carbon dioxide, expelled as a jet of black smoke. Repeat this "bellows breathing" two more times. Then, come out the way you came in, using your light to see your way, and take the waste container with you. When you are outside of your body, bury this container in the earth. Then, breathe out slowly and open your eyes.

Closing your eyes allows you to shut out the external world, permitting you to turn your senses inward to access the imaginal experience in a vivid manner. It is important to note that the senses are turned inward, for imagery practice is sense dependent; for, focusing inside to apprehend something is equivalent to apprehending something outside. The senses are required as the starting point to establish our encounter with any experience. Of course, with the imagery method we want to leave the habitual perceptions of everyday existence to participate in the non-habitual life-mode of inner life.

Some people may not feel comfortable shutting the eyes. It is not advisable to insist; however, I do feel this may limit the intensity of the inner experience.

Breathing out three times slowly is crucial. Long, slow exhalations have the effect of quieting us down inwardly, reducing anxiety, and creating a moment of relaxation when the attention can be placed squarely on the imagery process without distractions by tangential thoughts or by sorties into habitual fantasy life. There is also a physiological mechanism at play here: a nucleus in the brain called the Blue Nucleus is a group of cells that turns blue when it is actively engaged in sending neurotransmitter substance to various areas of the brain to enhance the functioning of those areas. What is of particular interest for us here are two such regions called the amygdala and the hippocampus. They are charged with mediating our emotional and thought life respectively. When they are in receipt of the neurochemical sent by the Blue Nucleus, they can process new data, allowing us to respond in new ways, not in the same reflexive habitual manner (Foote, Berridge, Adam, & Pirieda, 1991; Usher, 1999).

Most of the time the Blue Nucleus is deactivated and is actually pale in color, not blue. When this happens, no new data can be processed, and we are consigned to the same habitual activity. What makes the Blue Nucleus pale is a substance secreted by the adrenal gland called "nor-epinephrine." This chemical is activated in our usual, daily, chronically stressful, repetitive life situations. It is, perhaps, the most destructive chemical substance produced by the physical body.

How can we remove this toxic material, thereby resuscitating the Blue Nucleus's beneficial action? Two of the more significant ways available to us are:

1) imagery activity; and 2) long, slow exhalations coupled with normal—not exaggerated—inhalations. We have here physiological function—exhalation— and a mental function—imagery—acting in concert to create the possibility for change within us. Deep inhalation stimulates the adrenal gland, prompting an outpouring of adrenal chemicals that actually negate the effect we are trying to achieve (Porges, 1995a,b).

THE DISEASED AREA ITSELF

Initially, the patient generally is provided with a picture of the organ or region in question. Many people know little about the inside of their bodies. Not only do they not know what the organs look like, but they do not know where they are located. Once the picture is provided, imagery effectiveness is enhanced.

In addition to working on the diseased area itself, it is advisable to include a generalized cleansing exercise to create a clean field in which the healing is to take place. Some teachers of mental imagery techniques state that the organ in question should not be directly addressed, only the environment surrounding the organ. I disagree. The purpose of using imagery in the disease process is to create change directly in the organ. *Every* organ of the body has a brain which can take instruction and direction from the inner imagery intention. The existence of these brains is due to the migration of neural crest cells in early embryological development and is an established embryological fact (*Langman's Medical Embrylogy,* 2000). The implication for imagery therapy is that by ordering the brain of the organ to come into order, it in turn orders the organ to come into order. When we are in order we are healing.

In imagery work, it is also useful to be aware of a pattern of correlations. In the ancient spiritual tradition of the West there is the dictum "As above, so below." This is the law of analogy that forms the underpinning of how images are to be read and thereby understood. In terms of the body, one might understand that the upper and lower parts of the body correlate to each other with the diaphragm serving as the dividing line between the two. For instance, the fingers correlate to the toes, wrists to ankles, forearms to lower legs, and so on. Also, I have found correlation between the prostate gland and the sinuses around the eyes and nose. When the prostate is enlarged, the sinuses appear to be unusually stuffed. Thus, when I give imagery for prostate enlargement, I might give exercises as well for cleaning out the sinuses.

Awareness of these correlations is of inestimable value, for instance, in treating neurological problems. There is always an area of normal neurological functioning, even in those severe insults to the nervous system. Using imagery in these normal areas to create movement can result in a message sent to the impaired area to become activated. In imaginal therapy, movement means life, and imagery is the function that brings movement and life to one's being.

THE STRUCTURE OF IMAGERY

Composing imagery exercises is an art that enriches the process immensely. There are numerous points to bear in mind when creating imagery exercises that I have found helpful in their construction. Among the most important are these:

1. It is absolutely necessary to be familiar with anatomy and physiology. For instance, in the asthma exercise the bronchi and lungs are brought into play. Also, some understanding of asthma breathing has value, namely the need for that extra imaginal exhalation to release that last held bit of carbon dioxide. It may be helpful to also educate students (this term is preferable to "patient" or "client," because by *teaching* people they become their own healers) about their biology. As mentioned above, each person is given a picture (or computer graphic printout if that technology is available) of the anatomical area being worked on. The student looks at the picture for about 30 to 60 seconds. Afterwards he/she can close eyes and do the imagery exercise. The imagery experience is enhanced by first viewing the picture.

The knowledge of anatomy and physiology leads to constructing exercises specifically tailored for that student. In the asthma exercise, I indicate natural breathing by describing how the rib cage and diaphragm respond to expanding lungs. This gives a way to cue into an internal process to which the student has not paid attention and once the student focuses on it, he/she gains a greater sense of control over the process.

2. Imagery exercises have a threefold aspect to their usage that provides a useful orientation for their construction. Imagery exercises should contain three elements. They are: a) stimulation of conflict. That is, a slight shock should put the person in a confrontational position with the disturbance. This stimulation phase is to be followed by: b) a resolution of conflict in which the shock is quieted and the conflicted situation is overcome. This resolution is followed by: c) a sense of triumph, a real sense of victory and/or accomplishment.

Put in physiological terms, one begins by stimulating the sympathetic nervous system. Creating the shock mobilizes the fight-flight-fright system and prepares for the challenge about to be faced. The adrenal-pancreas-thyroid-pituitary axis is thrown into action. In the second phase, the parasympathetic nervous system is activated. This is the quieting system of the body and is intimately connected to the vagus nerve and its activity. This mother nerve sends branches to the heart, lungs, abdominal viscera, among other centers, to slow down physiological activity such as heart rate, respiration, blood pressure, intestinal peristalsis. It is here that the real forces are mobilized to handle the challenge, and the way is shown, via imagery function, how to effect change. Change is denoted by action. Without action no change is possible. In the therapy field, insight has been equated with change. However, in my experience, insight may be a preliminary to taking action, but it does not necessarily translate into action. In fact, the reverse is more apt to be the case. That is, action may trigger insight. I have compared both sides of the insight-action coin: I was a psychoanalyst trained to delay action until the reasons or the promptings underlying the action were clear. But I have switched from a psychological orientation to a phenomenological one—acting in accordance with the demands of the present without preliminary interpretation. I have found that action brings healing in a hurry! Action means movement, and movement means life!

Imagery creates an inner movement that brings life, reflected in the beneficial physiological and biological activity. Creating inner movement is a key to how imagery brings about results. In forming imagery exercises one must always keep the necessity for movement in mind. Images have to reflect motion. It is this *new* action that shows us the way to effect new behaviors (described below).

The next and final element in the process is the triumph. The triumphant aspect is tantamount to beginning the imprinting process that starts embedding this new possibility into one's biomental being. One is giving oneself a message that the challenge has been faced and conquered. It is a mental appreciation without arousing doubt (as many verbal ones do). One has mastered something in oneself by oneself for oneself and has, thus, reinforced one's self-authority. Here a synthesis is struck between sympathetic and parasympathetic activity as one comes away a more balanced and clear individual, self-empowered and more attuned to the present moment and the fullness of life.

The resolution and triumph is then repeated on a daily basis to create an imprinting into one's biomental being thereby creating a new habit. In effect, one is dosing oneself with a new medicine that is given three times a day at certain prescribed times for a period of 21 days. The best times for daily practice is early morning upon awakening: with the exception of having to urinate, nothing else comes first. Next is 5 to 6 P.M. The last time should be before going to bed. *All* practice is to be done sitting up straight in a chair, feet flat on the floor, arms on the arms of the chair, eyes closed, *always* breathing out long slow exhalations through the mouth and breathing in normally through the nose. The 21 days refers to the time it takes to break a habit and to create a new one. When you read the exercise, do it then, and start the next day to start counting 21 days. The total number of times you will have done the exercise is 64. Sixty-four is the number of life; for example, the DNA molecule is comprised of 64 strands; the *I Ching* (Chinese book of life) contains 64 hexagrams.

3. In constructing imagery exercises it is important to keep in mind that the way they are written have import. They are evocative (or not) of inner imagery. The more poetic the exercises are, the closer they are to the imagery process per se. I would like to pass along some pointers: Make sure that the exercise contains movement; the wording—like poetry—does not have to make logical sense; it is helpful to have movement words contain an "ing" ending, for example, climb*ing*, runn*ing*, walk*ing*. They prompt the inside to respond in an active fashion.

4. The sources for material for constructing imagery exercises are numerous. These sources are described in my book *Healing into Immortality* (Epstein, 1994). The student's conversation also is a good source of images. In the imaginal therapeutic process I conduct, the students' comments have no vital interest if the content refers to the past or the future, since both areas are illusory. They do not exist and only serve to account for the disturbing elements confronted in life at a particular moment. The therapist does not pay attention to the content of conversation, instead he/she is free to listen for the images used to describe the situation, internal or external. Almost invariably one will hear images used to describe a state of being. For instance, a depressed woman said: "I feel like I am in the bottom of a pit." An anxious man having difficulty at work said: "I feel like I'm strangling in the situation." Another anxious young man said: "I feel like I'm tied up in knots." These examples can be echoed a thousand-fold. A young woman who suffered from sacroiliac spasm said: "I bent over backwards to be patient and kind to this person who took advantage of me." When you hear these image words or phrases, they essentially dictate the imagery exercises. Making up exercises is an essential creative element in imaginal clinical work. Making them up "on the spot" in response to the student's suffering presents an interesting and enriching challenge.

In the case of the woman in the pit, I asked her to look around the bottom of the pit using a light, if she could not see clearly, to find something to help her escape. She discovered a ladder which she climbed and found a bright, sunny day in a beautiful landscape when she emerged. From this point on, the depressed state began to recede. In repeating the exercise she had to begin at the pit. The shock of the pit starts the threefold process of imagery experience described above. I asked the man "strangling in the situation" to see the strangulation. He saw a noose tied around his neck. He removed it and noticed not only a sense of relief but also a perceptible change in this breathing: deeper and slower. As he repeated this exercise over the ensuing days, he found a way to straighten out the job circumstances.

As one comes into balance through imagery experience, new ways of apperceiving and approaching life take shape and lead to new action or behaviors. The young man tied up in knots simply saw a rope full of knots that he methodically proceeded to untie. I asked him to sense and feel what was happening during this process. He reported afterwards—the reporting is done *after* the exercise is completed—that he felt a straightening of his spinal column and that he was standing more erect. He also felt a release of tension in his upper abdomen. He felt more in touch with an equilibrated, embodied self, and his entire mental and emotional outlook brightened. The woman who bent over backwards imaginally corrected that exaggeration by bending over forward to touch her toes with her hands without bending her knees. She found herself coming to a natural upright position and also becoming more "upright" in her relationship to that person whom she decided no longer to coddle or appease.

By following the direction coming from the student, one subscribes to a cornerstone of imaginal therapy: each one has the answer inside for healing. One merely reflects back the authenticity of that discovery. At the same time one is preserving that individual's freedom and autonomy emphasizing his/her own innate capacity and independence. This builds an inner sense of self-caring and self-empowerment. In effect, one is teaching the student to become his/her own healer. The clinician supplies the education, the student supplies his/her own self-heaing.

A closer examination of the structure of the imagery exercise described above reveals that it is not "scripted." That is, one is not told what has to happen at the conclusion of the exercise. The exercise emerges within the province of the individual's personal freedom, which must be honored. It is critical for the healing process that the therapist realizes that a person's freedom includes that of choosing to be well *or to be ill*. It is not for clinicians to insist that their students follow a preexistent standard of what has to be achieved and what must be shed. The choice is left up to the student, who opts to use or not use the tool(s) provided.

In the asthma exercise, light was used in two ways: 1) a light was taken along to see the way; 2) light came into the area to be healed. With respect to the first: bringing a light to examine an internal organ or any interior aspect of the body is most helpful. The illumination by the light has a salutary effect, revealing to the seeker an area usually shrouded in obscurity. This light is used to find the way to the area in question and to avoid disturbing any other structures along the way. It is valuable to use the light to examine the afflicted area from every angle. Often, such examination allays anxiety felt about the ailment as well as anxiety about directly confronting the diseased part and this is essential for healing. The general tendency in medical treatment is to treat sickness as an enemy to be avoided at all costs, and the goal is to eliminate pain as quickly as possible without examining its source. In my book *Healing Visualizations* (Epstein, 1989), pain relief through the imagery process is described, but this avenue is taken at the same time as considering the meaning of the pain. This process just does not happen when only immediate relief is sought through synthetic medication.

In regard to the second point: the direct relationship between light and healing cannot be stressed enough. Inner light drives out the darkness and introduces the domain of the holy into the healing process. It is worthy of note that the word *heal* comes from the same etymological root as the words *health, whole, holy*. To become whole is to become healthy. To become healthy requires that the healing process admit the holy. The holy comes as light entering from an invisible source promoting natural growth and sustenance, just as the visible sun creates a similar process in the external world. It is a common occurrence in imagery experience to spontaneously discover light, and to be bathed or immersed in light. Internally (and on the skin as well), light stimulates the growth of normal healthy cells and the repair of organs.

Using light of various colors can be significant. In the exercises presented here, white light was employed. For the brain and lungs, white light seems to have a powerful effect. Blue light is the healing color for the West and Middle East and green for the East. Red blood cells emit blue light; under electron microscopy the blue light shows up as halos around the red cells (*Blood,* 1985). In fact, *all* cells emit light, as do all organs. When cells and organs are dying, the light becomes extinguished. Blue light also naturally neutralizes the red of inflammation. Green light will still pain. Gold light gives life and vitality to organs. Violet light helps to regulate the insulin output of the pancreas. Blue-green light brings relief to the nasal region and sinuses.

The need for cleansing is of preeminent importance in healing. The way must be cleaned, room must be made, for something new to take place. The process of cleansing takes away clutter that gets in the way of change. Clutter can be understood on a mental level as old habits reflexively operating. No matter at what level—physical, emotional, mental, social, interpersonal, moral—some sort of contaminant has inserted itself into the garden of one's personal reality that needs to be removed.

When the contaminant enters, light is shut out or off, and light is necessary for life. One must allow light to enter, as it is the natural healing force, and cleansing prepares the way. This space I call the "space of freedom," where myriad options become possible. In the asthma exercise, cleaning out the mucus makes space available for a normal physiological exchange of gases. Then the restoration to a normal respiratory physiology becomes possible.

Habits, in my view, always are with us. The question is whether they are constructive or destructive. When an unproductive habit is rooted out, it is replaced by a productive one. By the repetition of an exercise, the imprinting pushes out the old habit, and allows the student to respond in new ways. In inner life, as in outer life, two objects cannot occupy the same space at the same time. Therefore, two habitual tendencies cannot coexist.

The new ways of responding eventually force out the old reflexive tendency. As this happens, one begins to feel the shift(s) taking place. Thus one may view physical illness as the building up of habit reflecting itself in a physical disturbance. The advent of the new habit brings with it the erosion of the old and with it the removal of the habit's physical reflection. For this reason, the student is asked to repeat the bellows breathing three times a day for up to 21 days.

Finally, the waste is buried in the earth after the student leaves the body. Whenever a person enters the body to work on a physical area, the exercise must end with a return to outside the body, exiting *by the same route* as was entered. In keeping to the same route, the overall physiological equilibrium of the body is maintained and the person returns to full waking-life consciousness which existed before the exercise without alteration, while the physiology of the diseased part has been repaired *at the same time.*

In many exercises used for affecting a disease process, some waste product is produced, which must be disposed. In cancer exercises, the debris created by breaking up the tumor may be removed, for example, by a river of white cells, or insects eating the tumor, or a tornado removing the cells. In the imagery portrayed in this chapter, the waste is sucked out and buried. Images of air, earth, fire, or water can be used as means of ridding oneself of the waste products. Remember, the removal of wastes is a decontamination and cleansing effort vital to the healing from illness.

CONCLUDING REMARKS

Mental imagery is a venerable and ancient tradition associated with healing in Western civilization. The imagery process has been and still is a significant form of practice in the Western spiritual tradition. It is germane to this tradition that the individual's freedom is maintained and preserved. Every effort is made to this end, realizing that every intervention or intrusion, no matter how innocent or brief, may coopt freedom. In my view, we are all 100 percent open to suggestion 100 percent of the time. The clinician should guard against exploiting that situation and should not trespass on the space of freedom. Teaching others how to use their minds to shape their realities and fulfill their possibilities honors that urge to freedom inherent in everyone. Once one understands how to use this powerful mind medicine tool, one no longer has to be dependent on the clinician. I have very successfully applied these principles in my practice, and hope that other clinicians will have the same experience.

REFERENCES

Achterberg, J., Dossey, B., & Kolkmeier, L. (1994). *Rituals of healing: Using imagery for health and wellness.* New York: Bantam Books.

Berridge, C. W., Adams, L. M., & Pirieda, J. A. (1985). *Blood.* Toronto: Torstar Books, 1998, plate pp. 33-34.

Epstein, G. (1994). *Healing into immortality.* New York: Bantam Books.

Epstein, G. (1989). *Healing visualizations: Creating health through imagery.* New York: Bantam Books.

Foote, D. L., Berridge, C. W., Adams, L. M., & Pirieda, J. (1991). Electrophysiological evidence for the involvement of the locus coeruleus in alerting, orienting, and attending. *Progress in Brain Research, 88,* 521-532.

Langman's Medical Embryology. (2000). T. W. Sadler & J. Langman (Eds.). Philadelphia: Lippincott Williams & Wilkins.

Porges, S. W. (1995a). Cardiac vagal tone: A physiological index of stress, *Neuroscience/Biobehavioral Review, 19*(2), 225-233.

Porges, S. W. (1995b). Orienting in a defensive world of our evolutionary heritage: A polyvagal theory of mammalian modification. *Psychophysiology, 32*, 301-318.

Sheikh, A. (Ed.). (2002). *Handbook of therapeutic imagery techniques.* Amityville, NY: Baywood.

Usher, M. et al. (1999). The role of locus coeruleus in the regulation of cognitive performance. *Science, 283*(5401), 549-554.

Viereck, G. S. (1929). What life means to Einstein. *The Saturday Evening Post,* October 26.

CHAPTER 19

Guided Imagery and Intuition

BELLERUTH NAPARSTEK

The discovery of the laws of nature requires first and foremost intuition . . .
logic comes after intuition.
                    Eugene Wigner (in Walsh & Shapiro, 1983, p. 260)

INTRODUCTION AND OVERVIEW

Guided imagery is an ideal vehicle for intuitive development. By its very
nature, it contains many of the elements that set the stage for accessing intuition. In
particular, guided imagery that focuses on opening the heart, evoking feelings of
love and gratitude, is an especially powerful and trustworthy vehicle for opening
intuitive ability (Naparstek, 1997).

When properly constructed and delivered, guided imagery alters consciousness; relaxes the body; turns attention inward; calms the environmental vigilance
of the ego; creates a sense of spiritual attunement; and drops awareness out of
analytic cognition and down into the clear, receptive state necessary for picking
up subtle signals (Naparstek, 1994). On a more physiological level, imagery
changes the biochemical mix in the bloodstream, lowers and coheres brain wave
frequencies, and amplifies the human energy field (McCraty, Atkinson, Tiller,
Rein, & Watkins, 1995).

And indeed, these very shifts are the focus of most intuition training
methodologies, developed by leaders in the field as diverse as Russell Targ,
Helen Palmer, Marilyn Schlitz, Norm Shealy, Henry Reed, Joe McMoneagle,
Deborah Rozman, and the Rev. Rosalyn Bruyere. Each of these intuition
teachers offers techniques designed to propel shifts in physiology, mood, cognition, perception, attitude, awareness, attentional focus, and spiritual attunement
(Naparstek, 1997).

Research in the field, interviews with nearly 50 intuitives, and clinical data from
psychotherapy combine to identify elements conducive to opening up intuitive
capacity. These are identified and juxtaposed against the basic characteristics
of guided imagery. An annotated guided imagery narrative follows, which

437

demonstrates the high compatibility of guided imagery for intuition development. The imagery is specifically designed to generate an intuition-rich experience.

CRITICAL SHIFTS

The Body: Relaxing Muscle Tension

Although people may find their intuition opened wide during adrenalized times of terror, fight-or-flight arousal, and other forms of excitement, lesser levels of fear and worry have the opposite effect, shutting down intuitive functioning. This is why relaxation exercises are commonly used as a preliminary means of moving into the necessary mind state to do intuitive work (Naparstek, 1997, pp. 53-54).

Indeed, the idea that relaxation is an intuition-liberating activity is well supported by the literature. Too much striving (Targ & Puthoff, 1974), too strong a need to succeed (Batcheldor, 1966), or too much of feeling responsible for outcome (Honorton & Schechter, 1986) will impede its appearance. Relaxation gently releases these obstacles.

During an experience of guided imagery, muscle tension softens, limbs become heavier, the voice drops lower, and breathing becomes slower, deeper, and steadier. As noted decades ago by consciousness pioneers Elmer and Alyce Green, brain waves slow down to at least alpha and often theta frequencies during guided imagery (Green & Green, 1977).

Medical research on imagery used with oncology, cardiac, migraine, surgery, angioplasty, and diabetes patients reveals outcomes of reduced pain, lowered anxiety, stabilized blood pressure, and reduced blood glucose levels (Naparstek, 1994, pp. 17-22), all of which can be causally related to heightened seratonin levels and a resultant sense of calm, peace and relaxation.

Cognition: Clearing and Stilling the Mind

Mental noise—analyzing, worrying, judging, remembering, anticipating, comparing, associating, and interpreting perceptual cues from the environment— creates a lot of internal busyness in the mind that tends to overwhelm the subtle, fleeting, fragmentary signals of intuition.

As a result, intuition development methods use meditative practices designed to still and clear the mind. One way to do this is through mindfulness and vipassana practices, where thoughts and perceptions are continually witnessed and released by a detached, observing part of the ego. This takes practice and discipline, but can result in a split-second ability to create a powerfully quiet backdrop for subtle, intuitive perception.

Another, less rigorous way to do this is to limit focus to just one thing or a very narrow band of things. Reciting mantras, repetitive motion, drumming, dancing, moving meditation, and automatic writing are some of the ways this is achieved. In addition, modern technology now offers Hemi-Sync headsets, isolation tanks, and various Ganzfeld methods to achieve the same ends (Broughton, 1991, pp. 99-105).

With guided imagery, narrowed focus can be achieved very easily through the use of evocative sensory and metaphoric images that can coax the mind out of its perpetual, cognitive multi-tasking. For many Westerners, this is a less demanding, more realistic alternative.

Awareness: Turning Attention Inward

Another highly desirable element for gathering intuitive information is a quality of deep inwardness, where external perception is temporarily turned off or, more accurately, set aside. Psi trainees learn the skill of disengaging their senses from the outside world and traveling to their own interior space.

The various Ganzfeld experiments of the seventies established the power of shutting off external signals, when Charles Honorton (1978) put subjects in a recliner, covered their eyes with pink-lit goggles and their ears with headsets issuing monochromatic sound. With the help of this paraphernalia, intuitive perception scores consistently improved (Honorton, 1978).

Stanley Krippner and Montague Ullman (1985) deftly substantiated the point by measuring ESP and precognition in the ultimate inward state of sleep. Their Maimonides Dream Lab studies demonstrated the viability of intuition during REM sleep, and underlined the vital assist to intuition that came from blocking out external perception and routine environmental scanning, particularly in the early stages of a trainee's skill development (Child, 1985).

The beauty of guided imagery is the way it so easily escorts awareness deep into the body, toward interior images and sensations. The imaginal realm is, by definition, an interior phenomenon. Indeed, most imagery designed for healing the body leans heavily on the kinesthetic sense, driving awareness deep into the body where the healing must occur (Naparstek, 1994). Because awareness is routinely turned inward during the experience of guided imagery, intuitive opening is effortlessly served.

Attitude: Intention without Striving

Although students of intuition are well advised to set their intention on opening up their intuitive capacity, they must learn to do so without the usual proactive fuss and forceful striving. Instead of making a tense effort, they learn to move into receptive mode, a state of open attention, relaxed expectation—what Elmer Green aptly termed "passive volition" (1977). This is arguably a key ingredient of the intuitive experience, and, for that matter, of all creative experience. The original meaning of the word "channeling"—now distorted beyond recognition—reflects the idea of becoming an open conduit through which information, intuition, energy, inspiration, and creativity can flow.

Kenneth Batcheldor's research (1966) proved the importance of passive volition by demonstrating what every artist and athlete knows—that when people try too hard, or feel too personally responsible for making something happen, they impede their abilities. He termed this phenomenon "ownership inhibition," and found it stood in the way of many a subject (Owen & Sparrow, 1976). Indeed, the effectiveness of such devices as the crystal ball or the tarot deck, aside from the way they redirect and narrow attentional focus, may be the way the mind is led to believe that the answers are coming from them and not the intuiter. This diminishes the impulse to try too hard.

Guided imagery is a pure form of passive volition, a virtual feast of intention without striving. One sits and conjures, in a state of open attention, adrift in the imaginal realm, envisioning and sensing the reality of the waking dream. In the words of Caroline Casey, it is a simple matter of "voting with the imagination" (Casey, 1997). Others with a religious orientation might call this prayer.

Emotion: Opening the Heart

The energy of the open heart, awash with feelings of love, gratitude, and peaceful joy, is fertile breeding ground for intuition, and at the same time creates a safe filter through which the intuitive information can be delivered with integrity and ethicality.

Empathy is the ultimate expression of ESP, precognition, and telepathy. When the heart is open, it becomes simple and natural to feel for others and apprehend their experience.

When the heart opens, the boundaries of the ego dissolve, and the sense of "self" becomes far broader and more inclusive. At its most intense, the open heart can include the entire universe, producing a mystical sense of timeless oneness. At these times, intuitive insight is wide and deep and noetic perception so transcends the limitations of the human mind that the experience is impossible to share in words (Naparstek, 1997).

According to noted researcher Richard Broughton, Director of the Institute for Parapsychology in Durham, North Carolina, and heir to the research files of the Rhine Institute, it is no secret among psi researchers that the best ESP results come from labs known for their compassionate, supportive, caring atmosphere (Broughton, 1991, pp. 132-137).

Even the exquisitely calibrated instruments at the Institute of HeartMath labs have attested to this when subjects were asked to focus on their hearts and generate feelings of "love and care." At the point where those efforts registered coherence in the measurable frequencies found in the brain, gut, and heart, this internal state of "liquid harmony" produces intuitive insight in the subjects being monitored (Rein, Atkinson, & McCraty, 1995).

There are several great traditions of loving-kindness meditation that produce these same effects, and most religious disciplines can point to one or two varieties they can claim.

Guided imagery is a secular way to achieve this openhearted state, and its nature is to do so readily. Since imagery that elicits feelings of love and gratitude will frequently result in heightened immune response, more stable blood pressure, improved surgical outcomes, and reduced stress, anger, and anxiety, it has been used and studied in many venues (Naparstek, 1994, pp. 17-22).

However, it often takes little more than having the subject relax, feel safe, settle in, and get sufficiently removed from cognitive thinking to become aware of feelings and sensations inside the body for the heart to open. Imagery deliberately designed to pump up feelings of love and gratitude can be very intense, powerful, and healing.

One example of such imagery can be found in the sample provided on the next page.

Spirit: Creating Sacred Space and Spiritual Attunement

Another key ingredient of most intuition training protocols is the idea of moving into sacred space—physically or metaphorically stepping across a boundary, into a non-ordinary space that represents the uncontaminated, clear, ego-less mind state.

This might be a specially designated physical area, marked by ritual objects endowed with symbolic meaning. It could be a statement of intention or a prayer voiced aloud. There might be symbolic gestures or a special way of sitting or standing (Naparstek, 1997, pp. 56-60).

One of the benefits of consistent posture, location, words, props, symbols, or images is the way they ultimately condition an automatic kick-in of intuition. Additionally, by stepping away from the demands of "self" and "ego," fewer personal filters pollute or distort the information. Projected wishes and fears are less likely to come into play if the ego has been dismissed. The primary goal, however, is simply to step back from everyday motivation and be ruled by higher intentions.

Imagery is easily employed to create sacred space. The imaginal border between ordinary and non-ordinary time and space might be created by an internal image of pulling aside a curtain; stepping across a threshold; turning on a switch; donning a ritual garment; stepping back into time and space; or moving down a stairway to deeper levels. It could be, as with the attached imagery sample, a feeling of being surrounded and protected by assistance from multiple realms. Imagery lends itself readily to conjuring up a sense of the sacred, and will sometimes appear to evoke it of its own accord.

Perception: Registering Subtle Data

Targ, Puthoff, and Harary established early on with their remote view-ing experiments at the Stanford Research Institute that ordinary subjects could be trained to become more intuitive (Targ & Harary, 1987; Targ & Puthoff, 1974). They concluded that what made the difference was training subjects to perceive and make note of subtle, fleeting signals—the kinds of things that are usually ignored—in a state of open attention. Once noted, subjects were instructed to leave the initial perception alone, trusting the raw data as it appeared, even when ambiguous, baffling, or apparently nonsensical. It was when subjects analyzed and tried to define their perceptions—termed "secondary elaboration" by the research team—that their accuracy went awry (Targ & Harary, 1987). Not surprisingly, in an exploration of traits of high psi scorers, it was found that people who scored well on psi tests were people who could tolerate ambiguity (Broughton, 1991, pp. 108-115).

Guided imagery favors this element as well. With the internal focus and attenuated, inner perception of guided imagery, there is greater ability to perceive the subtle, fleeting data that arises there. In addition, because the exercise of guided imagery is primarily a right-brained activity, secondary elaboration is not particularly in play. Cognitive activities, such as analyzing, categorizing, comparing, defining, are crowded out in favor of the experiential and the perceptual.

GUIDED IMAGERY FOR ENHANCING INTUITION: RECEIVING AN ANSWER AS A GIFT (© Naparstek, 1997)

What follows is a guided imagery narrative, usually delivered against a background of gentle, calming music (Kohn, 1995). It is presented in segments to reveal its underlying organization. The imagery is designed to elicit an intuitive answer to a quandary where cognitive approaches have afforded unsatisfactory solutions. The annotations highlight the ways that the imagery harnesses and employs the key elements presented in the preceding discussion.

Relaxing the Body and Clearing the Mind

See if you can position yourself as comfortably as you can . . . (non-directive language is used to ensure a sense of choice, safety and relaxation . . .) shifting your weight so you're allowing your body to be fully supported . . . (the beginnings of relaxing the body . . .) with your head, neck and spine straight . . . and gently allowing your eyes to close . . . (the syntax of these sentences encourages an attitude of receptivity as opposed to proactivity, as do words like "allowing" and "letting" . . .) letting your hands rest comfortably on your body . . . on your chest or midriff or abdomen . . . (this will become a consistent gesture that will serve as an anchor, conditioning the listener to relax when it is employed. . . .) so you can feel the rise of your body as you breathe in . . . and the way it settles back down as you breathe out . . . (using the breath as a device to promote relaxation and focus attention inside the body . . .).

Becoming more and more attuned to your breath as it moves in and out of your body . . . inhaling as fully and deeply as you comfortably can . . . all the way down into your belly if you can . . . and breathing out as fully and completely as you can . . . (encouraging abdominal breathing to deepen the relaxation . . .).

And this next time, as you're breathing in . . . see if you can imagine that the warm energy of your breath is going to any part of your body that's sore or tense or tight . . . and releasing the discomfort with the out-breath . . . so you can feel your breath going to all the tight, tense places.. warming and loosening and softening them . . . and then gathering up all the tension . . . and breathing it out . . . (deepening relaxation and interior focus even further by combining the breath with kinesthetic imagery . . .).

So that more and more, you can feel safe and comfortable . . . relaxed and easy . . . watching the cleansing action of the breath . . . (note the passive language and the increased shifting into receptive syntax and sentence structure . . .).

And any unwelcome thoughts that come to mind . . . those too can be sent out with the breath . . . released with the exhale . . . so that for just a moment the mind is empty . . . for just a split second, it is free and clear space . . . and you are blessed with stillness . . . (a mini-rendition of mindfulness meditation, where the breath is used as the device that clears the mind, another optimal condition . . .).

And any emotions that are rocking around inside . . . those too can be noted, and acknowledged and sent out with the breath . . . (using the breath to clear the emotions as well . . . a cleaner slate for what follows . . .) so that your emotional self can be still and quiet . . . like a lake with no ripples . . . (a visual image to potentiate the notion of stillness . . .).

Interior Focus on the Heart

And now, if you would . . . see if you can direct your attention inward . . . focusing your attention on your heart . . . (placing attention even more deeply inward and at the same time narrowing focus on the emotional nexus of the heart . . .) curious about how it feels in there . . . inside and all around your heart . . . (it is not unusual for this simple placement of attention on the heart to generate emotion) with all the gentle, curious focus you can bring to bear . . . just keeping your awareness there . . . connecting to the powerful rhythms of your heart . . . sensing it pulsing life and strength all through your body . . . (designed to support a sense of gratitude for the miracle of the body, in the service of further opening the heart). . . .

And now, see if you can imagine that you're actually breathing through your heart . . . (a device used by the Institute of HeartMath to add a potentiating, kinesthetic component to the imagery . . .), as if the breath were actually coming in through your heart . . . and breathing out through your heart . . . soft and warm and steady. . . .

So you can begin to sense a kind of warmth and fullness gathering all around and through your heart . . . all through your chest . . . very soft and rich and full . . . as you continue to focus your attention there . . . and breathe your breath there . . . right through the center of your heart . . . (underlining these images and ideas with repetition . . .)

Sacred Space and Opening the Heart

And now . . . see if you can become aware of the feel of the air around you . . . maybe sensing a subtle energy . . . a bristle of aliveness . . . like a gently vibrating cushion of energy . . . (the idea of protected space is introduced as a primarily kinesthetic image, which is more powerful and accessible than a strictly visual one . . .) softly surrounding and protecting you . . . maybe feeling it tingle on your skin . . . and perhaps even sensing its sparkling dots of dancing color (now visual) . . . or hearing its gentle, humming sound (auditory) . . . or catching the scent of something fresh and new around you . . . (olfactory . . .) and inside the cushion, you can feel safe and peaceful . . . (the emotional character of this image is now experienced, soon to be amplified further) . . . able to take in what is nourishing to you . . . but insulated from whatever you don't want or need . . . (this also defines the boundaries that contain the sacred space imagery). . . .

And now, if you would, see if you can imagine that this cushion of energy is drawing to it (still in passive, receptive mode, the action occurring by dint of the cushion) all the love and sweetness that has ever been felt for you by anyone at any time . . . (designed to generate feelings of love and gratitude in the recipient—this image opens the heart . . .) feeling it pull in all the caring, all the loving kindness that has ever been sent your way . . . every prayer and good wish . . . every smile and gesture of gratitude . . . (God is indeed in the details . . . specific details in the memory of a smile or a gesture are more powerful heart-openers than abstract ideas) . . . permeating and filling the field of energy all around you . . . pulling it all in like a powerful magnet . . . (a metaphor to underline the image . . .) calling every good wish home . . . and so increasing the powerful, protective field around you . . . (reminders of safety and protection allow the heart to remain open and open further. . .).

And perhaps even sensing the presence of those who've loved or nurtured you . . . (pumping up the love and gratitude even further . . .) those who love you now . . . or who will love you in the future (in case there is no one on the scene right now who qualifies for this role . . .) . . . just the ones you want with you . . . (a safety measure, in case someone shows up that the person doesn't want there . . . this permission to edit out unwanted visitors keeps the space relaxed and safe . . .) . . . alive or long gone . . . (this reminder that the visitors needn't be currently living is rarely necessary . . .) and sensing them around you now . . . perhaps even seeing a fleeting glimpse of somebody . . . catching an old, familiar scent (using all the senses, olfactory memory included . . .) . . . or hearing the rich timbre of a dearly loved voice . . . sensing a comforting presence by your side or just behind you . . . or feeling the soft, warm weight of a loving hand on your shoulder . . . (all these sensory images are designed to anchor the loving memories and further open the heart . . .).

There might even be a special animal . . . a dear old pet . . . (for those who have no supportive relationships to call upon, but can remember animals who sustained them . . .) . . . you might feel the presence of a special grandparent . . . a powerful ancestor whose banner you carry . . . (another, more abstract option for those without much experience of actual human support) or there might be guardian angels and guides . . . sweet spirits and magical beings . . . (spiritual visitors can fulfill the same purpose . . .) perhaps familiar, perhaps not . . . it doesn't matter . . . just so you feel their protection and support . . . those who believe in you . . . who love and support you . . . and guide you well. . . .

Subtle Perception in the Receptive State

One might lean into you . . . whispering words so close to your ear . . . that maybe you can feel the tickle of warm breath on your ear . . . (a space is left here for the open, receptive attention to subtle cues). . . .

Another, with a simple, gentle touch, might endow you with a certain feeling . . . a sense of something you need to know. . . .

And another might be carrying a gift for you . . . specially wrapped . . . offered with smiling eyes and loving hands . . . and you somehow know that under the wrapping there will be assistance from the highest place.. for your greatest good. . . .

And as you unwrap the gift . . . you might discover that what is under the wrapping makes sense to you.. or maybe it doesn't . . . it doesn't matter . . . (offering permission to let the images remain ambiguous and undefined) because you can keep it and hold it and examine it again and again . . . from every angle . . . until you know what you need to know . . . see what you need to see. . . .

Able to turn it in your hands . . . feel its texture . . . catch its scent . . . listen to its sound . . . yours to keep . . . and hold. . . .

Still aware of the presence of so many gathered around you . . . there to remind you of the assistance available to you all the time . . . even when you forget it's there . . . in the protective cushion of energy . . . sparkling, humming and dancing all around you. . . .

And you can feel the soft expansion, all around and through your heart . . . as you breathe in all the love and suport around you . . . (again strengthening the incorporation of the imagery by making it kinesthetic, placing it firmly in the body with the help of the breath . . .) and breathe out the richness of your gratitude . . .

taking in the nourishing power of all that protection and support . . . filling up with it . . . feeling the warmth of it spread all through your body . . . gently pulsing out from the center of your heart . . . and diffusing all through you . . . like ripples in a pond. . . .

And so . . . still aware of the warmth in the center of your chest . . . and the protection all around you . . . you can once again feel yourself in the center of your body . . . strong and peaceful and steady . . . aware of your hands, your feet, your breath in your belly . . . (more grounding in the body). . . .

And very gently, with soft eyes, allowing yourself to come back whenever you are ready . . . knowing in a deep place that you are better for this. . . .

And so you are.

CONCLUSION

Guided Imagery, by its very nature, contains most of the elements needed to promote the enhancement of intuitive capacity. Intuition development training requires the trainee to generate key shifts in body, cognition, awareness, emotion, attitude, perception and felt spiritual sense. Guided imagery, when constructed appropriately, creates the conditions for these shifts, and, as such, is a natural vehicle for unlocking intuitive ability.

REFERENCES

Batcheldor, K. (1966). Contributions to the theory of PK induction from Sitter-Group Work. *Journal of the American Society for Psychical Research, 78,* 1105-1122.

Broughton, R. (1991). *Parapsychology, the controversial science.* New York: Ballantine.

Casey, C. (1997). *Inner and outer space.* Boulder, CO: Sounds True Audio.

Child, I. (1985). Psychology and anomalous observations: The question of ESP in dreams. *American Psychologist, 40,* 1219-1230.

Green, E., & Green A. (1977). *Beyond biofeedback.* New York: Delacorte Press.

Honorton, C. (1978). Psi and internal attention states: Information retrieval in the Ganzfeld. In B. Shapin & L. Coly (Eds.), *Psi and states of awareness.* New York: Parapsychology Foundation.

Honorton, C., & Shechter, E. (1986). Ganzfeld target retrieval with an automated testing system: A model for Ganzfeld success. In D. Weiner & R. Nelson (Eds.), *Research in parapsychology.* Metuchin, NJ: Scarecrow Press.

Kohn, S. (1995). *Music from health journeys.* Akron: Image Paths.

Krippner, S., & Ullman, M. (1970). Telepathy and dreams: A controlled experiment with electro-encephalogram and electro-oculogram monitoring. *Journal of Nervous and Mental Diseases, 151,* 394-403.

McCraty, R., Atkinson, M., Tiller, W., Rein, G., & Watkins, A. (1995) Entrainment, coherence & autonomic balance: The effects of emotions on short-term power spectral analysis of heart rate variability. *American Journal of Cardiology, 76,* 1089-1093.

Naparstek, B. (1994). *Staying well with guided imagery.* New York: Warner Books.

Naparstek, B. (1997). *Your sixth sense: Unlocking the power of your intuition.* San Francisco: HarperCollins.

Owen, I., & Sparrow, M. (1976). *Conjuring up Philip.* New York: Harper & Row.

Rein, G., Atkinson, M., & McCraty, R. (1995). The physiological and psychological effects of compassion and anger. *Journal of Advancement in Medicine, 8,* 87-105.

Targ, R., & Harary, K. (1987). *The mind race: Understanding and using psychic abilities.* New York: Ballantine Books.

Targ, R., & Puthoff, H. (1974). Information transmission under conditions of sensory shielding. *Nature, 251,* 602-607.

Walsh, R., & Shapiro, D. H. (1983). *Beyond health and normality.* New York: Van Nostrand Rheinhold.

CHAPTER 20

Transpersonal Images: Implications for Health

WILLIAM BRAUD

The imagination of man can act not only on his own body, but even on others and very distant bodies. It can fascinate and modify them; make them ill, or restore them to health.

Ibn Sînâ (quoted in Regardie, 1974, p. 90)

THREE MODES OF KNOWING

In the Middle Ages, before the disciplines of theology, philosophy, and psychology had split and gone their separate ways, the metaphor of the *three eyes* frequently was used to describe different modes of knowing. Scholars, contemplatives, and visionaries such as Boethius, the Victorine mystics (Hugh of St. Victor, Richard of St. Victor, Thomas of St. Victor), Bonaventure, and others wrote of the *eye of the flesh* (or of the senses), the *eye of reason* (or of the mind), and the *eye of contemplation* (or of the heart or spirit) (Boethius, 524/1980; Bonaventure, 1259/1953; McGinn, 1995, 1996, 1998). Similar distinctions were made within the Islamic and Sufi traditions by al-Ghazzâlî, Ibn al-'Arabî, and others (Bruns, 1992; Corbin, 1981; Hollenback, 1996; Nasr, 1992; Schneck, 1980; Sells, 1996; Shah, 1964). These three modes of knowing correspond to, respectively, sensation and empirical knowing; thinking and rational knowing; and knowing directly and immediately through feelings, love, compassion, intuition, inspiration, revelation, and becoming or being what is to be known.

Different realms are accessible to the three eyes, and the reality status of what is "seen" through each eye differs from realm to realm. This reminds one of the different objects of knowing that inhabit Karl Popper's three worlds (of nature, of subjectivity, and of symbols and culture) (Popper, 1979, 1982; Popper & Eccles, 1983), to which George Zollschan (1989) added a separate and autonomous fourth world of inspiration—a fluid world of unbounded possibilities and no defined limits. A century earlier, William James (1890/1950) had proposed his own

448

version of the many worlds, listing seven of these—sensory qualities, physical things, abstract truths, widespread illusions or prejudices, supernatural and mythological worlds, worlds of individual opinion, and those of sheer madness and vagary. He suggested that "propositions concerning the different worlds are made from 'different points of view'; and . . . each world *whilst it is attended to* is real after its own fashion; only the reality lapses with the attention" (pp. 292-293). As we shall see later, *attention* and *intention* are key factors in determining what we may or may not know or accomplish within the various realms.

THREE MODES OF COMMUNICATING AND INFLUENCING

The three eyes is a useful metaphor for how and what we may know or perceive. We can extend the metaphor—to three mouths and three hands—in considering different modes of communication and influence. We can imagine sets of mouths and hands of the flesh, of the mind, and of the spirit.

We use *the mouth and hands of the flesh* to communicate with and influence ourselves, others, and the physical world in conventional, physical ways. In a health context, this corresponds to the *Era I medicine* described by Larry Dossey (1992, 1993, 1999). Here, health practitioners and clinicians prescribe mechanical, material, or physical interventions for their patients and clients. These take the familiar forms of mechanical adjustments, surgery, medicinal drugs, massage, physical regimens, and behavioral techniques, as well as the less familiar, but increasingly popular, alternative interventions of acupuncture, herbs, aromas, homeopathy, movements, sounds, and so on.

The mouth and hands of the mind correspond to the words, thoughts, feelings, emotions, images, memories, and expectations that we can use to communicate with our internal systems and influence our organisms. This is the realm of what Dossey has called *Era II medicine*, which emphasizes psychosomatic or mind-body interventions. These include most of the imagery approaches treated in this volume, along with related practices of relaxation, autogenics, hypnosis, psychophysiological self-regulation, biofeedback, psychoimmunological techniques, placebo effects, mental rehearsal, some forms of meditation and contemplation, cognitive therapies, and so forth (Dossey, 1992, 1993, 1999).

The mouth and hands of the spirit would correspond to more direct and immediate communications and interactions with other persons, as well as animate and inanimate systems, that distance or barriers might place beyond the reach of the other two sets of mouths and hands. These remote interactions—instances of Dossey's *Era III nonlocal medicine*—include diagnosis at a distance, distant healing, intercessory prayer, telesomatic events, forms of shamanic communication and healing, certain forms of what have come to be known as subtle energy effects, and, perhaps, noncontact therapeutic touch (Dossey, 1992, 1993, 1999).

Some of these interesting and important nonlocal interactions may be mediated or facilitated by transpersonal imagery.

TRANSPERSONAL IMAGERY

Jeanne Achterberg, in discussing the role of imagery in healing, distinguished two types of imagery. In *preverbal imagery*, the imagination acts upon one's own physical being to alter cellular, biochemical, and physiological activity. *Transpersonal imagery* "embodies the assumption that information can be transmitted from the consciousness of one person to the physical substrate of others" (Achterberg, 1985, p. 5). She suggested that the validation of transpersonal imagery must be sought in the more qualitative types of observational data gathered by anthropologists, theologians, and medical historians, and in intuitive philosophical speculation. Some of this anecdotal evidence for the existence and efficacy of transpersonal imagery will be presented in a later section of this chapter. We shall see that, in addition to the more naturalistic modes of inquiry that Achterberg suggests, experimental approaches also may be, and have been, used to validate the existence and functions of transpersonal imagery. First, however, it is important to describe in greater detail what is meant by "transpersonal imagery" and, indeed, by "transpersonal" itself.

In its most straightforward sense, transpersonal imagery is imagery that can exist or act *across* persons—i.e., from one person to another. Here, imagery could function as a bridge, connecting the conscious, imaginal content or activity of one person with the conscious or unconscious, physiological or psychological activities or experiences of another person.

There is another meaning of *trans*—as *beyond*—that is of great importance in the relatively young disciplines of transpersonal psychology and transpersonal studies. These fields of study explore experiences and processes that extend beyond the conventionally understood stages of personal development, beyond what is ordinarily understood as the individual ego or personality, beyond one's ordinary conditions of consciousness, and beyond the usual modes of knowing, being, and doing. Transpersonal experiences are those "in which the sense of identity or self extends beyond (trans) the individual or personal to encompass wider aspects of humankind, life, psyche or cosmos" (Walsh & Vaughan, 1993, p. 203). This emphasis does not exclude or invalidate the personal; rather, it places the personal in a larger context, and it recognizes that the transpersonal or the transcendent can be expressed *through* the personal—in still another meaning of *trans*. The emphasis on a beyond or a something more—which can be contrasted with a reductionistic, nothing-but mindset—is congruent with William James' (1902/1985) view that one can become conscious of and in touch with "a More" with which one is "conterminous and continuous" (p. 508) and that such forms of awareness are at the heart of what we today call spiritual experiences.

Although it is common to assign its earliest use to Stanislav Grof and Abraham Maslow in 1967 and 1968, the term *transpersonal* was used on earlier occasions by scholars and psychologists who contributed importantly to topics related to those addressed in this volume on healing images. Among these are William James [1905], Carl Jung [1917], Dane Rudhyar [1930], Eric Neumann [1954], and Ira Progoff [1955] (Boorstein, 1990; Sutich, 1976; Vich, 1988). Additionally, the subjects explored in transpersonal studies have considerable overlap with likely interests of readers of this volume—namely, the limitations of purely verbal, rational, and analytical modes of thought; consciousness and unusual states of consciousness; exceptional human experiences; creativity; our latent human potentials; inner wisdom; wholeness, health, and well-being; experientially-based therapies; and psychospiritual growth, development, and transformation. In addition to its more specific role in the context of transpersonal imagery, the transpersonal in general is relevant to our interests.

THE REALITY OF THE IMAGINAL

In transpersonal experiences, there can be an expansion of one's identity to include much more of the world, and there can be a greater appreciation of one's interconnectedness with all of nature. Some of these apprehensions may be represented in one's imagination and imagery. Are such awarenesses and images momentary illusions or ways of speaking, or is there some sense in which they partake of "reality"?

Certainly, perceptions and images can be illusory and have no correspondence with conventional reality. There is a tendency, especially among Western, Euro-centric thinkers, to attribute a status of unreality to all aspects of the imagination. The usual connotations of words such as *imaginary* or *fantasy* reveal such a mindset. However, there always has been a parallel stream of thought in which the transpersonal and the imaginal are considered *real*—although this reality may be of a different character than that of the physical entities with which we are familiar. A sampling of systems of thought in which a special reality is attributed to the imaginal realm would include shamanic worldviews (Hollenback, 1996; Peters, 1989; Walsh, 1989); the Tantric Buddhism of Tibet (Hollenback, 1996); descriptions of the spiritual and creative imagination in Ibn al-'Arabî and Suhrawardî, within mystical Islam (Corbin, 1981; Hollenback, 1996); the Western hermetic and magical traditions (Gray, 1975; Yates, 1964); various mystical traditions (Hollenback, 1996); and the views of Romantic poets such as Blake, Wordsworth, Coleridge, Keats, and Shelley (Bowra, 1961; Burnshaw, 1970). More recent and more familiar are many of the works of Carl Jung, James Hillman's archetypal psychology, Henry Corbin's writings on the imaginal faculty, Jess Hollenback's treatments of the empowered imagination, and Stanislav Grof's researches on the transpersonal realm, as revealed by imagery occurring in nonordinary states of consciousness (Avens, 1980; Corbin, 1972; Grof, 1972, 1973; Hillman, 1976, 1995; Jung, 1965).

Key considerations regarding different forms of imagery and their nature and "powers" have been provided by Henry Corbin (1972, 1981) in his elaboration of Ibn al-'Arabî's description of *himmah*—a kind of transfigured or empowered imaginal process or creative imagination, through which it becomes possible to directly perceive subtle or spiritual realities and to endow products of one's imagination and intention with a form of external reality, capable of being perceived by others—and by Jess Hollenback's (1996) treatments of *enthymesis* or empowered imagination, with properties identical to those of *himmah*. In these systems of thought, ordinary imagination may remain "local" in what it may know and accomplish. However, a special form of concentrated, empowered, transformed, or dynamized imagination can know and act veridically and nonlocally.

The imaginal is emphasized and is active in both the Era II and Era III categories of Dossey's schema. The validity (as an accurate means of knowing) and efficacy (in producing objectively measurable changes) of preverbal imagery have been demonstrated repeatedly in Era II contexts—through immunological, physiological, and behavioral studies of types well-documented in other chapters of this volume. The remainder of this chapter will explore indications of the reality, validity, and efficacy of transpersonal imagery in nonlocal, Era III contexts. The imagery to be discussed may be called "transpersonal" because it acts in a person other than the person who is its "source" (or because the imagery originates in a person other than the person in whom it is acting).

THE REACH OF THE IMAGINAL: ANECDOTAL EVIDENCE

Anecdotal accounts of the reach of the imaginal abound. We have received anthropological reports of distant knowing and distant imaginal influences, occurring under field conditions in many cultures and times (Angoff & Barth, 1974; Long, 1977; Van de Castle, 1977). With the increased interest in shamanic studies today, such reports have increased. Similar phenomena were noted commonly in 19th-century practices of mesmerism and hypnosis, in the forms of *community of sensation* and mental *suggestions at a distance* (Dingwall, 1968; Honorton, 1974, 1977). In health-related contexts, these effects have been reported in accounts of distant, mental, or spiritual healing and in accounts of remote diagnosis (Benor, 1993; Ehrenwald, 1977; Solfvin, 1984). In psychological situations, counselors and therapists have had experiences in which dreams or intuitive flashes provided specific diagnostic information, and in which preparatory or rehearsal efforts the night before important, upcoming sessions seemed to have already accomplished intended outcomes, distantly and mentally, even before the actual work of the sessions. In contexts of biofeedback and self-regulation training, curious correlations have been noted between the physiological activities and images of several clients practicing at the same time and between a client's physiological responses and the trainer's own reactions, images, and intentions—corresponding patterns that could not be explained in conventional terms. In psychoneuroimmunology investigations, the extreme specificity and rapidity of immunological changes, in response to specific forms of self-generated imagery, suggest the possibility of direct mental influences within one's own body (Braud, 1986). The diagnostic information that imagery can provide about one's internal bodily and psychological conditions also suggests the possibility of direct knowing effects above and beyond conventionally appreciated mechanisms of action (Achterberg, 1985).

USE OF IMAGERY IN NONLOCAL INTERVENTIONS: EMPIRICAL INVESTIGATIONS

The use of imagery in the nonlocal production of health-related outcomes, or of physiological or psychological changes with health-related potentials, has been documented not only in everyday life, field conditions, but also in carefully designed and executed laboratory studies. In this section, I will illustrate this approach by summarizing the methods and findings of an extensive research program in which my colleagues and I have been involved since 1977. This program involves laboratory experiments exploring what is now commonly known as "direct mental interactions with living systems" (DMILS). We have published seven major interim reports and reviews of these experiments (Braud, 1978a, 1990, 1993; Braud & Schlitz, 1983, 1989, 1991; Schlitz & Braud, 1997); interested readers are referred to these reports for specific details and additional information.

Methodological Safeguards

In these experiments, one person uses imagery as a vehicle for exerting a direct mental influence upon the objectively measured physiological activity of another person. The influencer and the influencee are situated in separate rooms, at a distance (20 meters or more) from one another, and the experimental protocol is designed to eliminate any conventional informational or energetic interactions between the two persons. Precautions are taken to prevent sensory cueing; these include the use of distant, closed rooms, auditory masking in the influencee's room, and a protocol that prevents auditory cueing. Influence periods are randomly interspersed among non-influence, control periods, and the influencee remains unaware of the precise beginning or sequence of these different types of periods. This design feature eliminates rational inference, expectation, and placebo-like confounds. It also guards against the possibility that the influencer and influencee may simply be responding to common external events or internal rhythms, and it rules out systematic, time-dependent artifacts such as adaptation or habituation to the environment or test conditions. Changes in the physiological activities of the influencee are monitored by electronic equipment, recorded in permanent form (as polygraph records and as digitized records in computer files), and blind-scored or computer-scored to prevent recording errors or motivated scoring errors. Results are statistically analyzed to determine the presence and magnitude of effects and to rule out coincidental, chance correspondences as viable explanations of any obtained outcomes. Replications are conducted to assure consistency and reliability.

General Procedures

The influencee and influencer are stationed in their separate rooms. The influencee is given general instructions and information about the study and is instrumented appropriately for the monitoring and recording of his or her psychophysiological activity. In most studies, electrodermal activity (EDA) is selected as the dependent variable for its ease of measurement, its sensitive reflection of sympathetic nervous system changes, and its reflection of emotional and psychological changes that are relevant to physical and psychological health and well-being (e.g., the measures can reflect levels of stress, anxiety, anger, or frustration, as well as general physiological or psychological overactivity, underactivity, and deviations from homeostasis or appropriate psychophysiological regulation). EDA is recorded continuously throughout a session, and the fluctuating, AC component of EDA (i.e., skin resistance responses, SRRs, corrected for a shifting skin resistance level, SRL, baseline or DC component), electronically integrated for each influence and non-influence period, serves as the specific physiological measure. In other studies, other response systems are measured. The influencee is asked to remain seated in a comfortable chair, in a dimly illuminated room, and maintain a moderate level of arousal—i.e., not to become overly excited or relaxed. The influencee is encouraged to let his or her cognitive activity be as freely variable as possible—i.e., not to cling to any particular mental content, but to let one's mentation flow freely, without attempting to control or guide it. The influencee also is asked to remain open to appropriate distant mental influences from the remote influencer. A session is typically 30 minutes or so in duration and consists of many sets of brief, interspersed influence and non-influence periods.

Transpersonal Imagery Components

In the separate influencer's room, an experimenter instructs the influencer regarding the distant mental influence procedures. A random process determines whether a given period is to be a non-influence, control period or an influence period. These periods typically are 30–60 seconds in duration. During a non-influence period, the influencer rests and attempts not to think about the influencee and to think about matters that are not related to the experiment. During influence periods, the influencer's aim is to either activate or calm the remotely situated influencee using appropriate mental imagery and intentions. If the protocol indicates an activation aim for a given period, the influencer attempts to activate the influencee using activating imagery and intentions. Three types of activation imagery strategies are used by the influencer.

1. The influencer uses activating mental imagery and self-regulation to produce a state of sympathetic autonomic arousal or activation in oneself, while intending and imagining the distant influencee's body mirroring these changes and also becoming activated. Imagery with exciting, energetic, or emotion-arousing content could be used—e.g., imagining that one is exercising vigorously, listening to energizing music, visualizing scary circumstances, imagining that one is laughing vigorously and is extremely joyful, imagining that one's own physiological activity is increasing (increased breathing, heart rate, blood pressure, muscle tension, etc.).

2. The influencer imagines the influencee encountering a situation or circumstance that, if actually encountered, would produce physiological activation or arousal. For example, one might imagine the influencee vigorously exercising, or encountering a scary situation, or engaging in some energetic activity. Along with this, one imagines and visualizes increases in the actual physiological activity that is being measured.

3. The influencer watches the feedback indicator (i.e., the polygraph record) and imagines and visualizes that indicator describing much activity (frequent and large deflections). Alternatively, one simply closes one's eyes and visualizes a very active polygraph record, filled with numerous, large-amplitude deflections, indicative of heightened influencee activity.

Any or any combination of these strategies can be used. Additionally, the influencer may try a given imagery strategy, observe its outcome (by means of the ever-available polygraph feedback record), stay with strategies that seem effective, or abandon seemingly ineffective strategies to shift to more effective ones. The influencer can use a trial and error approach to identify and tailor the most effective imagery strategies for oneself and one's influencee.

If the protocol indicates a calming aim for a given period, the influencer attempts to calm the influencee using calming imagery and intentions. Again, three types of imagery strategies are possible. Each of these is a complement of one mentioned above.

1. The influencer uses calming mental imagery and self-regulation to produce a state of sympathetic autonomic calmness, relaxation, and quietude in oneself, while intending and imagining the distant influencee's body mirroring these changes and also becoming very calm and relaxed. Imagery with relaxing, calming, tranquil content could be used—e.g., imagining that one is relaxing in a favorite location, visualizing oneself reclining comfortably and about to fall asleep, imagining soothing music, imagining extremely peaceful and tranquil circumstances, imagining that one's own physiological

activity is decreasing (decreased breathing, heart rate, blood pressure, muscle tension, etc.).

2. The influencer imagines the influencee encountering a situation or circumstance that, if actually encountered, would produce physiological deactivation, relaxation, and hypoarousal. For example, one might imagine the influencee at rest, relaxing, encountering a calming situation, or being present in a soothing, tranquil, pastoral setting. Along with this, one imagines and visualizes decrements in the actual physiological activity that is being measured.

3. The influencer watches the feedback indicator (i.e., the polygraph record) and imagines and visualizes that indicator describing greatly reduced (few and small deflections). Alternatively, one simply closes one's eyes and visualizes a very inactive polygraph record, having infrequent, small-amplitude deflections, indicative of reduced influencee activity.

In addition to these specific, process-oriented images, the influencer may engage in *goal-oriented imagery* of a more general and overarching sort. This would involve imaging and visualizing (and intending for) events that would be associated with a successful experiment outcome. Such events would include imagining the joy of the research personnel as they celebrate a positive outcome for a session or for the entire experiment, imagining a computer printing out significant findings, imagining reading a published report of positive findings of this session or this experiment, imagining how the outcome of the present session may contribute to the realization of some useful, health-related practical application of these principles, and so on.

Results Summary

Through the years, we have conducted 15 experiments in which "transpersonal imagery" and intentions were used in attempts to influence the ongoing EDA of a distant person. These studies provided statistically significant and reliable evidence for the existence of nonlocal, direct mental influences. The 15-study series yielded a combined, Stouffer z of 4.08, an associated p value of .000023, and a mean effect size d of +.29 (Braud & Schlitz, 1989). The EDA of influencees increased during periods in which remotely situated influencers used activating imagery, and decreased during periods in which calming, relaxing imagery was used, compared to appropriate control conditions. These experiments involved 323 separate sessions conducted with 271 different influencees, 62 influencers, and 4 experimenters. Subsequent to our 1989 report, 4 replication studies, involving a total of 75 additional experimental sessions, were attempted elsewhere. Updating our original work, in 1997, to include these replications yielded an overall $z = 4.82$, $p = .0000007$, and mean effect size $r = +.25$ (Schlitz & Braud, 1997).

We conducted additional experiments in which biological activities other than EDA were influenced, mentally and at a distance. The new response systems included: subtle muscular movements, muscular tremor, blood pressure, the spatial orientation of fish, the locomotor activity of small mammals, and the rate of hemolysis of human red blood cells, in vitro. Positive results were obtained for all of these new living systems, with the exception of muscular tremor. In 1991 we published a summary (meta-analysis) of all of our DMILS studies. The research program included 37 experiments, 655 sessions, 449 different influencees, 153 different influencers, and 12 different experimenters. The overall results, for all influenced living systems combined, yielded a combined (Stouffer) $z = 7.72$, $p = 2.58 \times 10^{-14}$, and a mean effect size $r = +.33$ (Braud & Schlitz, 1991).

In each of these studies, an influencer imagined and visualized the desired outcome activities occurring in the distant living "target systems." In the hemolysis study, for example, human red blood cells were osmotically-stressed by placing them in hypotonic saline solutions in test tubes in a distant room. The rate of cell destruction (hemolysis) was objectively monitored by a spectrophotometer interfaced with a computer. For influence periods (half of the set of hemolysis tubes), the remote influencers attempted to mentally "protect" the red blood cells by visualizing the cells with intact, resilient membranes that resisted the osmotic stress rather than bursting. Color slides of healthy, intact red blood cells were available to the influencers, should they choose to use this sensory aid to enhance their protective mental imagery. For non-influence, control periods (half of the set of hemolysis tubes), the influencers thought about matters unrelated to the experiment and did not entertain cell-related imagery. The experimenter who measured the hemolysis rates was blind as to whether or not remote influences were being attempted during the measurements. Hemolysis rate was significantly less during the periods of remote protective imagery than during control periods. There was a tendency, albeit a nonsignificant one, for greater remote hemolysis protection for one's own red blood cells than for another person's red blood cells (Braud, 1990).

In all of the studies mentioned above, imagery was used along with deliberate intentions for the distant, biological activities to change in particular ways. Following these studies, we conducted variations on these studies in which imagery was used in a different way, and in which directional intention was replaced by a "purer" form of *attention*. These studies also involved recording of EDA, but EDA now was used as an "unconscious" measure of the detection of remote staring. A person was stationed in a distant room, as before, and that person's ongoing, spontaneous EDA was monitored. A closed-circuit television camera was focused upon the person, allowing that person's visual image to be displayed on a television monitor in a distant room. On a random schedule, the observer either watched or did not watch the television image of the observee. During the watching periods, the observer attempted to deploy attention as fully as possible upon the person whose image was being viewed. During the nonwatching period, the observer did not view the image and attempted to think of things other than the experiment. Of course, the observees did not know whether they were being remotely viewed (stared at) or not, at any given moment. We conducted four experiments of this type in our own laboratory, and, subsequently, seven replication experiments were conducted elsewhere. In 1997, we reported a summary (meta-analysis) of all 11 of these experiments on electrodermal detection of remote staring. Overall, the 11 experiments involved 241 sessions and yielded a combined (Stouffer) $z = 3.87$, $p = .000054$, and an average effect size $r = +.25$ (Schlitz & Braud, 1997).

We have extended this work by conducting experiments in which persons used imagery and intention in attempts to facilitate the mental or psychological, rather than the physiological, activities of a distant person. In one study, we measured the self-reported vividness of mental imagery occurring during what might be described as a guided imagination exercise, using the Creative Imagination Scale (CIS) developed by Sheryl Wilson and T. X. Barber. For half of these persons, their imagery intensity was assessed under ordinary conditions. For the other half, imagery was assessed while a distant "helper" was generating similar imagery (augmented by sensory aids) and intending to assist the first person's imagery, mentally and at a distance. The vividness and realism of imagery was significantly greater when the imager was being mentally and distantly assisted by the similar, concurrent imagery of another person (Braud & Jackson, 1983). The imagers were, of course, "blind" as to whether or not this remote imagery aid was in effect. This study can be understood as one in which nonlocal, transpersonal imagery was used to facilitate local, preverbal imagery.

Most recently, we have found that similar remote, mental assistance can be effective in helping persons concentrate and focus their attention on a centering object in a meditation-like setting. Fewer distractions to concentration were reported by persons who were being mentally assisted by the concurrent, focused attention of another, distant person (Braud, Shafer, McNeill, & Guerra, 1995).

Influences "Across Time"

In the studies described above, process-oriented and goal-oriented imagery and intentions acted nonlocally with respect to space—a person's direct mental influence was monitored in a distant living system. We have also conducted sessions in which the to-be-influenced living system was distant in *time*. The procedures and analysis methods for these temporally nonlocal experiments are similar to those of the concurrent influence studies, with the important exception that the activity of the living "target" system is monitored and recorded *before* the influence attempts are made. Any systematic results in such experiments must involve time-displaced influences. Although such outcomes would appear impossible, given our conventional apprehensions of time and of causality, there are, nonetheless, both theoretical and empirical supports for such outcomes. The issues and studies in this area are too complex to be treated in this chapter, and so the reader is referred to a recently published paper that describes these studies in detail (Braud, 1999, 2000). For present purposes, I will simply indicate that there exists both anecdotal and laboratory evidence that supports the possibility of apparently "backward-acting," time-displaced, direct mental influences of living systems. Our imaginal processes appear to be capable of exerting objectively measurable influences not only upon present, distant biological and physical systems, but also upon the past and future activities of these systems.

Size of Effect and Replicability

Probability values and effect sizes were reported above. Another way of estimating the strength of these effects is to calculate the actual percentage of events or activities that change in association with these direct mental interventions. In various reported aggregations of these studies, the average influence has ranged from 4 percent or 8 percent in certain electrodermal influence studies, to 80 percent, 90 percent—and even 100 percent—changes in individual sessions. In special experiments, remote, direct mental influence effects on EDA did not differ appreciably from the size of deliberate, self-regulation effects on these same activities (Braud & Schlitz, 1983). Expressed in either probability, effect size, or percent change terms, these effects are far from negligible. While it is true that these effects do not always occur or replicate, their reproduction records are far from unacceptable, can compare favorably with the replication records of other behavioral or biomedical findings, and are not atypical of events that are newly being explored and about which the essential factors necessary for their production are not yet fully known or understood.

ROLE OF IMAGERY IN NONLOCAL KNOWING: EMPIRICAL INVESTIGATIONS

The studies summarized above explored processes that could be considered models, analogs, or scaled-down versions of nonlocal imaginal *interventions* that may occur in everyday life. In addition to these, there have been numerous laboratory studies of processes equivalent to nonlocal imaginal *diagnosis*. In these studies, imagery can serve as a vehicle for veridical perception or knowledge of physical, biological, or psychological events that distance and other barriers have placed beyond the reach of the conventional senses. There are extensive empirical studies of remote knowing through imagery. Because these are so numerous, and in order not to duplicate materials presented in Belleruth Naparstek's chapter, I will limit my discussion to some of my own research and theorizing in this area.

Our access to information or circumstances beyond the reach of our conventional senses can be revealed in many ways. This "knowing" can be expressed in clear, information-rich thoughts—as when the name of an illness or condition comes to mind. Equally unambiguous are specific bodily changes or conditions that are felt or exhibited, and that correspond clearly and closely to those of a distant person; these could be described as empathic or telesomatic indicators (Dossey, 1993; Schwarz, 1967). Other expressions can take the form of behavioral, perceptual, or memory-related changes that betray a knowing that has not yet reached our conscious awareness; these are the psi-mediated instrumental responses (PMIR)—e.g., finding ourselves at the right place at the right time, and thereby avoiding an accident or gaining access to needed information—that have been well-described and studied by Rex Stanford (1974a, 1974b). Knowledge of events beyond sensory range also can be indicated by subtle physiological changes, of which we may be unaware; by a diffuse awareness too vague to be articulated; or by a direct experience of "knowing" that also is difficult or impossible to put into words. Perhaps most commonly, our knowledge of distant or otherwise inaccessible events is expressed by imagery that bears some resemblance to the distant event or circumstance.

Methods and Findings

In order to qualify imagery as transpersonal—in the senses we have been using in this chapter—it is necessary to distinguish images that carry information about distant circumstances or events from other forms of imagery. Some of the latter include imagery that might arise naturally regardless of distant events, images that might be triggered by some common, conventional event that influences both the distant event and the person generating the imagery, and images that may correspond to the distant, to-be-known events only through chance or coincidence. Our experimental designs allow us to make these distinctions through the use of sensory shielding, truly random selection of the events to be known, blind evaluation of imagery correspondences with the true target event versus randomly selected non-target "decoys," and statistical analyses that compare obtained results with theoretically or empirically derived baselines.

We have conducted experiments in which spontaneously arising imagery, in suitably prepared individuals, could be shown to correspond to distant, randomly-selected target events. These events could be randomly selected pictures or objects, or their representations in the thoughts, images, and sensations of other persons. In some cases, the research participants were in ordinary states of consciousness (in remote viewing studies); in other cases, the participants were studied under the more imagery-rich conditions provided by relaxation, autogenic, sensory restriction (*Ganzfeld*), or hypnotic induction procedures, or during guided imagery, "waking dream," or nocturnal dream conditions (Braud, 1978b, 1981). In these, and in many related studies, transpersonal imagery can be demonstrated to have a veridical, *noetic* character—allowing accurate access to information temporarily unavailable to the conventional senses.

In principle, the focus of this imagery could be "targeted" to physical or psychological conditions of distant persons, for purposes of remote or augmented diagnosis. For example, in one test session a participant was asked to describe the health condition of an absent "target person." The participant described a young girl with blonde hair in ringlets, a metal brace on one of her legs, her heart "blown up, like a big red balloon," and the unusual circumstance of her heart displaced to the "wrong" side of the body. Each of these images corresponded perfectly to the conditions of the target person. Such accurate correspondences of "local" imagery with remote realities have been observed in countless formal and informal experiments.

MODULATING FACTORS

Although considerable uncertainty and mystery continue to exist with respect to the nature of these transpersonal imagery effects, and the conditions that influence them, we are able to make certain generalizations about the factors that seem to facilitate or impede their occurrence. These empirical generalizations are based upon our own research, conducted over a span of 30 years, and upon a huge database of similar research findings reported by others (Braud, 1991; Broughton, 1991; Edge, Morris, Rush, & Palmer, 1986; Krippner, 1977-1982, 1984-1994; Kurtz, 1985; Radin, 1997; Wolman, 1977).

Physical Facilitators and Inhibitors

Transpersonal imagery effects, in both their influential/intervention and noetic/diagnostic forms, have not been shown to be influenced importantly by physical factors. Factors such a distance, time, physical barriers, and the physical nature of the events to be known or influenced do not appear to play critical roles in transpersonal imagery outcomes. One factor that does seem important is the amount of free variability that is inherent in the system to be influenced. Random or labile physical systems that are relatively free from internal or external constraints or structure seem most amenable to being influenced through transpersonal imagery.

Three additional, possible physical correlates have been suggested. A tantalizing one, in terms of potential medical applications, is that water that has been "treated" through transpersonal imagery or related intention techniques may be physically altered. Such treated water appears to have decreased hydrogen bonding, compared to untreated, control water (Schwartz, De Mattei, Brame, & Spottiswoode, 1990). To the extent that changes in hydrogen bonding characterizes either disease conditions or therapeutic agents, this possible mode of action of nonlocal influence may provide a useful entry point for health applications.

Two other physical factors have recently been found to correlate with the likelihood or accuracy of nonlocal knowing, and these are, indeed, curious ones. One is the degree of activity in the earth's geomagnetic field. A decrease in this ambient activity (equivalent to a reduction in the amount of "noise" in the earth's electromagnetic "atmosphere") is associated with increased effectiveness of nonlocal knowing, both in the laboratory and in spontaneous occurrences in everyday life (Persinger, 1989; Spottiswoode, 1990). The other recently identified physical variable is the local sidereal time at the site at which a nonlocal knowing experiment is being conducted (Spottiswoode, 1997). It remains to be seen how well these unusual findings hold up to future replications and how these curious relationships might be understood.

Physiological Facilitators and Inhibitors

Although the nonlocal knowing effects we have been considering probably can occur in any physiological state, they appear to occur most readily or most accurately—or, at least, are most readily *noticed* or *detected*—under conditions of reduced muscular activity, reduced sympathetic autonomic activation, relatively reduced arousal, and a freeing of the brain (of the knower) from heavy information-processing demands (Braud, 1981, 1991). There also are indications—not as definitive as the foregoing—that heightened sympathetic nervous system arousal (in the influencer) may be associated with the production of some forms of nonlocal influence effects (Braud, 1985).

Complementary principles may apply to what is to be known or what is to be influenced. For example, heightened physiological arousal (which could be associated with increased *need*) in one person may make that person or that person's circumstances more discernable to others via the latter's nonlocal knowing. A person whose internal systems are relatively quiet and relatively free from internal or external structure or energetic- or information-handling demands may be more susceptible to nonlocal influence than would overly structured, constrained, or burdened physiological systems. This is an analog of the physical indeterminacy, randomness, or lability mentioned, above, as a physical facilitator.

Psychological Facilitators and Inhibitors

It is in the psychological area that we have learned most about facilitating and inhibiting factors. Many of the psychological facilitators of transpersonal imagery effects are closely related to, or may be variations of, faith, hope, and love, and many of the inhibitors are related to the opposites of these three virtues. Space permits only a brief mentioning of these factors here; more extended treatments are available elsewhere (Braud, 1991; Schmeidler, 1988; Wolman, 1977). Psychological facilitators of transpersonal imagery effects include: attitudes of belief, confidence, trust, hope, expectation of a successful outcome, the presence of strong motives and incentives, need, positive dispositions, caring, and a reduction in egocentric motives, strivings, or involvements. Psychological inhibitors include: attitudes of disbelief, distrust, doubt, suspicion, absent or negative expectations of success, increased egocentric motivation or too-effortful striving, and the absence of sufficient need, motivation, or purpose for the task at hand.

Additional psychological facilitators include: psychological comfort and absence of stress; freedom from distractions or "psychological noise"; conditions of relaxation and quietude; ability to direct attention inwardly and access inner processes; ability to control, deploy, and concentrate attention, generally; ability to generate and to detect imagery; ability to reduce "left-hemispheric," analytical thought and to increase "right-hemispheric," synthetic, and intuitive modes of mentation; ability to engage in a form of volition and intention that is more "passive" and less effortful (this is akin to wishing, rather than willing); freedom from excessive cognitive structure or information-handling demands; the presence of openness; and the absence of defensiveness (Braud, 1975; Stanford, 1977). Additional psychological inhibitors would include the absence or opposites of the facilitators just listed.

Also important to the occurrence of these transpersonal imagery effects is the preparedness, adequateness, and predisposition of the participant. The most effective participant would be one who is familiar with the imaginal world, skilled in negotiating this realm, and skilled in the use of creative imagination. Training in active imagination, psychophysiological self-regulation, concentration, meditation, and related psychospiritual practices may be useful preparations for engaging in transpersonal imagery exercises and nonlocal knowing and influence attempts.

IMPLICATIONS AND POTENTIAL APPLICATIONS

The most obvious health-related implications and potential practical applications of nonlocal knowing and influence mediated by transpersonal imagery are in the areas of diagnosis and intervention in instances of physical and psychological health disturbances. Just as *preverbal* imagery may serve these functions within a given individual—as a large extant literature and many of the chapters of this volume clearly indicate—so, too, may images provide diagnostic information and serve an influential, intervention function with respect to *other* individuals. These complementary functions may already be present, in various and unknown degrees, even in the more local, personal uses of imagery. In learning more about, and possibly influencing, one's own bodily and psychological circumstances, imagery may act *directly*, as well as through its conventionally understood mediating channels of neurological and immunological secretions and processes (Braud, 1986). The direct action of imagery may even be present in the familiar processes of volitional action, memory, perception, and so on.

A similar mix of local and nonlocal effects may be present in any and all diagnostic and healing interventions provided by health practitioners, and may, indeed, be an important component of the mysterious art of healing. The nonlocal working of imagery, in this fashion, may be a crucial aspect of such common phenomena as accurate and useful intuitions about a patient or client, the efficacy of therapeutic touch and similar techniques, quick and accurate diagnoses by physicians or therapists, physicians' bedside manners, the ways in which voiced (or unvoiced) prognoses fulfill themselves, effective nonspecific influences of medical or therapeutic interactions, spontaneous remissions, and placebo effects. If this is the case, then we could make greater use of our knowledge of the facilitators and inhibitors of transpersonal imagery in order to amplify any of the processes just mentioned, for the increased benefits of our patients, our clients, and ourselves.

The experiments summarized earlier in this chapter, along with many similar ones of other investigators, help us disentangle nonlocal from local aspects, and they provide indications of what is possible when the nonlocal aspect is acting alone. These experiments already have indicated that, even when acting in this "purer" form, the active and creative imagination—in its modes of imagery and intention—is able to provide accurate knowledge about, and influence, physical, physiological, and psychological circumstances that constitute or are related to health issues. For example, in our own work, we have found evidence for direct mental influences upon autonomic nervous system activity of distant persons, and upon rate of hemolysis of human red blood cells. In one study, we found that these remote mental influences were greater for persons who had a greater "need" to be influenced—i.e., for persons with overly active autonomic activity (Braud & Schlitz, 1983). In other experiments, persons were able to remotely help others focus their attention, helping them calm and focus their wandering thoughts—an outcome that could have well-being implications in the psychological realm. Although these are basic research studies, conducted in the laboratory, already they involve actual forms of healing. Other forms of direct, imagery-mediated, remote healing effects or healing analog effects have been well-documented elsewhere (Benor, 1993; Solvfin, 1984). So, we have both direct evidence of remote healing, as well as many more instances of influences that can indicate this possibility more indirectly and in an "in principle" form. Similar evidence—some direct, some indirect—exists for the reality of the diagnostic modes of these effects (Shealy & Myss, 1988).

The important next steps in these areas are to explore more thoroughly what may or may not be accomplished through transpersonal imagery. What are the ranges and limits of such effects? What else can we learn about the factors that make these effects more or less likely? Surely, there are spectra of magnitudes of effect, loci of action, and purposes for which these knowings and influences may occur. It would be unwise to overestimate what might be accomplished through these means, and it would be equally unwise to underestimate the power of imaginal, adjunctive techniques. Even small remote mental influences upon the more labile, more susceptible earliest stages or seed moments of illnesses or of health—in both physical and psychological areas—can become amplified and blossom into much larger, later outcomes with definite health relevance. Research in the area of chaos studies has shown that the later, very large-scale activities of certain animate and inanimate systems can be extraordinarily sensitive to very slight changes in initial conditions (Briggs & Peat, 1989; Gleick, 1987). The imaginal processes treated in this chapter may be capable of exerting comparably large, later effects through their initial, subtle influences in critical stages of the developmental processes of symptoms and syndromes—both physiological and psychological, both harmful and healthful. Specific examples of actual and hypothetical health applications, especially in the context of time-displaced, direct mental influences, have been described elsewhere (Braud, 2000).

Conventional physical and psychological techniques, including thoughts and preverbal forms of imagery, may be applied "locally"—i.e., within oneself—for harmful, as well as for healthful, purposes. The field of psychosomatic medicine is devoted largely to learning about and alleviating ways in which our thoughts, feelings, and images can foster illness. The incidence of iatrogenic illnesses and disorders illustrates how conventional techniques can be misused, when applied to others. Like conventional Era I and Era II techniques, it is likely that Era III nonlocal techniques might also be applied in ways that could be harmful, as well as healthful, to others. In considering potential practical applications of imagery-mediated direct mental influences, it would be unwise for us to ignore possible "negative" applications—be these intentional or unintentional. A survey of a range of actual and potential negative nonlocal influences has been provided by Larry Dossey (1997); it would be good for practitioners to be aware of these.

Perhaps the most important implication of this transpersonal imagery work is what might be termed *dyadic co-doing*. In any dyadic situation in which one person is helping another person change some aspect of mind or body—e.g., teacher-student, physician-patient, therapist-client, trainer-trainee dyads—if the "leader" in the dyad actively produces the desired physical and psychological changes in herself or himself, using active, creative imagination in the form of imagery and intentions, filling oneself in actuality and in imagination, with these desired qualities may directly facilitate similar desired changes in the "follower" in the dyad. These intention- and imagery-produced and mirrored changes may occur in addition to those accomplished in a more mediated fashion through teachings, instructions, exercises, or other conventional interventions. One may actualize a beneficial change or emphasis in another by realizing and embodying such a change in oneself, with the help of imagery, intention, and other forms of the active and creative imagination. Such dyadic co-doing effects are, undoubtedly, already occurring, spontaneously, in many dyadic situations in which the requisite facilitating conditions are present. These effects might be enhanced through deliberate and focused attention and intention.

At a more conceptual, theoretical level, the findings reviewed in this chapter have important implications for our understanding of the imagination. In unbroken traditions, going back to early Greek and Persian thinkers, there have been treatments of the imaginal or the imagination as a special and powerful human faculty with noetic and creative properties of its own (Avens, 1980; Corbin, 1972).

In these traditions, the active and creative imagination has been viewed as a bridge or intermediary between the sensory realm (of the body) and the intellectual realm (of the mind), between the conscious and the unconscious, between mind and matter, and between possibility and actuality. The imagery effects noted in this chapter are consistent with such a view. Increasing interest and recent developments in the areas of transpersonal psychology, consciousness studies, the efficacy of prayer, the role of spirituality in health, alternative medical and psychological interventions, and the new positive psychology movement within the American Psychological Association (Seligman & Csikszentmihalyi, 2000) all promise to cast new light on the nature and power of the imagination and of the imaginal realm.

The perceptive reader probably noticed a drift from the use of *imagery*, earlier in this chapter, to *imaginal* or *imagination* in later parts of the chapter. It is never clear whether the effects attributed to imagery are really due to the imagery, per se, or to the specific or generalized intentions that lie behind the images. Perhaps it is intention and focused attention that truly are responsible for both local and nonlocal "imagery" effects. Perhaps images are simply clothed intentions— specific intentions or focused attentions that have been dramatized or personified in imagery forms. *Imaginal* and *imagination* are more generic and can contain both images and the intentions and other mental processes that lie behind or are associated with imagery. A shift from imagery to imagination may serve us well as we continue to explore this realm wherein different possibilities emerge.

REFERENCES

Achterberg, J. (1985). *Imagery in healing: Shamanism and modern medicine* (p. 5). Boston: Shambhala/New Science Library.

Angoff, A., & Barth, D. (1974). *Parapsychology and anthropology*. New York: Parapsychology Foundation.

Avens, R. (1980). *Imagination is reality: Western nirvana in Jung, Hillman, Barfield, and Cassirer*. Irving, TX: Spring Publications.

Benor, D. J. (1993). *Healing research: Holistic medicine and spiritual healing*. Munich, Germany: Helix Verlag.

Boethius. (1980). *The consolation of philosophy* (V. E. Watts, Trans). New York: Penguin. (Original work written 524)

Bonaventure. (1953). *The mind's road to God* (G. Boas, Trans.). New York: Liberal Arts Press. (Original work written 1259)

Boorstein, S. (1990). Introduction. In S. Boorstein (Ed.), *Transpersonal psychotherapy* (pp. 1-5). Palo Alto, CA: Science & Behavior Books.

Bowra, C. M. (1961). *The romantic imagination*. New York: Galaxy/Oxford University Press.

Braud, W. G. (1975). Psi-conducive states. *Journal of Communication, 25*, 142-152.

Braud, W. G. (1978a). Allobiofeedback: Immediate feedback for a psychokinetic influence upon another person's physiology. In W. Roll (Ed.), *Research in parapsychology 1977* (pp. 123-134). Metuchen, NJ: Scarecrow Press.

Braud, W. G. (1978b). Psi conducive conditions: Explorations and interpretations. In B. Shapin & L. Coly (Eds.), *Psi and states of awareness* (pp. 1-41). New York: Parapsychology Foundation.

Braud, W. G. (1981). Lability and inertia in psychic functioning. In B. Shapin & L. Coly (Eds.), *Concepts and theories of parapsychology* (pp. 1-36). New York: Parapsychology Foundation.

Braud, W. G. (1985). ESP, PK, and sympathetic nervous system activity. *Parapsychology Review, 16*, 8-11.

Braud, W. G. (1986). PSI and PNI: Exploring the interface between parapsychology and psychoneuroimmunology. *Parapsychology Review, 17*(4), 1-5.

Braud, W. G. (1990). Distant mental influence of rate of hemolysis of human red blood cells. *Journal of the American Society for Psychical Research, 84*, 1-24.

Braud, W. G. (1991). Implications and applications of laboratory psi findings. *European Journal of Parapsychology, 8*, 57-65.

Braud, W. G. (1993). On the use of living target systems in distant mental influence research. In L. Coly & J. D. S. McMahon (Eds.), *Psi research methodology: A re-examination* (pp. 149-188). New York: Parapsychology Foundation.

Braud, W. G. (1999). Transcending the limits of time. *Inner Edge, 2*(6), 16-18.

Braud, W. G. (2000) Wellness implications of retroactive intentional influence: Exploring an outrageous hypothesis. *Alternative Therapies in Health and Medicine, 6*(1), 37-48.

Braud, W. G., & Jackson, J. (1983). Psi influence upon mental imagery. *Parapsychology Review, 14*, 13-15.

Braud, W. G., & Schlitz, M. (1989). A methodology for the objective study of transpersonal imagery. *Journal of Scientific Exploration, 3*, 43-63.

Braud, W. G., & Schlitz, M. J. (1983). Psychokinetic influence on electrodermal activity. *Journal of Parapsychology, 47*, 95-119.

Braud, W. G., & Schlitz, M. J. (1991). Consciousness interactions with remote biological systems: Anomalous intentionality effects. *Subtle Energies: An Interdisciplinary Journal of Energetic and Informational Interactions, 2*, 1-46.

Braud, W. G., Shafer, D., McNeill, K., & Guerra, V. (1995). Attention focusing facilitated through remote mental interaction. *Journal of the American Society for Psychical Research, 89*(2), 103-115.

Briggs, J., & Peat, F. D. (1989). *Turbulent mirror: An illustrated guide to chaos theory and the science of wholeness.* New York: Harper & Row.

Broughton, R. S. (1991). *Parapsychology: The controversial science.* New York: Ballantine.

Bruns, G. L. (1992). *Hermeneutics ancient and modern.* New Haven, CT: Yale University Press.

Burnshaw, S. (1970). *The seamless web.* New York: George Braziller.

Corbin, H. (1972). *Mundus imaginalis*, or the imaginary and the imaginal. *Spring*, 1-19.

Corbin, H. (1981). *Creative imagination in the Sûfism of Ibn 'Arabî* (R. Manheim, Trans.). Princeton, NJ: Princeton/Bollingen.

Dingwall, E. (Ed.). (1968). *Abnormal hypnotic phenomena* (4 vols.). London: Churchill.

Dossey, L. (1992). Era III medicine: The next frontier. *ReVision, 14*(3), 128-139.

Dossey, L. (1993). *Healing words: The power of prayer and the practice of medicine.* New York: HarperCollins.

Dossey, L. (1997). *Be careful what you pray for . . . you just might get it: What we can do about the unintentional effects of our thoughts, prayers, and wishes.* New York: HarperCollins.

Dossey, L. (1999). *Reinventing medicine.* New York: HarperCollins.

Edge, H. L., Morris, R. L., Rush, J. H., & Palmer, J. (1986). *Foundations of parapsychology.* New York: Routledge & Kegan Paul.

Ehrenwald, J. (1977). Parapsychology and the healing arts. In B. Wolman (Ed.), *Handbook of parapsychology* (pp. 541-556). New York: Van Nostrand Reinhold.

Gleick, J. (1987). *Chaos: Making a new science.* New York: Viking.

Gray, W. G. (1975). Patterns of Western magic. In C. T. Tart (Ed.), *Transpersonal psychologies* (pp. 431- 472). New York: Harper & Row.

Grof, S. (1972). Varieties of transpersonal experiences: Observations from LSD psychotherapy. *Journal of Transpersonal Psychology, 4*(1), 45-80.

Grof, S. (1973). Theoretical and empirical basis of transpersonal psychology and psychotherapy: Observations from LSD research. *Journal of Transpersonal Psychology, 5*(1), 15-53.

Hillman, J. (1976). *Re-visioning psychology.* New York: Harper & Row.

Hillman, J. (1995). *The thought of the heart and the soul of the world.* Woodstock, CT: Spring.

Hollenback, J. B. (1996). *Mysticism: Experience, response, and empowerment.* University Park, PA: Pennsylvania State University Press.

Honorton, C. (1974). Psi-conducive states of awareness. In E. Mitchell (J. White, Ed.), *Psychic exploration: A challenge for science* (pp. 616-638). New York: Putnam.

Honorton, C. (1977). Psi and internal attention states. In B. Wolman (Ed.), *Handbook of parapsychology* (pp. 435-472). New York: Van Nostrand Reinhold.

James, W. (1950). *The principles of psychology* (vol. 2, pp. 292-293). New York: Dover. (Original work published in 1890)

James, W. (1985). *The varieties of religious experience* (p. 508). New York: Penguin. (Original work published in 1902)

Jung, C. G. (1965). *Memories, dreams, reflections.* New York: Vintage.

Krippner, S. (Ed.). (1977-1982). *Advances in parapsychological research* (Vols. 1-3). New York: Plenum.

Krippner, S. (Ed.). (1984-1994). *Advances in parapsychological research* (Vols. 4-7). Jefferson, NC: McFarland and Company.

Kurtz, P. (Ed.). (1985). *A skeptic's handbook of parapsychology.* Buffalo, NY: Prometheus.

Long, J. (Ed.). (1977). *Extrasensory ecology: Parapsychology and anthropology.* Metuchen, NJ: Scarecrow Press.

McGinn, B. (1995). *The foundations of mysticism.* New York: Crossroad.

McGinn, B. (1996). *The growth of mysticism.* New York: Crossroad.

McGinn, B. (1998). *The flowering of mysticism.* New York: Crossroad.

Nasr, S. H. (1992). *Science and civilization in Islam.* New York: Barnes & Noble Books.

Persinger, M. (1989). Psi phenomena and temporal lobe activity: The geomagnetic factor. In L. Henkel & R. Berger (Eds.), *Research in parapsychology 1988* (pp. 121-156). Metuchen, NJ: Scarecrow Press.

Peters, L. (1989). Shamanism: Phenomenology of a spiritual discipline. *Journal of Transpersonal Psychology, 21*(2), 115-137.

Popper, K. R. (1979). *Objective knowledge.* Oxford: Clarendon.

Popper, K. R. (1982). *Unended quest.* Glasgow: Collins.

Popper, K. R., & Eccles, J. C. (1983). *The self and its brain.* London: Routledge & Kegan Paul.

Radin, D. (1997). *The conscious universe: The scientific truth of psychic phenomena.* New York: HarperCollins.

Regardie, I. (1974). *The philosopher's stone.* Saint Paul, MN: Llewellyn Publications.

Schlitz, M., & Braud, W. (1997). Distant intentionality and healing: Assessing the evidence. *Alternative Therapies in Health and Medicine, 3*(6), 62-73.

Schmeidler, G. R. (1988). *Parapsychology and psychology: Matches and mismatches.* Jefferson, NC: McFarland & Company.

Schneck, G. (1980). Three forms of knowledge. In *Visits to Sufi centers: Some recent research papers on Sufis and Sufism* (pp. 32-35). London: Society for Sufi Studies.

Schwartz, S., De Mattei, R. J., Brame, E. G., & Spottiswoode, S. J. P. (1990). Infrared spectra alteration in water proximate to the palms of therapeutic practitioners. *Subtle Energies, 1*(1), 43-72.

Schwarz, B. E. (1967). Possible telesomatic reactions. *Journal of the Medical Society of New Jersey, 64*(11), 600-603.

Sells, M. (1996). Bewildered tongue: The semantics of mystical union in Islam. In M. Idel & B. McGinn (Eds.), *Mystical union in Judaism, Christianity, and Islam* (pp. 87-124). New York: Continuum.

Seligman, M., & Csiksentimihalyi, M. (2000). Positive psychology: An introduction. *American Psychologist, 55*(1), 5-14.

Shah, I. (1964). *The Sufis.* Garden City, NY: Doubleday.

Shealy, C. N., & Myss, C. M. (1988). *The creation of health: Merging traditional medicine with intuitive diagnosis.* Walpole, NH: Stillpoint.

Solfvin, J. (1984). Mental healing. In S. Krippner (Ed.), *Advances in parapsychological research* (Vol. 4), pp. 31-63). Jefferson, NC: McFarland and Company.

Spottiswoode, J. (1990). Geomagnetic activity and anomalous cognition: A preliminary report of new evidence. *Subtle Energies, 1,* 91-102.

Spottiswoode, J. (1997). Apparent association between effect size in free response anomalous cognition experiments and local sidereal time. *Journal of Scientific Exploration, 11,* 109-122.

Stanford, R. G. (1974a). An experimentally testable model for spontaneous psi events. I. Extrasensory events. *Journal of the American Society for Psychical Research, 68,* 34-57.

Stanford, R. G. (1974b). An experimentally testable model for spontaneous psi events. II. Psychokinetic events. *Journal of the American Society for Psychical Research, 68,* 321-356.

Stanford, R. G. (1977). Conceptual frameworks of contemporary psi research. In B. Wolman (Ed.), *Handbook of parapsychology* (pp. 823-858). New York: Van Nostrand Reinhold.

Sutich, A. J. (1976). The emergence of the transpersonal orientation: A personal account. *Journal of Transpersonal Psychology, 8*(1), 5-19.

Van de Castle, R. (1977). Parapsychology and anthropology. In B. Wolman (Ed.), *Handbook of parapsychology* (pp. 667-686). New York: Van Nostrand Reinhold.

Vich, M. A. (1988). Some historical sources of the term "transpersonal." *Journal of Transpersonal Psychology, 20*(2), 107-110.

Walsh, R. (1989). What is a shaman? Definition, origin, and distribution. *Journal of Transpersonal Psychology, 21*(1), 1-11.

Walsh, R., & Vaughan, F. (1993). On transpersonal definitions. *Journal of Transpersonal Psychology, 25*(2), 199-207.

Wolman, B. (Ed.). (1977). *Handbook of parapsychology.* New York: Van Nostrand Reinhold.

Yates, F. A. (1964). *Giordano Bruno and the hermetic tradition.* London: Routledge & Kegan Paul.

Zollschan, G. K. (1989). Varieties of experienced "reality" as reverberations from four worlds. In G. K. Zollschan, J. F. Schumaker, & G. F. Walsh (Eds.), *Exploring the paranormal: Perspectives on belief and experiences* (pp. 48-76). Dorset: Prism.

CHAPTER 21

Death Imagery: Confronting Death Brings Us to the Threshold of Life[1]

ANEES A. SHEIKH AND KATHARINA S. SHEIKH

There is an old story that Plato, on his deathbed, was asked by a friend if he would summarize his great life's work, the *Dialogues*, in one statement. Plato, coming out of a reverie, looked at his friend and said, "Practice Dying." (Keleman, 1974, p. 1)

The enigma of death has invited a broad range of speculation, and reactions to death range from profound terror to ecstatic bliss. For instance, for Robert Browning, death is the "black minute"; for Soren Kierkegaard, it evokes the "fear of nothingness"; and for John White, it represents the "mortal terror of oblivion." Others view death more dispassionately: Hindus think of it as endless rebirth; Hans Christian Anderson calls it "the unwritten story"; and Rainer Maria Rilke describes it as the "side of life averted from us." Then there are those who embrace death enthusiastically: It is "welcome relief" to Socrates, the "ideal abode" to Plato, the "enlightenment" or the "supernatural brilliance" to Buddhists, the "touch of God's fingers" to Alfred Tennyson, "completeness" to Rabindranath Tagore, and the "just way" to James Riley (Blazer, 1978). In *The Prophet*, Kahlil Gibran describes death as deliverance from a shackled existence:

For what is it to die but to stand naked in the wind and to melt in the sun?
And what is it to cease breathing, but to free the breath from its restless tides,
    that it may rise and expand and seek God unencumbered?
Only when you drink from the river of silence shall you sing.
And when you reach the mountain top, then you shall begin to climb.
And when the earth shall claim your limbs, then shall you truly dance.
(Gibran, 1923, p. 81)

---

[1]We gratefully acknowledge Karen Beeuwsaert's help with some of the research for this chapter.

CONFRONTING DEATH: ONLY WHEN YOU DRINK
FROM THE RIVER OF SILENCE SHALL YOU SING

Generally, Western cultures have regarded death as an unpleasant reality, which is not an integral part of life, but exists outside of it or, at least, on its fringes. Death has been hidden from view or treated as another disease to be overcome (Aguilar & Wood, 1976; Braga & Braga, 1975; Paz, 1961). And yet since ancient times, death has been the main source of inspiration for philosophers, writers, artists, and composers. Michelangelo remarked, "No thought exists in me which death has not carved with his chisel," and Thomas Mann felt that "without death there would scarcely have been poets on earth" (Kübler-Ross, 1975, p. 2). In *Doctor Zhivago,* Boris Pasternak views virtually all human activity as an effort at coming to terms with death:

> Now what is history? It is the centuries of systematic explorations of the riddle of death, with a view to overcoming death. That's why people discover mathematical infinity and electromagnetic waves, that's why they write symphonies. . . . Man does not die in a ditch like a dog—but at home in history, while the work toward the conquest of death is in full swing; he dies sharing in this work. (1958, p. 10)

There is general agreement among world religions that a meaningful life is possible only after death has been accepted as a basic condition of life (Long, 1975). The goal is not simply to view death as the final act in life, but to welcome it as a persistent ingredient in the entire process of life. By recognizing the finiteness of one's existence, one is permeated by the urgency to cast off those extrinsic roles and to devote every day to growing as fully as possible (Levitan, 1985; Sheikh, Twente, & Turner, 1979).

Thus the acceptance of death brings one to the threshold of living authentically. This thought is a cornerstone of existential philosophy. Herman Feifel (1961, p. 71) says, "Life is not genuinely our own until we renounce it." Rollo May maintains, "With the confronting of non-being, existence takes on vitality and immediacy, and the individual experiences a heightened consciousness of himself and his world, and others around him" (May, 1958, p. 47). Irvin Yalom (1980, p. 163) feels that "by keeping death in mind one passes into a state of gratitude for the countless givens of existence." Santayana (see Yalom, 1980, p. 163) remarks, "The dark background which death supplies, brings out the tender colors of life in all their purity," and Nietzsche (1974, p. 37) states:

> Out of such abysses, from such severe sicknesses, one returns newborn . . . with a more delicate taste for joy, with a more tender tongue for all good things, with merrier senses, with a second dangerous innocence in joy.

Literature is replete with examples of individuals who underwent extensive personal transformation due to their close brush with death. Max Frisch's (1957) Faber in *Homo Faber,* Tolstoy's Pierre in *War and Peace,* and Ivan Ilyich in the

Death of Ivan Ilyich are obvious examples. Another striking and well-known illustration is the repentant Ebenezer Scrooge. We may forget that his cold heart was not melted simply by the warmth of the Christmas Spirit—to that it had proven itself totally impervious. What transformed Scrooge was the encounter with his own death. The Ghost of Christmas Yet to Come used a potent form of death imagery therapy: Scrooge had the opportunity to witness his own death, to overhear acquaintances dismiss lightly his passing, and to observe strangers quarreling over his worldly possessions. Then Scrooge attended his own funeral, and, finally, in the last scene preceding his transformation, he examined the inscription on his tombstone (Yalom, 1980).

DEATH IMAGERY: AN OVERVIEW OF ANCIENT AND MODERN APPROACHES

It has become apparent that many thinkers agree that learning to die is a prerequisite to living meaningfully. While the time when death is imminent can be a fertile period of personal growth, we should not and must not wait until then to learn the lessons of death. For centuries, and in several cultures, variations of the experience of death in imagination have been effectively used. These death imagery techniques provide the opportunity to confront death and to come to terms with it. This section reviews a number of such approaches.

Death Imagery in Ancient Initiatory Experiences

As Metzner (1986) points out, death-rebirth fantasy and associated ritual practices have been an essential component of initiatory experiences in several traditional cultures. For example, the training of shaman-healers involved sloughing off all old attachments and old ways of living. "Sometimes the older shaman, while instructing the apprentice, would symbolically 'kill' the apprentice. This was then followed by a restoration or reconstitution . . . into a new more power-filled form, endowed with healing and magical abilities" (Metzner, 1986, p. 146). This aspect of shamanic training is very similar to the process of *mortificatio* in alchemy which has a literal meaning of "killing" or "dead-making." *Mortificatio* involved conscious and intentional attempts to reduce ego attachments through symbolic meditations and visualization that stressed "darkness, defeat, torture, mutilation, death and rotting," followed by positive images of "growth, rejuvenation, fruiting, ripening, and rebirth" (Metzner, 1986, p. 146).

Death-rebirth imagery and rituals are also very common in the initiation rites of numerous tribes around the world. Neale (1969, pp. 169-170) describes one such initiation ritual:

> After the older men have prepared a sacred place in the bush, the mother brings her son to the edge of the village. She does not know the content of the rites. She has heard only rumors about death and manhood. She does know

that occasionally a child fails to return. The little boy knows the same. Both are filled with excitement and pride, but also with great anxiety. The men rush forward and force the boy away from his mother. She weeps and wails over the forthcoming death of her son. He is taken to a hut where he lies down on his back with his arms crossed over his chest. He is covered with a rug and told not to utter a sound. During the coming days, he may be symbolically burned by a fire, buried in a shallow pit, be ritually dismembered, or have a tooth knocked out. All these things—the separation from his mother, the darkness, and the physical dangers—are symbolic experiences of death. The boy is told that the gods are killing him. He does not know for sure whether he will literally survive or not. By means of this first half of the puberty ritual, the world of the child and his personality are destroyed.

The second half of the ritual takes place over an extended period of time. The boy meets his god and receives his name. After this he may have to be fed by a guardian for as much as six months, for newborn infants cannot feed themselves without help. During this time he is instructed and trained to meditate on his experiences. By story, dance, and pantomime, he is introduced to the gods, the history of the tribe, and to the way he is to live. Finally, the boy is returned to the community to take his place as a new person in a new world. The boy and his mother may not acknowledge each other for some time to come. After all, her son has died, it is a strange adult who returned to the village. In the spiritual sense, the boy does not know his mother. His old world and old self have been destroyed. Death has led to rebirth and a new creation.

Buddhist Meditation on Death

This type of meditation is very commonly used by Buddhist monks. The monk sits down in the graveyard or crematorium and reflects upon the corpses or ashes, and he even imagines his own body to be among these remains. This exercise renders him more profoundly aware of the brevity and uncertainty of life and the inevitability of death. He realizes that human beings and their objects of pleasure do not endure for long. This insight prompts him to abandon all ambition to shape the world in accordance with his wishes. "And, with the passing of the habit of living a life of willfulness (and its offspring, anxiety and fear) will come automatically a peace of mind and tranquility which will abide unaltered in all conditions of life and all states of mind" (Long, 1975, p. 69).

Many Buddhist teachings concerning death are contained in *The Tibetan Book of the Dead*. It presents not only the most effective method of "living toward death," but also contains instructions on how to die well (Evans-Wentz, 1960). The dying person is advised to remain calm and alert in the face of death and to shun distraction and confusion. He/she is reminded too that his/her life-forces are about to disengage themselves from the body and that he/she should focus upon this event. He/she is then prepared for the meeting with death by its description: death is the "brilliant light of Ultimate Reality" or "the luminous splendor of the colorless light of Emptiness." The moribund should immerse himself/herself in that supernatural brilliance, sloughing off all belief in an individual self and realizing that the "boundless light of this true Reality" is his/her own true self (Evans-Wentz, 1960; Long, 1975; Rahula, 1959; Robinson, 1970).

Sufi Contemplation upon Death

The Sufis, in keeping with the Prophet Mohammed's advice, "Die before you are dead," have given great importance to the contemplation of death. They reflect upon the inevitable future decay and disintegration of all living beings, and upon the fact that their own bodies soon will be nothing but rotten flesh and dry bones upon which worms will feed. Thus they achieve the awareness of the impermanence of temporal life. For the Sufis, this meditation on death is a vital step toward beatitude—the ultimate goal of all spiritual striving. Death represents the dismemberment of the present imperfect state, which then renders possible the rebirth of a personality with spiritually healthy and stable traits.

The devastation of winter makes way for the renewal of spring. Similarly the old self must die before it can be reborn. After longings for material riches and bodily pleasures, ambivalence toward others and, above all, egoism are seen in the correct light and abandoned, rebirth is bound to occur (Ajmal, 1979, 1989).

As Andrew Harvey (1994) writes, "Our life is constantly tempting us to identify ourselves with it. Everytime we identify ourselves with it, we fall prey to the illusion of separation from other people, we fall prey to the illusion of time and the illusion that we are dying. It is only by dying to that illusion that we can enter reality" (p. 291). He urges, "Transfigure this life into a slaughterhouse of the ego. Burn away the false self and radiate . . . love, knowledge, bliss, and joy to everyone. When you *are*, you will never die, because there is only *Being*" (p. 295).

Practicing Death

In the *Republic,* Plato maintains that there are four stages of cognitive development: 1) during the first stage one perceives only shadows and other superficial or insubstantial things; 2) the second stage is marked by the perception of the reality of physical objects; 3) the third stage is characterized by the capacity for abstract mathematics and deductive reasoning; 4) the fourth stage involves the experience of the forms, the eternal archetypes or potentials, that structure all thought and perception. Plato argues that these forms are truly known only by the experience of the highest level of reality, after all physical and mental activity ceases. In the dialogues, such as *Phaedo, Meno, Theaetetus,* and *Phaedrus,* he equates "true knowledge, knowledge of the Forms, with knowledge of the world experienceable 'after death'" (Shear, 1978). In *Phaedo,* he states unequivocally that the philosopher's true method, the method of gaining knowledge of the Forms, consists of practicing death, that is, giving the soul the opportunity to become accustomed "to withdraw from all contact with the body and concentrate itself by itself . . . alone by itself" (*Collected Dialogues of Plato*, edited by Hamilton & Cairns, 1973).

Koestenbaum's Exercises

Koestenbaum (1976) describes several death and immortality exercises which he feels are very effective. Some he has developed and others he has taken from Herman Feifel and Robert Kastenbaum. One exercise consists of composing your own obituary. This act leads you to face the crucial question of what it means to be a human being, and what is involved in passing the time on earth well, and most importantly, what it means to be *you*. Other exercises described by Koestenbaum are: 1) imaging that you are attending your own funeral and overhearing a friend speak frankly about the significance of your life; 2) experiencing a rebirth fantasy; 3) writing a script for your own death, describing *how, when,* and *where* it took place; 4) reading a vivid and moving account of the death of a 6-year-old abandoned child and, subsequently, completing seven sentences. Koestenbaum maintains that these exercises help to courageously face the reality of your own death and thus to make crucial discoveries.

Koestenbaum (1976) also presents an immortality exercise which has the form of a guided daydream or fantasy. First, he asks the subject to imagine that he/she is a dying patient in the hospital. Then he presents a sequence of thoughts that occur immediately before death. He tells the individual that all worldly things are receding into a meaningless distance, and that he/she now feels more "like a god in outer space observing life than a human being participating in the affairs of the world" (p. 189). Suggestions of this nature are followed by induced images in which the person accepts death, feels at peace, experiences himself/herself as a part of the universal scheme, and has a sense of the eternal nature of consciousness. Koestenbaum claims that this exercise can lead to a premonition of the experience of immortality. "The key dynamism bringing about this realization is relinquishing the sense of being an individual" (p. 189).

Stephen Levine's Work on Conscious Living and Conscious Dying

Levine's work (1972, 1979, 1984, 1989) shows that it is only by opening to the reality of death that one can make living a conscious process of growth. His books "demonstrate a remarkable ability to articulate for Western audiences the value of meditation practice in confronting and accepting death. From the point of view of Eastern psychology, particularly Buddhist psychology, real acceptance and understanding of death, illness, and suffering must move beyond mere intellectual speculation and abstraction. Experience is the only teacher. Openness to the fullness of experience is developed through the consistent practice of meditation" (Kruck & Sheikh, 1991, p. 46). Levine offers a series of excellent imagery-based meditational/experiential exercises toward this end. These include:

Letting the mind float in the heart, losing self-image, self-forgiveness and forgiving others, loving kindness, grief meditation, pain and healing meditation, meditation on heavy emotions, meditation on death and dying, moment of death meditation, and *after death meditation.* "Regardless of an individual's theoretical or theological background, Levine provides an outline for rethinking the presuppositions upon which our attitudes toward death and dying are based" (Kruck & Sheikh, 1991, p.66). He presents an alternative approach that rests on the idea that life and death are complementary dimensions of a single integrated process. For a detailed discussion of his techniques the reader is referred to other sources (Levine, 1972, 1979, 1984, 1989; Kruck & Sheikh, 1991).

Grieving Through Imagery

In our society, the grief-stricken often are discouraged from facing the reality of death by relatives and friends who take over for them and invite them to be mere observers. Consequently, it becomes difficult for the bereaved to come to grips with the death of their loved ones (Nichols & Nichols, 1975). Recently several clinicians have suggested imagery techniques that, in combination with other therapeutic interventions, reconstruct death-related events, and thus facilitate the grieving process (Aguilar & Wood, 1976; Droege, 1987; Melges, 1982; Melges & DeMaso, 1980; Morrison, 1978; Ramsay & Noorbergen, 1981; Volkan, 1975; Williamson, 1978). Melges and DeMaso (1980), for example, believe that unresolved grief reactions generally persist due to the obstacles that inhibited the grieving process at the time of the loss. When the bereaved is given an opportunity to relive, revise, and revisit scenes of the loss in present-time imagery, and thus remove these obstacles, grief resolution is facilitated. Following is a case history provided by Melges and DeMaso (1980, p. 58).

> A 27-year-old, married mother of two children, became acutely incapacitated with an uncanny fear of death when, shortly after her husband's grandmother died, she revisited the same cemetery where her stepfather was buried three years previously. She had idealized her stepfather as being a "perfect man." During the re-grief therapy, when she was reliving seeing her stepfather's body in the funeral home, she became aware of her anger toward him for having sexually played with her as a girl but she could not express this anger in the relived-remembered scene because her mother, from whom they had kept the secret, was there at the funeral home. The therapist asked her to revise the scene, removing the mother along with all other people, and encouraged her to express her anger and feelings. With the scene thus revised, she gave full vent to her anger and her guilt for having to carry this secret for so long. After that, she felt free to express her love for him, which she had refused to do during his terminal illness. She also acknowledged her complicity in the sexual activities, and then forgave him and subsequently felt he understood and forgave her for not caring for him during his terminal illness. With her guilt and anger dismantled, she felt immediately relieved, no longer "haunted" by the death phobia.

Although techniques such as those described by Melges and DeMaso are not concerned directly with the issue of one's own death, they nevertheless are bound to lead one to confront it. Morrison (1991) offers a note of caution that "imagery techniques may not be appropriate for those therapists who have not carefully analyzed their own imagery" and that therapists "should be aware that directed imagery can occasionally provoke traumatic emotional reactions in clients, and they must be ready for them" (pp. 90-91).

Death Imagery Technique

In an article published in 1979, Sheikh, Twente, and Turner report death imagery techniques that they developed. One can use these procedures to attain mere relaxation, or relaxation may be considered as only the first step in therapy. For relaxation purposes, the subject is asked to take a few deep breaths and lie down. Then he/she is given the following instructions:

> Imagine that you are dead. You have lost all your ability to counter the force of gravity and are completely immobilized and inactive. All your muscles, even all your body cells are pulled down by gravity. You no longer have to struggle, be tense, and spend energy to stay alive. You no longer have to direct your thinking or censor your thoughts. The thoughts come and go as they like. As your "dead" body is pulled more and more by the force of gravity, you have a feeling that you are shedding off your body. Your thoughts scatter and all the verbal chatter and commotion vanish into thin air. As you shed your body, you become a weightless, bodiless, pure consciousness. There is stillness and quiet and a benign indifference of nature. (Sheikh et al., 1979, p. 154)

Often the subject initially experiences some anxiety; however, this soon gives way to feelings of deep relaxation and a sense of being at peace with the world. During this relaxed state, long forgotten memories, particularly of unfinished issues pertaining to parents, often surface spontaneously. They provide significant material for meaningful therapy. For continuing therapy, specific imagery procedures have been developed. These include: 1) visualizing, confronting, and finally saying farewell to all those individuals, alive or dead, with whom the subject had significant emotional contact; 2) visualizing himself/herself as an infant, as a child, as an adolescent, and as he/she is now, and saying goodbye to all these aspects of development; 3) finishing in imagery, the unfinished tasks that arise in associated memories. After the completion of the unfinished business and the farewell process, the subject is directed to experience a departure from his/her body.

Hypnotic Death and Suicide Rehearsal

Levitan (1985) developed a hypnotic death rehearsal technique initially to help patients faced with imminent death. However, since then he has been using it to assist clients with concerns about the death and dying process. It is very similar to the death imagery technique discussed above but differs in the sense that "the therapist is continually involved in reframing and interpreting the visualized images reported by the subject. The principal objective of this hypnotic death rehearsal is to demystify the death experience and allow the patient to approach it with familiarity and confidence" (Levitan, 1991, p. 96). A variation of this, the hypnotic suicide rehearsal, aims at focusing "subjects to critically evaluate the consequences of death by suicide and hopefully eliminate magical thinking in this regard" (p. 96). For further details of these techniques, the reader is referred to other sources (Levitan, 1985, 1991).

Perinatal Experiences and Holotropic Therapy

Grof and Halifax (1977) provide a description of experiences related to the events immediately preceding, accompanying, and following birth that their subjects had during psychotherapy under the influence of LSD. They term these as perinatal experiences. These experiences largely pertain to the problems of biological birth, physical pain, suffering, disease, agony, aging, and death. The encounter with suffering and agony, Grof and Halifax state, ends in an experience of complete annihilation on all levels, including physical, emotional, intellectual, moral, and transcendental.

> This is usually referred to as an "ego death": it seems to involve instantaneous destruction of all the previous reference points of the individual. The experience of total annihilation is often followed by a vision of blinding white or golden light and a sense of liberating decompression and expansion. The universe is perceived as indescribably beautiful and radiant; individuals feel cleansed and purged, and talk about redemption, salvation, or union with God. (Grof & Halifax, 1977, p. 51)

Grof and Halifax (1977) claim that people return from the perinatal experience with the confidence that they have "confronted the ultimate crisis" and achieved deep understanding into the nature of death and dying. They "discover the importance of accepting, surrendering, and relinquishing" (p. 52). Despite its intimate connection with the experience of biological birth, Grof (1985) emphasizes that "the perinatal process transcends biology and has important psychological and spiritual dimensions. It should not therefore be interpreted in a concretistic and reductionistic fashion" (p. 100).

Recently Stanislav Grof and Christine Grof have developed a procedure called holotropic therapy or holonomic integration that they claim achieves the same goals without the use of drugs. Holotropic therapy consists of a combination of intense breathing, music, and focused body work. Further details of this procedure are available elsewhere (Grof, 1985).

Other Related Techniques

Yalom (1980) reviews a number of, what he calls, "artificial aids" to counteract the individual's persistent denial of death.

(1) *The Line of Life*. In this simple yet profound exercise the subject is asked to draw a straight line on a blank sheet of paper. One end of this straight line represents his/her birth and the other his/her death. Then the subject is asked to draw a cross on the line to indicate the point where he/she is now and then to meditate upon this for a brief period.

(2) *Calling Out*. This technique is employed with large groups who are then divided into smaller groups. "Each individual's name is written on a slip of paper, placed in a bowl, and then randomly chosen and called aloud. An individual whose name is called stops talking and turns his back to the others" (Yalom, 1980, p. 174). Yalom reports that this exercise has helped many individuals enhance their awareness of the precarious nature of existence.

(3) *Life Cycle Group*. This procedure was used by Elliot Aronson and Ann Dreyfus at the National Training Laboratory summer program at Bethel, Maine. In this program, the participants focused on main issues in each developmental stage.

> In the time devoted to old age and death, these participants spent days living like old people. They were instructed to walk old, to dress old, to powder their hair and attempt to play elderly people they have known well. They visited a local cemetery. They walked alone in a forest, imagined passing out, dying, being discovered by friends, and being buried. (Yalom, 1980, p. 175)

(4) *Death Awareness Workshops*. A number of workshops have focused on the issue of encountering one's death. Yalom reports one which was conducted by W.M. Whelan. It consisted of one 8-hour 8-member group session in which:

> (1) Members complete a death anxiety questionnaire and discuss anxiety-provoking items, (2) Members, in a state of deep relaxation, fantasize in great detail, with awareness of all five senses, their own (comfortable) death, (3) Members are asked to construct a list of their values and then asked to imagine a situation in which a life-saving nuclear fallout shelter is able to save only a limited number of people: each member has to make an argument, on the basis of his or her value hierarchy, why he or she should be saved, (4) Again in a state of deep muscle relaxation, the members are asked to fantasize their own terminal illness, their inability to communicate, and, finally, their own funerals. (Yalom, 1980, p. 175)

(5) *Interaction with the Dying*. Yalom (1980) reports that in group sessions, patients suffering from catastrophic illness often display much affect and wisdom. In order to expose the everyday psychotherapy clients to the wisdom of the dying, Yalom, at times, invited the former to observe group sessions of the latter, or he introduced a seriously ill patient into the group psychotherapy sessions of regular patients. Yalom describes several salutary effects of these interventions.

Yalom suggests that if we as psychotherapists accept the notion that the awareness of our death can be the catalyst for personal change, then we should attempt to use all opportunities to facilitate this process. In addition to providing the structured exercises, we should help clients recognize the reminders of the fragility of life that surround us, such as, birthdays, anniversaries, children leaving for college, serious illness, and the death of loved ones. Since most of these experiences are painful, we as therapists can easily make the mistake of focusing primarily on the alleviation of pain and miss this opportunity to nudge the patient along on the quest for wisdom and peace (Yalom, 1980).

POSSIBLE BENEFITS OF DEATH IMAGERY WORK

Whether one examines the death imagery experiences of the shamans, the near-death experiences reported by Moody (1975), Ring (1980, 1984), and others (Metzner, 1986), the perinatal experiences under the influence of LSD (Grof & Halifax, 1977), or the recent death imagery work by clinicians, they all appear to be overwhelmingly health giving and life transforming. The benefits mentioned in the literature range anywhere from deep relaxation to metaphysical awakening. This section briefly surveys a number of beneficial effects of death imagery.

Deep Relaxation

It has been reported that dying in imagination often turns out to be a deeply relaxing experience (Sheikh, Twente, & Turner, 1979). In the beginning, subjects might experience increased anxiety, particularly those who find even the mention of death threatening. This reaction, however, tends to give way to a feeling of deep relaxation: a fully conscious, dreamlike state which is profoundly soothing at both the physical and mental level. Preliminary laboratory work indicates a slowing down of the heartbeat, flattening of the galvanic skin response, and escaping of trapped air from the body. During death imagery, spontaneous remission of some minor psychosomatic symptoms has been noted, and George Twente (1979) has encountered cases of defecation and sexual orgasm. All of these changes can be considered as objective indicators of a deeply relaxed state of mind and body. At times, the relaxed state produced by death imagery verges on the religious. Koestenbaum (1976) describes it thus:

I felt suddenly and inexplicably that the burden and weight of living had been lifted. I felt supported. The burden of living was no longer mine alone. I sensed a current stronger than me and one in which I am only a part and which supports me as the sea supports a ship. . . . At that brief moment it became intuitively clear to me that the religious position that there is a God, that I can participate in His life, and that I am not really different from God but a part of Him, made sense. I felt that my body was supported by nature, so my individual awareness was supported by a cosmic consciousness. . . . Did I at that moment lose my freedom? No, but I did lose the sense that I was a capillary cut off from the universal bloodstream. I had a sense of continuity with all of Being, rather than the sense of separation and alienation. (pp. 117-118)

Finishing the Unfinished Business

As one gives in to death imagery and enters a relaxed state, unresolved situations from the past as well as from the current scene often make their appearance spontaneously and almost beg to be reexperienced and resolved. This unfinished emotional business more often than not relates to one's parents and potentially can be resolved through continued image therapy. One kind of unfinished situation that often emerges during death imagery is unresolved grief. At times spontaneous regrieving in imagery clears the air. In other cases, the therapist may have to intervene and manipulate certain images (see Dr. Morrison's chapter in this book).

Out-of-Body Experience

Some subjects experience a pleasurable and profoundly relaxing feeling of shedding their body. The reports include feelings of well-being, of vitality, of the freedom which perhaps a bird experiences when it is let out of its cage, and feelings of ecstasy. For example, one subject reported that she became lighter and lighter and finally floated away from her body. Suddenly she was adrift in a quiet world of blue-white light. Initially, her body tugged at her and tried to bring her back, but she did not want to come back, for she sensed that out there lay peace. In the beginning, as she floated, she had the shape of a ball, but as she traveled she began to expand and assume new shapes. Suddenly, she separated into a million little particles, mixing with the light and energy and feeling very exhilarated. As she moved farther and farther away from earthly existence, time became meaningless and a feeling of peace engulfed her. The after-effects of this experience were very positive. The subject reported that all her senses became very acute, that she felt spiritually revived and totally at peace with her life (Sheikh et al., 1979).

It should be noted that we have no reason to believe that these out-of-body experiences are an indication of *actual* projection of the psychic self which enables the person to perceive events in a far-off location. But subjects do feel that they are doing so.

Ehrenfeld (1974) speculates that out-of-body feelings occur because of the need to believe that consciousness survives death. Palmer (1978) remarks: "Because of our religious upbringing (whether we accept it intellectually or not) death means possibility, or at least the hope that our soul is real and will leave the body to carry on in another state. Therefore, a psychological set favoring out-of-body experiences is present in this 'real-life' situation" (see Neher, 1980, p. 194).

Arguments and speculations aside, the fact remains that a large number of people are capable of having profound experiences of this type and that they find them exhilarating and deeply therapeutic. It would be worthwhile to conduct systematic research aimed at mapping the various parameters of such experiences and discovering their correlates, antecedents, and consequences.

Here and Now: Importance of the Moment

As someone once remarked, "If the stars came out only once in a lifetime, all of us would be out to see them and would be left speechless by the grandeur of that sight . . . but when they shine every night we go for months without ever looking up" (Adams, Otto, & Cowley, 1984, p. 131).

We often live in anticipation of tomorrow or in reminiscence of yesterday, and meanwhile each day is lost. Martin Buber spoke about "infusing the routines of everyday life with the breath of eternity." He conveyed a sense of the breadth and depth that could be ours if we would give up the preoccupation with the past and develop the skill of sensing fully all that is available to us at any moment (Adams, Otto, & Cowley, 1984, p. 131).

Alan Watts (1968, 1972) remarked that people who constantly are searching for health, beauty, and fulfillment fail to grasp that they already exist on an intriguing globe floating in a fascinating universe. We have been told by numerous traditions, that facing the inevitability of death can lead to the realization that the meaning of life is close at hand. It can foster a new appreciation for the value of time and the beauty and sanctity of life (Barrett, 1988; Butler, 1963; Cumming & Henry, 1961; Sheikh et al., 1979). Dostoevski writes in *The Idiot:*

> This man had once been led out with the others to the scaffold and a sentence of death was read over him. . . . Twenty minutes later a reprieve was read to them, and they were condemned to another punishment instead. Yet the interval between those two sentences, twenty minutes or at least a quarter of an hour, he passed in fullest conviction that he would die in a few minutes. . . . The priest went to each in turn with a cross. He had only five minutes more to live. He told that those five minutes seemed to him an infinite time, a vast wealth . . . "What if I were not to die? What if I could go back to life—what eternity! And it would all be mine! I would turn every minute into an age; I would lose nothing, I would count every minute as it passed. I would not waste one." (quoted in Barrett, 1962, p. 140)

Death and Creativity

Being aware and open to the reality of death appears to be linked to all that we value in human experience, including love and creativity. With regard to creativity, Rollo May wrote:

> Creativity is a yearning for immortality. We know that each of us must develop the courage to confront death. Yet we also must rebel and struggle

against it. Creativity comes from this struggle—out of the rebellion the creative act is born. (May, 1975, pp. 31-32)

Studies by Goodman (1975) suggest that the fear of death and creativity are significantly related. Creative individuals appear to be able to overcome their fear of death by viewing life in terms of 100-to1000-year perspectives. On the other hand, those who see life in terms of 2-to10-year perspectives demonstrate greater concern about death.

The intricate connection between death and creativity is also confirmed by the frequent manifestation of previously dormant creative talents in individuals who narrowly escaped death. Such people undergo the profound experience of rebirth: they now reassess the meaning of life and often struggle to express creative energies which lay buried. The patient who gained a reprieve from death may channel all energy into writing some wonderful verses or working out a new scientific theory (Garai, 1988).

Death and Love

The close relationship between death and love is clear on many levels. Perhaps the most dramatic illustrations are found in the reproductive cycle of some animals. The male bee dies after he has inseminated the queen. The female praying mantis bites off the male's head as he copulates, and as soon as she is inseminated, she eats the male to provide nourishment for the young.

In literature, death and love have always been inseparable. Italian writers commonly play upon the words *amore* (love) and *morte* (death). Mythologies of various cultures portray the sex act as death and rebirth; for, the ability for surrendering one's self must precede the spontaneity of orgasm (May, 1968).

On the psychological plane, passionate love is inevitably accompanied by the spectre of death. The lover must grapple with the painful possibilities of the death of the relationship, the death of the beloved, his/her own death, and the death of the offspring. Love heightens the lover's vulnerability and sense of mortality, but the realization of the precarious nature of life also leads to increased reverence for life and more genuine living. As Stephen Levine (1982, p. 99) observes:

> If our only spiritual practice were to live as though we were already dead, relating to all we meet, to all we do, as though it were our own final moments in the world, what time would there be for false games or falsehoods or posturing . . . Only love would be appropriate, only the truth.

Essence versus Accessory Attributes

Perls visualized the accessory attributes as an edifice constructed of four layers. The first two layers consist of the role-playing which we have found useful in everyday life—to please others and to motivate them to support us. Many live out their lives without ever penetrating beyond these outer layers. The third layer envelops the sense of emptiness—the very feeling most people like to keep at a distance with frantic everyday routines. The fourth layer is one which is most difficult to penetrate—it consists of our terror of dying which is an inescapable and everpresent undercurrent. Only after we have grappled with this condition can we proceed to the center of this edifice and recognize our authentic self (Becker, 1973).

Awareness of death through imagery can spontaneously lead us to sift our essence from accessory attributes. This process has been termed *disidentification*. Assagioli (1965) attempted to help his clients reach their core of pure consciousness by encouraging them to imagine shedding their bodies, emotions, desires, and eventually their intellect.

Yalom employs a structured disidentification exercise which takes only about 30 to 45 minutes. In a quiet setting, Yalom asks the participants to list, on separate cards, eight important responses to the question "Who am I?" He then asks them to arrange the cards in order of importance, placing the cards which come closest to expressing their essence at the bottom. Next, Yalom asks the participants to meditate on what it would be like to give up the attribute described on the top card. After 2 to 3 minutes, he asks them to proceed to the next card and so forth, until they have shed all eight attributes (Yalom, 1980). Yalom feels that disidentification is an effective mechanism of change. The awareness of death brings about a shift in perspective from which the person can easily distinguish between core and accessory attributes.

Along the same vein, Metzner (1986) has found that self-knowledge is the ultimate reward bestowed on those who confront their own death. The self that the individual had thought he/she was, dies; and the true self emerges into prominence. All ego concerns and petty interests dissolve into insignificance in the light of the real self, which is nothing less than a spark from the eternal source of life.

Other Possible Effects

Several other beneficial effects of confrontation with death have been reported in the literature. These include: 1) a change of attitude toward dying, including a loss of fear; 2) belief in the survival of consciousness after biological death; 3) diminished earthly ambitions; 4) increased reverence for life; 5) stimulated interest in philosophy, religion, and mysticism; and 6) an altered perception of time.

CONCLUDING REMARKS

Throughout the ages, all major spiritual and philosophic traditions have stressed the importance of dealing with death; and, as the preceding pages indicate, recently a number of other lines of inquiry have reaffirmed this view. There appears to be general agreement across subjects and across approaches, concerning the consequences of a confrontation with death. They are reported to be overwhelmingly positive and can even be self-transcending and life-transforming. This emerging consensus invites us to speculate that perhaps "we all harbor functional matrices in our unconscious mind that contain an authentic encounter with death . . . human beings not only know intellectually that they will die, they also possess subliminal knowledge of what it feels like to experience death" (Grof & Halifax, 1977, p. 9).

Recent attempts to induce the experience of death and rebirth through imagery-related approaches under relatively controlled conditions are expected to lead to a deeper understanding of the process of death and the consequences of confronting it. Without a doubt, the study of the death experience is of crucial importance in the understanding of psychological processes. No genuine comprehension of religion, mysticism, or mythology is possible without intimate knowledge of the death experience (Grof, 1985; Grof & Halifax, 1977). A profound symbolic confrontation with death can contribute to better emotional and psychological functioning and a satisfying adjustment to life. Feifel maintains that "only by integrating the concept of death into the self does an authentic and genuine existence become possible" (1961, p. 65).

In short, embracing the inevitability of death is a prerequisite for personal evolution, and in broader terms, it is death which makes cosmic evolution possible. As the 13th century Persian poet-philosopher Rumi says:

> I died a mineral, and became a plant.
> I died a plant, and rose an animal.
> I died an animal and I was a man.
> Why should I fear? When was I less by dying? (Nicholson, 1978, p. 103)

REFERENCES

Adams, R. S., Otto, H. A., & Cowley, A. S. (1984). *Letting go: Uncomplicating your life.* New York: Science and Behavior Books.

Aguilar, I., & Wood, V. N. (1976). Therapy through death ritual. *Social Work,* January, 49-54.

Ajmal, M. (1979). *Sufi contemplation upon death.* Unpublished paper. National Institute of Psychology, Islamabad, Pakistan.

Ajamal, M. (1989). *Death imagery in Sufism.* Unpublished manuscript. National Institute of Psychology, Islamabad, Pakistan.

Assagioli, R. (1965). *Psychosynthesis: A collection of basic writings.* New York: Viking.

Barrett, W. (1962). *Irrational man.* New York: Anchor Books.

Barrett, D. (1988). Dreams of death. *Omega, 19*(2), 95-101.

Becker, E. (1973). *The denial of death.* New York: Free Press, A Division of Macmillan.

Blazer, J. A. (1978). The concept of death as a factor in mental health. *Psychology, 15* (1), 68-77.

Braga, J. L., & Braga, L. D. (1975). Foreword. In E. Kübler-Ross (Ed.), *Death: The final stage of growth*. New Jersey: Prentice Hall.

Butler, R. N. (1963). The life review: An interpretation of reminiscence in the aged. *Psychiatry, 119,* 721-728.

Cumming, E., & Henry, W. E. (1961). *Growing old.* Illinois: Free Press.

Droege, T. (1987). *Guided grief imagery: A resource for grief ministry and death education.* New York: Panlist Press.

Ehrenfeld, J. (1974). Out-of-the-body experience and the denial of death. *Journal of Nervous and Mental Disease, 159,* 227-233.

Evans-Wentz, W. Y. (1960). *The Tibetan book of the dead.* New York: Oxford Universities Press.

Feifel, H. (1961). Attitudes toward death: A psychological perspective. In R. May (Ed.), *Existential psychology.* New York: Random House.

Frisch, V. M. (1957). *Homo Faber.* Frankfurt: Suhrkamp Verlag.

Garai, J. (1988). *Birth, death, and rebirth as archetypes of the creative experience.* Unpublished manuscript.

Gibran, K. (1923). *The Prophet.* New York: Alfred A. Knopf.

Goodman, L. (1975). *Winning the race with death.* Paper presented as part of a symposium on "Fear, Death, and Creativity," American Psychological Association, Chicago.

Grof, S. (1985). *Beyond the brain: Birth, death, and transcendence in psychotherapy.* Albany, NY: State University of New York Press.

Grof, S., & Halifax, J. (1977). *The human encounter with death.* New York: Dutton.

Hamilton, E., & Cairns, H. (Eds.). (1973). *Collected dialogues of Plato.* New Jersey: Princeton University Press.

Harvey, A. (1994). *The way of passion: A celebration of Rumi.* New York: Tarcher/ Putnam.

Keleman, S. (1974). *Living your dying.* New York: Random House.

Koestenbaum P. (1976). *Is there an answer to death?* New Jersey: Prentice-Hall.

Kruck, J. S., & Sheikh, A. A. (1991). Images of life and death: An overview of Stephen Levine's work on conscious living and conscious dying. In A. A. Sheikh & K. S. Sheikh (Eds.), *Death imagery: Comforting death brings us to the threshold of life.* Milwaukee, WI: American Imagery Institute.

Kübler-Ross, E. (Ed.). (1975). *Death: The final stage of growth.* New Jersey: Prentice-Hall.

Levitan, A. A. (1985). Hypnotic death rehearsal. *American Journal of Clinical Hypnosis, 27*(4), 211-215.

Levitan, A. A. (1991). Hypnotic death rehearsal. In A. A. Sheikh & K. S. Sheikh (Eds.), *Death imagery: Comforting death brings us to the threshold of life.* Milwaukee, WI: American Imagery Institute.

Levine, S. (1972). *Death row: An affirmation of life.* San Francisco: Glide Publications.

Levine, S. (1979). *A gradual awakening.* New York: Anchor Press/Doubleday.

Levine, S. (1982). *Who dies? An investigation of conscious living and conscious dying.* New York: Anchor Books/Doubleday.

Levine, S. (1984). *Meetings at the edge.* New York: Anchor Press/Doubleday.

Levine, S. (1989). *Healing into life and death.* New York: Doubleday.

Long, J. B. (1975). The death that ends death in Hinduism and Buddhism. In E. Kübler-Ross (Ed.), *Death: The final stage of growth.* New Jersey: Prentice Hall.

May, R. (1958). The origins and significance of the existential movement in psychology. In R. May, E. Angel, & H.F. Ellenberger (Eds.), *Existence: A new dimension in psychiatry and psychology.* New York: Simon & Schuster.

May, R. (1968, February). The daemonic: Love and death. *Psychology Today, 1*(9), 16-25.

May, R. (1975) *The Courage to create.* New York: W. W. Norton.

Melges, F. T. (1982). *Time and the inner future: A temporal approach to psychiatric disorder.* New York: Wiley.

Melges, F. T., & DeMaso, D. R. (1980). Grief resolution therapy: Reliving, revising, and revisiting. *American Journal of Psychotherapy, xxxiv,* 51-61.

Metzner, R. (1986). *Opening to inner light.* Los Angeles: Jeremy P. Tarcher.

Moody, R. A. (1975). *Life after life.* New York: Bantam.

Morrison, J. K. (1978). Successful grieving: Changing personal constructs through mental imagery. *Journal of Mental Imagery, 2,* 63-68.

Morrison, J. K. (1991). The clinical use of imagery to induce psychotherapeutic grieving. In A. A. Sheikh & K. S. Sheikh (Eds.), *Death imagery: Confronting death brings us to the threshold of life.* Milwaukee, WI: American Imagery Institute.

Neale, R. E. (1969). *In praise of play.* New York: Harper & Row.

Neher, A. (1980). *The psychology of transcendence.* New York: Prentice-Hall.

Nichols, R., & Nichols, J. (1975). Funerals: A time for grief and growth. In E. Kübler-Ross (Ed.), *Death: The final stage of growth.* New Jersey: Prentice-Hall.

Nicholson, R. A. (Trans.). (1978). *Rumi: Poet and mystic.* London: Unwin Paperbacks.

Nietzsche, F. (1974). *The gay science.* New York: Random House.

Palmer, J. (1978). ESP and out-of-body experiences: An experiential approach. In D. S. Rogo (Ed.), *Mind beyond the body.* New York: Penguin.

Pasternak, B. (1958). *Doctor Zhivago.* New York: Pantheon.

Paz, O. (1961). *The labyrinth of solitude.* New York: Grove.

Rahula, W. (1959). *What the Buddha taught.* New York: Grove.

Ramsay, R. W., & Noorbergen, R. (1981). *Living with loss.* New York: William Morrow.

Ring, K. (1980). *Life at death.* New York: Coward, McCann & Geoghegan.

Ring, K. (1984). *Heading toward omega.* New York: William Morrow.

Robinson, R. H. (1970). *The Buddhist religion: A historical introduction.* Belmont, CA: Dickenson.

Shear, J. (1978, September). *Plato, Piaget, and Mararishi on cognitive development.* Paper presented at the American Psychological Association Convention, Toronto.

Sheikh, A. A., Twente, G. E., & Turner, D. (1979). Death imagery: Therapeutic uses. In A. A. Sheikh & J. T. Shaffer (Eds.), *The potential of fantasy and imagination.* New York: Brandon House.

Twente, G.E. (1979). Personal Communication.

Volkan, V. D. (1975). "Regrief" therapy. In B. Schoenberg (Ed.), *Bereavement: Its psychological aspects.* New York: Columbia University Press.

Watts, A. (1968). *The meaning of happiness.* New York: Harper & Row.

Watts, A. (1972). *The book on the taboo against knowing who you are.* New York: Random House.

Williamson, D. S. (1978, January). New life at the graveyard: A method of therapy for individuation from a dead former parent. *Journal of Marriage and Family Counseling,* 93-101.

Yalom, I. D. (1980). *Existential psychotherapy.* New York: Basic Books.

CHAPTER 22

Imagery and Spiritual Development

BONNEY GULINO SCHAUB AND
RICHARD SCHAUB

I think it not improbable that man, like the grub that prepares a chamber for the winged thing it never has been but is to be—that man may have cosmic destinies that he does not understand.

Oliver Wendell Homes (in Walsh & Shapiro, 1983, p. 273)

Spiritual development is an issue of emerging interest in the helping professions (Burkhardt & Jacobson, 1999; Chandler, Holden, & Kolander, 1992). Increasingly, health professionals are utilizing practices that have spiritual origins (Schaub, 1995), and major medical centers, such as Harvard Medical School, are holding extensive conferences on spirituality and healing. The paradigm of wellness across the lifespan espoused by the American Counseling Association (Myers, 1992) includes spiritual development as a key concept. Religious or spiritual problems have been included as a condition in the Diagnostic and Statistical Manual, Fourth Edition (DSM-IV) (Lukoff, Lu, Turner, & Gackenbach, 1995).

Spirituality can be studied from many perspectives, including faith development (Fowler, 1981), religious development (Genia, 1995), transpersonal levels of development (Wilber, Engler, & Brown, 1986), the development of "greater knowledge and greater love" (Chandler, Holden, & Kolander, 1992), the clinical practicality of spiritual consciousness (Schaub & Schaub, 1997), and East-West cross-cultural stages of spiritual development (Wilber, 1999).

In Wilber's synthetic model (1999a), he argues that human development can be broadly categorized as pre-egoic (a "prepersonal" sense of self), egoic (a personal sense of self), and trans-egoic (a transpersonal or spiritual sense of self). He seeks to integrate the western psychological tradition of ego study with the world's spiritual traditions of trans-egoic study.

TRADITIONAL MODELS OF SPIRITUAL DEVELOPMENT

There are of course many religion-based and traditional models of spiritual development. For example, Mevlana Jelaleddin Rumi (1207-1273), the great Islamic poet and philosopher, referred to three stages (Thackston, 1994):

1. The Primitive Man—the materialist, who serves no God and is concerned only with the present time.
2. The Immature Man—the religious person, who serves only God and is concerned only with future time.
3. The Mature Man—the person who learns how to see the invisible hidden in the visible, who serves God by loving people, and is not concerned with time.

Another traditional example is Dante (1265-1321), the author of one of the acknowledged masterpieces of world literature, *The Divine Comedy*. Dante described the realms of hell, purgatory, and paradise as three levels of human nature that can be explored and experienced by any "pilgrim," i.e., anyone willing to make the journey. The nine circles of hell are characterized by souls who willfully repeat life-destroying patterns and refuse to learn. The mountain of purgatory is characterized by souls who willingly work on healing their emotional limitations. Paradise is characterized by souls who are learning how (through wisdom and contemplation) to tolerate the light of God, i.e., enlightenment. Dante's view of spiritual development was the gradual liberation of a person's free will to consciously choose to leave hell, to climb Purgatory, and to study the way into the higher consciousness of Paradise. Strikingly, the climb up the mountain of purgatory is guided by visual and auditory inner images that activate higher qualities and potentials in the pilgrim, thereby allowing him to climb the mountain with greater and greater ease.

Both Rumi (Islam) and Dante (Catholicism) honored their religious tradition and at the same time advocated that each individual, regardless of background, has the developmental possibility of spiritual wisdom.

The universal humanism of their outlook can serve as a guideline for today's professional. The health professional works with a diverse population in a secular setting and cannot ethically apply religiously based spirituality to their clients and patients. Instead, the professional must seek out non-sectarian methods of evoking their clients' spirituality in the process of healing. The knowledge treasures of the world's spiritual traditions can serve as an inspiration to the health professional, but the actual application of methods must meet a contemporary, secular, scientific standard. For one example of an approach that meets this standard, we turn to the imagery work of the Italian psychiatrist, Roberto Assagioli (1888-1974).

ASSAGIOLI'S USE OF IMAGERY IN SPIRITUAL DEVELOPMENT

According to Grof and Grof (1989), the classic modern work on spiritual development and spiritual crises is Assagioli's 1933 essay, "Self-Realization and Psychological Disturbances." A posthumous collection of Assagioli's essays, Transpersonal Development (1991), elaborates on his study of the modern person's process and problems of spiritual development.

In all of his work, Assagioli was concerned with the potentials of the person beyond the socially conditioned personality. Along with Jung, he pioneered in Europe what later became transpersonal psychology in the United States. His main theme was that higher potentials exist in each person, and that the activation of these potentials brings wisdom into the mind, peace into the body, and joy into the emotions. With such positive benefits, Assagioli considered it obvious that the higher consciousness of humanity should be studied and activated. Imagery was his primary method to accomplish this.

IMAGERY AND SPIRITUAL EXPERIENCES

Assagioli identified the cross-cultural images that are known to activate spiritual energies and emotions. These include images of ascent, descent, expansion, awakening, light-enlightenment, fire, empowerment, love, wisdom, path-pilgrimage, transmutation, new birth-regeneration, liberation, resurrection-return (Assagioli, 1965). Rather than wait for these images to possibly appear in the dream life of his clients, Assagioli advocated the active use of these images in order to activate higher consciousness and spiritual development.

In the three case studies that follow, we can see how spiritual images reduce suffering and increase peace and spiritual knowledge. In Charles' case, imagery activated his spirituality as he went through the dying process. In Laurie's case, imagery helped her expand her capacity for compassion and wisdom in the face of fears of loss. In Tom's case, imagery helped him experience an expansion of consciousness, placing his emotional struggle into a much greater perspective.

CASE STUDY: CHARLES

Charles was terminally ill from AIDS. The AIDS virus had by now led to neurological damage. Charles was unsteady on his feet and his speech was beginning to slur. His memory was slipping away from him.

This case study describes an imagery session with Charles. The session took place in his apartment as he was lying in bed in severe discomfort from skin rashes and from the side effects of his medications. Under these circumstances, it would be hard to imagine how imagery could help. In fact, this single session provided

Charles with a higher vision that helped him throughout the dying process. The imagery therapist was a holistic nurse trained in Clinical Imagery.

Charles knew the nurse well and trusted her as much as he trusted anyone. This certainly contributed to the depth of the experience. The nurse asked Charles to close his eyes and follow her voice. The nurse asked him, despite the severe itching, to try to bring his attention to his nostrils. She then talked to him about how to follow his breathing. She suggested that he not try to do anything special to it—not to try to make it rhythmic, not to try to make it more noticeable. Instead, just let it be the way it is. She then asked him to imagine that each breath had the potential to take him deeper and deeper into calmness—as he gave permission to his breath to do this for him. [Note: This is a standard relaxation technique in imagery and hypnosis.]

The nurse noticed that Charles' chest was in a slower breathing pattern. This suggested that Charles was responding to her directions and was experiencing a more relaxed, more inwardly absorbed state. The nurse next suggested that he continue to follow his breathing and to listen to her at the same time. The nurse talked slowly about the fact that in all times and in all cultures, people have prepared themselves for inner work in exactly the same way Charles was now doing. She spoke further about imagery as an ageless practice for realizing inner wisdom. She then wondered if Charles could begin to imagine someone in another time and culture following his breath and going toward wisdom, just as Charles was doing now.

The nurse saw Charles' chest slow down even more. Her own personal experience in imagery told her that at that moment Charles had deeply let go. She said nothing else. She silently meditated by his bedside, keeping her eyes open to observe any changes in him.

Twenty-five minutes passed. The nurse felt a peace palpable in the room. Charles slowly opened his eyes. He began to tell the nurse what he had experienced:

> I felt my body sink deep in the bed. I felt a great heaviness and peace. The itching was gone, and it's still gone. I saw an image of a young man. I saw him become ill, and saw his flesh begin to fall off him, until he became a skeleton.
>
> Then his flesh reappeared, and his life force returned. He was the same healthy young man I first saw. Soon, the flesh began to come off him again, his life force left him, and he became a skeleton again. At that point, I saw an old man behind him, and I realized that as the old man moved his hand to the left, the flesh came off the young man, and as the old man moved his hand to the right, the life came back to the young man. I watched this with great feelings of peace. I felt something very important was being taught to me. I can't even say the peace was in me, because by the time I was watching this I had absolutely no sense of my body at all. My body was gone. My body had dropped away. I was free, I was floating free. I had no fear at all. I was free.

Charles closed his eyes and sank back into peace. The nurse sat quietly, not wanting to say anything.

When the nurse visited Charles a week later, he had invited three friends to be at the session. He wanted them to experience the imagery so that they could learn it and practice it with him whenever they visited. Charles felt he had found a way to help himself.

In a month, Charles could no longer manage at home. He was hospitalized, and after a few days he stopped communicating. He was not in a coma, but his attention was definitely elsewhere. Visitors would talk to him, not get a reply, and then leave. The nurse visited him, and the same process happened. Everyone began to accept this as either a neurological and/or emotional consequence of his dying process.

The nurse found out from his friends that Charles had made them promise to guide him to his inner wisdom if he was near death. Finding this out, the nurse intuited that Charles was not communicating because he was determined to keep his consciousness focused inward. The friends had agreed to the promise, but they all felt embarrassed about the thought of guiding Charles in the hospital room with other patients and other visitors around.

One evening, his friend, Paul, was visiting him at the hospital. As Paul was about to leave, the floor nurse told Paul that this was probably Charles' last night. Charles' vital signs and her long clinical experience told her so. Paul became upset and started toward the elevator to go outside. He suddenly remembered the promise to Charles—to guide him to inner wisdom in the event he was about to die.

Paul went back to the hospital room. There was Charles, still uncommunicative. His silence had continued throughout his hospitalization. Feeling self-conscious, Paul leaned close to Charles' ear and began to instruct him on the imagery process he learned from the nurse. Charles continued to lie there, unresponsive. Nevertheless, Paul continued to guide Charles to follow his breathing, and to begin to imagine a wisdom figure from another time and place also following his breath, to imagine both Charles and the wisdom figure meditating together, and to be open to any communication from the wisdom figure.

Paul finished the guiding. To Paul's great surprise, Charles spoke. Charles said, "Don't worry—Charles is already gone." Paul began to both cry and feel happy. He did not know what was happening to him. He felt the need to go outside for some fresh air. Charles died 30 minutes later" (Schaub & Schaub, 1997).

In a clinical situation in which curing was not possible, the imagery worker had provided Charles with a way to enter the dying process with inner peace and greater wisdom.

CASE STUDY: LAURIE

The images from sacred art have always been utilized to give people direct mental-emotional-energetic experiences of spiritual knowledge.

In imagery class, I am asked to go through a collection of images and to pick one for reflection. I find myself drawn to the Catholic sacred image of Mary holding her crucified son, Jesus, in her arms. I'm first drawn to the Virgin Mary's face. It is the face of a young girl not past adolescence. Soft, delicate, yet serenely sad, wise beyond her years, yet innocent and confused by the situation she is in.

My eyes survey the rest of the sculpture. The soft, translucent white of the marble, the folds of drapery and the large figure of the dead Christ draped across Mary's lap. This lifeless body is much too large to be Mary's child. I've seen this image many times—why are there tears in my eyes? I'm drawn back to Mary's delicate face. Why is she so young and innocent? Certainly Michelangelo knew how to sculpt an older woman. No, there is a reason she appears like this. Suddenly I understand. This image is about a human experience. The death of a child. Is a person ever old enough to not be totally vulnerable to this loss?

When I first became a mother, I remember being frightened by the intensity of my protective instincts and the degree to which thoughts of my son being harmed terrified me. I feel joined to Mary's face. I can see myself and all mothers. My tears continue. The image expands to connecting with the universal fear of death and loss. Can spirituality offer me solace in the face of loss of a child? I think about how angry I get when I hear pat answers to the question, Why? Don't tell me about karma, or God's Will, or that it's part of a lesson. Those answers bypass the sorrow, my experience of grief. This Pieta image is different. It honors the absence of an answer. Somehow that look of innocence is so compelling. She needs compassion. She's just a child in the face of the mystery of loss. This allows me to gain strength from the shared human experience. I am not alone.

In this moment, I understand the power of the image to transcend time and space—to draw me to a place of truth. Michelangelo was only 25 when he created this work. What did he know about losing a child? Yet somehow he created the Pieta—his genius and inspiration coming from a source that is timeless and universal. It emerges from the ground of being and includes me in it. (Schaub, 1999)

The interaction between the client and a powerful spiritual image provided her with a new philosophical and emotional strength to reduce her fears.

CASE STUDY: TOM

Tom wanted to use imagery to transform his habitual critical attitudes toward others. The imagery worker could have used a variety of cognitive-behavioral imagery techniques, but instead choose to experiment with the spiritual symbol of ascent. The imagery worker's thinking was that a symbol of ascent could serve as a "higher" perspective for Tom. As we see in Tom's description of the imagery session, the ascent symbol became the activator of a transpersonal experience.

A deep desire of mine has to become a more loving and accepting person towards others. I came across this process of imagery and spiritual symbols. So I gave it a try.

My therapist asked me to close my eyes and settle my body in my chair. Slowly, I brought my awareness to my breathing and noticed its slow rhythmic pattern. The effects of this alone gave me a sense of relief and calm. I put in my imagination the suggestion to have an image of ascent, and I waited with an open attitude.

I begin to see in my mind an ancient Mayan Temple. It was long deserted and overgrown. I approached it with anticipation.

When I got to the top, I had a breathtaking view of the surrounding valley. As I turned, I see a huge fire on the temple top. The flame must be six feet in diameter and spitting flames 30 feet into the air. I moved closer and noticed a wooden bench situated there that seemed to indicate that I should sit down. As I sat and gazed into the fire, I saw a flaming figure emerge from within the depths. This figure consisted not of flesh and bones but simply fire. He stepped onto a plank and stood about four feet from where I was sitting.

I went into conversation with him. One of my intentions of this imagery session was to talk about my desire to be more loving and accepting of others. The first thing he reminded me of was that my acceptance of others was also the work of accepting myself. I told him that I wanted to be able to look at people in my life, strangers included, and be able to see them with love and compassion. How do I do this, I asked?

He stated I could use the image of the acorn and its development to a mighty oak. I took this to mean holding people with a larger view than what I see in them in the moment. *To trust in the unseen potential.*

I called up images of different people in my life. I experienced myself feel differently towards them. I felt subtle shifts of attitudes. Small amounts of love and acceptance began to bubble up from within. Just to make sure, I chose a complete stranger I had seen on the street. I chose the kind of person I often write off with judgements and stereotypes. I stayed with it and recalled my inner guide's words.

I also did something unique in this process. An idea dawned on me to leave my body and to merge into the inner guide so that I could look out through his eyes. A wonderful thing began to happen. I found myself filling with thoughts of compassion. I couldn't sustain it very long but I had an experience of what I was hoping for.

I thanked the inner guide for this experience. He invited me to come with him on a short journey. Eagerly I followed him. He jumped into the fire and disappeared. When I entered the flame, I felt my body burn off. It didn't hurt at all. My sense of my body disappeared and I experienced myself in a state of pure awareness. All I saw now was a blue light like at the bottom of a candle's flame. I stared at it for what seemed like an eternity. What followed were several bursts of light waves emanating from within the blue flame. It looked like something from a Star Trek movie. There was a gigantic wave of light that went out from this tiny blue flame and traveled to the ends of universe and further. I could see it with my own eyes. The next thing I know I entered into the flame and "caught a ride" on the next wave.

When I arrived at the farthest reaches of the universe, I could still see the blue flame of the candle. My awareness of myself was so incredibly expanded. I was able to be aware of being at both places in the exact same moment. How long I stayed in this awareness is hard to tell. I somehow brought myself back to the blue flame and then reemerged at the top of the Mayan Temple. The inner guide was gone at this point. I knew that I had touched a higher wisdom. (Thompson, 1999)

As Assagioli (1965) notes, ascent is one of the images that can evoke transpersonal-spiritual knowing and feeling. Tom's experience pointed him toward wanting to know more about the transpersonal dimension of awareness latent in each of us.

SUMMARY

Ancient traditional practices and modern scientific research verify imagery's effectiveness for inner transformation. In this article, three clients underwent positive spiritual experiences through the direct impact of inner imagery work. Spiritual experiences have a natural ability to encourage each person to want to know more, which in turn generates new development of the mind and heart. As more people experience higher vision and higher understanding, the world will become a saner place. Imagery contributes to this advancement of human nature.

REFERENCES

Assagioli, R. (1965). *Psychosynthesis.* New York: Penguin.

Assagioli, R. (1991). *Transpersonal development.* London: HarperCollins.

Burkhardt, M., & Jacobson, M. (1999). Spirituality and health. In B. Dossey, K. Keegan, & C. Guzzetta (Eds.), *Holistic nursing: A handbook for practice* (3rd Edition, pp. 91-121). Gaithersburg, MD: Aspen Publishers.

Chandler, C., Holden, J., & Kolander, C. (1992). Counseling for spiritual wellness: Theory and practice. *Journal of Counseling and Development, 71*(2), 168-175.

Fowler, J. (1981). *Stages of faith: The psychology of human development and the quest for meaning.* San Francisco: Harper & Row.

Genia, V. (1995). *Counseling and psychotherapy of religious clients. A developmental approach.* Westport, CT: Praeger.

Grof, C., & Grof, S. (1989). *Spiritual emergency: When personal transformation becomes a crisis.* Los Angeles: Jeremy Tarcher, Inc.

Lukoff, D., Lu, F., Turner, R., & Gackenbach, J. (1995). Transpersonal psychology research review: Researching religious and spiritual problems on the Internet. *The Journal of Transpersonal Psychology, 27*(2), 153-170.

Myers, J. (1992). Wellness, prevention, development: The cornerstone of the profession. *Journal of Counseling and Development, 71*(2), 136-139.

Schaub, B. (1999). Personal communication—letter.

Schaub, B., & Schaub, R. (1997). *Healing addictions: The vulnerability model of recovery.* Albany, NY: Delmar.

Schaub, R. (1995, Spring). Alternative health and spiritual practices. *Alternative Health Practitioner, 1*(1), 35-38.

Thackston, W. (1994). *Signs of the unseen: The discourses of Jalaluddin Rumi.* Putney, VT: Threshold.

Thompson, S. (1999). Personal communication—letter.

Walsh, R., & Shapiro, D. (1983). *Beyond health and normality.* New York: Van Nostrand Rheinhold.

Wilber, K. (1999). Spirituality and developmental lines: Are there stages? *Journal of Transpersonal Psychology, 31*(1), 1-10.

Wilber, K. (1999a). *Integral psychology.* Boston: Shambhala.

Wilber, K., Engler, J., & Brown, D. (1986). *Transformations of consciousness.* Boston: Shambala.

Contributors

JEANNE ACHTERBERG, Ph.D. is Director of Research at North Hawaii Community Hospital in Kamuela, Hawaii, and is also on the faculty of Saybrook Institute in San Francisco. She is internationally recognized for her innovative work on imagery and healing and has published over 100 papers and six books. Her book, *Imagery in Healing: Shamanism and Modern Medicine* has been acclaimed as a classic in the field of mind-body studies. Other books include: *Woman as Healer* and *Rituals for Healing: Using Imagery for Health.*

SHEILA M. BAER, M.S. is pursuing her doctoral studies in clinical psychology at Marquette University where she received her master's degree in 1999. She has conducted research on various aspects of psychotherapy and has a long-standing interest in the power of the mind which she plans to pursue further after completing her Ph.D.

HEIDI BECKMAN, Ph.D. obtained her doctoral degree in clinical psychology from Marquette University in August 2000. She is currently a postdoctoral fellow at the University of Kansas School of Medicine–Wichita, involved in clinical work in the areas of acute adolescent psychopathology and consultation-liaison services, along with medical education and applied research. She recently received a grant from the medical school to examine how anxiety manifests itself differently in various eating disorder diagnostic groups.

DANIEL M. BERNSTEIN, Ph.D. received his doctoral degree from Simon Fraser University in Vancouver, Canada. Currently, he is a post-doctoral fellow at the University of Washington. His doctoral work explored the relationship between remembering and believing. He has also investigated issues regarding sleep and dreams, visual information processing, and the cognitive impact of mild traumatic brain injury.

WILLIAM BRAUD, Ph.D. Formerly on the staff of the University of Houston and the Mind Science Foundation in San Antonio, Texas, is currently Professor and Research Director at the Institute of Transpersonal Psychology in Palo Alto, California where he conducts research in the areas of exceptional human experiences, consciousness studies, transpersonal studies, spirituality, and expanded research methods. Dr. Braud has also done very significant work on the influences of relaxation, imagery, positive emotions, and intentions on health and well-being.

PAT M. COOK, M.A. is the founder and Director of the Open Ear Center for Music in Healing in Washington State and editor of the *Open Ear Journal*. She is a teacher, clinician, and pioneer in the use of cross-cultural sound and music in health care. Pat has traveled extensively throughout the world, recording and participating in healing rituals that employ music. She is a Fellow of the Association for Music and Imagery and is currently completing her doctorate in music education and ethnomusicology at the University of Washington. Her publications include: *Shaman, Jhankari, and Nele: Music Healers of Indigenous Culture*.

BARBARA M. DOSSEYY, Ph.D., R.N., M.S., H.N.C., F.A.A.N. is Director of Holistic Nursing Consultants, Santa Fe, New Mexico, and is internationally recognized as a pioneer in the holistic nursing movement. She has received many awards and is a seven-time recipient of the *American Journal of Nursing* (AJN) Book of the Year Award. She has authored or co-authored 19 books with the most recent being *Florence Nightingale: Mystic, Visionary, Healer; Holistic Nursing: A Handbook for Practice;* and *AHNA Standards of Holistic Nursing Practice*.

JANE G. DRESSER, M.N., M.Ed. is a Clinical Nurse Specialist and Advanced Practice Nurse Prescriber in a private practice. She holds degrees in nursing from Florida State University and the University of Florida, and a degree in Counseling Psychology from the University of Houston. Her practice and research interests have focused on severe and persistent mental illnesses with an emphasis on the treatment of borderline personality disorder.

GERALD N. EPSTEIN, M.D. is a psychiatrist in private practice in New York and an Assistant Clinical Professor at Mount Sinai Hospital. He founded the American Institute for Mental Imagery where he trains health professionals and conducts research in mind-body medicine. Dr. Epstein studied with Colette Aboulker-Muscat, a renowned teacher and mystic in Jerusalem, and he is the author of a number of books including: *Waking Dream Therapy, Healing Visualizations, Healing into Immortality,* and *Climbing Jacob's Ladder*.

MARY JANE ESPLEN, Ph.D., R.N. is a Clinical-Scientist within the Psychotherapy Division of the Department of Psychiatry at the University of Toronto. Her Ph.D. work involved a study of guided imagery in bulimia nervosa and she completed a post-doctorate in psycho-oncology. Dr. Esplen has conducted studies investigating the use of imagery in individual as well as in group psychotherapy. She has recently received a Research Scientist Award from the National Institute of Canada for her research on interventions for individuals with a predisposition to cancer.

SHIRIN EZAZ-NIKPAY, M.Sc. Following her undergraduate psychology degree at Goldsmiths College, University of London, United Kingdom, pursued her interest in alternative healing methods during her master's degree in medical anthropology at Brunel University, Middlesex, United Kingdom. She is now training to become a gestalt psychotherapist at the Therapeutisches Institut in

Berlin, Germany, and is currently working as a psychosocial consultant for refugee families and children with mental health problems.

HOWARD HALL, Ph.D., Psy.D. holds two doctorate degrees in psychology, a Ph.D. from Princeton University in experimental psychology and a Psy.D. from Rutgers University in clinical psychology. He has been on the faculty at the Pennsylvania State University and is currently on faculty at the Case Western Reserve University School of Medicine, Department of Pediatrics, and also holds a staff position at Rainbow Babies and Children's Hospital, Cleveland, Ohio. Dr. Hall teaches clinical hypnosis at national workshops. For the past two decades Dr. Hall has conducted and published pioneering work on the effects of hypnosis, imagery, and relaxation on immune responses. He is a Senior Fellow of Kairos Foundation for research in the field of consciousness and healing.

COLLEEN HEINKEL is currently Associate Editor of Prehospital and Disaster Medicine and Executive Director of the World Association of Disaster and Emergency Medicine, an international organization committed to the improvement of emergency and disaster response through research and worldwide exchange of information. She is currently completing a doctoral degree in clinical psychology at Marquette University with an emphasis on behavioral medicine and holds a research position in the Department of Emergency Medicine at the University of Wisconsin–Madison.

AMY HOFFAMAN, M.S. is currently completing her doctoral work in clinical psychology at Marquette University. Her research interests include physiological psychology, stress, and alternative treatment modalities for stress-related health problems. For her dissertation, she is studying the effects of mindfulness meditation on stress, anxiety, and depression. She plans to pursue a career as a health psychologist.

LESLIE KOLKMEIER R.N., M.Ed. spent over 25 years in the health field. Moving from bedside nursing to teaching and finally to private practice focusing on biofeedback and applied psychophysiology, she recently retired to a farm in Wisconsin. She is active in the fiber arts and writing, and utilizes her skills with her hospice patients.

JOHN P. KROP, L.C.S.W. is a retired psychotherapist. He was Director of the Center for Human Communication in Los Gatos, California and taught at John F. Kennedy University, University of San Francisco, and School voor Imaginatie in Amsterdam. He studied with Fritz Perls, Virginia Satir, Richard Bandler, John Grinder, and Alexander Lowen. His method of working called Action Therapy is documented in a series of videotapes available in the United States (VHS) at Envision Video Productions 1-800-219-6674; and in Europe at the School voor Imaginatie, Amsterdam 20 6731395.

ROBERT G. KUNZENDORF, Ph.D. is a Professor of Psychology at the University of Massachusetts Lowell, Research Associate in Psychiatry at Harvard Medical School, co-editor of the journal *Imagination, Cognition and Personality,* and Past President of the American Association for the Study of Mental Imagery.

Dr. Kunzendorf has published four edited books and over 75 articles, which focus on conscious reality-testing, and various aspects of the mind-body problem.

ROBERT G. LEY, Ph.D. received his doctoral degree in clinical psychology from the University of Waterloo in Waterloo, Ontario. He is Professor in Clinical Psychology at Simon Fraser University in Vancouver and has a private practice in clinical and forensic psychology. Dr. Ley has a long-lasting research and clinical interest in emotions, imagery, brain laterality, and psychopathology and is the author of numerous journal articles and book chapters.

BELLERUTH NAPARSTEK, L.I.S.W., B.C.D. is a nationally recognized innovator in the field of guided imagery, and the creator of Time Warner's best-selling, 52-title *Health Journeys* guided imagery audio series. She is the author of *Staying Well with Guided Imagery,* a widely used primer for medical professionals and health consumers and *Your Sixth Sense* that explores the connection between imagery and intuition and has been translated into Spanish, Italian, Portuguese, Slovenian, Polish, Turkish, and Chinese. She has helped to make guided imagery part of mainstream healthcare by persuading several big insurance companies and hundreds of hospitals and clinics to consider imagery as a viable healing tool.

DAVID PINCUS, Ph.D., completed his doctoral work in clinical psychology at Marquette University. He has previously published an integrated family systems theory based on principles from nonlinear dynamical systems theory, and his doctoral thesis expands this theory to small groups. His future professional plans include providing psychotherapy, research, consulting and professional training in the area of non-linear dynamics and psychology. He is currently completing a year-long clinical internship with Shasta County Mental Health, Redding, California.

MICHELLE ROSENFELD, M.S. is currently working toward her Ph.D. in clinical psychology at Marquette University. She has done research in the area of eating disorders and psychotherapy outcomes and has practicum experience in the areas of therapy, assessment, and consultation. Michelle has employment experience in pediatric neuropsychological assessment and educational assessment and currently works as an assessment specialist in a behavioral health hospital where she does level of care assessments and consults with two local emergency rooms.

LINDA G. S. RUSSEK, Ph.D. is President of the Family Love and Health Foundation. She received her Ph.D. from the United States International University in 1978. For 20 years she was a Research Psychologist at the Harvard University Student Health Services and Director of the Harvard Mastery of Stress Follow-Up Study with her late father, Dr. Henry I. Russek, who was Director of the New York Meetings of the American College of Cardiology. She is the co-author of *Living Energy Universe, Discovering the Living Soul,* and *The G. O. D. Hypothesis* with Gary E. Schwartz.

TULSI SARAL, Ph.D. is a Professor of Clinical Psychology at the University of Houston-Clear Lake where he teaches courses in Group Psychotherapy, Transpersonal Therapy, and Sex Therapy. Dr. Saral is licensed as a Clinical Psychologist in the State of Illinois and as a Marriage and Family Therapist in Texas. He is a Diplomat of the American Board of Sexology and a Fellow of the American Academy of Clinical Sexologists. Dr. Saral is a Past President of the American Association for the Study of Mental Imagery and has published extensively on the various aspects of imagery and communication.

BONNEY GULINO SCHAUB, M.S., R.N., C.S. is co-founder of the New York Psychosynthesis Institute and on the faculty of the Italian Society for Psychosynthesis Psychotherapy in Florence. She is co-director of Clinical Imagery and Clinical Meditation Certification Program at the Institute and a leader, teacher, and author in the holistic nursing movement.

RICHARD SCHAUB, Ph.D. has trained hundreds of helping professionals internationally in the clinical applications of imagery and meditation. He is co-author of *Healing Addictions: The Vulnerability Model of Recovery,* and is publisher of the newsletter, *Ocean of Being: Discoveries in Human Potential.* He is in private practice in New York City and in Huntington, Long Island.

K. DAVID SCHULTZ, Ph.D., A.B.P.P. is a licensed psychologist with a private practice providing clinical psychotherapy services, leadership training, and organizational consultation services to individuals, families, schools, human service agencies, and other community service organizations. He is an Assistant Clinical Professor of Psychiatry at the Yale University School of Medicine and a Diplomat in Clinical Psychology of the American Board of Professional Psychology.

GARY E. SCHWARTZ, Ph.D. is Professor of Psychology, Medicine, Neurology, Surgery, and Psychiatry, Director of the Human Energy Systems Laboratory, and Director of the Bioenergy Core, the Pediatric Alternative Medicine Center, at the University of Arizona. He was an Assistant Professor at Harvard for five years. He was a Professor of Psychology and Psychiatry at Yale University, Director of the Yale Psychophysiology Center before moving to Arizona in 1988. He has published more than 300 scientific papers, including six papers in the journal *Science,* co-edited 11 academic books, and recently written *The Living Energy Universe; Discovering the Living Soul;* and *The G. O. D. Hypothesis,* with Linda G. S. Russek, Ph.D.

ANEES A. SHEIKH, Ph.D. is Professor and former Chair of the Department of Psychology at Marquette University and Clinical Professor of Psychiatry and Behavioral Medicine at the Medical College of Wisconsin. Through his guided imagery workshops, he has trained thousands of health professionals around the world. Dr. Sheikh has published numerous journal articles, book chapters, and 13 books on imagery and related topics. He was the founding editor of *The Journal of Mental Imagery.* Dr. Sheikh is Past President of the American

Association for the Study of Mental Imagery and is internationally recognized for his contributions to the field of imagery.

KATHARINA S. SHEIKH, M.A. is the President of the Institute for Human Enhancement and also teaches German and French at Divine Savior Holy Angels High School. Educated in Germany, France, Canada, and the United States, she holds graduate degrees from the University of Toronto and Marquette University. She is the co-editor of *Imagery in Education, Healing East and West,* and *Death Imagery.*

MERVIN R. SMUCKER, Ph.D. is Associate Clinical Professor and Director of Cognitive Behavioral Training in the Department of Psychiatry at the Medical College of Wisconsin, where he is involved in ongoing clinical research in the area of trauma. Dr. Smucker previously trained and worked with Aaron T. Beck, M.D. at the University of Pennsylvania Medical School for six years, where he served as Director of Education and Clinical Training at the Center for Cognitive Therapy. He has conducted workshops and seminars throughout the world. Author of many published articles in the area of imagery and trauma, Dr. Smucker has recently published a book on his imagery-based treatment for trauma victims: *Cognitive Behavioral Treatment for Adult Survivors of Childhood Trauma: Imagery Rescripting and Reprocessing.*

JAN TAAL, Drs. is Trainer-Director of the School for Imagery in Amsterdam in the Netherlands. He is a clinical psychologist, health-care psychologist, and psychosynthesis psychotherapist. He has a rich experience in teaching imagery and in the clinical application of imagery in a wide range of contexts, including working with the severely traumatized.

MAX VELMANS, Ph.D. is currently a Reader in Psychology at the University of London. He has around 60 publications on consciousness, including *Understanding Consciousness* (shortlisted for the 2001 British Psychological Society Book Award), *The Science of Consciousness,* and *Investigating Phenomenal Consciousness.* In 1987 he founded a mind/body special interest group within the British Psychological Society and in 1997 co-founded the BPS Consciousness and Experiential Psychology Section. He is a frequent speaker at national and international conferences in this area.

TONYA WACHSMUTH-SCHLAEFER, M.S. obtained a master's degree in Clinical Psychology from Marquette University. Currently, she develops and implements home therapy programs for children with autism, using a variant of Applied Behavior Analysis. Her clinical and research areas of interest include autism, imagery, and children.

JO M. WEIS, Ph.D. received her doctorate at Marquette University and completed a post-doctoral fellowship at the Medical College of Wisconsin in Medical Rehabilitation Psychology. She is currently a faculty member in the Department of Psychiatry at the Medical College of Wisconsin, in addition to her private practice at Cognitive Therapy and Consulting Services in Milwaukee,

Wisconsin. Her program of research focuses on clinical interventions in the treatment of trauma.

SVEN VAN DE WETERING is currently working as a part-time faculty member in the Psychology Department at the University College of the Fraser Valley, while also completing his doctoral dissertation at Simon Fraser University in Vancouver, Canada. His present research focuses on the communication of attributions and the effects of that communication on prejudice. He has also written about the application of evolutionary theory to the human sciences.

BEVERLY HABECK YAHNKE, Ph.D. is a Christian Psychologist in private practice. Her clinical setting invites clients to bring the resources of their faith with them into the therapeutic process. Her current areas of research and inquiry include Christian spiritual disciplines, soul care and the implications of one's faith for healing. She is a graduate of Marquette University where she earned her degree in Educational Psychology.

Index

Appetite, nicotine and, 225
Ibn al-Arabî, 448, 451, 452
Archetypal psychology, 451
Aristotle, 13–14
Aronson, Elliot, 480
Arrhythmias, 38, 305–306
Art, spiritual development and sacred, 493–494
Arthritis, 38
Ascent symbol, spiritual development and, 494–496
Ascetic practices, 9–10, 44
Asclepius, 13–14
Assagioli, Roberto, 18, 490–491
Association for Music and Imagery Journal, 126
Asthma, 40, 56, 433
Attentional-perceptual dynamics, pain and, 184–185
Attention deficit disorder (ADD), 129–130
Auditory stimulation programs, 129–131
  See also Music
Authentic living, death imagery and, 472
Autobiographic imagery, sex therapy and, 266, 269
Autogenic training, 408
Autonomic nervous system (ANS), 55, 145, 151
Aversive imagery, 241–242, 246–247, 350
Awareness and intuitive functioning, 439
Axis-I/II disorders, pain and, 179, 186
Ayurveda medicine, 422

Babylonia, 408
Bachelard, Gaston, 3
Bair, J. H., 38
Balance and Renaissance physicians, 15
Balance and Tibetan Buddhist medicine, 11
Barber, T. X., 458
Batcheldor, Kenneth, 440
Beck, Judith, 350
Beck Depressive Inventory, 363, 365

Behavioral interventions/issues/theories
  depression, 345, 348, 353–354, 361, 364, 370–372
  historical background, 350
  obesity, 237–240
  pain, 180–182
  post-traumatic stress disorder, 386–389
  responses associated with imagery, 151–152
  weight management, 237–240
Beliefs, pain and, 182–183
Benson, Herbert, 147, 414
Beta brainwaves, 133
Bible, the, 7
Bidirectional linkages, 72–73
Binet, Alfred, 17
Biochemical theories of depression, 345, 346
Bioelectromagnetics, 96
Biofeedback
  cardiovascular system, 34, 38
  defining terms, 38
  effectiveness of, individual differences in, 39
  electromyography, 319
  first experiment employing, 38
  global influence of consciousness, 55
  physiological change due to, 408
  transpersonal images, 452–453
Biofeedback and Self-Regulation, 39
Biological theories of depression, 345, 346
Biological theories of obesity, 238–239
Biomedical accounts of mind-body unity, 53, 57
Biopsychosocial model of depression, 346, 347
Biopsychosocial models, pain and, 191
Blood flow, 35
Blood pressure, 34, 301–302, 415–416
Blue light as healing color, 434
Blue Nucleus and neurotransmitter substances, 428–429
Body, imaginary inventory of the, 21
Body chemistry, 35–36
Body imagery, sex therapy and, 267–270, 272

Live events, depression and attributions
of, 369
Living systems theory, 93
See also Dynamical energy systems
theory
Love
death imagery, 484
dynamical energy systems theory, 92,
107–110
meditation, 441
Sufism, 8
Lown, Bernard, 27
Lymphocytes, 37, 79, 80, 416

Magical healing methods, 20
Magnetic energy, 97–98
Magnetic resonance imaging (MRI), 75,
228
Maine Medical Center, 149
Makahu imagination and Kahuna healers
of Polynesia, 5–6
Mandala device in Tantric yoga, 10–12
Mantras and Tibetan medicine, 12
Marital therapy, depression and, 346,
348
Maslow, Abraham, 451
Matthew-Simonton, Stephanie, 37,
409–411
McClelland, David, 41
McCulloch, Warren, 101
McMoneagle, Joe, 437
Meaning to life, instinctively finding,
147–148
Mechanistic physiopathology as dominant
approach to disease, 15
Medical College of Ohio, 149
Medications, depression and, 346
Medications, pain, 181
Medicine
ERA III nonlocal, 449
Tibetan Buddhist, 10–12
traditional healing practices,
cross-cultural, 422–423
Western, historical perspectives on,
12–16

Meditation
adrenocortical activity, 33
cardiopulmonary responses, 31–32
death imagery, 474–475
electrodermal changes, 32
electroencephalography, 32–33
loving-kindness, 441
music, 116
research and methodological flaws,
30–31
Tibetan medicine, 11–12
See also Relaxation exercises
Melanoma, 80
Melatonin, meditation and, 33
Melody, 121
Memory
anxiety, 354
depression, 369
dynamical energy systems theory, 92,
100–107
episodic, 102, 211–213
false, 385
post-traumatic stress disorder, 384
systemic, 105
transitory, 101
Menninger Foundation, 414
Meno, 475
Mesmerism, 452
Mesocorticolimbic dopamine pathway,
smoking cessation and, 225–226
Metabolic perspectives on obesity, 239
Metaphors
communicating/influencing, three
modes of, 449
depression, 361
eating disorders and, 285–286
knowing, modes of, 448
Meta-psychology of healing, cancer and,
421–425
Meyer, Adolf, 29
Michelangelo, 472
Migraines, 35, 38
Mind-body unity, 53, 57
See also Causation, the problem of
mental; Inner wisdom; Physiological
consequences of imagery related
approaches